Rehabilitation in
SPORTS
MEDICINE

a comprehensive guide

Rehabilitation in SPORTS MEDICINE

a comprehensive guide

Paul K. Canavan, MA, PT, ATC, CSCS
Director of Physical Therapy and Rehabilitation
Center for Sports Medicine
Pennsylvania State University
University Park, Pennsylvania

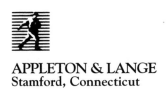

APPLETON & LANGE
Stamford, Connecticut

Prentice Hall International (UK) Limited, *London*
Prentice Hall of Australia Pty. Limited, *Sydney*
Prentice Hall Canada, Inc., *Toronto*
Prentice Hall Hispanoamericana, S.A., *Mexico*
Prentice Hall of India Private Limited, *New Delhi*
Prentice Hall of Japan, Inc., *Tokyo*
Simon & Schuster Asia Pte. Ltd., *Singapore*
Editora Prentice Hall do Brasil Ltda., *Rio de Janeiro*
Prentice Hall, *Upper Saddle River, New Jersey*

Library of Congress Cataloging-in-Publication Data

Rehabilitation in sports medicine : a comprehensive guide / edited by
    Paul K. Canavan.
        p.   cm.
    ISBN 0-8385-8313-X (alk. paper)
    1. Sports injuries—Patients—Rehabilitation.   I. Canavan, Paul
K.
RD97.R436   1998
617.1′027—dc21   97-17095

Acquisitions Editor: Michael P. Medina
Development Editor: Kathleen McCullough
Production Editor: Lisa M. Guidone
Designer: Mary Skudlarek

ISBN 0-8385-8313-X

9 780838 583135   90000

Contents

Contributors

Joi Augustin, MS, RD
Nutritionist
Frances Stern Nutrition Center
New England Medical Center
Boston, Massachusetts

Kevin Black, MD
Associate Professor
Department of Orthopaedics
Team Physician
Hershey Bears Hockey Club
Hershey Medical Center
Hershey, Pennsylvania

Turner A. "Tab" Blackburn, Jr., MEd, PT, SCS, ATC
Co-Director
Berkshire Institute of Orthopaedic and Sports
   Physical Therapy
Adjunct Assistant Professor
University of St. Augustine
Wyomissing, Pennsylvania

Robert D. Bronstein, MD
Attending Orthopedist
Strong Memorial Hospital
Professor
Division of Athletic Medicine
Department of Orthopaedics
University of Rochester School of Medicine
   and Dentistry
Rochester, New York

Paul K. Canavan, MA, PT, ATC, CSCS
Director of Physical Therapy and Rehabilitation
Center for Sports Medicine
Pennsylvania State University
University Park, Pennsylvania

Terri Chmielewski, MA, PT
Physical Therapy Coordinator
Healthsouth Sports Medicine Rehabilitation Center
Birmingham, Alabama

Andrew J. Cosgarea, MD
Orthopaedic Consultant
Athletic Department
Assistant Professor
Department of Orthopaedic Surgery
Sports Medicine Center
Ohio State University
Columbus, Ohio

Kenneth E. DeHaven, MD
Professor and Associate Chair
Director of Athletic Medicine
University of Rochester School of Medicine and Dentistry
Rochester, New York

Craig Denager, PhD, PT, ATC
Physical Therapist and Athletic Trainer
Center for Sports Medicine
Associate Professor
Departments of Orthopaedic/Rehabilitation
   and Kinesiology
Pennsylvania State University
University Park, Pennsylvania

Noel D. Duncan, PhD
Department of Physiology
University of Melbourne
Australia

Johanna Dwyer, DSc, RD
Director
Frances Stern Nutrition Center
New England Medical Center
Professor of Medicine and Community Health
Tufts University Schools of Medicine and Nutrition
   Science and Policy
Boston, Massachusetts

Gregory P. Ernst, PT
Lieutenant Commander
Medical Service Corps
U.S. Navy
Doctoral Candidate
University of Virginia
Charlottesville, Virginia

Judy Goffi, MS, RD
Nutritionist
Frances Stern Nutrition Center
New England Medical Center
Boston, Massachusetts

J. Allen Hardin, MS, PT, ATC
Physical Therapist and Director of Clinical Research
Berkshire Institute of Orthopaedic and
    Sports Physical Therapy
Wyomissing, Pennsylvania

Fred S. Harman, MS
Center for Sports Medicine
Pennsylvania State University
University Park, Pennsylvania

John Heil, PhD
Director of Sports Psychology Program
Department of Psychological Medicine
Lewis-Gale Clinic
Roanoke, Virginia

Jacob Heydemann, MD
El Paso Orthopaedic Surgery Group
El Paso, Texas

Shepard Hurwitz, MD
Director
Division of Foot Surgery
Associate Professor
Department of Orthopaedics
University of Virginia
Charlottesville, Virginia

Robert G. Kelly, PT, ATC
Coordinator of Sports Medicine Physical Therapy
Team Physical Therapist
Hershey Bears Professional Hockey Club
Pennsylvania State Sports Medicine at the
    Milton S. Hershey Medical Center
Hershey, Pennsylvania

William J. Kraemer, PhD
Director of Research
Center for Sports Medicine
Professor of Applied Physiology
Pennsylvania State University
University Park, Pennsylvania

John G. Lachacz, PT, OCS, ATC
Director of Physical Therapy
Froedtert Hospital
Medical College of Wisconsin
Milwaukee, Wisconsin

Becca Main, BS
Head Coach Field Hockey
Quinnipiac College
Hamden, Connecticut

Jerry Martin, MS, CSCS
Head Strength Coordinator
Division of Athletics
University of Connecticut
Storrs, Connecticut

Jill Merchant, MS, RD
Frances Stern Nutrition Center
New England Medical Center
Tufts University School of Nutrition Science
    and Policy
Boston, Massachusetts

Michael Meese, MD
Orthopaedic and Sports Medicine Associates
Clinical Instructor
Department of Orthopaedic Surgery
University of Medicine and Dentistry of
    New Jersey–New Jersey Medical School
Newark, New Jersey

Alan Peppard, MS, PT, ATC
Director of Sports Physical Therapy
University Sports Medicine
University of Rochester School of Medicine
    and Dentistry
Rochester, New York

Margot Putukian, MD, FACSM
Team Physician
Primary Care Sports Medicine
Center for Sports Medicine
Pennsylvania State University
University Park, Pennsylvania

Lee H. Riley III, MD
Assistant Professor
Department of Orthopaedic Surgery
    and Neurosurgery
Johns Hopkins School of Medicine
Baltimore, Maryland

Wayne J. Sebastianelli, MD
Director Athletic Medicine/Team Orthopaedic Surgeon
Center for Sports Medicine
Pennsylvania State University
Associate Professor
Department of Orthopaedics/Rehabilitation
Penn State/Hershey Medical Center
University Park, Pennsylvania

Sok Yi, MD
Chief Resident
Department of Orthopaedic Surgery
University of Virginia
Charlottesville, Virginia

Wayne Stokes, MD
Assistant Professor and Team Physician
Center for Sports Medicine
Pennsylvania State University
University Park, Pennsylvania

Pietro M. Tonino, MD
Chief
Section of Sports Medicine
Assistant Professor
Department of Orthopaedic Surgery
Loyola University Medical Center
Forest, Illinois

Michael L. Voight, DPT, SCS, OCS, ATC
Co-Director
Berkshire Institute of Orthopaedic and
    Sports Physical Therapy
Adjunct Assistant Professor
University of St. Augustine
Wyomissing, Pennsylvania

Kevin E. Wilk, MA, PT
National Director
Research and Clinical Education
Healthsouth Rehabilitation Corporation
Adjunct Assistant Professor
Marquette University–Program in Physical Therapy
Birmingham, Alabama

Craig C. Young, MD
Medical Director of Sports Medicine
Assistant Professor of Orthopaedic Surgery and
    Community and Family Medicine
Medical College of Wisconsin
Milwaukee, Wisconsin

David Yukelson, PhD
Sport Psychology Specialist
Academic Support Center for Student-Athletes
Pennsylvania State University
University Park, Pennsylvania

Louie Zuniga, MS, PT
Director
El Paso Physical Therapy Services
Clinical Instructor
Texas Tech University Health Science Center
El Paso, Texas

Preface

Rehabilitation in Sports Medicine: A Comprehensive Guide was developed for many reasons. Over the past several years and having had many conversations with various health care professionals, including physical therapists, athletic trainers, primary care physicians, strength and conditioning coaches, orthopedic surgeons, and researchers in the field of exercise and sport science, I realized that there was a significant need for a comprehensive reference book that included surgical and nonsurgical treatment approaches for common sports-related injuries. I also realized a reference book that would answer the most often asked questions about nutrition, strength training, psychology, and rehabilitation following athletic injury was needed.

I found many well-written books in the current sports medicine literature; however, many of them do not stress or even mention the importance of the roles of strength and conditioning, prevention of injuries, nutrition, psychology, rehabilitation procedures, and physiologic factors in sports training. This book provides a reference guide for the above-mentioned subjects as well as surgical and nonsurgical rehabilitation of common injuries.

Athletic injuries affect many people other than the athlete involved. The support structure that an athlete has from family, teammates, coaches, and friends, as well as the support from the rehabilitation team, is paramount to foster an optimal environment in which the athlete can progress. One of the biggest factors in rehabilitation is the compliance, dedication, determination, and drive of the injured individual. An injured athlete with a chronic injury and/or a significant acute injury should be promptly referred to a physician. A comprehensive evaluation of the injured athlete is the essential first step in the rehabilitation process. The physician makes an accurate diagnosis by means of a history physical evaluation and appropriate diagnostic tests. Also, the etiology of the injury must be determined. It is an injustice to treat the athlete just symptomatically and not problematically. Educating oneself as to the demands of an individual's sport and the position he or she plays is necessary in order to develop a time and criteria-based rehabilitation program.

Obtaining an individual's complete medical history is crucial in establishing the etiology of their condition. The evaluation must look at intrinsic as well as extrinsic factors that could be associated with the injury. Intrinsic factors include flexibility, strength, age, muscular weakness, muscle imbalance, muscular endurance, cardiovascular fitness, bony alignment, surface structure, and menstrual irregularities. Extrinsic factors include shoewear, orthotics, practice and conditioning programs, playing surface, and equipment. Identifying common injuries, determining the mechanisms of injury, and teaching athletes modified techniques may help to prevent some types of injuries.

Some athletes suffer repetitive stress injuries, such as stress fractures, shin splints, shoulder impingement syndrome, and tendinitis. Injuries of this nature can be prevented. Many of these injuries are due to an athlete's body not being in optimal condition to withstand the stresses placed on it by hard pre-season practices or due to the length of the season. Many athletes lose strength at the end of their season compared with the beginning. An in-season and off-season strength and conditioning program is essential for injury prevention. One must look at current and past research in the field to be able to modify and enhance treatment and rehabilitation of injuries in general.

The health care professional should gain the support and confidence of the coach as well as the athlete throughout the rehabilitation. Over the years, I have seen many instances of delayed referrals of injured athletes by the athletic trainer to the primary care physician or to another health care provider. This may be because the athletic trainer is very busy, has too much "pride," or for other reasons. The primary goal of providing quality care for the injured athlete and returning him or her to competition in a timely and safe manner must always be kept in mind.

In order to be an effective health care professional, one needs to think of the four Cs:

1. *Communication.* Talk to and, more importantly, listen to the patient-athlete. The importance of obtaining a good medical history is paramount in identifying the cause or possible causes of an athlete's injury. Also, explain the situation to the athlete in a clear manner so that he or she un-

derstands what needs to be done and how to do it quickly, safely, and efficiently in order for him or her to go back to participating in their sport. Communication within the rehabilitation team is also very important. Increased communication between people of different disciplines results in increased respect for each other's profession. However, as in any profession, some individuals are better prepared to deal with various aspects of the rehabilitation based on their experience and skill.

The rehabilitation team is analogous to a bicycle chain: if one link sticks or is broken, then the bike does not move well, or move at all. It is also important to realize that as health care professionals we are here for the patients and that they are not here for us.

2. *Comfort.* Make the patient feel at ease. This is especially important with an athlete who has a "serious" injury in which he or she will be out of participation for an extended period of time or one who is in a lot of pain. Make the injured athlete know that you are giving him or her your full attention.

3. *Confidence.* Let the athlete know that you have worked with people with similar injuries and they have been helped. By establishing comfort and communication with the athlete, their confidence in you as a professional improves. Again, support from the coach is also beneficial.

4. *Compliance.* Know an individual's tendencies to do too little or too much. Knowledge of the need for the amount of supervised rehabilitation and training is also very important. Ask the patient-athlete what equipment and facilities he or she has access to. Also, knowing such things as how much time a person will devote to the exercises or if he or she will take medication at appropriate times has a significant bearing on the amount and type of treatment provided. Making the rehabilitation process fun by varying exercises and making some exercises into a "game" also improves compliance.

The goal of this book is to provide a comprehensive reference guide for medical professionals and others who deal with injured athletes in the treatment of common athletic injuries. It gives the reader information that will help develop an individualized rehabilitation program in a complete manner and answer many questions in regard to many different aspects of sports medicine.

Paul K. Canavan, MA, PT, ATC, CSCS

Foreword

Sports participation in the United States continues to grow at a phenomenal rate, and with this growth in participation, the sports medicine field has experienced a similar rate of expansion. Athletic injuries are an unfortunate but all-too-common consequence of sports participation, and today's sports medicine professional must meet the challenge to provide competent care in the prevention, treatment, and rehabilitation of athletic injuries.

Competent care consists of the ability to make an accurate diagnosis of injury and provide initial treatment. This is followed by instituting a rehabilitation program designed to return the athlete to preinjury levels of conditioning and skill. The rehabilitation program should be specific to the needs of the individual, progressive in nature, and functional to the demands of the sport or activity. Finally, attention should be given to the prevention of injury or reinjury through the adherence of sound physiologic training principles and execution of proper exercise techniques.

The sports medicine professional may be one member of a health care team. This team may be composed of health care specialists whose complimentary skills combine to provide an effective, integrated approach to injury treatment and rehabilitation. These specialists may include and not be limited to the athletic trainer, physical therapist, sports and conditioning specialist, sports psychologist, nutritionist, and physician.

Rehabilitation in Sports Medicine: A Comprehensive Guide will serve as a valuable reference source to aid the sports medicine professional in the treatment of athletic injuries. An integrated approach to injury care is presented, blending the various disciplines of the sports medicine field to provide a total care package. Good reading!

Kevin Moody
Director of Sports Medicine
U.S. Olympic Training Center
Lake Placid, New York

Time is at a premium throughout the year for a coach. A support network of quality health care professionals plays a vital role in preparation of a team. The pertinent information regarding the time frame of when an injured athlete will be able to compete is essential with practice and game preparation. As in the coaching profession, health care professionals need to identify strengths and weaknesses of athletes. From this determination, development and implementation of a plan are very important. One or several injured athletes can have a positive or negative impact on the team as a whole. Health care providers can have a positive influence.

Rehabilitation in Sports Medicine: A Comprehensive Guide provides the health care professional with an appreciation for many who contribute to the rehabilitation of injured athletes.

Joseph V. Paterno
Head Football Coach
Pennsylvania State University
University Park, Pennsylvania

Successful *and* safe return of the injured athlete to competition typically requires the combined efforts of many individuals who are involved in their treatment and rehabilitation process. Effective communication and coordination within this "team" greatly enhances the process and permits the athlete to proceed with confidence. Successful sports medicine programs have long recognized this to be a critical component of their success.

Until now, there have been few opportunities to find published resources that sufficiently emphasize this element of coordination of the talents of physicians, physical therapists, trainers, strength and conditioning coaches, and researchers in the rehabilitation process. This book is organized to provide this perspective and emphasis from recognized experts in the field, which makes it a unique contribution to sports medicine literature.

Kenneth E. DeHaven, MD
Professor and Associate Chair
Director of Athletic Medicine
University of Rochester School of Medicine
and Dentistry
Rochester, New York

Acknowledgments

I would like to thank Kathleen McCullough, Managing Editor of Development at Appleton & Lange, for her hard work to make this book possible. My gratitude also goes to Edward H. Wickland, Jr., Vice-President and Publisher at Appleton & Lange, for his continued faith in the project. The support from my family was instrumental during the process of putting together this book. In addition, I would like to thank Tanya Confer for her assistance in the clinic and her support. Finally, I would like to thank all the contributing authors for their fine efforts.

Chapter 1

Strength and Conditioning: Developing a Plan

Jerry Martin and Paul K. Canavan

One of the major goals in the development of a year-round strength and conditioning program is to help the athlete increase muscular strength, power, endurance, and decrease the chances of injury. In order for the program to be beneficial to the athlete, a basic understanding of the anatomy and physiology of the neuromuscular and cardiovascular systems must be established. Just as importantly, is the understanding that certain adaptations need to occur within these systems that will help make the athlete successful in his or her specific sport. Accordingly, it should be clear that these adaptations will only occur through specific manipulations in the strength and conditioning program.

Consistent training with proper variation within the prescribed basic principle of resistance training will allow for optimal gains in strength according to each individual's genetic potential. As with any training modality (speed, strength) the limiting factors of performance may be genetic (fiber typing) or may be limited by decisions of the athlete (poor nutrition). The strength and conditioning professional, as well as the athlete, must understand that the ultimate limiting factor for athletic performance is genetics.

As an individual starts to train, the initial strength gains are great due to the untapped potential that's available. The initial strength gains of the athlete during the beginning phases of a strength training program are strictly due to psychomotor learning. During the first few weeks of resistance training, the body learns the basic skills needed to perform the exercise task. New motor pathways are recruited and the athlete becomes more efficient at the exercise.

As training continues, the body "learns" the exercise tasks and becomes efficient in its movements. Once these initial strength gains have past, future gains will be based on different factors such as muscle hypertrophy (increasing the muscle cross-sectional area). At this point, it is important that the strength and conditioning professional refine the program to optimize the effort put forth by the athlete. When starting a strength and conditioning program it is important to understand the total spectrum of the training process.

FLEXIBILITY TRAINING

Flexibility is an important element of athletic performance and may also aid in injury prevention.[1,2] When assessing the needs of an athlete, the range of motion (ROM) in the specific sport movement must be determined. A variety of levels of flexibility are needed by participants of different sports as well as different positions of the same sport.[3] The overall flexibility of a gymnast may seem more important for his or her sport than that of a hammer thrower in track and field. The throwing arm of a baseball pitcher may seem to need more ROM than that of his or her nonthrowing arm. It is important to realize that flexibility is sport specific.

Flexibility is the range of possible movement in a joint and its surrounding muscles; it is also referred to as static flexibility. Dynamic flexibility refers to the resistance of a joint during movement.[4] Young people tend to be more flexible than older people, and females more flexible than males. Active persons tend to be more flexible than inactive ones.[5]

Several factors limit the ROM at the joint. The bony structure of the joint and the interface between the two articulating surfaces can prevent excessive ROM at different joints. The soft tissues that surround the joint, such as muscles, tendons, fascia, ligaments, and skin also restrict joint motion. Therefore, the soft tissue around the joint must be progressively stretched in order to increase specific joint flexibility. Once optimal flexibility is reached by the athlete, the athlete should maintain that flexibility through proper warm-up, flexibility, and weight training techniques. Pain can also limit motion.

Stretching should be done before practice or competition. Stretching may aid in injury prevention by increasing core temperature and ease of movement. Stretching also allows time for the athlete to prepare mentally for competition.[6] The amount of stretching should be a matter of overall need for flexibility of the sport, flexibility of the athlete, and the possibility of external environmental temperatures. Postpractice or postcompetition stretching may also facilitate a decrease in postexercise soreness. For those who lack proper flexibility for their sport, stretching exercises can be done throughout the day during free time and may not only be athletically beneficial but relaxing as well.[7]

WAYS TO STRETCH

Prior to stretching a "warm up" exercise must be performed for over 5 minutes in duration. This can be a light jog or stationary bike for example. Active stretch occurs when the athlete supplies the force of the stretch. For example, in a seated position on the ground the athlete supplies the force for the forward lean in order to stretch the hamstrings and the low back.

A passive stretch occurs when a partner or a device provides the force to the target area. An example of this type of stretch is when lying on the back with one leg extended, a cord is placed around the heel and the leg is pulled toward the upper body to stretch the hamstrings.

Static stretch is a constant one in which the end position of the ROM is held for a period of time (10 to 30 seconds). This type of stretching is easily learned. Since it is done under a controlled manner, the stretch reflex is not enacted.

Ballistic stretching involves the same movements of the static stretching but incorporates a bouncing action at the end point of the ROM. Ballistic stretching may cause injury to muscle if it is done to a sight of a previous injury. Excessive force or bouncing may elicit a strong stretch reflex, which in turn may cause injury.

Dynamic stretch involves flexibility of sport-specific movements. That is to say specific movements associated with the sport are done at greater ROM than a normal "stretch." This type of stretching may not only be specific to the sport but may also be specific to the position played by the athlete.

The muscle most directly involved in bringing about a movement around a joint is called the prime mover or the agonist. A muscle that can slow down or stop the movement is called the antagonist. The antagonist assists in joint stabilization and in breaking the limb towards the end of a fast movement, protecting ligamentous and cartilaginous joint structures from sustaining potentially destructive forces. Proprioceptive neuromuscular facilitation (PNF) combines the contraction and relaxation techniques of both the agonist and the antagonist muscles. This technique causes neural responses that inhibit the contraction of the muscle that is being stretched. There is a decrease in resistance and an increase in ROM.[8] It is important to note that all stretching activity has the possibility of injury, but as long as each technique is performed in a precise manner the chances of injury are unlikely.

STRENGTH

During training both acute and chronic physiologic changes occur. An acute response to exercise occurs as an almost immediate response to the stress placed on the system. An example of this is an increase in heart rate during the performance of a submaximal lift for a 20 repetition max (20 RM). A chronic change occurs when the body responds to an exercise stimulus over a period of time. An example is an increase in the cross-sectional area of the specific muscle to resistance training. This chronic change is due to the exercise stress and is referred to as *training adaptation.*

One of the most basic adaptations that occurs with resistance training is an increase in muscle mass. This increase in cross-sectional area is referred to as hypertrophy. An increase in the cross-sectional area gives the athlete the potential to generate more force. Muscle hypertrophy does not occur uniformly between fast-twitch and slow-twitch muscle fiber. It has been shown that fast-twitch muscle fibers respond greater to hypertrophy than slow-twitch muscle fiber.[9] It can be presumed that a person with a relative low proportion of fast-twitch muscle fibers will have a limited potential to develop a substantial increase in muscle mass. Several recent studies have shown that females can improve their cross-sectional muscle area through resistance training as well.[10] However, the difference between genders, as well as differences between an individual's specific muscle hypertrophy, depends on a number of different factors. These factors include hormonal excretions such as testosterone and human growth hormone, as well as hormonal ratios.

Testosterone is an androgen with masculizing effects on the body. Testosterone is closely involved with the growth and development of males throughout puberty and is responsible for the development and maturation of male sex organs and secondary sexual characteristics.[11]

The interest of testosterone in the field of strength and conditioning is its effect on muscle cell growth.[12] The increase in the musculature appears to be its effects on protein synthesis.[13] Testosterone is reported to enhance glycogen synthesis and to increase red cell mass by increasing erthropoietin levels.[12]

A single training session of resistance exercise has been demonstrated to increase the peripheral concentrations of testosterone above resting levels. As long as the intensity of the exercise session is relative to the lifter's experience, there doesn't seem to be any difference in the magnitude of the hormonal response.[14] However, changes in the testosterone secretions may differ and may be related to the design of the exercise format. Theses design variables include rest periods between sets and the percentage of an individual's maximum weight that is lifted.

Human growth hormone is a polypeptide hormone secreted in a pulsated fashion by the anterior pituitary gland. Human growth hormone has a number of various physiologic roles in the human body, such as increasing protein synthesis and mobilizing free fatty acids for use as an energy source.[15]

This particular hormone can be affected by the duration and intensity of exercise. Weight training exercise has a positive influence in increasing postexercise levels of human growth hormone. This is especially true if the exercise bout includes the use of large muscle masses and short rest periods (under 3 minutes) between sets.[16]

The initial gains that accompany resistance training within the first few weeks with very little increase in muscle mass suggest that other factors instead of shear cross-sectional area must not be the only factor in determining muscular strength. It is believed that neural factors play an important role in increasing strength during the first 3 to 5 weeks of training.[17] This neuromotor learning phase teaches one's skeletal system "how to perform" the exercise. After this short period of time, muscle hypertrophy becomes one of the leading factors in the development of further strength increases.

Further studies have suggested that a more efficient order or pattern of recruitment of the muscle fibers may be responsible for the increase in force production.[18] Another neural factor that may increase force production is the increased synchronization of motor unit firing. A motor unit is a single motor neuron and all of the muscle fibers that it innervates. This unit is the basic functional entity of muscular contraction. Muscular control is also based on the number of muscle fibers per motor unit.

Muscles that need precise control, such as the eye, may have only one muscle fiber per motor unit. However, at the other end of the spectrum, muscles that perform less precise movements, such as the quadriceps, may have several hundred muscle fibers served per motor unit. It seems logical that the greater the synchronization, the greater number of motor units firing, creating the greatest amount of force production. However, it appears that some muscles can be maximally activated during voluntary effort; others cannot.[19]

Inhibition of muscle contraction by reflex protective mechanisms such as the Golgi tendon organs, might be necessary to prevent the muscles from exerting more force than the bones and connective tissues can tolerate. Training may gradually reduce or counteract these inhibitory impulses, allowing the muscle to reach greater levels of strength. A resistance training program in which the antagonists muscles are contracted immediately prior to the performance of an exercise is more effective than a program in which precontraction of the antagonists is not performed.[20] This precontraction in some way partially inhibits the neural self-protective mechanisms, allowing for a more forceful contraction. This can be of importance when creating an exercise program. For example, an exercise program can be created to combine antagonists muscle groups with agonists muscle groups. A chest and back combination can be beneficial for creating maximal force production as compared with performing chest exercises solely separate from back exercises.

A combination chest and back exercise session consists of exercising the major muscle groups of the chest by using such exercises as the bench press, incline press, and the dumbbell fly. By referring the chest muscles as the agonist muscle group, the exerciser would perform one set of the chest exercises followed by one set of a back exercise or antagonist muscle group. These exercises for the back could include bent over row, lat pull down, and the seated row. These exercises can be alternated until the desired number of sets is completed by each muscle group.

Another agonist and antagonist combination would be the quadriceps and hamstring muscle group. To exercise the quadriceps, the leg extension machine is ideal for quadriceps isolation. This exercise is immediately followed by exercising the hamstrings with a leg curl exercise.

By alternating these chest and back and quadriceps and hamstring exercises, or in this instance agonist and antagonist muscle groups, the exerciser is able to generate a more forceful contraction and thus is able to apply a greater stress to the desired exercise area.

Finally do not underestimate the level of fear when starting a resistance training program with a beginning lifter. Inhibitory mechanisms are excited when a person is new to certain lifts. In the eye of the beginner, it may be a dangerous and injury-producing environment. As the lifter becomes experienced in training, these fears seem to subside as well as some of the inhibitory responses, both physically and psychologically.

Importance of Certification

With the age of "athletic strength and conditioning" in full bloom, there is a need to set certain standards. These standards, although different within each health profession, must still be met by all parties in each specific field. This includes the area of strength and conditioning. The strength and conditioning professional must be abreast of the newfound enthusiasm for recreational as well as specific athletic strength and conditioning. What was once a luxury, having a strength and conditioning professional at the professional sport level, is now becoming the norm at all major colleges and most high school settings. With this boom in specific strength and conditioning, responsibilities, expectations, and *results* are demanded along with the validity, competency, and liability that goes along with the profession.

The importance of knowledge in the professional area is vital. One way a person is recognized as a professional is by certification. The only strength and conditioning association that is currently accredited by the National Commission for Certification Agency is the National Strength and Conditioning Association's Certified Strength and Conditioning Specialist (CSCS). These guidelines for base knowledge and competency were set forth by the National Organization for Competency Assurance.[21] It is this accreditation that the general public or athlete uses when acquiring a knowledgeable and competent professional in the coaching techniques of enhancing sport performance.

CONDITIONING

There are two major anaerobic sources of energy (ATP-PC and lactic acid) and one source of aerobic energy (oxidative). Knowledge of these energy sources and their interactions among each other is important to the overall success of a quality conditioning program. Anaerobic energy production is essential for the maintenance of high-intensity exercise when the demand for ATP is greater than what can be produced aerobically. At the onset of high-intensity exercise, ATP is mostly derived anaerobically, which provides up to 80 to 90 percent of the total ATP required due to the short supply of oxygen. In order to further meet the energy demands of the muscles, the cardiovascular system increases its oxygen delivery. However, since the ATP demand is so much greater than what can be supplied by the aerobic energy system, the anaerobic system further supplies the ATP to

continue the exercise bout until temporary system fatigue is reached. The appropriate contributions of anaerobic and aerobic sources of ATP production during high-intensity exercise lasting around 3 minutes are:

Anaerobic Aerobic

80 percent	20 percent in the initial 30 seconds
45 percent	55 percent from 60 to 90 seconds
39 percent	70 percent from 120 to 180 seconds[22]

ATP-PC Source

When ATP is broken down, ATP-PC, the energy result, is used to cause a muscle contraction. ATP-PC is stored within the muscle itself and does not require oxygen to release this energy; thus this substance is readily available for immediate use at the muscle site. Another advantage is that the ATP-PC source has a large power capacity. It is capable of giving the muscle a large amount of energy over a very short period of time. Due to these characteristics, the ATP-PC source is the primary energy source for high-intensity, short-duration power events. These events include maximal lifts, 40-yard sprints, shotput, and high jump among others. However in an all out effort the ATP-PC energy source will be exhausted in 30 seconds or less.[23]

Lactic Acid Source

Stored within the muscle itself is the carbohydrate glycogen. This substance is composed of sugar molecules referred to as glucose. The energy necessary to create a muscle contraction is derived by splitting glucose molecules, creating the compound pyruvate, and thus releasing energy. Again, no oxygen is required for this process to take place, hence this process is referred to as anaerobic glycolysis. However, the body creates more lactic acid than it is able to form into energy. This buildup of lactic acid has several side effects. One side effect is that in a high enough concentration, nerve endings become affected, causing pain. Also as the concentration of lactic acid increases, blood pH becomes more acidic, interfering with the binding of calcium with troponin.[24] This interference with calcium affects the contractile ability of the muscle; the amount of energy that can be obtained from the lactic acid source is limited due to this side effect.

The lactic acid source is a major supplier of energy during maximal muscular effort lasting approximately 1 to 3 minutes in length. Examples of such maximal efforts are the 400 and 800 meter sprints in track.

Oxygen Source

The aerobic energy source uses oxygen in the production of ATP and is therefore an aerobic energy source. This oxygen system metabolizes carbohydrates and fats.

Protein can also be used to generate ATP, but this is usually during long-term starvation or during extremely long intense exercise bouts when carbohydrates are not replenished. The maximal amount of energy that can be produced via the oxygen system is limited by how much the body can obtain and utilize oxygen (cardiovascular system). The ability of the body to obtain and utilize oxygen is expressed as VO_2 max. This term can be expressed in relative terms when assessing VO_2 max according to body weight as VO_2/kg/min/L. This places everyone on a similar scale relative to body weight. In doing this, the strength and conditioning professional and sport coach has a quantified means to measure the aerobic capacity of athletes.

The aerobic system cannot produce the ATP needed per unit of time in order to perform high-intensity, maximal performances. On the other hand, due to the availability of carbohydrates and fats, and the lack of waste products, the aerobic energy system can supply virtually an unlimited amount of ATP over an extended period of time as long as the intensity of the effort is low enough. Therefore, it is the body's system of choice for long duration, low-intensity activity such as marathon running, distance swimming, and prolonged cycling.

TRAINING THE ENERGY SYSTEMS

To train athletes as individuals, as a group, or as a team, a basic form of work terminology must be established. The following are some related terms that may help in the communication and physical development of athletes.

- *Work interval*. The part of the training session that is constituted by the time (30 seconds) and/or the training distance (200 m).
- *Training intensity*. The relationship between the specific training distance and the percentage of the athlete's best time. For example, if an athlete's best time for 200 m is 26 seconds and the training intensity is 80 percent, the athlete would run for a training session 200 m at 31.2 seconds. The training distance remains the same but the time factor is different. Therefore training intensity can be expressed as a percentage of maximal performance. A further example is 200 m at 26 seconds equals maximal performance, 80 percent equals 31.2 seconds, 70 percent equals 33.8 seconds, 60 percent equals 36.4 seconds, and so on. Training intensity can also be a percentage of maximal heart rate where maximum heart rate is expressed as 220 minus age equals age-related maximal heart rate.
- *Recovery interval*. This is the period of time between work intervals. The recovery interval can include some active recovery such as slow walking. Recovery intervals can be a specific time or expressed as a certain percentage of the athlete's age-related maximal heart rate. For example, recover to 65 percent of one's age-related maximal heart rate before starting the next work interval.
- *Work-rest interval*. This is the time ratio between the work interval and the rest interval. Interval training can be used to increase the efficiency of the phosphagen, glycolytic, or oxidative energy systems. If the goal is speed endurance, the work-rest interval should be quite long, for example 1:5 or 1:6. If the goal of the training program is endurance, the work-rest interval should be shorter, for example 1:1 or 1:2. Here would be a good opportunity to use heart rate monitors.

  Instead of using time as a factor, heart rate can be used to judge the intensity of the run and the proper amount of rest for each individual athlete. An example of this is to have the athlete run multiple 400 meters during their training sessions. The athlete has to exceed 180 heartbeats per minute during the work phase. This is approximately 90 percent of maximum heart rate for the college age male. For the rest phase, when the athlete heart rate returns to 140 beats per minute (about 70 percent of maximum heart rate), they proceed to run the next 400 meters. Depending on each individual's fitness level, rest periods between running bouts may be long, if they are in poor condition, or it may be short, showing signs of good conditioning.
- *Repetition*. One work interval and one rest interval is considered one repetition.
- *Set*. A group of work–rest intervals. Five 100-m sprints with five rest intervals in succession would be considered one set.
- *Training time*. The time of the work interval. This is based on the percentage of intensity and the athlete's best time. Training can vary with the specific needs of the athlete or the sport. If the athlete's best time in the 200 m is 26 seconds, and the training intensity is 80 percent of maximum, the athlete's training time would be 31.2 seconds in the 200 m.

Overtraining

The development of maximal athletic performance is dependent on a carefully designed and implemented total training program. The art of developing such a program is based on how much stress is needed to improve a positive adaptation compared to applying too much stress that in turn associates itself with a decrease in training adaptation and therefore poor athletic performance.

Overtraining is a general term used to define both the process of training excessively and the fatigue that may develop. It is the process of training at volumes and intensities that are too extreme for the present physical and mental state of the athlete.

Overtraining is characterized by physiologic and psychological symptoms, as well as a decrease in athletic performance. Due to the number of symptoms associated with overtraining, it is a complex problem. In a survey of overtrained athletes, it was found that 77 percent were involved in sports requiring high levels of strength, speed, or coordination.[25] It has also been suggested that explosive, nonendurance type athletes develop symptoms associated with altered sympathetic system function while endurance athletes developed symptoms associated with altered parasympathetic system function. Since the differences in adaptations in aerobic and anaerobic training are specific to the demands of the specific activities, the physiologic factors contributing to overtraining for elite performance could be quite different.

The overtraining symptoms that an athlete develops are specific to the type of training they encounter. Athletes whose sport performance includes large quantities of intense anaerobic exercise where speed, strength, and coordination are important, seem to develop sympathetic overtraining characteristics. The sympathetic overtraining syndrome shows an increase in sympathetic activity in the resting state that contributes to the following symptoms: increased heart rate, decreased lean body mass, decreased appetite, disturbed sleep, decreased performance, decreased recovery after exercise, increased irritability and emotional liability, loss of training and competitive desire, increased resting blood pressure, increased incidence of injuries and infections, and decreased maximal plasma lactate level during exercise.[26]

When large amounts of aerobic training are performed, the athlete seems to develop in a manner opposite to the sympathetic overtraining syndrome, the parasympathetic overtraining syndrome. The parasympathetic overtraining syndrome in the resting state contributes to the following symptoms: low resting heart rate, early fatigue, decreased performance, quick recovery of heart rate after exercise, more sleep than usual, demented counterregulatory capacity against hypoglycemia, and depression.[26]

It seems that overtraining varies among individual athletes according to sport and present psychological and physiologic states. Highly motivated athletes seem to be at a higher risk for overtraining than other athletes.

Perhaps the most effective tool used by the strength and conditioning professional to help prevent overtraining is the careful planning and monitoring of all training sessions. This, along with knowledge of the makeup of individual athletes, assists in early recognition of overtraining symptoms. Hopefully, with minimal restoration time, the athlete will again be competing and training at optimal levels.

PLYOMETRICS

Plyometric refers to exercises that enable a muscle to produce maximal force in as short a time as possible. Plyometrics are most notably performed using the lower body muscles; however, there are some exercises that incorporate the use of the upper body. Plyometrics uses the natural elastic properties of the muscles and the connective tissues to produce a maximal force either linear, vertical, lateral, or combination thereof. This eccentric elongation to concentric contraction of muscles and connective tissues is referred to as the stretch shortening cycle.[27] Plyometric exercise utilizes the force of gravity (stepping off a box) to store energy (eccentric load) and uses that stored energy to immediately react (concentric contraction) in a dynamic nature (jumping off the ground). It must be understood that due to the tremendous momentum shifts that take place from eccentric to concentric movements, tremendous stress is place on the musculoskeletal system of the body. Knowing this, a strength base needs to be developed before the implementation of a plyometrics program.

Athletes selected for plyometric training should complete a basic strength program over a period of several weeks or even months. Athletes in poor condition, especially in strength, are not viable candidates to take part in plyometric training. An estimated minimum strength level 1.5 to 2.5 times body weight in the free weight squat has been recommended for safe participation in lower body plyometric drills.[28] For upper body drills, the ability for athletes to bench press their weight (above 90 kg) and 1.5 times for smaller athletes (below 90 kg) is a reasonable guideline for moving to more advanced upper body plyometrics.[29]

Plyometric exercises are especially useful in sports that require speed and strength.[30] Those sports that require the need to exert a maximal force at a high speed include track and field, football, basketball, baseball, and volleyball. Plyometrics for the lower body include box jumps, bounding, hopping, and depth jumps.[31] Those exercises that increase speed and strength development for the upper body include medicine ball throws, catches, and several variations of push-ups.

Training drills that incorporate the stretch-shortening cycle can improve gross motor skills for sport movements. The careful selection, proper teaching by a qualified strength and conditioning professional, loading, and progression of plyometrics can minimize problems as well as maximize performance.

ACUTE PROGRAM VARIABLES

Acute program variables describe the combinations of training possibilities. The proper decisions that must be made by the strength professional are reflective on a number of different factors. Those factors can be personal reasons (philosophy) or somewhat uncontrolled circumstances (facilities). One factor is administrative concerns, which will be discussed later.

Choice of Exercise

Based on observation and a needs analysis, exercises should be chosen that stress the appropriate muscles and joint actions associated with the specific sport. Exercises should be broken down into two main categories: structural, which are multijoint in nature, and body part, which are single-joint movements.

Structural exercises reflect a holistic approach and incorporate the balance and coordination of many muscles working together to accomplish a successful lift. It is important to incorporate structural lifts into a program if the sport in question uses whole body movement such as basketball, football, track and field, and volleyball. These movements may need more technical expertise and greater coaching time; however, once learned, they offer the advantage of greater overall stress to the body by incorporating greater involvement of muscle mass. These exercises are advantageous when it is necessary to train many athletes and time is a limiting factor. Some common structural exercises are bench press, parallel squat, power clean, and the shoulder press.

Number of Sets

The number of sets should be chosen based on factors related to muscle size, muscle group, injuries associated with the sport, and required training results. An individual will show a faster rate of gains when doing multiple sets versus a single-set system.[32] The entire principle of multiple sets is based on stress adaptation. As the muscle adapts, a more pronounced or different stress must be applied to continue positive gains. Single-set exercises may be beneficial for those just starting an exercising program where multiple sets are too taxing for the body.

Rest Period

The amount of rest allowed between sets determines the recovery process and the energy sources that are available for the next set. Since the ATP-PC system is so powerful, it is needed for any maximal or near maximal efforts. To replenish this energy source, a recovery period of 2 to 3 minutes is needed between exercise bouts. If exercise intensity is high and recovery between sets is less than 1 minute, the lactic acid energy source is placed under great amounts of stress and its concentrations become quite high in the blood plasma. However, it can be the decision of the strength and conditioning professional that this is a needed stress applied to the body since the sport (basketball) depends on the tolerance of lactic acid in the blood system. Other athletes may also depend on the lactic acid energy source for their sport, such as 400 and 800 m sprint athletes and wrestlers. There are times in the training program when the athlete may either need a total recovery of the energy system or an incomplete energy recovery between sets to create the appropriate stress on the body during the training bout.

Loading Needs

Load can be determined by a number of factors. One factor is a repetition max (RM) scheme. This means that a 6-RM load is defined as the most weight an athlete can successfully lift for six repetitions. A 10-RM is defined as the most weight an athlete can lift successfully for ten repetitions.

Another means to calculate load is by using a percentage of a 1 RM. After an athlete performs a 1 RM, a percentage is taken from that max and used in a training session. For example, if an athlete's 1 RM for a given exercise is 300 pounds, 60 percent of that 1 RM would be 180 pounds. For the next training session the athlete uses 60 percent of his or her 1 RM (180 pounds) for a given number of repetitions (15 repetitions). This type of formulation depends on a maximum lifting test in all of the exercises. This can be too time consuming.

A third means to determine on athlete's maximal lifts is through a predicted maximum formula. Table 1-1 is used to determine the athlete's maximum weight by the number of repetitions he or she can achieve at a submaximal load.

It is generally assumed that the higher the repetitions involved in the exercise program, the lower the load is to be lifted. As the athlete trains at the higher repetition end of the spectrum, 20 repetitions or higher, strength gains and power gains will be nominal. However, the athlete can benefit through this type of training by increasing overall endurance. As the training repetitions become lower (six repetitions or less) and the load increases, strength and power simultaneously increase yet overall muscle endurance decreases.

Speed of Exercise

Specific adaptations are also associated with specific speeds of movement.[33] In order to increase strength at a high speed, the velocity of movement of the exercise must also be high. Fast explosive exercises such as the Olympic lifts (snatch, clean and jerk), where speed of movement is emphasized, results in a substantial improvement in

TABLE 1–1. PREDICTED MAXIMUM CHART

Weight Used	Repetitions Completed								
	2	3	4	5	6	7	8	9	10
100	106	109	112	115	118	121	124	127	130
105	111	114	118	121	124	127	130	133	137
110	117	120	123	127	130	133	136	140	143
115	122	125	129	132	136	139	143	146	150
120	127	131	134	138	142	145	149	152	156
125	133	136	140	144	148	151	155	159	163
130	138	142	146	150	153	157	161	165	169
135	143	147	151	155	159	163	167	171	176
140	148	153	157	161	165	169	174	178	182
145	154	158	162	167	171	175	180	184	189
150	159	164	168	173	177	182	186	191	195
155	164	169	174	178	183	188	192	197	202
160	170	174	179	184	189	194	198	203	208
165	175	180	185	190	195	200	205	210	215
170	180	185	190	196	201	206	211	216	221
175	186	191	196	201	207	212	217	222	228
180	191	196	202	207	212	218	223	229	234
185	196	202	207	213	218	224	229	235	241
190	201	207	213	219	224	230	236	241	247
195	207	213	218	224	230	236	242	248	254
200	212	218	224	230	236	242	248	254	260
205	217	223	230	236	242	248	254	260	267
210	223	229	235	242	248	254	260	267	273
215	228	234	241	247	254	260	267	273	280
220	233	240	246	253	260	266	273	279	286
225	239	245	252	259	266	272	279	286	293
230	244	251	258	265	271	278	285	292	299
235	249	256	263	270	277	284	291	298	306
240	254	262	269	276	283	290	298	305	312
245	260	267	274	282	289	296	304	311	319
250	265	273	280	288	295	303	310	318	325
255	270	278	286	293	301	309	316	324	332
260	276	283	291	299	307	315	322	330	338
265	281	289	297	305	313	321	329	337	345
270	286	294	302	311	319	327	335	343	351
275	292	300	308	316	325	333	341	349	358
280	297	305	314	322	330	339	347	356	364
285	302	311	319	328	336	345	353	362	371
290	307	316	325	334	342	351	360	368	377
295	313	322	330	339	348	357	366	375	384
300	318	327	336	345	354	363	372	381	390
305	323	332	342	351	360	369	378	387	397
310	329	338	347	357	366	375	384	394	403
315	334	343	353	362	372	381	391	400	410
320	339	349	358	368	378	387	397	406	416

(Continued)

TABLE 1-1. (*Continued*)

Weight Used	Repetitions Completed								
	2	**3**	**4**	**5**	**6**	**7**	**8**	**9**	**10**
325	345	354	364	374	384	393	403	413	423
330	350	360	370	380	389	399	409	419	429
335	355	365	375	385	395	405	415	425	436
340	360	371	381	391	401	411	422	432	442
345	366	376	386	397	407	417	428	438	449
350	371	382	392	403	413	424	434	445	455
355	376	387	398	408	419	430	440	451	462
360	382	392	403	414	425	436	446	457	468
365	387	398	409	420	431	442	453	464	475
370	392	403	414	426	437	448	459	470	481
375	398	409	420	431	443	454	465	476	488
380	403	414	426	437	448	460	471	483	494
385	408	420	431	443	454	466	477	489	501
390	413	425	437	449	460	472	484	495	507
395	419	431	442	454	466	478	490	502	514
400	424	436	448	460	472	484	496	508	520
405	429	441	454	466	478	490	502	514	527
410	435	447	459	472	484	496	508	521	533
415	440	452	465	477	490	502	515	527	540
420	445	458	470	483	496	508	521	533	546
425	451	463	476	489	502	514	527	540	553
430	456	469	482	495	507	520	533	546	559
435	461	474	487	500	513	526	539	552	566
440	466	480	493	506	519	532	546	559	572
445	472	485	498	512	525	538	552	565	579
450	477	491	504	518	531	545	558	572	585
455	482	496	510	523	537	551	564	578	592
460	488	501	515	529	543	557	570	584	598
465	493	507	521	535	549	563	577	591	605
470	498	512	526	541	555	569	583	597	611
475	504	518	532	546	561	575	589	603	618
480	509	523	538	552	566	581	595	610	624
485	514	529	543	558	572	587	601	616	631
490	519	534	549	564	578	593	608	622	637
495	525	540	554	569	584	599	614	629	644
500	530	545	560	575	590	605	620	635	650

maximal power output. This not only occurs due to muscle hypertrophy, but also because of the maximal rate at which force can be developed. It also seems that any training velocity increases strength at that specific training velocity but also increases strength at lower velocities.[34]

Proprioceptors are unique sensory receptors located inside muscles, joints, and tendons that monitor the length and tension of the musculotendonous complex.[35] These receptors provide information to the central nervous system concerning the position of body parts in three-dimensional space. This body awareness is referred to as kinesthetic sense, and is essential for executing coordinated movements and maintaining muscle tone and posture. This "specificity of training" mimics similar sport movements (vertical jump) with resistant training movements (hang snatch), thus providing a positive relationship between weight training exercises and improved sport performance.[36]

NEEDS ANALYSIS

The first step to start a strength and conditioning program is the development of a needs analysis. A needs analysis is done by assessment of the biomechanical and physiologic needs of both the sport and the individual athletes who participate in that sport.

The first question in the *needs analysis* requires an examination of the muscles and joints associated with the specific sport and an understanding of their particular movements and associated stresses. For example, sports that require high-velocity sprinting would depict a need for exercises for the hamstrings, quadriceps, and gluteals. It is critical to understand how these muscles interact with each other and their combined stresses on the hip, knee, and ankle. A physiologic analysis allows the creation of a program that addresses the components of strength and flexibility, power, endurance, and speed associated with the particular sport.

Video Analysis

It is important to take the time to evaluate such specific aspects of movement and to quantify the muscles, angles, velocities, and forces involved. One way that a sport can be biomechanically analyzed is through videotape. Some major questions can be answered through this medium. These questions include the joint range of motion (ROM), the pattern of joint movements, and the velocity of the limb around its joint. Videotape can also help to analyze the physiologic needs of particular positions. The analysis also gives a chance to see how muscles work kinematically. The following procedures may answer some of the previous questions about a specific sport and its needs.[37]

- Select a videotape of an athletic contest, most notably a game instead of a practice session.
- Select a movement that is intense in nature and critical to the total performance of the athlete. An example of this is the drive of the hips and legs in the triple jumps or the landing of the pitchers front leg on the mound.
- Identify the joints that are susceptible to the greatest amounts of force. Focus on common areas of injury such as particular muscles or joints. A good example of this is the ankle, knee, and hips of the triple jumper and the shoulder of the baseball pitcher.
- Determine the contraction modes (concentric, eccentric, and isometric) of the movement and their sequence. An offensive lineman in football starts from an isometric stance to an explosive, propulsive, concentric movement of the quadriceps. A basketball player jumping for a rebound goes from eccentric to concentric with the quadriceps. A baseball pitcher goes from accelerating the baseball to decelerating the arm during the follow through phase of the pitching arch, from concentric to eccentric.
- For each joint involved, determine its range of motion. Check to see if the joint is going through a full ROM, if the contraction mode is always the same, or if it is constantly changing.
- Try to determine the interaction of the total body within the specific sport skill. An example of this is in the sprinting movement, the coordinated motion of the leg with the motion of the arms. Another example is how the leg drive interacts with the forehand swing in the tennis athlete.
- Select exercises that closely match the limb ranges and angular velocities, making sure that the exercises are appropriately concentric, isometric, or eccentric. As an example, in the jump of a basketball player for a rebound, there is a propulsive concentric contraction of the quadriceps, driving the body upwards followed by a forceful eccentric elongation to help decelerate the body on landing. This is biomechanically similar to the hang clean exercises in the weight room.
- It is advised to make the exercise the most difficult at the point in the ROM where intensity during the athletic performance is the greatest. This can be accomplished by a number of different methods. One method is by adding resistance manually by use of an experienced spotter, where during that particular ROM the spotter applies more resistance to the barbell. Also, by applying the principle that the greatest resistance to movement around a body joint occurs when the weight is horizontally farthest from the joint (midpoint in the barbell curl due to the increase of the arm resistance from the joint), gravity has its greatest effect in this position as well. This can be modified by simply changing the point of peak tension to which the exercise is done (from a standing barbell curl to a preacher barbell curl). Tension of the muscle can also be increased by attempting to increase the velocity of movement of the weight as the limb travels through the target angle. Finally, short ROM exercises can be incorporated with heavier weights to specifically target those areas where the greatest amounts of force are required. For example, doing quarter squats, where heavy weight could be used for high jumpers where knee flexion and extension and hip flexion and extension are very limited in their specific events.

PERIODIZATION

When creating programs for a group of individuals such as a team, the strength and conditioning professional must be aware enough to adjust the program for each person's tolerance level. Knowing this level through performance testing can achieve optimal results and reduce the chance of injury or overtraining. Progression in resistance training should follow a staircase effect. As an individual starts a training session with a certain amount of strength, that strength decreases due to fatigue by the end of the training session. However, with proper recovery, the athlete will begin the following training session at a slightly higher level of strength. This staircase process will repeat for each training session. The challenge for both the athlete and the strength and conditioning professional is to vary program variables in an organized fashion to continue this staircase effect through the career of the athlete. Periodization is this gradual changing or manipulation of specificity, intensity, and volume of training to achieve peak levels of performance for the most important competitions such as end-of-season championships. Training programs usually shift from high-volume, low-intensity general exercises to a low-volume, high-intensity specific exercise training program.[38] These training time segments are referred to as cycles or phases, and are broken up usually according to the level of athletic competition. A macrocycle is as long as 4 years (Olympic competition) or as short as a couple of months (multisport athlete in high school). Each macrocycle is broken up into two or more mesocycles that revolve around dates of major competitions or competitive seasons. For ease of administration, these mesocycles may evolve themselves around the school calendar, which has its own preseason, in-season, and off-season periods. Each mesocycle is then divided into smaller periods of training that include a hypertrophy and endurance phase, strength phase, power phase, competition phase, and transition phase.[39]

Hypertrophy and Endurance Phase

The hypertrophy and endurance phase occurs during the beginning of the off-season programming.[40] It is usually associated with low-intensity (power output), high-volume training (high number of repetitions) and acquisition of technique (teaching). The primary goal for this phase of training is to increase total muscle mass while enhancing muscle endurance. Exercises are usually nonspecific to the sport yet are implemented to develop a base of fitness. Repetitions of exercises are around 10 to 12 RM repetitions, with the number of sets being one to three per exercise. The conditioning program is aerobic in nature to increase overall general conditioning and to decrease the total body fat of the ath-

lete if necessary. For example, a sprinter may start this phase of conditioning doing longer distance training in order to increase overall conditioning level and to decrease body fat. This in turn can make the athlete a more prolific sprinter during the competition phase.

Strength Phase

In this phase, intensity and load gradually increase to around 80 percent of the athlete's maximum. The repetitions of the exercises are within the 5- to 8-RM range, and the number of sets per exercise is within the 3- to 5-set range. The exercises themselves are more sport specific. The purpose of this phase is to develop strength in the athlete. Technical coaching is still important, since there is an implementation of different exercise movements as well as increases in loads. Conditioning becomes of more moderate distances while there is an increase in overall intensity. Interval training can be implemented with the beginning of athletic drills and agility. Testing of overall strength is important as a marker for the implementation of plyometric training (squatting 150 percent of your body weight for typical college male athlete).

Power Phase

The intensity of weight training increases to 90 percent or more of 1 RM during the power phase. The repetitions of the structural exercises are from 1- to 5-RM range. The exercises are specific to the event or sport that the athlete participates in. The number of sets are within the 3 to 5 range per structural exercise. The power exercises play an important role in the continuing development of speed and strength (power). Conditioning intensity will continue to increase with work intensity near or at contest pace. Advanced plyometrics, speed development, and specific athletic drills play a more important role in the overall development of the athlete.

Competition Phase

The competition phase is that time where the athlete peaks for the competitive season. During this phase, it is difficult to manipulate the program variables due to the differences of the sport seasons. An example of this is the college basketball season where the athletes may be in competition for 4 months, compared to the Olympics where the competitive event may only last a few days or maybe just one day. Whatever the case, the athlete should be in the best possible condition both mentally and physically. The strength program is of high intensity with the repetitions being between 1 and 5 RM of the sport-specific exercises. The conditioning program is again sport-specific training with near or at pace level with full recovery between intervals.

Transition Phase

The transition phase is marked by either a period of low volume and low intensity or a period of active rest with activity being recreational, light, and unsupervised. During periods of prolonged strenuous training, athletes cannot achieve best performance results for two main reasons. First, it takes time to adapt to the training stimulus. Second, hard training work induces fatigue that builds over time. Thus, a period of relatively easy (low volume, low intensity) training is needed to realize the effect of the previous hard training sessions. Adaptation occurs mainly when the load being lifted is different than the "normal" load lifted.[41] This principle effect of adaptation is called delayed transformation, and the process is referred to as tapering. This transition phase can be used between phases in general but is most noticeable right before the major competition.

ADMINISTRATIVE CONCERNS

No matter how knowledgeable strength and conditioning professionals are, there are limitations to what they can do. Those limitations may be due to factors that are not in their control. Some factors to be aware of, even before the development of an exercise program, are time, space, number of athletes, equipment, and practice demands of the athlete.

In the educational setting, an athlete has many obligations, including practice, classes, homework, competition, eating, and sleeping. Because of this, the strength and conditioning professional has to devise a program that will improve the athlete's performance but at the same time understand the other commitments and responsibilities. Examples of time and exercise management are limiting rest periods between sets, development of an exercise program that incorporates multijoint exercises, and creation of an atmosphere in the strength facility that promotes work instead of a social environment.

In general, there should be 100 square feet of room per athlete in the weight facility. When space is a problem, a solution can be the development of a circuit training program, where a high volume of athletes can train in a short period of time. Circuit training is a work to rest interval where each athlete exercises at a specific exercise station for a set period of time (40 seconds). When the work time has expired, each athlete then moves to the next preappointed station to rest (20 seconds) until the work interval starts again.

Develop a priority listing of those sports which have the potential to gain the most from an exercise program. Use outside areas as a place to do manual resistance exercises or body weight training (pull-ups, push-ups, sit-ups). These ideas can help when space is a limiting factor and there are many athletes to contend with.

Equipment can also be a limiting factor out of the strength and conditioning professional's control. If new equipment can be ordered, get equipment that has the ability to do a number of different exercises. One idea is to use a power rack as a contained area where different exercises can be done from the same power rack using a multiadjustable bench. Some exercises that can be done from this configuration are the bench press, incline press, seated press, squat, and push press.

Adaptations to resistance training are specific to the type of exercises being performed as well as the specific conditioning factors involved. Explosive training evokes increases in muscular power (speed and strength). Traditional heavy training with conventional exercises creates mainly size and strength. However, neither type of training enhances aerobic power. Aerobic conditioning increases aerobic power but does not in itself enhance strength or muscle size.

TESTING

Those individuals who have an interest in personal fitness through the demands of professional sport athletic performance must have a means to critique physical changes. These changes can be monitored through testing. A test is simply a means of assessing someone's ability in a particular task. Test results provide a variety of information to strength and conditioning professionals. Testing can reveal strength and conditioning status, athletic talent, possible health risks, and specific performance weaknesses, and can also serve as a basis for developing individual exercise programs and as a motivator to athletes.

A test must fulfill three requirements to produce an acceptable means of evaluation. These requirements are validity, reliability, and objectivity.[42]

Validity

Validity is a degree to which a test measures the characteristics it is intended to measure.[43] There are four types of validity: construct validity, predictive validity, content validity, and concurrent validity. To better understand these four traits of validity, consider the 40-yard dash test for speed for a football running back.

Construct validity is the degree to which a test measures some part of a whole skill or an abstract trait. In this case, the 40-yard sprint measures a trait commonly used in football, sprinting speed. Predictive validity is the degree to which one measure can predict performance based on another measure. The player with a faster 40-yard sprint time would theoretically have an advantage in the sport of football when compared to a player with a slower 40-yard sprint time. Content validity is a technique based on the subjectively established fact that the test measures the wanted content. The 40-yard sprint test is an accepted standard to measure speed, an important asset in the sport of football. Concurrent validity is the degree to which scores on a test correlate with scores on the accepted standard. If an athlete has a low time in the 40-yard dash test, it is accepted that he or she is faster than an athlete with a higher time (slower speed) in the same test measured in the same manner.[42]

Reliability

Reliability refers to the degree of consistency that a test measures what it's suppose to measure. It is the repeatability of the test.[42,44] This means that an athlete who hasn't changed any physical factors will have the same scores with a reliable test if the test is repeated. There are some factors that can negatively effect reliability such as lack of consistency of the athlete being tested, failure of the calibration of the testing instrument, or the inability for the instrument to measure accurately. If the testers do not consistently follow standardized testing procedures, the test marks can show a measurement error that will adversely affect the reliability of the test.

Objectivity

Objectivity is the degree to which multiple tests agree with the magnitude or scoring of the test.[44,45] To keep objectivity high, the tester should be familiar with testing instrumentation; otherwise an error in scoring can result.

In all possible scenarios, the same tester should test all athletes who participate in the same test; this may relieve any tester bias. If this is impossible, it is important that all testers use the same protocols when testing subgroups. This allows for the resultant measurements to be compared more accurately; thus the degree of objectivity remains high.

Test Selection

When selecting tests, the strength and conditioning professional must have the knowledge and experience of sport. In choosing an appropriate test for running ability in basketball, the strength and conditioning professional must not only understand the metabolic properties associated with the sport (ATP-PC glycolytic, oxidative), but should understand the physical demands (strength).

The test should not only be valid, reliable, and objective, but must appeal to the competitive nature of the athlete so that he or she puts forth a maximal effort. The test should also show some economic value and be simple to administrator. This assures a rapid and efficient means to test large groups without expensive drawn-out procedures. When selecting tests, special considerations should be noted:

- *Age-related factors.* Tests that are valid to college-age athletes may not be appropriate for adolescents or preadolescents due to age or inexperience.
- *Sex-related factors.* While some performance testing may be appropriate for assessing upper body strength (pull-ups) for males, it may not be appropriate for females due to the lack of upper body mass.
- *Experience-related factors.* Advanced tests may be appropriate to those athletes with certain maturity or experience levels but may not be suitable for novices (one-legged consecutive plyometric hops).
- *Environmental factors.* Some tests may be adversely affected by heat, cold, high altitude, and humidity.
- *Position within a sport.* The 40-yard dash test may be a valid and a reliable test for the skill positions in football but may not be for linemen. In that instance, a 10-yard dash may be a more pertinent test to measure their specific performance needs.
- *Unbiased test.* An unbiased test is one that takes into account the strength and metabolic needs of the specific training sessions. It would be unfair to test athletes in the 12-minute run for their aerobic capacity if their only training sessions have been anaerobic in nature.

To determine which tests should be used, the strength and conditioning professional needs to know the parameters of fitness needed to be successful in the given sport. A sample of certain components of tests is given in Table 1–2.[46]

To determine athletic performance levels, the strength and conditioning professional must use valid, reliable, and objective tests. The skills needed for good performance as well as energy systems that are required

TABLE 1–2. TESTS USED TO DETERMINE ATHLETIC FITNESS

Component	Test
Speed	20, 40, 100-yard dashes
Strength	Bench press, parallel squat
Muscle endurance	Timed sit-ups, timed push-ups
Explosive power	Vertical jump, standing broad jump, two-hand medicine ball put
Quickness and agility	20-yard shuttle, T-test
Flexibility	Sit and reach, shoulder elevation
Cardiorespiratory endurance	1.5-mile run, 12-minute run
Anaerobic endurance	Basketball line drill, 300-yard shuttle
Body composition	Skinfold measurements

From Graham J,[46] with permission.

to compete successfully should be analyzed. The test administrators need a complete understanding of all testing procedures and an unbiased attitude to all athletes when testing. All athletes should be informed of the objectives of the test and should be well motivated. Tests should be given from least fatiguing, most coordinated movements, to the most fatiguing, gross motor movements, with ample rest between tests. By providing valid tests with a high degree of reliability and objectivity three to four times a year, the athlete and the strength and conditioning professional will have the basis for evaluating the performance of the athlete and the effectiveness of the strength and conditioning program. The tests can also be a motivating factor for athletes to improve. The results can be shared with the athlete and coach and modifications can be made for each individual based upon his or her needs.

ROLE OF THE STRENGTH AND CONDITIONING PROFESSIONAL IN REHABILITATION

The successful rehabilitation of an injured athlete requires a multitude of professionals. These professionals, through a joint effort, can guide the athlete through a comprehensive rehabilitation process. The sports medicine team can consist of a physician, athletic trainer, physical therapist, and a strength and conditioning professional. A more advanced team can include a sport psychologist, nutritionist, and an orthopedic surgeon.

As soon as a medical evaluation is completed, the strength and conditioning staff is in contact with the other rehabilitation team members to determine the extent of the injury and the limitations that are placed on the athlete. For this process to take place, an understanding of each team members' responsibility and area of expertise should be understood. This shared knowledge and communication is the foundation of a good sports medicine team.

Routine testing done by the strength and conditioning professional can help in establishing the preinjury status of the athlete. The information is shared with the rest of the rehabilitation team to help guide the rehabilitation process.

The continuation of normal resistance training exercises, even at different intensities and loads, not only maintains the athlete's strength and conditioning parameters but also has a neural crossover effect to help build strength in the injured area.[47] Strength training can also have positive psychological benefits to athletes. Overall, strength and conditioning are integral parts of a preventive and sport enhancement program. Utilization of professionals who are knowledgeable in conditioning can help the transition of an injured athlete back to successful competition.

REFERENCES

1. Beaulieu JE. *Stretching for All Sports*. Pasadena: Athletic Press; 1980.
2. Walker SH. Delay of twitch relaxation induced by stress and stress relaxation. *J Appl Physiol*. 1961;16:801–806.
3. Anderson B, Beaulieu JE, Cornelius WL, et al. Flexibility. *NSCA J*. 1984;6:10–12.
4. Fox EL. *Sport Physiology*. Philadelphia: Saunders; 1979.
5. Getchell B. *Physical Fitness: A Way of Life*. New York: Wiley; 1979.
6. Allerheiligen WB. Stretching and warm-up. In: Baechle TR, ed. *Essentials of Strength Training and Conditioning*. Champaign, IL: Human Kinetics; 1994:289–313.
7. Prentice WE. Flexibility: Roundtable. *NSCA J*. 1984; 6:10–22, 71–73.
8. Hatfield BD, Brody EB. The psychology of athletic preparation and performance: The mental management of physical resources. In: Baechle TR, ed. *Essentials of Strength and Conditioning*. Champaign, IL: Human Kinetics; 1994: 163–187.
9. Hather BM, Tesch PA, Buchanan P, Dudley GA. Influence of eccentric actions on skeletal muscle adaptations to resistance training. *Acta Physiol Scand*. 1991;143:177–185.
10. Staron RS, Malicky ES, Leonardi MJ, et al. Muscle hypertrophy and fast fiber type conversions in heavy resistance trained women. *Eur J Appl Physiol*. 1989;60:71–79.
11. Hoffman J. Testosterone: A review of physiological effects and exercises responses. *NSCA J*. 1992;14:10–17.
12. Mooradian AD, Morely JE, Korenman SG. Biological actions of androgens. *Endocr Rev*. 1989;8:1–28.
13. Griggs RC, Kingston W, Jozefowicz RF, et al. Effects of testosterone on muscle mass and protein synthesis. *J Appl Physiol*. 1989;66:498–503.
14. Fahey TD, Rolph R, Moungmee P, et al. Serum concentrations, body composition and strength of young adults. *Med Sci Sports Exerc*. 1976;8:31–34.
15. Stone MH. Human growth hormone: Physiological functions and ergogenic efficacy. *NSCA J*. 1995;17:72–74.
16. Kraemer WJ, Machitellim L, Gordon SE, et al. Hormonal and growth factor responses to heavy resistance training protocols. *J Appl Physiol*. 1990;69:1442–1450.
17. Moritani T, DeVries HA. Neural factors versus hypertrophy in the time course of muscle strength gain. *Am J Phys Med Rehabil*. 1979;82:521–524.
18. Dudley GA, Harris RT. Neuromuscular adaptations to conditioning. In: Baechle TR, ed. *Essentials of Strength Training and Conditioning*. Champaign, IL: Human Kinetics; 1994:12–18.
19. Belanger AY, McComas AJ. Extent of motor unit activation during effort. *J Appl Physiol*. 1981;51:1131–1135.
20. Caiozzo VJ, Laird T, Chow K, et al. The use of precontractions to enhance the in vivo force velocity relationship. *Med Sci Sports Exerc*. 1983;14:162.

21. Bachele TR. National guidelines for certification programs. *NSCA J.* 1995;17:48-49.
22. Friedman JE, Neifer PD, Dohm GL. Regulation of glycogen resynthesis following exercise. *Sports Med.* 1991; 11:232-243.
23. Meyer RA, Terjung RL. Differences in ammonia and adenylate metabolism in contracting fast and slow muscle. *Am J Physiol.* 1979;237:c11-c18.
24. Nakamura Y, Schwartz S. The influence of hydrogen ion concentration calcium binding and release by skeletal muscle sacroplasmic reticulum. *J Gen Physiol.* 1972;59:22-32.
25. Fry RW Morton AR, Garcia-Webb P, Keast D. Monitoring exercise stress by changes in metabolic and hormonal responses over a 24-hour period. *J Appl Physiol.* 1991; 63:228-234.
26. Lehmann M, Dickhutn H, Gendrisch G, et al. Training-overtraining. A prospective, experimental study with experienced middle and long-distance runners. *Int J Sports Med.* 1991;12:444-452.
27. Jones NL, McCartney N, McComas AJ, eds. *Human Muscle Power.* Champaign, IL: Human Kinetics; 1986:27-39.
28. Bielik E, et al. Roundtable: Practical considerations for utilizing plyometrics, part 1. *NSCA J.* 1986;8:14-22.
29. Wathan D. Literature review: Explosive/plyometric exercises. *NSCA J.* 1993;15:17-19.
30. Lundin P. A review of plyometric training. *Track Field Q Rev.* 1989;89:37-40.
31. Chu DA. *Jumping into Plyometrics.* Champaign, IL: Leisure Press; 1992:1-12.
32. McDonagh MJN, Davies CTM. Adaptive responses of mammalians skeletal muscle to exercise with high loads. *Eur J Appl Physiol.* 1984;52:139-155.
33. Moffroid MT, Wipple RH. Specificity of speed of exercise. *Phys Ther.* 1970;50:1693-1699.
34. Hakkinen K, Komi PV, Alen M. Effect of explosive type strength training on isometric force and relaxation time, electromyographic and muscle fiber characteristics of leg extensor. *Acta Physiol Scand.* 1985;125:587-600.
35. Baechle TR, ed. *Essentials of Strength Training and Conditioning.* Champaign, IL: Human Kinetics; 1994.
36. Canavan PK, Garrett GE, Armstrong LE. Kinematic and kinetic relationships between an Olympic-style lift and the vertical jump. *J Strength Condition Res.* 1996;10:127-130.
37. Fleck SJ, Kraemer WJ. *Designing Resistance Training Programs.* Champaign, IL: Human Kinetics; 1987.
38. Gambetta V. Concept and application of periodization. *NSCA J.* 1991;13:64-65.
39. Wathen D, Roll F. In: Baechle TR, ed. *Essentials of Strength Training and Conditioning.* Champaign, IL: Human Kinetics; 1994.
40. Charniga A, Gambetta V, Kraemer W, et al. Periodization, part 1. *NSCA J.* 1993;15:57-76.
41. Zatsiorsky VM. *Science and Practice of Strength Training.* Champaign, IL: Human Kinetics; 1995:108-135.
42. Baumgartner T, Jackson A. *Measurement for Evaluation in Physical Education and Exercise Science.* Dubuque: Brown; 1987.
43. Hastad DN, Lacy AC. *Measurement and Evaluation in Contemporary Physical Education.* Scottsdale, AZ: Gorsuch; 1989.
44. Johnson B, Nelson J. *Practical Measurements for Evaluation in Physical Education.* 2nd ed. Minncapolis: Burgess; 1974.
45. Semenick D. Selecting appropriate tests; organizing testing procedures; testing protocols and procedures. In: Baechle TR, ed. *Essentials of Strength Training and Conditioning.* Champaign, IL: Human Kinetics; 1994.
46. Graham J. Guidelines for providing valid testing of athlete's fitness levels. *NSCA J.* 1994;16:7-14.
47. Wathen D. Athletic rehabilitation: The role of CSCS. *NSCA J.* 1989;11:29-34.

Nelson and associates investigated changes in bone density of inactive postmenopausal women compared to postmenopausal women performing weight-bearing exercise for 1 year and found improved bone density in the exercisers and bone loss in the nonexercisers.[12]

SPECTRUM OF ACTIVITY

Optimal dietary recommendations for individuals engaged in sports differ depending on the extent of physical activity and exercise. These differences are most apparent for water, energy, carbohydrate, and electrolytes. A wide range of types of athletic activity is discussed in this chapter. It is important to distinguish between the many degrees of activity performed, because they place different demands on the body's metabolic and fluid balance systems.

For the purpose of defining nutritional needs related to sports, the following classification of athletes by the extent of their exertion is useful.

- *Recreational athletes.* Athletes following previous American College of Sports Medicine (ACSM) guidelines, who exercise 3 to 5 times per week within their target heart rate ranges (THR), which are 70 to 85 percent of maximum heart rate (MHR) and equivalent to working out at 60 to 80 percent Vo_2 max.[13] Exercise duration can be 30 to 60 minutes total or pieced together throughout the day according to the latest ACSM recommendations.[14] Also, "weekend warriors" who exercise at least three sessions per week fit into this category.
- *Competitive athletes.* Athletes in training can be further stratified according to type of sport. Endurance athletes are individuals who engage in vigorous activity for more than 1 to 1.5 hours per day, 5 to 7 days per week. Ultra-endurance athletes exercise vigorously for 3 or more hours per day. Examples of these two categories of athletes are cross-country high school and college runners, competitive marathoners, distance swimmers, triathletes, and duathletes. Individuals who lift weights for over 1 hour per day, 5 to 6 days per week represent another type of competitive athlete with differing nutritional needs. And, lastly, the team sports athletic group includes individuals who mix vigorous endurance and sprint activities. For nutritional recommendations, this group includes those who train six or more times per week for more than 1 hour per session. Long-lasting vigorous activities like rowing, swimming, cross-country running, and cycling are team sports that have nutritional requirements similar to the endurance athlete. Activities such as football, wrestling, hockey, and gymnastics, where athletes engage in multiple quick bouts of strenuous exercise, are classified as team sports. Other team sports are those requiring strenuous exertion for somewhat extended periods (greater than 45 minutes). Examples are hockey, soccer, basketball, and track and field.

BODY WEIGHT AND BODY COMPOSITION

Recommendations for Body Weight and BMI

A healthy body weight is that which is associated with improved sports performance and decreased morbidity and mortality.[15] In the United States, desirable weights or the average weights for minimal mortality are presently derived from insurance data on weight and longevity. Usual weights in the U.S. population may be too high; however, actuarial data also have their limitations. Frame size was not actually measured. An effort was made to develop recommendations on frame based on data from other populations, and these were then applied to individuals who had been weighed when they were insured many years previously. This was the genesis of the frame size in the 1983 Metropolitan Life Insurance Company Tables of ideal weight for height that were predictive of lowest mortality. Also, average weights for minimal mortality are not necessarily optimal with respect to least morbidity; such weights may be lower.

There is some evidence that average to moderately below average weights are correlated with decreased mortality. In the American Cancer Society's long-term perspective study (1959 to 1972), those groups with weights within normal limits or 80 to 90 percent of average weights had the lowest mortality rates. Men and women greater than 130 to 140 percent of average weight had mortality rates that were 50 percent higher.[16]

Body mass index (BMI) is a single value that expresses weight to height. It is used in many standards for obesity and leanness. The formula is BMI = weight (kg)/height (m)^2. The 1995 Dietary Guidelines for Americans at all ages suggests a healthful range for BMI to be from 19 to 25.[17] Very low (less than 15th percentile) and very high BMI are associated with health risk.[18] Two analyses, in 1984 and 1988, of groups of U.S. Army trainees revealed that incidence of sports injury was higher among those with BMIs in both the highest (BMI greater than 28 for men and BMI greater than 24 for women) and lowest (BMI less than 21 for men and BMI less than 20 for women) quartiles.[19] Similar trends were evident in a study on long-distance runners done by Marti and colleagues.[20]

For adolescents, BMI calculated within chronologic age groups is an effective measure for determining overweight status.[21] The Expert Committee on Clinical Guidelines for Overweight in Adolescent Preventive Services has published recommendations for BMI standards to screen adolescents at risk for being overweight and for those who are already overweight.[22] According to the standards designed by this committee, adolescents with BMIs greater than or equal to the 95th percentile (greater than 30 kg/m^2) are considered overweight, and those with BMIs between the 85th and 95th percentiles are at risk for becoming overweight.[23]

For both young and older adults, desirable body weights were defined until recently as a BMI between 18 and 25 at age 21, and allowance was made for gains of 5 to 10 pounds later in life.[24] The 1989 Dietary Guidelines for BMI were 19 to 25 for individuals 19 to 34 years of age, and 21 to 26 for those over age 35 (see Fig. 2-1), based on work done at the National Institute on Aging.[25] The lower range for persons over 35 years in the 1995 Dietary Guidelines differs from the earlier guidelines because of the greater emphasis it places on decreased morbidity. When individuals exceed a BMI of 25, weight reduction may be called for, depending on other risk factors and conditions present. At a BMI of 27, almost all individuals could gain health benefits from a reduction of body weight. For athletes who have a larger muscle mass, the percent of body fat is a better predictor and should determine need for weight loss. Modest weight losses of 5 to 10 percent of body weight or 1 to 2 BMI units (BMI units are approximately 2.2 kg or 6 lbs) can have lasting benefits, if sustained, in previously overweight persons. Higher weights and BMI within each healthy weight range are for individuals with increased muscle and or bone mass such as football or baseball players.

The 1995 Dietary Guidelines for Americans have evolved to include emphasis on physical activity along with diet modification recommendations to achieve or maintain a healthy body weight focusing on finding energy balance between food intake and activity level. To decrease energy intake, the 1995 Dietary Guidelines suggest that people choose a variety of high-nutrient, low-calorie foods, decrease fat intake, eat more fruits, vegetables, and grains as illustrated in the Food Guide Pyramid pattern (see Fig. 2-2), and decrease intake of sweets, as well as lessen or avoid alcohol consumption.[26]

Weight Loss and Obesity Treatment

Obesity treatment is multifaceted and should include "self-monitoring, goal-setting exercise, nutrition education, stress management, and social support," according to the Food and Nutrition Board.[27] Nutrition, physical activity, behavior modification, pharmacologic therapy, surgery, and combinations of these represent the many weight loss approaches available today. Physical activity

and exercise are also considered critical in weight management and prevention of weight regain following weight loss.[27] Physical activity and exercise increase total daily energy expenditure, help to maintain or increase fat-free mass, and enhance loss of body fat. Thus, they are useful parts of a weight management plan.[28-31] When very low calorie reducing diets (less than 800 calories per day) are undertaken without exercise, there is a risk of greater losses of fat-free mass.[32] Therefore, it is essential to include physical activity with a low-calorie diet that is customized to individual health and behavior modification needs. Furthermore, it is important to realize that significant weight loss will not occur from exercise alone; nutritional and behavioral interventions are needed as well.[33] Performing aerobic exercise while dieting can increase adherence to nutritional changes.[34] It also predicts long-term weight loss and successful weight maintenance.[35] Athletes who have gained weight secondary to long-term injuries should follow the general recommendation of not exceeding 1 to 2 pounds of weight loss per week on weight-reducing regimens. This will preserve fat-free mass.

During the weight maintenance phase after weight reduction, a physically active life promotes positive nitrogen balance, improved glucose tolerance, and maintenance of lowered weights. Exercise induced thermogenesis is sustained after exercise at least until the muscle has recovered.[36-43] Exercise also transiently raises energy expenditure at rest. Although this may not be enough to cause weight loss in the absence of a hypocaloric diet, it nevertheless helps. Other health benefits of exercise include a decreased risk of degenerative disease and depression.

Body Composition

The BMI is the simplest screening tool for determining weight status. However, assessment of weight or weight for height using BMI is misleading in certain circumstances, particularly in athletes with large muscle mass. For example, athletes such as football and baseball players or short distance runners may have high BMIs, but their body fat may be within the normal range. More accurate assessment of body composition permits quantification of various tissue components, risk assessment, and more highly specific recommendations.

At any given BMI, a central body fat distribution also predicts increased risks to health within each gender. Abdominal fat (as assessed by a high waist circumference) is associated with higher health risks than excess gluteal fat in regions below the waist (as assessed from hip circumference).[44,45] These patterns of fat distribution are commonly referred to as "apple" (android or upper abdominal) verses "pear" (gluteal, lower, or gynoid) body shapes. The gynoid or lower body fat distribution (low

Weigh Your Risk with BMI

Your weight may put you at risk for certain medical problems.
Body mass index (BMI) is a height-weight calculation that helps to determine if you are at risk. Weight-related illnesses include diabetes, heart disease, certain cancers, stroke, and high blood pressure. Please talk to your physician to determine if you are in danger of developing health problems and what you can do to reduce your risk.

How to use this chart:
1. Look down the left column to find your height (*measured in feet and inches*).
2. Look across that row and find the weight nearest your own.
3. Look to the number at the top of the column to identify your BMI.
4. If your number is 27 or greater, you may be at risk.

WEIGHT (*In Pounds*)

BMI ►	19	20	21	22	23	24	25	26	27	28	29	30	35	40
4'10"	91	96	100	105	110	115	119	124	129	134	138	143	167	191
4'11"	94	99	104	109	114	119	124	128	133	138	143	148	173	198
5'	97	102	107	112	118	123	128	133	138	143	148	153	179	204
5'1"	100	106	111	116	122	127	132	137	143	148	153	158	185	211
5'2"	104	109	115	120	126	131	136	142	147	153	158	164	191	218
5'3"	107	113	118	124	130	135	141	146	152	158	163	169	197	225
5'4"	110	116	122	128	134	140	145	151	157	163	169	174	204	232
5'5"	114	120	126	132	138	144	150	156	162	168	174	180	210	240
5'6"	118	124	130	136	142	148	155	161	167	173	179	186	216	247
5'7"	121	127	134	140	146	153	159	166	172	178	185	191	223	255
5'8"	125	131	138	144	151	158	164	171	177	184	190	197	230	262
5'9"	128	135	142	149	155	162	169	176	182	189	196	203	236	270
5'10"	132	139	146	153	160	167	174	181	188	195	202	207	243	278
5'11"	136	143	150	157	165	172	179	186	193	200	208	215	250	286
6'	140	147	154	162	169	177	184	191	199	206	213	221	258	294
6'1"	144	151	159	166	174	182	189	197	204	212	219	227	265	302
6'2"	148	155	163	171	179	186	194	202	210	218	225	233	272	311
6'3"	152	160	168	176	184	192	200	208	216	224	232	240	279	319
6'4"	156	164	172	180	189	197	205	213	221	230	238	246	287	328

HEIGHT

AT RISK

Figure 2–1. Dietary guidelines. (Modified with permission from George Bray, MD.)

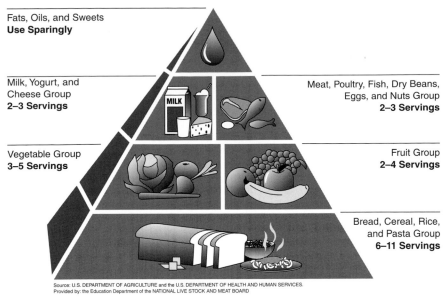

Fats, Oils, and Sweets
Use Sparingly

Milk, Yogurt, and
Cheese Group
2–3 Servings

Meat, Poultry, Fish, Dry Beans,
Eggs, and Nuts Group
2–3 Servings

Vegetable Group
3–5 Servings

Fruit Group
2–4 Servings

Bread, Cereal, Rice,
and Pasta Group
6–11 Servings

The **Food Guide Pyramid** emphasizes foods from the five food groups shown in the three lower sections of the Pyramid. Each of these food groups provides some, but not all, of the nutrients you need. Foods in one group can't replace those in another. No one food group is more important than another—for good health, you need them all.

How Many Servings Do You Need?

The **Food Guide Pyramid** shows a range of servings for each food group. The number of servings that are right for you depends on how many calories you need. Calories are a way to measure food energy. The energy your body need depends on your age, sex and size. It also depends on how active you are.

In general, daily intake should be:

- 1,600 calories for most women and older adults;
- 2,200 calories for kids, teen girls, active women and most men; and
- 2,800 calories for teen boys and active men.

Those with lower calorie needs should select the lower number of servings from each food group. Their diet should include 2 servings of meat for a total of 5 ounces. Those with average calorie needs should select the middle number of servings from each food group. They should include 2 servings of meat for a total of 6 ounces. Those with higher calorie needs should select the higher number of servings from each food group. Their diet should include 3 servings of meat for a total of 7 ounces. Also, pregnant or breastfeeding women; teens; or young adults up to age 24 should select 3 servings of milk. The amount of food that counts as one serving is listed below. If you eat a larger portion it is more than one serving. For example, a slice of bread is one serving, so a sandwich for lunch would equal two servings.

For mixed foods, estimate the food group servings of the main ingredients. For example, a large piece of sausage pizza would count in the bread group (crust), the milk group (cheese), the meat group (sausage) and the vegetable group (tomato sauce). Likewise, a helping of beef stew would count in the meat group and the vegetable group.

What Counts as a Serving?

Bread, Cereal, Rice & Pasta Group	Vegetable Group	Fruit Group	Milk, Yogurt & Cheese Group	Meat, Poultry, Fish, Dry Beans, Eggs & Nuts Group	Fats, Oils & Sweets
1 slice bread	½ cup chopped raw or cooked vegetables	piece fruit or melon wedge	1 cup milk or yogurt	2½ to 3 ounces cooked lean beef, pork, lamb, veal, poultry or fish	use sparingly
1 tortilla	I cup raw, leafy vegetables	¾ cup fruit juice	1½ ounces natural cheese		
½ cup cooked rice, pasta or cereal	¾ cup vegetable juice	½ cup chopped, cooked or canned fruit	2 ounces process cheese	Count ½ cup cooked beans or 1 egg or 2 tablespoons peanut butter or ⅓ cup nuts as 1 ounce of meat	
1 ounce ready-to-eat cereal	½ cup scalloped potatoes	¼up dried fruit	2 cups cottage cheese		
½ hamburger roll, bagel or English muffin	½ cup potato salad		1½ cups ice cream or ice milk		
3-4 plain crackers (small)	10 French fries		1 cup frozen yogurt		
1 pancake (4-inch)					
½ croissant (large)					
½ doughnut or danish (medium)					
¹⁄₁₆ cake (average)					
2 cookies (medium)					
¹⁄₁₂ pie (2-crust, 8")					

Lean Meat Choices

Beef	Pork	Lamb	Veal
Round Tip	Tenderloin	Loin Chop	Cutlet
Top Round	Boneless Top Loin Chop	Leg	Loin Chop
Eye of Round	Boneless Ham, Cured		
Top Loin	Center Loin Chop		
Tenderloin			
Sirloin			

Figure 2–2. Food guide pyramid with suggestions for daily food choices. (Copyright 1993 by the National Live Stock and Meat Board.)

waist to hip ratio [WHR]) has been associated with less health risk. WHR or waist and hip circumferences can be used to get a rough measure of upper versus lower types of fat distribution. Waist to hip ratios of greater than 1 in men and greater than 0.9 in women indicate increased health risk[46] or an "apple" shape. One recent expert group recommended WHR less than 0.9 for men and WHR less than 0.8 for women as most desirable for heart health.[47]

Individual assessment of body composition for athletes utilizes standards derived from populations of similar physical activity level, age, and gender. In Table 2–1, average percent body fat for both athletes and nonathletes are provided.

Precise measurement of body composition is difficult and costly, but research techniques are continuously being refined and improved upon to maximize accuracy and minimize time and expense. Some of the most common procedures at present to estimate percent body fat

and amount of lean tissue (muscle, bone, water) are described in Table 2–2. Many indirect methods are available to estimate total body water (TBW), and from this measurement, an estimate of body fatness can be derived.

There are many myths about body composition, some of which are summarized in Table 2–3. Athletes need to be aware of the reality behind various claims and should look to health care professionals, such as exercise physiologists, physicians, or registered dietitians, for factual information.

Body weight, body mass index, and body composition can affect physical capacity. Lean body mass appears to be especially important. In studies of fit military personnel, those who are overfat and underweight (equivalent to having low levels of fat-free mass) have lower lifting performance capabilities than those who are overweight without being overfat. Correlations between body composition and performance vary, depending on the measure of performance that is being assessed. The ability to perform sit-ups, for example, correlates more with percent fat than with fat-free mass. Excessive fat appears to act as a mechanical obstacle while performing this test.[48] Running performance is affected in healthy individuals when they wear shoulder harnesses and weight belts, suggesting that fat weight impedes performance.[49] Others have found that muscular strength and endurance capacities decrease with increased body weight, and that lean body mass is the most highly correlated predictor of run times and aerobic capacity.[50] Increased lean body mass improves many aspects of performance. Excess fat beyond a healthy amount hinders performance by adding weight and requiring more work for equivalent tasks.

TABLE 2–1. BODY FATNESS RANGES OF ATHLETES AND NONATHLETES

Population Sector	Average Percent Body Fat	
	Men	*Women*
Athletes < 40 years old		
Anaerobic[a]	10–17	8–13
Aerobic[a]	13–27	13–27
Distance runners[b]	5–12	10–20
Gymnastics[b]	3–6	8–18
Wrestling	6–16	
Swimming	4–10	14–25
Volleyball	10–15	20–23
Basketball	7–12	18–27
Football	9–19[c]	
U.S. Army Trainees (average age = 20)[d]	2.13–36.12	15.8–42.6
Nonathletes by Age Group		
Ages 6–22[e]	10–15	16–26
Ages 23–44	11–24[f]	25–33[g]
Ages 45–54[h]	26	34
Ages 55–64[h]	25	42
Ages 65–78[h]	30	43

[a] Economos CD, Bortz SS, Nelson ME. Nutritional practices of elite athletes. *Sports Med.* 1993;16:381–399.
[b] Tufts University, contractor for USDA HNRC. Body fat values in athletes and Vo₂ max.
[c] Range varies according to position.
[d] Jones BH, Bovee ME, Knapik JJ. Associations among body composition, physical fitness and injury in men and women Army trainees. In: Marriot BM, Grunstop SJ, eds. *Body Composition and Physical Performance.* Washington, DC: National Academy Press; 1992.
[e] Lohman TG. Applicability of body composition techniques and constants for children and youths. *Exc Sport Sci Reviews.* 1986;14:325–357.
[f] Myhre LG, Kessler WV. *J Appl Physiol.* 1966;21:1251.
[g] Chen KP. *J Formosan Med Assoc.* 1953;52:271.
[h] Frontera WR. *J Appl Physiol.* 1991;71:644–650.

DIETARY RECOMMENDATIONS FOR ACTIVE PEOPLE

General Dietary Recommendations

Recreational and competitive athletes who train 1 hour or less per day should follow the Dietary Guidelines for Americans and use the Food Guide Pyramid for general guidelines.[51] Athletes who exercise for greater than 1 hour per day may require increased amounts of energy (calories), carbohydrate, protein, and fluids to meet increased demands of training. General guidelines are for a moderately low fat (20 to 30 percent of total calories), high carbohydrate (55 to 65 percent of total calories) diet in most circumstances regardless of caloric intake.[52,53]

The USDA's Food Guide Pyramid (see Fig. 2–2)[54] is a pictorial diagram that illustrates an eating pattern for general health, but it can be adapted for athletes. Suggested numbers and sizes of servings recommended

TABLE 2–2. BODY COMPOSITION: METHODS OF MEASUREMENT

Method of Assessment	Principle and Procedures	Equipment Needed	Advantages	Disadvantages
Anthropometry, skinfolds, skeletal diameters, girth, and body girths	Different equations using skinfold and/or girth measures to estimate body fat. These are based on measures of subcutaneous fat at selected sites used to project total body fat. Waist-to-hip girth ratios (WHR) are used to predict placement of body fat.	Skinfold calipers (Skyndex, Lange, Harpenden). Measuring tape. Pertinent nomograms and equations.	Practical for screening large populations. Waist circumference adjusted for age showed strong estimate of body fat with minimal bias.[a] Low cost. Portable equipment. Less invasive than most techniques.	Requires training and experience. Consistency of measurement depends on level of experience. Can have high degree of measurement error. Multiple spot skinfolds needed to estimate total body fat more accurrately. Accurate and consistently placed girth measures are difficult. Invasive. Time consuming.
Hydrostatic weighing	Based on principle that fat density $<$ water density $<$ density of bone and muscle, % body fat is calculated from body density = weight in air/(wt in air − wt in water/water density) − residual lung volume. Percent fat (495/body density) − 450[b]	Large water tank with underwater chair designed for weighing is suspended from scale with secure cable.	Body density measures are more accurate than anthropometric measures.[b] Very repeatable (variability $<$ 1.3%).[c,d] Often used as standard to evaluate other techniques.	Not cost effective. Large equipment and laboratory setting needed. Difficult for subject to perform.
Bioelectrical impedance analysis	Measure of conductivity is used to estimate TBW. Fat-free mass with its higher electrolyte content is more conductive than fat.[e]	2-needle electrodes attached to wrist and ankle bioimpedance machine to measure voltage between electrodes.	Reasonably noninvasive, fast, and simple. Good predictor of body fat.[f]	Variations in hydration status can alter results. Expensive equipment.
Near infrared interactance (NIR) (Futrex 5000)	Near-infrared spectroscopy used to measure deflection of light at muscle belly. Sex, wt, ht, and exercise level used with infrared readings to calculate % body fat.	Fiber-optic probe (wand). Optical standard armband.	Portable. Easy-to-use. Very fast. Noninvasive	Greatest errors at extremes of body fatness.[f] Shown to be less accurate than skinfold measures.[g] Not well correlated with underwater weight (UWW) values.[h] Activity levels highly variable among individuals and this changes body fat estimate considerably.[i]
Magnetic resonance imaging (spin-echo and inversion recovery)	Magnet and radio waves used to create an energy field to be transferred into highly visible image. Cross-sectional images of abdomen can be used to assess intra-abdominal fat.	Magnetic resonance scanner.	Can differentiate intra-abdominal and subcutaneous areas of fat.[j] No radiation hazard.	Very expensive. Highly specialized personnel needed.
CT (computer tomography) scan	3-dimensional cross-sectional view of selected body structure.	X-ray machine, computer tomography scanner.	Can distinguish between subcutaneous and intra-abdominal fat.	Subjects exposed to radiation. Expensive.

(Continued)

TABLE 2–2. *(Continued)*

Method of Assessment	Principle and Procedures	Equipment Needed	Advantages	Disadvantages
Deuterium-labeled water	Measures TBW through ingestion of deuterium oxide and subsequent measures of saliva, blood, or urine.	Deuterium oxide laboratory analysis.	Repeatable and comparable to UWW.[k] Salivary and urine measures are noninvasive.	Invasive. Extensive procedures to obtain fluids needed to measure TBW. Potential side effects of large isotope dose. High cost of isotopic water ($500–$1000 per trial).

[a] Equations from Lean MEJ, Han TS, Deurenberg P. Predicting body composition by densitometry from simple anthropometric measurements. *Am J Clin Nutr.* 1996;63:4–14.
    BD = 1.1674 − (0.00125 × waist[cm]) − (0.000231 × age).
    BF% = (0.567 × waist[cm]) + (0.101 × age) − 31.8.
[b] Marcus J, ed. *Sports Nutrition: A Guide for the Professional Working with Active People.* Chicago: American Dietetic Association; 1986.
[c] Behnke AR, Feen BG, Welham WC. The specific gravity of healthy men. *JAMA.* 1942;118:495–498.
[d] Oppliger RA, Looney MA, Tipton CM. Reliability of hydrostatic weighing and skinfold measurements of body composition using generalizability study. *Hum Biol.* 1987;59:77–96.
[e] *Body Composition Assessment in Youth and Adults.* Report of the Sixth Ross Conference on Medical Research. Columbus, OH: Ross Laboratories; 1985.
[f] Wilmore KM, McBride PJ, Wilmore JH. Comparison of bioelectric impedance and near-infrared interactance for body composition assessment in a population of self-perceived overweight adults. *Int J Obesity.* 1994;18:375–381.
[g] Israel RG, Houmard JA, O'Brien KF, et al. Validity of a near-infrared spectrophotometry device for estimating human body composition. *Res Q Exerc Sport.* 1989;60:379–383.
[h] Davis PG, Van Loan M, Holly RG, et al. Near infrared interactance vs hydrostatic weighing to measure body compostition in lean, normal, and obese women. *Med Sci Sports Exerc.* 1989;21:S100. Abstract.
[i] McLean KP, Skinner JS. Validity of Futrex-5000 for body composition determination. *Med Sci Sports Exerc.* 1992;24:253–258.
[j] Terry JG, Hinson WH, Evans GW, et al. Evaluation of magnetic resonance imaging for quantification of intraabdominal fat in human beings by spin-echo and inversion-recovery protocols. *Am J Clin Nutr.* 1995;62:297–301.
[k] Bartolli WP, Davis JM, Pate RR, et al. Weekly variability in total body water using H_2O_2 dilution in college-age males. *Med Sci Sports Exerc.* 1993;25:1422–1428.

per day and examples of each type of food are shown to assist in food selection and portioning for a healthy eating pattern. Following this diagram, energy intakes for recreational athletes and the average American range from 1600 to 2800 calories. For other populations of athletes, the pyramid can be used, but recommendations need to be tailored to meet individual nutritional needs. For instance, ultra-endurance and endurance athletes may need to alter the number of servings shown in the pyramid to meet their increased needs because they spend so much time and energy exercising. A college swimmer may practice for 5 hours a day; he or she will need to consume an additional 1800 to 3750 calories, depending on the intensity of the workout, to maintain energy balance. From this added expenditure alone, an athlete could more than double the suggested number of servings at each level of the pyramid in some cases. In practice, however, doing so would create a diet that was too bulky. In that case, sources of concentrated energy could be added to meet caloric needs.

Energy Recommendations

The energy intake that is required for energy balance and optimal performance varies widely according to physical activity and exercise, as shown in Table 2-4. Energy needs can range from 32 to 50 calories per kg.[55,56] This wide range is due partly to the energy expenditure of

exercise itself.[57] Research shows ultra-endurance athletes or young adults may consume greater than 50 kcal/kg per day. On a hard training day or competitive day, which may have twice the usual amount of exercise, actual dietary intakes may be much higher.[58] Other factors involved are anthropometric measurements (especially weight since it affects the energy costs of moving the body), age, sex, and environmental factors such as exercising in very cold climates.

Fat-free mass, especially skeletal muscle, increases with most types of exercise and tends to decrease with age. As a result of decreases in physical activity, disuse atrophy, and disease, lean body mass often declines with aging. Perhaps the most common cause of declines in fat-free mass (and consequently in resting metabolism) is a decreasing level of physical activity, which is present in both males and females with increasing age.[59,60] On average, fat-free mass decreases 2 to 3 percent every 10 years beginning in early adulthood.[61] This decline means that dietary intakes must be nutrient-dense with respect to protein, vitamins, and minerals to meet the recommendations for optimal health and performance at lower energy intakes.

Conversely, fat-free mass increases with growth, so that younger athletes who are growing need more energy. Children and adolescents need more calories per kilogram than adults for growth. The adolescent growth spurt is particularly demanding in this regard. Children often need

TABLE 2–3. THE TRUTH ABOUT BODY COMPOSITION

Body Composition Myths	The Reality Is. . .
Fat can be changed to muscle.	• Fat and muscle are two different tissues within the body; muscle tissue can be lost and is difficult to restore. Fat can be lost and is not difficult to regain. • Exercising specific areas, such as performing abdominal tucks on a regular basis, tones muscle in that area, but fails to reduce abdominal fat unless combined with negative energy balance. • Creating an energy deficit between intake and output through diet and aerobic exercise promotes subcutaneous fat reduction all over the body.
Dropping weight quickly does not affect strength.	• Rapid weight loss through a variety of methods promotes loss of lean body mass (water, muscle, bone), in turn reducing strength. • Slower losses of 1 to 2 lb per week encourages fat loss rather than loss of lean tissue, therefore preserving strength.
Loading up on amino acids will build muscle.	• Adequate protein (amino acids) can be achieved through diet alone. • There is no benefit of taking protein supplements over foods that naturally contain protein. • Many amino acid supplements actually contain small amounts of amino acids as compared to protein-containing food.
Overweight = overfat.	• Athletic individuals occasionally may have BMIs greater than healthy ranges due to an abundance of lean body mass (LBM) without being overfat. • Before assuming a competitive athlete is overweight, a complete assessment of fatness, body composition, and BMI should be made.

to eat small, frequent meals to meet their energy needs, and this can be a challenge if they are involved in sports.

Men have proportionally more metabolically active fat-free mass than women, and this means that they have increased resting metabolic rates. Because women have lower resting energy needs, their caloric intakes for weight maintenance are lower than that of men of the same weight and activity levels. The Harris–Benedict[62] and Cunningham[63] equations adjust for gender in determining estimated daily energy expenditure. Increases or decreases in fat-free mass may also be important deter-

minants of energy needs and performance of persons engaged in various sports.

Sports performed in various environments can also affect energy needs. Thermogenesis and the demands of exercise in very cold conditions or at very high altitudes increase energy output, and therefore energy needs.[64] Exercising in extremes of heat and humidity affects fluid needs more than energy needs.

Other metabolic conditions can also affect energy expenditure. An athlete who is HIV positive or has AIDS will have much higher energy and protein needs to avoid

TABLE 2–4. MACRONUTRIENT NEEDS OF ATHLETES

Activity Type	Energy Needs[a]	Carbohydrate[b]	Protein	Fat and Cholesterol
Ultraendurance and endurance (>1 hr/day)	2000–6000 kcal/day[c,d]	55–70% of calories (6–10 g/kg wt) 25–30 g dietary fiber/day	1.0–1.4 g/kg[e]	<30% kcal from fat 10% or less saturated fat 10% monounsaturated fat 10% polyunsaturated fat <300 mg cholesterol
Other strenuous team sports and competitive strength training (>1 hr/day)	1800–4000 kcal/day[f]	55–70% of calories (6–10 g/kg wt) 25–30 g dietary fiber/day	1.0–1.8 g/kg[e]	Same as above
Recreational and some competitive athletes (female ballet dancers and gymnasts)	1600–2800 kcal/day[g]	60–65% of calories Moderate intake of simple sugars 25–30 g dietary fiber/day	0.8 g/kg for adults and older adolescents	Same as above

[a] To determine more accurate energy needs consult a Registered Dietitian.
[b] Carbohydrate needs vary substantially with stage of activity (see carbohydrate sections of text for specific variations in needs).
[c] Horton E. Metabolic fuels, utilization, and exercise. *Am J Clin Nutr.* 1989;49:931–932.
[d] Durnin J. The energy cost of exercise. *Proc Nutr Soc.* 1985;44:273.
[e] Lemon P. Do athletes need more dietary protein and amino acids? *Int J Sport Nutr.* 1995;5:S39–S61.
[f] Food and Nutrition Board. *Recommended Dietary Allowances.* 10th ed. Washington, DC: National Academy of Sciences; 1989.
[g] USDA. *USDA food guide pyramid.* USDHHS, Human Nutrition Information Service, August 1992, leaflet no. 572.

additional declines in immune system function due to undernutrition and loss of fat-free mass. Malabsorption and frequency of infection put added demands on the HIV-positive athlete. Special attention needs to be given to individual athletes with decreased appetite and gastrointestinal complications to ensure adequate dietary intake to prevent or slow loss of lean tissue.

Hemiplegics and partially paralyzed persons form a unique class of athletes with increased energy demands due to training combined with decreased energy demands secondary to loss of movement in some parts of the body.[65] Exercise can help prevent unwanted weight gain and somewhat offset the need for low-calorie diets in such individuals. Dietary studies have shown the diets of hemiplegics to be high in fat and low in carbohydrate, like those of some athletes.[66] Consistent aerobic exercise can decrease the risk of heart disease in this high-risk population[67] by increasing HDL.[68-70]

During pregnancy, energy needs increase because of development of the placenta and fetus as well as increased blood volume and body fat in the mother (see Table 2-5).[71] In the first trimester, there is little change in energy requirements. In the second and third trimesters, an estimated (net) 300 more calories per day is recommended for appropriate weight gain after adjusting for usual physical activity levels. Optimal weight gain over the course of pregnancy is based largely on prepregnancy weight or BMI. Adequate caloric intake for weight gain can be a concern for certain pregnant athletes. Most athletes cease competition or heavy training in the second trimester, but those who continue with their doctor's consent will need more calories.

For lactation, an additional 500 calories per day on average is recommended. Energy needs of lactation vary with the amount of milk produced.[72] Many women return to competition and heavy training by 6 to 8 weeks

TABLE 2–5. RECOMMENDED DAILY ALLOWANCE RANGES SELECTED NUTRIENTS[a]

Nutrient	Males 15+	Females 15+	Pregnant or Lactating
Protein (g)	59–63	44–50	60–65
Vitamin D (µg)	5–10	5–10	10
Vitamin E (mg)	10	8	10–12
Vitamin C (mg)	60	60	70–95
Thiamin (mg)	1.2–1.5	1.0–1.1	1.5–1.6
Riboflavin (mg)	1.4–1.8	1.2–1.3	1.6–1.8
Calcium (mg)	800–1200	800–1200	1200
Phosphorus (mg)	800–1200	800–1200	1200
Iron (mg)	10–12	10–15	15–30

[a] Needs vary according to age.
From Food and Nutrition Board. *Recommended Daily Allowances.* 10th ed. Washington, DC: National Academic of Sciences, 1989. With permission.

postpartum (again, this should be only with a doctor's consent), and they will need more calories.

Carbohydrate

Carbohydrate should make up the majority of food energy in a healthy diet. Between 55 and 70 percent of caloric intake should be in the form of carbohydrate for different types of athletes (see Table 2-4).[73,74] This percentage will vary with the level of total energy intake. Recreational athletes will obtain ample amounts of carbohydrate by following the serving recommendations outlined in the Food Guide Pyramid. Competitive athletes with high caloric intakes may consume only 55 to 60 percent of total calories as carbohydrate if they ingest 6 to 10 g carbohydrate per kilogram body weight (approximately 450 to 800 g per day).[75,76]

Carbohydrate in Athletic Performance

Carbohydrate is an extremely important nutrient that improves athletic performance and increases time to fatigue (that is, the time before fatigue occurs) in some types of exercise. Depending on the type, intensity, and length of activity, the proportions of carbohydrate and fat that are oxidized during exercise vary.[77] Muscle glycogen, blood glucose, plasma free fatty acids, and muscle triglycerides are the major fuel sources of exercising skeletal muscle.[78,79] During low-intensity (40 to 60 percent VO_2 max) activity (such as walking, less than 4 mph), or low-impact aerobics, an exercising individual relies on fat for about half of this fuel need. At increased intensities (60 to 85 percent VO_2 max) of exercise, such as sprinting or weightlifting, mobilization of free fatty acids is inhibited, and carbohydrate stores, in the form of muscle or liver glycogen, serve as the major fuel for such activity.[80] For endurance athletes, training can increase fat utilization and slow time to glycogen depletion. Thus, highly trained endurance athletes can burn more energy as fat than untrained athletes.

Glycogen levels of both skeletal muscle and the liver are directly correlated with sports performance, and these in turn depend in part on carbohydrate in the diet. When liver and muscle glycogen stores are exhausted, fatigue results and performance suffers.[81,82] Performance in endurance activities is enhanced with a high-carbohydrate diet because it maximizes glycogen stores.[83,84] Aside from dietary intake of carbohydrate, training status is the other major determinant of muscle and liver glycogen levels.[85,86] Both are under the athlete's control. Liver glycogen serves the primary function of keeping optimal levels of glucose in the blood. This is especially important for sustenance of brain cells, which preferentially oxidize glucose. Thus, adequate blood glucose levels are essential for normal central nervous system function.[87] During endurance events, an athlete must consume enough carbohydrate to maintain or replenish liver glycogen. Transient changes in alertness may occur as a result of the very low blood sugar levels that could develop if liver glycogen stores are depleted.

Before Competition

For events lasting more than 90 minutes, a diet adequate in carbohydrate is an effective method of increasing glycogen stores to above-normal levels before a competitive event if the athlete rests. This form of modified carbohydrate loading is safe to do many times throughout the year without health risk.[88] Note that current recommendations for this practice no longer include the previously recommended carbohydrate-depletion period, because there is a risk of hypoglycemia without a worthwhile countervailing benefit. Tapering down on activity levels for 3 successive days with 1 to 2 days of rest prior to the event is necessary to maximize glycogen stores. Many athletes who compete will choose two to three events per year to taper off their exercise levels and will gradually reduce their total training time per day over 2 to 3 weeks. This allows for a more complete muscle rest. Athletes need less food energy when resting after they have decreased their energy output in physical activity.

A high carbohydrate diet eaten 3 to 6 hours before competition provides additional performance benefits beyond those involved in carbohydrate loading and provision of carbohydrate supplements during exercise.[89,90] This meal should provide 200 to 350 g carbohydrate to maximize liver and muscle glycogen levels. A precompetition meal that is based on these suggestions is shown in Appendix 2–1.

During Competition

Carbohydrate ingestion during prolonged activities (greater than 90 min) improves performance.[91] It helps maintain plasma glucose levels throughout activity, keeps glucose oxidation at a maximum (1 g/min), and prolongs the time to fatigue. Two protocols are currently recommended: ingest 40 to 75 g simple sugar per hour while active or ingest 200 g simple sugar if exercise has gone on a long time (2.25 hours).[92] However, consumption of carbohydrate during activity is limited in its benefits. More than 75 g of carbohydrate replacement per hour is no more beneficial than 40 to 75 g.[93] Moreover, supplementation once fatigue has occurred is not helpful to performance.[94]

Unfortunately, carbohydrate consumption during the event is also not without its problems. Gastrointestinal distress and time taken out of an event to consume carbohydrate sources are two negative consequences that must be weighed against benefits in each situation. Carbohydrate in the form of a diluted beverage would be effective in both fluid replacement and carbohydrate ingestion during exercise. Beverages that are greater than

8 to 10 percent carbohydrate by weight may cause a delay in fluid absorption,[95] so choice of beverages less than 8 to 10 percent are desirable. Carbohydrate needs during exercise can also be met with solids such as bagels, bananas, and sports bars. However, water replacement is needed as well.

After Event

High carbohydrate intakes during the recovery period increase muscle glycogen concentration to above normal levels. This phenomenon is referred to as supercompensation,[96] and this practice improves performance.[97,98] Glycogen repletion can occur in 24 hours following a long endurance competition if intake of carbohydrate is adequate.[99] This is why a diet high in carbohydrate rather than protein or fat is important for athletes. Some athletes fail to recover or fully replete glycogen stores, and this decreases performance. Recovery recommendations are shown in Table 2–6, and an example of a postcompetition diet is shown in Appendix 2–1.

Dietary Carbohydrates: Simple and Complex Sources

Carbohydrates are classified as either simple or complex. Complex carbohydrates are polysaccharides, many sugar units linked together in long chains. Simple sugar units are monosaccharides (glucose, fructose, and galactose) and disaccharides (sucrose, maltose, and lactose). Simple carbohydrates as well as complex carbohydrates are important as sustenance before and after sporting events. Simple carbohydrates are often better tolerated during events.

If a competitive athlete wishes to increase his or her carbohydrate intake prior to a race, during an event, or during the glycogen repletion phase, foods and beverages high in simple sugars (such as high-fructose corn syrup or cane sugar containing beverages) may aid in meeting calorie requirements and hasten absorption for quick energy. While the individual is replenishing glycogen, taking in simple sugars may in fact be more effective at increasing glycogen concentrations than ingesting starchy foods high in complex carbohydrates.[100]

Glucose substrates are oxidized directly by muscle, while other forms of simple sugars such as fructose and lactose are transformed into glucose by the liver. Sucrose provides the same health and metabolic benefits as glucose.[101] In general, different forms of simple sugars have similar effects on performance, hydration, increasing plasma glucose, and maintaining carbohydrate oxidation.[102-104] Therefore, fructose has no specific advantages over sucrose.

Milk, milk products, calcium-fortified soy milk, and frozen yogurt are examples of high-carbohydrate foods that contain simple sugars and that are produced in low-fat varieties. These foods also represent good sources of

TABLE 2–6. FLUID REPLACEMENT GUIDE FOR DIFFERENT ATHLETIC ACTIVITIES

Activity Type	Approximate Time of Event	Intensity (Vo_2 Max)	Recommended Fluid Intakes[a,b]	Potential Problems[c]
• Track and field events • Many team competitions: hockey, basketball, baseball, football • Wrestling, tennis, and gymnastics matches • Rowing races • Aerobics and dance	<1 hour	75–130%	**0–15 minutes prior to event:** 300–500 mL of beverage, 6–10% carbohydrate (CHO)	Decreased time and desire to drink Decreased rate of gastric emptying with increased exertion
• Marathon at elite speed • Most triathlons • Distance swimming • Tennis matches • Soccer	1–3 hours	60–90%	**Before:** 300–500 mL water **During:** 800–1600 mL/hr, cool, 6–8% CHO drink with 10–20 mg NaCl	Hyperglycemia Hypohydration/hypovolemia Hyperthermia Depletion of glycogen
• Other marathoners • Ultramarathons and triathlons • Long cycling events • Hiking with heavy pack	>3 hours	30–70%	**Before:** 300–500 mL water **During:** 500–1000 mL/hr, cool, 6–8% CHO drink with 20–30 mg NaCl	Hyperglycemia Hypohydration/hypovolemia Hyperthermia Depletion of glycogen Hyponatremia
Recovery period		Cooling down	**After:** Ingest beverage to provide 50 g CHO per hour usually for 3–4 hours (total 7–10 g/kg) Glycogen stores replaced in 24 hours postevent. Ingest 30–50 mg NaCl	Replacement of fluid and electrolytes Replenishing glycogen stores

[a] American College of Sports Medicine recommends that runners replace fluids at a rate of 100–200 mL/2–3 km.
[b] Coyle and Montain, who acknowledge variability in water and electrolyte losses dependent on exertion and sweat rate, recommend ingesting 625–1250 mL/hr of exertion.
[c] Thirst sensation not good indicator for amount of fluid replacement needed to prevent dehydration, especially at higher intensities of exercise.
From Gisolfi CV, Duchman S. Guidelines for optimal replacement beverages for different athletic events. *Med Sci Sport Exerc.* 1992;24:679–687. With permission.

calcium, riboflavin, and protein with varying amounts of lactose. Lactose-intolerant individuals or those athletes who experience gastrointestinal upset from lactose ingestion prior to an event may consider lactose-free products, such as Lactaid or soy milk. Cheese contains little to no carbohydrate and a large percentage of calories from fat, and therefore is less desirable in these respects.

Vegetables contain little carbohydrate, some protein, and many vitamins and minerals, such as beta-carotene, vitamin C, iron, and potassium. Most vegetables contribute high amounts of fiber without much calories, making them an insignificant source of carbohydrate for athletes. Exceptions are vegetable juices (mixed vegetable or carrot juice) that provide about half the calories of fruit juice, mostly as carbohydrate.

Fruit juices provide carbohydrate (also simple sugar), vitamin C, and often potassium, but no protein. A good low-cost alternative to sports drinks is diluted half strength 100 percent fruit juice, which provides about 6 percent carbohydrate in solution with more vitamins and minerals and similar amounts of potassium than most sports drinks. Fruits are also a good source of carbohydrate (mainly sim-

ple sugars), vitamins, and minerals. As with vegetables, they contain variable amounts of fiber that can be filling.

Grains, breads, cereals, and other starches, including starchy vegetables such as peas, corn, and potatoes, should make up most of the carbohydrate in athletes' diets. These are mostly composed of complex carbohydrates, and they provide B vitamins such as thiamin. Whole grain products such as whole wheat bread, brown rice, or bulgar are higher in fiber and provide more iron and zinc than enriched grain products. Fiber is not recommended in large amounts in precompetition meals due to its increased bulk and slowing effect on gastrointestinal absorption. However, for most active individuals during most of their training programs, a diet high in fiber, providing 25 to 30 g per day, is advisable. Fiber is also helpful in weight loss and maintenance programs since it promotes the feeling of fullness, contributes no food energy, and is found largely in fruits, vegetables, and whole grains, which are typically low in fat and high in vitamins and minerals.

It may not be possible to ingest very high percentages of complex carbohydrate on a very high calorie diet due to the bulk of many of these foods. For instance, 65 percent of a 5000-calorie diet in the form of mostly complex carbohydrates is equivalent to 10 cups juice, 2 cups yogurt, 8 cups pasta (1 pound), 3 cups of rice, and 7 slices of bread in a day. Balancing complex carbohydrates with greater amounts of simple sugars becomes more necessary as energy intake increases significantly. For example, by adding 2 sports drinks, a gel packet, and 500 calories from high-calorie sweet snacks, the other needed carbohydrate calories can be met with 6 cups juice, 1 cup yogurt, 6 cups pasta, 2 cups rice, and 5 slices of bread.

A low-fiber alternative can be simple carbohydrate sources such as sugars, honey, fat-free sweets (fig bars) and sports drinks, bars, and gels, which provide more carbohydrate per unit volume but insignificant amounts of vitamins and minerals. As long as athletes meet vitamin and mineral needs, simple carbohydrate may supplement extra needed calories.

In assessing the benefits of simple versus complex carbohydrate sources in the diet, several goals must be considered. If an individual is following a diet combined with physical activity to maintain a healthy body weight or to lose weight, concentrated sweets should be limited. They are typically very calorie dense with low nutrient value. For example, a snack consisting of a bag of jellybeans provides about 200 calories more than an equally sized bag of pretzels.

Fat

Fat has many vital functions in the body that are often be overlooked by individuals aiming for optimal fitness and a very low fat diet. Fat provides structure to cell membranes, it cushions and protects internal organs, it is involved in hormone production, and it provides fuel for energy storage in adipose and muscle tissue. Essential fatty acids and fat-soluble vitamins (vitamins A, D, E, and K), which are necessary for many physiologic functions, are dependent on adequate dietary fat. The National Academy of Sciences reports that 3 to 6 g of linoleic acid (essential fatty acid) each day is required to prevent fatty acid deficiency.[105] Most people will ingest adequate essential fatty acids in a mixed diet. For vegetarians or people on very low fat diets, essential fatty acid needs could be achieved by consuming one tablespoon or approximately 15 g of corn, safflower, or soybean oil a day.

In contrast, overconsumption of fat poses many health risks, namely cardiovascular disease, obesity, and some cancers. According to the most recent national survey data, the average American consumes 34 percent of total calories from fat.[106] Among elite athletes in training for aerobic activities, the average fat intake in terms of percent of total daily calories probably ranges from 20 to 40 percent for males and 26 to 38 percent for females.[107] The American Heart Association (AHA), the American

Dietetic Association (ADA), and the American Cancer Society (ACS) recommend all adults should lower their total fat intake to less than 30 percent of calories. Of this 30 percent, it is further recommended that less than 10 percent of calories come from saturated fat, primarily found in fatty cuts of meats and poultry, whole-fat dairy products, butter, and tropical oils. The majority of fat in the athlete's diet, then, should be from sources which contain polyunsaturated or monounsaturated fat, such as vegetable oils, seeds, and nuts.

For most active adults, the recommendations for fat intake made by the AHA, ADA, and the ACS are appropriate. Athletes may typically consume a similar amount of total grams of fat as less active individuals. However, they may have a much lower percent of calories coming from fat. This is because they may be eating a diet with much higher amounts of carbohydrate and their total energy intakes are higher. Nevertheless, athletes should be aware of the sources of hidden fats, preferred types of fats, and low-fat cooking methods, and be able to select low-fat foods when dining out. Registered dietitians specializing in sports nutrition work with clients to help clarify this information and provide individualized dietary guidelines to help clients optimize their exercise performance and nutritional status. Some general guidelines are listed in this section.

Guidelines for choosing low-fat foods

1. Hidden fat can add to excess fat intake. Be moderate in the consumption of sweets or bakery items such as muffins, scones, cookies, cakes, or pies.
2. Limit fried foods in which total fat is high such as fried fatty meats, donuts, chips, french fries, or onion rings.
3. Limit added fats like gravy, whipped cream, butter, margarine, sour cream, or cream cheese.
4. Choose unsaturated fat over saturated fat by using vegetable oils (olive, safflower, or canola) instead of butter when cooking.
5. Choose low-fat and nonfat dairy products to reduce saturated fats.
6. Remove or trim meats and poultry of visible fat to reduce total fat and saturated fat. Also select the leanest cuts.
7. Broil, boil, grill, steam, stir fry, or pan fry in small amounts of oil instead of frying.
8. Balance your diet by mixing a high-fat meal with two low-fat meals so that your daily average calories from fat is below 30 percent.

Fat Metabolism

Stored fat provides for practically a limitless fuel source during exercise, even in the leanest of athletes. When an individual is eating adequate calories and is at rest, the substrates for energy production are usually 60 percent fat, 40 percent carbohydrate, and a trace of protein. As the intensity of exercise (or percent Vo_2 max) increases, the percent of energy produced from fat decreases because fat oxidation requires more oxygen. At mild exercise intensity or 50 percent of Vo_2 max, the fuel mix is 50 percent fat, 50 percent carbohydrate, and a trace of protein. During high-intensity, short-duration exercise, carbohydrate provides 95 percent of the energy and fat only 5 percent.[108]

Aerobic conditioning increases the rate of fat metabolism during exercise. This results from many physiologic and hormonal adaptations that occur in response to aerobic conditioning. Endurance training results in an increase in cardiac output that enables the individual to supply more oxygen to exercising muscles. There is also a rise in the number of mitochondria in trained muscles, which in turn increase the oxidative enzyme content. With an increase in oxidative enzymes, the trained person can metabolize fat at a higher rate than the less active individual, and this can prolong endurance through a glycogen-sparing effect.[109]

The enhanced metabolism of fat by a trained individual is apparent in a reduced respiratory quotient at the same level of exercise effort, a lower rate of metabolizing muscle glycogen, and a reduced production of lactate.[110] These training effects contribute to increased endurance because they prolong the time to fatigue or reduction of muscle glycogen. This glycogen sparing effect has led some to claim that there are performance-enhancing benefits to a high-fat diet. However, there have been no valid, replicated studies to support this theory,[111] and the health hazards of a high-fat diet are well established. Furthermore, it is well established that endurance athletes train and compete at an exercise intensity between 65 and 75 percent of their Vo_2 max.[112] At intensities above 70 percent Vo_2 max, carbohydrates, not fatty acids, are the preferred energy substrate.[113] Therefore, the evidence available to date supports maintaining a diet high in carbohydrate and low in fat, especially for endurance athletes.

Protein

Different athletic training programs may increase the dietary protein requirements of the body to values greater than the recommended dietary allowances (RDA) by increasing protein turnover rates. However, these changes in protein needs are minimal and are definitely attainable through food intake alone with appropriate diet planning.

Protein requirements of athletes who exercise 1 hour or less per day are similar to the recommended daily allowance for the general adult population of 0.8 g/kg body weight per day. For some athletes, 0.8 g protein/kg per day is too low to meet needs.[114] Specific recommendations based on athletic type are shown in

Table 2–4. Protein needs for more intense athletes can range from 0.94[115] to 1.37[116] g/kg per day or even as high as 1.2 to 1.4 g/kg per day in endurance athletes and 1.4 to 1.8 g/kg per day in strength trainers.[117] The American Dietetic Association recommends 1.0 g protein/kg per day. Figures are provided in terms of grams per kilogram because protein needs directly correlate with fat-free mass. Protein recommendations of 12 to 15 percent of caloric intake can be too high or too low depending on variables such as body composition and total energy expenditure.

Most Americans consume a diet adequate in protein containing approximately 1.0 g/kg per day.[118] However, those who consciously limit intakes of high-protein foods such as meat, fish, poultry, pork, and dairy products can decrease their dietary intake of protein significantly if these reductions are not compensated for with other protein-containing foods. Lacto-ovovegetarians (those that eat dairy) and vegans (nonanimal product eaters) can also meet protein needs without supplementation if their diets are properly planned to contain ample amounts of high-quality vegetable proteins. For example, the combination of two–thirds cup cooked whole grain rice with a half cup of cooked lentils provides about the same amount of complete protein as an ounce of meat.

A common interpretation by individuals interested in "bulking up" is that more protein will result in an accumulation of greater muscle mass. Athletes typically ingest 1.2 to 2.0 g protein/kg per day.[119,120] Protein is not the only, or even the most significant, nutrient to ensure muscle deposition.[121,122] Total energy intake to create positive nitrogen balance is also necessary for muscle hypertrophy. By having enough food and energy supplied through the diet, the body can utilize protein for muscle building versus use of muscle as energy for bodily functions. Weight resistance training is the most important factor.

Micronutrients

Vitamins and minerals perform a multitude of functions in the body without directly contributing energy. As metabolic cofactors, energy constituents, and catalysts, these micronutrients are required for energy production, cell respiration, various carbohydrate, protein, and fat metabolic pathways, and red blood cell production.

Most athletes who consume large amounts of energy can meet vitamin and mineral suggestions in the recommended dietary allowances (see Table 2–5) from food alone.[123] However, some researchers contend that highly active athletes may require B vitamins, vitamin C, and various minerals in greater amounts than the RDAs for these nutrients.[124-126] Despite increased needs in some athletic populations, an extensive review on vitamin and mineral status in athletes notes that most studies show no difference in micronutrient status between athletes and untrained persons studied as controls.[127] One study that looked at ultramarathoners' intakes revealed ample vitamin and mineral intakes.[128] Thus, athletes who consume a balanced diet consisting of large amounts of calories to meet increased energy needs are likely to ingest enough micronutrients to meet increased demands arising from exercise. Other athletes on strict caloric restrictions or engaged in rapid weight reduction (wrestlers making weight) are possibly at risk for nutrient deficiencies as well as dehydration. If a chronic negative energy and nitrogen balance exists, inadequate micronutrient intake potentially exists as well.[129] In these cases, a vitamin and mineral supplement may be needed to prevent deficiencies.

Despite adequate vitamin and mineral intakes among most athletes, the average prevalence of use of supplements among athletes is estimated at 46 percent with women and elite athletes supplementing more than men and college or high school athletes.[130] Unfortunately, consumption of fortified foods and specially formulated foods that contain significant amounts of added micronutrients are not typically figured into the equation in such prevalence estimates. These foods may also contribute significantly to an individual's nutrient intake, so it is important to clearly state recommendations to avoid oversupplementation. Supplement use, like the use of fortified foods, nutritional bars, and drinks, should not be condemned. However, in most cases it is not necessary. On the other hand, if a nutrient deficiency exists, supplementation to achieve normal levels can improve performance. But if serum levels and stores of a nutrient are already adequate, supplementation has not been shown to improve performance.[131] Also, overdosing of certain nutrients is potentially toxic and it could increase competitive inhibition, which can counteract goals of supplementation by inhibiting absorption of nutrients. For example, excess calcium can interfere with iron absorption. Consequences of supplementation in amounts significantly above recommended levels could harm performance and contradict injury prevention goals.

Vitamins and minerals that are of particular interest in athletic populations secondary to function and implications for injury prevention and rehabilitation are individually discussed next.

Vitamin D, Calcium, and Phosphorus

Vitamin D, calcium, and phosphorus status in part determine an individual's bone health. Vitamin D, a fat-soluble vitamin required for mineral balance and skeletal formation, is found in vitamin D fortified milk, tuna, salmon, and sardines. Skin exposure to sunlight results in vitamin D production by the body. Calcium, a mineral necessary for bone formation and maintenance, regulation of heartbeat, nerve transmission, and blood clot formation, is found in highest amounts in milk and milk products, calcium-fortified orange juice, and dark leafy greens.

Phosphorus, which is found in varying amounts in most foods, is an important component of bone as well. Dietary intake of these three micronutrients largely affects bone density, a critical marker for skeletal injury risk. Incidence of fracture is indirectly correlated with bone density.

Calcium balance is affected by a variety of factors. Amenorrhea (cessation of menstrual periods), which is common in very lean female athletes (high incidence in ballet dancers[132,133] and competitive runners), causes hormonal imbalances that lead to bone loss and decreases in bone mass.[134] Incidence of stress fractures is higher in amenorrheic athletes, making amenorrhea an additional injury risk factor.[135-137] The stress of some athletic training regimens on the body has been shown to cause menstrual abnormalities[138,139]; however, it is also common in females with eating disorders and very low body fatness. The minimum body fat to initiate menarche is 17 percent, and to keep menses regular is 22 percent according to Frish and McArthur.[140,141]

Other factors that affect calcium balance are genetics, age, gender, activity level, and usage of estrogen replacement therapy or birth control pills. Exercise, especially strength-bearing activity, promotes mineralization and helps to maintain bone mass with aging, thus decreasing fracture incidence.[142] Factors that improve calcium balance and bone mineralization throughout the life span can prevent or delay the onset of osteoporosis. Postmenopausal estrogen replacement therapy, premenopausal use of birth control pills, and adequate dietary calcium with or without supplementation are associated with improved bone density.

Iron

The primary nutrient deficiency in the United States is iron-deficiency anemia, which can depress exercise performance.[143-145] Low iron intake, blood loss, increased hemolysis, poor iron absorption, increased needs for iron, excessive blood donations, or a combination of these factors can contribute to iron deficiency.[146-148] Athletes, especially females, commonly have low iron status.[149] According to one review, substandard ferritin concentration is prevalent in 37 percent of female athletes compared to only 23 percent in untrained females.[150] Endurance athletes are at greater risk if occult gastrointestinal bleeding occurs as a result of heavy training programs. Without adequate iron stores, hemoglobin levels do not reach their full potential, which decreases VO_2 max potential. If mild iron deficiency exists, foods rich in iron such as lean meat, fish, poultry, and iron-fortified grains should be recommended. If levels do not normalize from dietary manipulations, short-term iron supplementation to achieve normal hemoglobin levels should be considered. No improvement occurs with iron supplementation if levels are already normal.

B-complex Vitamins

Thiamin, riboflavin, and niacin are essential cofactors for enzymes involved in energy metabolism. Both thiamin and riboflavin needs increase with increasing caloric intake. Thus, athletes with high energy demands require higher amounts of these nutrients. High amounts of thiamin are present in lean pork, lean meats, and whole grains. Riboflavin is highest in low-fat milk, milk products, and enriched grains. Fish, poultry, and peanut butter contain large amounts of niacin.

Antioxidants

Other vitamins being actively researched for protective benefits related to chronic disease prevention and exercise performance are the antioxidants, vitamins C and E. These vitamins have been shown to decrease lipid peroxidation, but without improving exercise performance.[151,152] The theory behind antioxidants is their ability to prevent or repair free radical damage caused by oxidation. Vitamin E has shown a protective benefit against oxidative muscle damage.[153] Claims have been made by some investigators that vitamin E needs may be increased with increased training secondary to oxidative stress and free radical production from exercising muscles to exhaustion. Rich sources of vitamin E are wheat germ, nuts, vegetable oil, leafy greens, and egg yolks.

Vitamin C can potentially prevent onset of upper respiratory infections,[154] but more research is needed to confirm these findings. Vitamin C is high in fruits and vegetables, especially oranges, broccoli, and green pepper. Today, there is some concern that the established RDA for vitamin C is not high enough. Recommendations to raise the RDA to 200 mg from the current level of 60 mg per day have been suggested by some scientists.[155] Such a recommended amount could be ingested by eating 1 orange, 1 cup of strawberries, and two thirds of a cup of cooked broccoli in a day.

Currently, due to inconclusive evidence of benefit from large doses of antioxidant vitamins, the current RDA (8 to 10 mg vitamin E and 60 mg vitamin C) is recommended, and these levels can be achieved through ingestion of antioxidant-rich fruits and vegetables and plant oils. Supplementation is not necessary to get adequate amounts of these vitamins.

FLUID AND ELECTROLYTE RECOMMENDATIONS FOR ACTIVE PEOPLE

Fluid needs vary with size, body composition, caloric intake, dietary composition, environmental conditions, and activity levels. Daily fluid requirements consist of insensible water losses plus any additional water needed to digest food components and excrete dietary waste. For example, high-protein diets, which are also usually high in electrolytes, increase fluid needs secondary to the kidney's increased urine production as a response to higher urea and solute loads. The basic fluid requirement, or recommended allowance, for adults is 1 mL of water per calorie of energy expenditure at usual levels of physical activity.[156] Additional fluid needs are contingent on losses, whether from exercise or other causes such as sweating, fever, vomiting, or diarrhea.

With increased muscular movement, the body's metabolic rate increases along with enhanced energy oxidation, which is accompanied by much excess heat. The rise in core body temperature occurs secondarily. Sweating occurs to remove most of this additional heat from the body via evaporative cooling. In some activities, such as wet suit surfing, heat is removed by the insulating properties and cold temperature of the water. Sweating rates vary according to environmental conditions, clothing, fitness level, intensity, type and duration of activity, and hydration status. The tremendous variability in the rate of fluid loss creates difficulty in determining exactly what the standards should be for fluid replacement. However, some general recommendations for different conditions will be described. Heat loss is most efficient when sweat is able to fully evaporate off the skin's surface. Large amounts of fluid and electrolytes are lost in sweating, with an estimated one to five times more fluid exiting plasma into sweat than into any other fluid space in the body.[157]

Highly fit individuals with increased aerobic fitness levels or those who are acclimated to hot climates have more efficient bodily cooling systems than their less fit and less acclimated peers. These trained individuals minimize their core temperature by increasing heat and water loss during exertion.[158] Untrained individuals dissipate sweat at a lower rate.[159] Therefore training can increase sweat rates by 10 to 20 percent, or about 200 to 300 mL/hour more than the untrained state.[160] Trained individuals therefore require more fluids.

Sweat is a hypotonic solution that contains sodium, potassium, magnesium, and chloride.[161] Sodium and chloride, the major ions of extracellular fluid, serve regulatory functions such as maintaining water and osmotic pressure equilibrium among the extracellular and plasma compartments. Thus, it is important to have adequate amounts of sodium and chloride to replace water losses during prolonged intense activity to ensure adequate hydration without causing electrolyte imbalances such as hyponatremia or hypernatremia. Potassium and magnesium are the major cations in the intracellular compartment. Potassium, the dominant electrolyte in terms of amounts, functions in water, acid–base balance, and osmotic pressure balance. It is positively correlated with muscle mass and is necessary for building muscle. Magnesium is lost in sweat, but is preserved well by the kidneys; thus, intake of it is not a predominant concern before, during, or after exercise.

It is important to consistently maintain adequate hydration. Individuals who are sufficiently hydrated can withstand higher core temperatures. Hypohydration, not aerobic fitness levels, is the primary culprit in most athlete-related heat illness cases.[162] If athletes are exercising at high intensities, it is vital to consciously replace fluids before, during, and after bouts of activity (as outlined in Table 2-6). Thirst sensation is suppressed during vigorous activity,[163] at the very time when fluids are depleted most quickly. Therefore, the athlete must remember to drink even when he or she is not thirsty.

When exercising in hot climates, water losses may reach 3 to 4 L per hour and as high as 10 L in a day. Losses are higher in hot, dry than in hot, wet environments.[164] Humid environments promote increased water retention on the skin and have higher vapor pressures opposing evaporation of sweat, making cooling the body more difficult and less efficient. If an athlete is exercising in hot and humid environments, frequent (every 15 minutes) intakes of 4 to 6 ounces of fluid are recommended.[165]

Exercising in cold temperatures at high altitudes creates increased water loss via respiration, independent of activity level. During usual respiration, an average man expires about 200 mL of water per day under normal conditions, 350 mL of water per day in dry climates, and up to 1500 mL of water per day in cold weather at high altitudes.[166] Therefore, on top of losses from exercise, an athlete working out under a combination of these conditions may need an additional 6 to 7 cups (1440 to 1680 mL) of fluid per day to replace respiratory losses.

The body must maintain optimal blood volume if arterial pressure and body temperature are to be regulated during physical activity.[167-170] Water must be replaced to prevent dehydration. Dehydration is associated with decreased muscular strength, lessened endurance, increased cramps and muscular exhaustion, and greater likelihood of heat-related illness.[171-173] Active individuals should try to keep fluid consumption in line with fluid losses. That is, they should replace fluid at the rate they lose it, or attempt to replete 80 percent of lost fluid during exercise (1 pound weight loss is equal to approximately 15 ounces water or 454 mL).[174] The general rule for water replacement is to drink 16 ounces of water (480 mL) for every pound of weight lost during exercise.[175] More specific fluid replacement guidelines pertaining to different physical activity variables are outlined in Table 2-6.

SPECIAL CONSIDERATIONS: ERGOGENIC AIDS

Finding the perfect ergogenic (performance enhancing) aid is every athlete's dream. Of all the performance enhancers, certainly water and carbohydrate have been well demonstrated to be important. Caffeine, a stimulant found naturally in coffee, some carbonated cola beverages, chocolate (in smaller amounts), and in some over-the-counter medications, improves endurance performance by exerting a lipolytic effect that spares muscle glycogen. Psychologically, caffeine improves performance by prolonging the onset of mental fatigue and boredom during long bouts of exercise.[176] Nervousness and sleep deprivation may occur as a result of very high caffeine intakes. Since caffeine has shown performance benefit, the U.S. Olympic Committee established standards to regulate caffeine consumption before and during competition (urine levels must be less than 12 mg/dL).

Carnitine is a performance enhancer of questionable efficacy. Its function is to transport free fatty acids into the mitochondria, where they are oxidized. It is contended that a possible ergogenic effect is in carnitine's physiologic role of free fatty acid transport. It is hypothesized that additional carnitine could spare muscle glycogen and therefore enhance performance. Since carnitine is synthesized in the human body in the presence of lysine and methionine,[177] and is found in animal foods, additional benefits from supplementation are unlikely.

Coenzyme Q10 (CoQ10) is a substance that facilitates oxidative metabolism in the mitochondria. Despite the effective use of CoQ10 in cardiac patients to improve oxygen uptake,[178] evidence in human subjects has shown no improvement in athletic performance while taking CoQ10 supplements.[179]

Medium-chain triglyceride (MCT) oil is also advertised as having ergogenic potential; however, physiologically there are no grounds for this argument. Unless an athlete suffers from fat malabsorption, which is very rare in the general population, MCT oil would provide no benefit over other sources of fat in the diet or in supplemental foods such as sports bars.

The ergogenic claims for chromium picolinate are that it will increase glucose tolerance in athletes and improve both carbohydrate and fat metabolism. If chromium status is normal, no additional performance benefit has been proven by supplementation with chromium. Good dietary sources that have high bioavailability for chromium include wheat germ, apples, mushrooms, and American cheese.

Many other ergogenic aids are promoted to the public, such as choline, bee pollen, lecithin, and various herbal remedies such as green tea, Ma Huang (ephedrine), and ginseng. Evidence is inconclusive concerning benefits of these products. At present their use is not recommended.

Sports bars, drinks, and gels are tasty and convenient but not necessarily effective as performance enhancers. Depending on the type of athlete and his or her energy, carbohydrate, fluid, and electrolyte needs, different sports products could be helpful (see Tables 2-7 and 2-8). However, it is important to limit the car-

TABLE 2–7. NUTRIENT CONTENT OF SPORTS DRINKS (8 OZ) AND SPORTS GELS (1 PACKET)

Sports Drink or Gel	Calories	Carbohydrate (g)	Carbohydrate (%)	Potassium (mg)	Sodium (mg)
10-K	60	15	6	30	55
Daily's 1st Ade	60	15	7	25	55
Hydra Fuel	66	16	7	50	25
Exceed	68	17	7.2	56?	66
Max	70	17	7.5	0	15
R.P.M.	70	17	7.6	70	0
PowerAde	67	17	8	33	73
All Sport	70	17	8	55	55
Snapple Snap-Up	80	20	8	49	58
Carbo Plus	60	15	16	100	5
Sports Pep Pocket (1.25 oz)[a]	100	25	100	80	50
GU (1.1 oz)[a]	100	25	100	n/a	n/a
Leppin Sport Squeezy (1 oz)[a]	70	17	971	n/a	8
Gatorade ReLode (0.75 oz)[a]	80	20	100	n/a	25

[a] Recommend drinking 8–10 oz water just before or after consuming gel pack.
N/A, not available.
Information from respective manufacturers.

bohydrate concentration of beverages to 6 to 8 percent to allow for efficient gastrointestinal absorption. Drinks have the advantage over bars and gels in providing fluids. If an athlete uses a sports bar or gel for energy, consuming additional water is crucial to prevent dehydration.

Other food constituents can be used to supplement an athlete's diet if more calories are needed. Frappes, fruit shakes, and powdered drink beverages such as instant breakfast mixes, which are added to milk, can be consumed to provide additional energy to meet daily demands.

SPECIAL PROBLEMS

Eating Disorders

Eating disorders are more prevalent in athletic than nonathletic populations, especially among women. Athletes with eating disorders either starve themselves intentionally to reduce their weights by 15 to 25 percent (anorexia nervosa) or rid themselves of excess calories by vomiting following a binge (bulimarexia). Prevalence of anorexia is 4 to 14 percent in athletes while it is only 3 to 5 percent in the general population.[180,181] Others gorge and binge and suffer from bulimia. Bulimia rates are estimated at 14 percent in male athletes and 35 percent in female athletes.[182] An estimated 5 to 20 percent of college women have bulimia.[183] Restrictive eating associated with anorexia, bulimarexia, or thirsting in athletes (usually resulting in BMIs beyond lower normal limits) have risks similar to those of rapid weight loss methods. Anorexics run the risk of glycogen depletion and problems related to bone mass depletion such as amenorrhea and dehydration. Bulimics are more likely to maintain an average weight. However, water and electrolyte imbalances can occur from practices such as laxative or purgative abuse (bingeing and vomiting) or compulsively exercising as a form of purging. Having an eating disorder may drastically reduce both physiologic and mental stamina in sports. Moreover, anorectics are subject to increase risk of injury in cases when amenorrhea is persistent or BMI is below 19. Individuals who are suspected of having an eating disorder should be referred to a registered dietitian, a psychiatrist, and his or her primary physician, and must be followed by this multidisplinary team.

Weight (Fat-free Mass) Maintenance

Maintaining a healthy body weight following weight loss, during a recovery period from injury, or during a modified off-season training regimen can be difficult, given the remarkable decreases in caloric expenditure that can ensue when athletes become sedentary. With the changing needs each of these situations involve, appropriate dietary manipulations must be made to best stabilize current weights at healthy levels.

Rapid weight loss (greater than 2 lb per week) is very difficult to maintain and signifies mostly loss of water weight or lean body mass. Rapid weight loss can lead to dehydration or loss of fat-free mass, and both are detrimental to athletic performance.

Following injuries, such as breaks in bones and muscle tears, energy, protein, calcium, and other nutrients are involved in the healing process. For example, the college swimmer who burns 2500 calories per day from training workouts alone will have a significant drop in energy needs if an injury occurs and he or she abruptly stops training. If the injury is severe, protein demands will increase secondary to healing with an increase in needs of up to 50 percent of the RDA. However, this may not be too different from his or her protein needs for endurance training. In any event, most Americans eat enough protein to accommodate these needs. In summary, an athlete in this situation or a similar one would need to focus more on consuming nutrient-dense (high amounts of protein, vitamins, and minerals per calorie) food to create a diet higher in protein, vitamins, and minerals in relation to reduced calorie needs.

During off-season months, athletes can have difficulty maintaining usual body weights that are optimal for their event. A marathoner who would benefit from maintaining a weight toward the lower extreme of his or her

TABLE 2–8. NUTRIENT CONTENT OF VARIOUS SPORTS BARS

Sports Bar	Calories	Carbohydrate (g)	Protein (g)	Fat (g)	% Calories from Carbohydrate : Protein : Fat
Ultra Fuel	490	100	15	3	82:12:6
Exceed	280	53	12	2	76:17:7
Clif Bar	250	50	5–6	3	80: 9:11
Body Bar	219	50	6	0	89:11:0
BTU Stoker	250	47	10	3	73:16:11
Cross Trainer	245	46	11	<2	75:18:7
Hot Stuff	270	46	15	2	68:22:7
EdgeBar	240	46	10	<2	77:17:6
Forza Bar	233	45	11	1	77:19:4
Super Protein Bar	250	45	13	2	72:21:7
Diet Fuel	180	44	15	1	62:33:5
PowerBar	225	42	10	2	75:17:8
CytoBar	235	42	12	2	71:21:8
Pure Power	240	42	12	3	70:20:11
Pro-Sports	240	40	15	<2	67:25:8
Tiger Sport	230	40	11	3	70:19:11
Time Bar	235	40	8	<2	68:14:8
Yohimbe Bar	241	37	6	4	61:10:15
Calcium Almond Blitz (+1200 mg calcium)	150	29	2	2	78:6:12
Fin Halsa	170	28	11	2	65:25:10
Beta Bar	230	23	13	10	38:23:39
Perfect Protein Bar	190	21	12	7	43:25:32
Tiger's Milk	160	20	6	7	47:14:37
PR Bar	186	19	14	6	41:30:30
Balance Bar	180	13.5	18	6	30:40:30

Information from manufacturers.

ideal weight range needs to decrease calories significantly following the repletion of glycogen stores when rest is imperative. Wrestlers who constantly diet to "make weight" may also face problems of weight gain in the off season when energy expenditures decline and energy intake does not.

Weight Gain

An uncommon but nevertheless pressing problem that affects some athletes (mainly children and adolescents) is the inability to increase weight, specifically fat-free mass. Highly active individuals with high metabolic rates during phases of rapid growth can have trouble meeting increased energy needs. Weight gain tactics, such as amino acid overloading and steroid abuse, are inappropriate, expensive, and in the case of steroid use, prejudicial to health.

Amino acid overloading is not proven effective for enhancing weight gain or muscle mass. Most Americans already consume adequate protein. The major issue for

athletes who need to gain weight is to achieve a state of positive nitrogen balance, which can only be achieved if adequate energy is ingested to exceed daily demands including energy burned during exercise and needed for growth if applicable. Steroid use is not authorized in competitive sports without a medical indication (such as disease requiring steroid treatment) because its health risks outweigh the potential benefits.

CONCLUSIONS

Improved endurance, strength, and Vo_2 max, and reduction of injury and some chronic disease risks, are all associated with good nutritional status and a physically active lifestyle. Appropriate nutrition is essential to meet the needs of all types of athletes, from those individuals who walk for a half hour per day to ultra-endurance athletes who train 3 hours per day. Just as amounts of exercise vary tremendously between individuals, their corresponding nutritional needs differ in many ways.

The information outlined in this chapter must be individualized to accommodate an athlete's age, gender, body anthropometrics, and environmental conditions in addition to his or her training program. To ensure the realization of all the potential benefits of sound nutrition in relation to sports, the advice of a registered dietitian specializing in the needs of athletes is a very important supplement to any athlete's training program.

Acknowledgments

We acknowledge with thanks the partial support of the Gerber Foundation for Dr. Dwyer's contribution.

REFERENCES

1. Powell KE, Thompson PD, Caspersen CJ, Kendrick JS. Physical activity and the incidence of coronary heart disease. *Ann Rev Public Health.* 1987;8:253–287.
2. National Cholesterol Education Program. Second *Report of the Expert Panel on Detection, Evaluation, and Treatment of High Blood Cholesterol in Adults.* National Institutes of Health, National Heart, Lung, and Blood Institute. September, 1993. NIH pub. no. 93-3095.
3. Tsopanakis C, Kotsarellis D, Tsopanakis AD. Lipoprotein and lipid profiles of elite athletes in Olympic sports. *Int J Sports Med.* 1986;7:316–321.
4. Berg A, Keul J. Influences of maximum aerobic capacity and relative body weight on the lipoprotein profile in athletes. *Atherosclerosis.* 1985;55:225–231.
5. Gordon R, Castelli WP, Hjortland MC, et al. High density lipoprotein as a protective factor against coronary heart disease. The Framingham study. *Am J Med.* 1977; 62:707–713.
6. The fifth report of the Joint National Committee on Detection, Evaluation, and Treatment of High Blood Cholesterol. *Arch Intern Med.* 1993;153:154–182.
7. Campaigne BN, Lampman RM. *Exercise in the Clinical Management of Diabetes.* Champaign, IL: Human Kinetics; 1994.
8. Helmrich SP, Ragland DR, Leung RW, Paffenbarger RS. Physical activity and reduced occurrence of non-insulin-dependent diabetes mellitus. *N Engl J Med.* 1991;325:147–152.
9. Powell KE, Caspersen CJ, Koplan JP, Ford ES. Physical activity and chronic diseases. *Am J Clin Nutr.* 1989;49 (suppl 5):999–1006. Review.
10. Cordain L, Latin RW, Behnke JJ. The effects of an aerobic running program on bowel transit time. *J Sports Med* 1986;26:101–104.
11. Kriska AM, Sandler RB, Cauley JA, et al. The assessment of historical physical activity and its relation to adult bone parameters. *Am J Epidemiol.* 1988;127:1053–1063.
12. Nelson ME, Fiatarone MA, Morganti CM, et al. Effects of high-intensity strength training on multiple risk factors for osteoporotic fractures. A randomized controlled trial. *JAMA.* 1994;272:1909–1914.
13. American College of Sports Medicine. *Guidelines for Exercise Testing and Prescription.* 4th ed. Philadelphia: Lea & Febiger; 1991.
14. Pate RR, Pratt M, Blair SN, et al. Physical activity and public health. A recommendation from Centers for Disease Control and Prevention and the American College of Sports Medicine. *JAMA.* 1995;273:402–407.
15. Dwyer J. Policy and healthy weight. *Prev Med.* 1996; 25:1–4.
16. Lew EA, Garfinkel L. Variations in mortality by weight among 750,000 men and women. *J Chron Dis.* 1979; 32:563–576.
17. U.S. Department of Agriculture. Committee by the Agricultural Research Service. Dietary Guidelines Advisory Committee. *Report of the Dietary Guidelines Advisory Committee on the Dietary Guidelines for Americans,* 1995.
18. Manson JE, Willett WC, Stampfer MJ, et al. Body weight and mortality among women. *N Engl J Med.* 1995; 333:677–685.
19. Jones BH, Manikowski R, Harris JA, et al. Incidence of and risk factors for injury and illness among male and female Army basic trainees. Report no. T 19/88. Natick, MA: U.S. Army Research Institute of Environmental Medicine; 1988.
20. Marti B, Vader JP, Minder CE, Abelin T. On the epidemiology of running injuries. The 1984 Bern grand-prix study. *Am J Sports Med.* 1988;16:285–294.
21. Himes JH, Dietz WH. Guidelines of overweight in adolescent preventive services: Recommendations from an expert committee. *Am J Clin Nutr.* 1994;59:307–316.
22. Himes JH, Dietz WH. Guidelines of overweight in adolescent preventive services: Recommendations from an expert committee. *Am J Clin Nutr.* 1994;59:307–316.
23. Must A, Dallal GE, Dietz WH. Reference data for obesity: 85th and 95th percentiles of body mass index (wt/ht^2) and triceps skinfold thickness. *Am J Clin Nutr.* 1991; 53:839–846. Correction: *Am J Clin Nutr.* 1991;54:773.
24. Consensus panel addresses obesity question. *JAMA.* 1985;254:1878.
25. Committee on Diet and Health, Food and Nutrition Board. *Diet and Health: Implications for Reducing Chronic Disease Risk.* Washington, DC: National Academy Press; 1989.
26. U.S. Department of Agriculture, Human Nutrition Information Service. *Food Guide Pyramid.* August 1992, leaflet no. 572.
27. Thomas PR, ed. *Weighing the Options, Criteria for Evaluating Weight-management Programs.* Washington, DC: Food and Nutrition Board, Institute of Medicine; 1995.
28. Dwyer JT, Lu D. Popular diets for weight loss from nutritionally hazardous to healthful. In: Stunkard AJ, Wadden TA, eds. *Obesity: Theory and Therapy.* 2nd ed. New York: Raven; 1993.
29. Institute of Food Technologists' Expert Panel on Food Safety and Nutrition. Human obesity. *Contemp Nutrition.* Princeton, NJ: 1993;18:7–8.
30. Thomas PR, ed. *Weighing the Options, Criteria for Evaluating Weight-management Programs.* Washington, DC: Food and Nutrition Board, Institute of Medicine; 1995.

31. Whatley JE, Poehlman ET. Obesity and exercise. In: Blackburn GL, Kanders BS, eds. *Obesity: Pathophysiology, Psychology and Treatment*. New York: Chapman & Hall; 1994.

32. Pavlou KN, Steffee WP, Lerman RH, Burrows BA. Effects of dieting and exercise on lean body mass, oxygen uptake, and strength. *Med Sci Sports Exerc*. 1985; 37:758-765.

33. Zelasko CJ. Exercise for weight loss: What are the facts? *J Am Diet Assoc*. 1995;95:1414-1417.

34. Racette SB, Schoeller DA, Kushner RF, Neil KM. Exercise enhances dietary compliance during moderate energy restriction in obese women. *Am J Clin Nutr*. 1995; 62:345-349.

35. Pavlou KN, Krey S, Steffee WP. Exercise as an adjunct to weight loss and maintenance in moderately obese subjects. *Am J Clin Nutr*. 1989;49:1115-1123.

36. Brehm B, Gutin B. Recovery energy expenditure for steady state exercise in runners and nonexercisers. *Med Sci Sports Exerc*. 1986;18:205-210.

37. Kaminsky LA, Whaley MH. Effect of interval-type exercise on excess postexercise oxygen consumption (EPOC) in obese and normal weight women. *Med Sci Sports Exerc*. 1993;2:106-111.

38. Gore CJ, Whithers RI. The effect of exercise intensity and duration on the oxygen deficit and excess post-exercise oxygen consumption. *Eur J Appl Physiol Occup Physiol*. 1990;60:169-174.

39. Kaminsky LA, Padjen S, LaHam-Saeger J. Effect of split exercise sessions on excess postexercise oxygen consumption. *Br J Sports Med*. 1990;24:95-98.

40. Bahr R. Excess postexercise oxygen consumption—magnitude, mechanisms, and practical implications. *Acta Physiol Scand*. 1992;(suppl 605):1-70.

41. Howley ET, Glover ME. The calorie costs of running and walking one mile for men and women. *Med Sci Sports Exerc*. 1974;6:235-239.

42. Melby CL, Lincknell I, Schmidt WD. Energy expenditure following a bout of non-steady state resistance exercise. *J Sports Med Phys Fit*. 1992;32:128-135.

43. Chad RE, Quigley BM. Exercise intensity: Effect on postexercise O_2 uptake in trained and untrained women. *J Appl Physiol*. 1991;70:1713-1719.

44. Bouchard C, Bray GA, Hubbard VS. Basic and clinical aspects of regional fat distribution. *Am J Clin Nutr*. 1990;52:946-950.

45. Seidell JC, Cigolini M, Charzewska J, et al. Measurement of regional distribution of adipose tissue. Presented at the First European Congress on Obesity, June 1988, Stockholm.

46. Going S, Going J. (Body) composition 101. *Diabetes Forecast*. May 1993:33-36.

47. National Cholesterol Education Program. *Highlights of the Report of the Expert Panel on Detection, Evaluation and Treatment of High Blood Cholesterol in Adults*. Bethesda: National Institutes of Health; 1987. DHHS pub no. (NIH) 88-2926.

48. National Academy of Sciences, Institute of Medicine. Body Composition and Physical Performance. Washington, DC: National Academy Press; 1992:95.

49. Cureton KJ, Sparling PB, Evans W, et al. Effect of experimental alterations in excess weight on aerobic capacity and distance running performance. *Med Sci Sports Exerc*. 1978;10:194-199.

50. Harman E, Sharp M, Manikowski R, et al. Analysis of muscle strength data base. *J Appl Sports Sci Res*. 1988;2:54. Abstract.

51. U.S. Senate Select Committee on Nutrition and Human Needs. *Dietary Goals for the U.S.* 2nd ed. Washington, DC: Government Printing Office; 1977.

52. U.S. Department of Agriculture, Committee by the Agricultural Research Service. Dietary Guidelines Advisory Committee. *Report of the Dietary Guidelines Advisory Committee on the Dietary Guidelines for Americans*, 1995.

53. U.S. Department of Agriculture, U.S. Department of Health and Human Services. Human Nutrition Information Service. *USDA Food Guide Pyramid*. August 1992, leaflet no. 572.

54. U.S. Department of Agriculture, U.S. Department of Health and Human Services, Human Nutrition Information Service. *USDA Food Guide Pyramid*. August 1992, leaflet no. 572.

55. Marcus J, ed. *Sports Nutrition: A Guide for the Professional Working With Active People*. Chicago: American Dietetic Association; 1986.

56. Brotherhood J. Nutrition and sports performance. *Sports Med*. 1984;1:350-389.

57. Holt WS. Nutrition and athletes. *Am Fam Physician*. 1993;47:1757-1764.

58. Economos CD, Bortz SS, Nelson ME. Nutritional practices of elite athletes. *Sports Med*. 1993;16:381-399.

59. McGandy RB, Barrows CH Jr, Spanias A, et al. Nutrient intakes and energy expenditure in men of different ages. *J Gerontol*. 1966;21:581-587.

60. Elmstahl S. Energy expenditure, energy intake and body composition in geriatric long-stay patients. *Comp Gerontol*. 1987;A1:118-125.

61. National Research Council. *Recommended Dietary Allowances*. 10th ed. Washington, DC: National Academy Press, 1989.

62. Harris JA, Benedict FG. *A Biometric Study of Basal Metabolism in Man*. Philadelphia; Lippincott; 1919:227. Carnegie Institute (Washington) pub no. 279.

63. Cunningham JJ. A reanalysis of the factors influencing basal metabolic rate in normal adults. *Am J Clin Nutr*. 1980;33:2372-2374.

64. Thomas CD, Baker-Fulco CJ, Jones TE, et al. *Nutritional Guidance For Military Field Operations in Temperate and Extreme Environments*. Natick, MA: U.S. Army Research Institute of Environmental Medicine; June 1993. USARIEM technical note 93-8.

65. Kearns PJ, Thompson JD, Werner PC, et al. Nutritional and metabolic response to acute spinal-cord injury. *JPEN*. 1992;16:11-15.

66. Levine AM, Nash MS, Green BA, et al. An examination of dietary intakes and nutritional status of chronic healthy spinal cord injured individuals. *Paraplegia*. 1990;30:880-889.

67. Zlotolow SP, Levy E, Bauman WA. The serum lipoprotein profile in veterans with paraplegia: The relationship to

nutritional factors and body mass index. *J Am Paraplegia Soc.* 1992;15:158-162.

68. Gordon R, Castelli WP, Hjortland MC, et al. High density lipoprotein as a protective factor against coronary heart disease. The Framingham study. *Am J Med.* 1977;62:707-713.

69. Tsopanakis C, Kotsarellis D, Tsopanakis AD. Lipoprotein and lipid profiles of elite athletes in Olympic sports. *Int J Sports Med.* 1986;7:316-321.

70. Berg A, Keul J. Influences of maximum aerobic capacity and relative body weight on the lipoprotein profile in athletes. *Atherosclerosis.* 1985;55:225-231.

71. Food and Nutrition Board. *Recommended Dietary Allowances.* 10th ed. Washington, DC: National Academy of Sciences; 1989.

72. Food and Nutrition Board. *Recommended Dietary Allowances.* 10th ed. Washington, DC: National Academy of Sciences; 1989.

73. Position of the American Dietetic Association and the Canadian Dietetic Association: Nutrition for physical fitness and athletic performance for adults. *J Am Diet Assoc.* 1993;93:691-696.

74. American College of Sports Medicine. *Guidelines for Exercise Testing and Prescription.* Philadelphia: Lea & Febiger; 1991.

75. Coyle EF. Substrate utilization during exercise in active people. *Am J Clin Nutr.* 1995;61(suppl):968S-979S.

76. Costill DL. Carbohydrates for exercise: Dietary demands for optimal performance. *Int J Sports Med.* 1988;9:1-8.

77. Knogh A, Lindhard J. Relative value of fat and carbohydrate as a source of muscular energy. *Biochem J.* 1920;14:290-298.

78. Coyle EF, Coggan AR, Hemmert MK, Ivy JL. Muscle glycogen utilization during prolonged strenuous exercise when fed carbohydrate. *J Appl Physiol.* 1986;61:165-172.

79. Romijn JA, Coyle EF, Sidossis L, et al. Regulation of endogenous fat and carbohydrate metabolism in relation to exercise intensity. *Am J Physiol.* 1993;265:E380-E391.

80. Hagerman FC, ACSM. Energy metabolism and fuel utilization. *Med Sci Sports Exerc.* 1992;24(suppl 9):S309-S314.

81. Coyle EF. Substrate utilization during exercise in active people. *Am J Clin Nutr.* 1995;61(suppl):968S-979S.

82. Burke LM, Read SD. Sports nutrition. Approaching the nincties. *Sports Med.* 1989;8:80-100.

83. Christensen EH, Hansen O. Arbeitsfahigkeit und Ehrnahrung. *Scand Arch Physiol.* 1939;81:160-175.

84. Brewer J, Williams C, Patton A. The influence of high carbohydrate diets on endurance running performance. *Eur J Appl Physiol.* 1988;57:698-706.

85. Williams C. Carbohydrate needs of elite athletes. *World Rev Nutr Diet.* 1993;71:34-60.

86. Nilsson LH, Hultman E. Liver glycogen in man—the effect of total starvation or a carbohydrate-poor diet followed by carbohydrate refeeding. *Scand J Clin Lab Invest.* 1973;32:325-330.

87. Williams C. Carbohydrate needs of elite athletes. *World Rev Nutr Diet.* 1993;71:34-60.

88. Sherman WM, Costill DI, Fink WJ, Miller JM. The effect of exercise and diet manipulation on muscle glycogen and its subsequent use during performance. *Int J Sports Med.* 1981;2:114-118.

89. Neufer PD, Costill DL, Flynn MG, et al. Improvements in exercise performance: Effects of carbohydrate feedings and diet. *J Appl Physiol.* 1987;62:983-988.

90. Wright DA, Sherman WM, Dernbach AR. Carbohydrate feedings before, during, or in combination improve cycling endurance performance. *J Appl Physiol.* 1991;71:1082-1088.

91. Coggan AR, Coyle EF. Carbohydrate ingestion during prolonged exercise: Effects on metabolism and performance. *Exerc Sports Sci Rev.* 1991;19:1-40.

92. Coggan AR, Swanson SC. Nutritional manipulations before and during endurance exercise: Effects on performance. *Med Sci Sports Exerc.* 1992;24:S331-S335.

93. Mitchell JB, Costill DL, Houmard JA, et al. Influence of carbohydrate dosage on exercise performance and glycogen metabolism. *J Appl Physiol.* 1989;67:1843-1849.

94. Coggan AR, Coyle EF. Reversal of fatigue during prolonged exercise by carbohydrate infusion or ingestion. *J Appl Physiol.* 1987;63:2388-2395.

95. Hoffman CJ, Coleman E. An eating plan and update on recommended dietary practices for the endurance athlete. *J Am Diet Assoc.* 1991;91:325-330.

96. Bergstrom J, Hultman E. Muscle glycogen synthesis after exercise: An enhancing factor localized to the muscle cells in man. *Nature.* 1966;20:309-310.

97. Pizza FX, Flynn MG, Duscha BD, et al. A carbohydrate loading regimen improves high intensity, short duration exercise performance. *Int J Sport Nutr.* 1995; 5:110-116.

98. Bergstrom J, Hultman E. Muscle glycogen synthesis in relation to diet studied in normal subjects. *Acta Med Scand.* 1967;182:109-117.

99. Coyle EF. Substrate utilization during exercise in active people. *Am J Clin Nutr.* 1995;61(suppl):968S-979S.

100. Roberts KM, Noble EG, Hayden DB, et al. Simple and complex carbohydrate-rich diets and muscle glycogen content of marathon runners. *Eur J Appl Physiol.* 1987;57:70-74.

101. Murray R, Paul GL, Seifert JG, et al. The effects of glucose, fructose, and sucrose ingestion during exercise. *Med Sci Sports Exerc.* 1989;21:275-282.

102. Coggan AR, Coyle EF. Carbohydrate ingestion during prolonged exercise: Effects on metabolism and performance. *Exerc Sports Sci Rev.* 1991;19:1-40.

103. Massicotte D, Peronnet F, Brisson G, et al. Oxidation of a glucose polymer during excrcise: Comparison of glucose and fructose. *J Appl Physiol.* 1989;66:179-183.

104. Murray R, Paul GL, Seifert JG, et al. The effects of glucose, fructose, and sucrose ingestion during exercise. *Med Sci Sports Exerc.* 1989;21:275-282.

105. Food and Nutrition Board. *Recommended Dietary Allowances.* 10th ed. Washington, DC: National Academy of Sciences; 1989.

106. Centers for Disease Control and Prevention. Daily dietary fat and total food-energy intakes—NHANES III, phase 1, 1988-91. *JAMA.* 1994;271:1309.

107. Economos CD, Bortz SS, Nelson ME. Nutritional practices of elite athletes. *Sports Med.* 1993;16:381-399.

108. Fox EL. *Sports Physiology.* 2nd ed. Philadelphia: Saunders; 1984.

109. Fox EL. *Sports Physiology.* 2nd ed. Philadelphia: Saunders; 1984.

110. Gollnick PD. Metabolism of substrates: Energy substrate metabolism during and as modified by training. *Fed Proc.* 1985;44:353-357.

111. Sherman WM, Leenders N. Fat loading: The next magic bullet? *Int J Sport Nutr.* 1995;5:S1-S12.

112. Sherman WM, Lamb DR. Nutrition and prolonged exercise. In: Lamb DR, Murray R, eds. *Perspectives in Exercise Science and Sports Medicine.* Volume 1, *Prolonged Exercise*, Carmel, IN: Benchmark 1988;213-280.

113. Coyle EF, Coggan AR, Hemmert MK, Ivy JL. Muscle glycogen utilization during prolonged strenuous exercise when fed carbohydrate. *J Appl Physiol.* 1986;61:165-172.

114. Food and Nutrition Board. *Recommended Dietary Allowances.* 10th ed. Washington, DC: National Academy of Sciences; 1989.

115. Paul GL. Dietary protein requirements for physically active individuals. *Sports Med.* 1987;8:154-176.

116. Butterfield G, Cady C, Moynihan S. Effect of increasing protein intake on nitrogen balance in recreational weight lifters. *Med Sci Sports Exer.* 1992;24:S71. Abstract.

117. Lemon P. Methods of weight gain in athletes. *Sports Sci Exchange Roundtable.* 1995;6:21.

118. American Dietetic Association. Position of the American Dietetic Association: Nutrition for physical fitness and athletic performance for adults. *J Am Diet Assoc.* 1987; 87:933-939.

119. Hoffman C, Coleman E. An eating plan and update on recommended dietary practices for the endurance athlete. *J Am Diet Assoc.* 1991;91:325-330.

120. Neilman D. *An Introduction to Fitness and Sports Medicine.* Palo Alto: Bull; 1990:221-270.

121. Paul GL. Dietary protein requirements for physically active individuals. *Sports Med.* 1987;8:154-176.

122. Butterfield G, Cady C, Moynihan S. Effect of increasing protein intake on nitrogen balance in recreational weight lifters. *Med Sci Sports Exer.* 1992;24:S71. Abstract.

123. Economos CD, Bortz SS, Nelson ME. Nutritional practices of elite athletes. *Sports Med.* 1993;16:381-399.

124. Belko AZ. Vitamins and exercise—an update. *Med Sci Sport Exerc.* 1986;19(suppl):S191-S196.

125. Niemen DC, Gates JR, Butler JV, et al. Supplementation patterns in marathon runners. *J Am Diet Assoc.* 1989; 89:1615-1619.

126. Clarkson PM, Haymes EM. Trace mineral requirements for athletes. *Int J Sport Nutr.* 1994;4:104-119.

127. Fogelholm M. Indicators of vitamin and mineral status in athletes' blood: A review. *Int J Sport Nutr.* 1995; 5:267-284.

128. Singh A, Evans P, Gallagher KL, Deuster PA. Dietary intakes and biochemical profiles of nutritional status of ultramarathoners. *Med Sci Sport Exerc.* 1993;25:328-334.

129. Fogelholm M. Indicators of vitamin and mineral status in athletes' blood: A review. *Int J Sport Nutr.* 1995; 5:267-284.

130. Sobal J, Marquart L. Vitamin/mineral supplement use among athletes: A review of the literature. *Int J Sport Nutr.* 1994;4:320-334.

131. Keith RE. Vitamins in sport and exercise. In: Wolinsky I, Hickson JF, eds. *Nutrition in Exercise and Sport.* Boca Raton: CRC Press; 1989.

132. Calabrase LH, Kirkendall DT. Nutritional and medical considerations in dancers. *Clin Sports Med Sci.* 1983;2:539.

133. Benson JE, Geiger CJ, Eiserman PA, Wardlaw GM. Relationship between nutrient intake, body mass index, menstrual function, and ballet injury. *J Am Diet Assoc.* 1989;89:58-63.

134. Drinkwater BL, Nilson K, Chesnut CH III. Bone mineral content of amenorrheic and eumenorrheic athletes. *N Engl J Med.* 1984;311:277.

135. Lloyd T, Triantafyllou SJ, Baker ER, et al. Women athletes with menstrual irregularity have increased musculoskeletal injuries. *Med Sci Sports Exerc.* 1986;18:374-379.

136. Marcus M, Cann C, Madvis P, et al. Menstrual function and bone mass in elite women runners. *Ann Intern Med.* 1985;102:158-168.

137. Kadel NJ, Tietz CC, Kronmal RA. Stress fractures in ballet dancers. *Am J Sports Med.* 1992;20:445-449.

138. Baker ER. Menstrual dysfunction and hormonal status in athletic women: A review. *Fertil Steril.* 1981;36:325-328.

139. Feicht CB, Johnson TS, Martin BJ, Wagner WW. Secondary amenorrhea in athletes. *Lancet.* 1978; 2:1145-1146.

140. American College of Sports Medicine. Position statement on proper and improper weight loss programs. *Med Sci Sports Exerc.* 1983;15:ix-xiii.

141. Frisch RE, McArthur JW. Menstrual cycles: Fatness as a determinant of minimum weight for height necessary for their maintenance of onset. *Science.* 1974; 185:949-951.

142. Nelson ME, Fiatarone MA, Morganti CM, et al. Effects of high-intensity strength training on multiple risk factors for osteoporotic fractures. A randomized controlled trial. *JAMA.* 1994;272:1909-1914.

143. McDonald R, Keen C. Iron, zinc, and magnesium nutrition and athletic performance. *Sports Med.* 1988;5:171-184.

144. Edgerton V, Ohira Y, Hettiarachchi J, et al. Elevation of hemoglobin and work tolerance in iron-deficient subjects. *J Nutr Sci Vitaminology.* 1981;27:77-86.

145. Anderson H, Barkve H. Iron deficiency and muscular work performance: An evaluation of cardio-respiratory function of iron deficient subjects with and without anemia. *Scand J Lab Invest.* 1970;25(suppl 144):1-39.

146. Siegel A, Hennekens C, Solomon H, Van Boeckel B. Exercise-related hematuria: Findings in a group of marathon runners. *JAMA.* 1979;241:391.

147. Stewart J, Alhquist D, McGill D, et al. Gastrointestinal blood losses and anemia in runners. *Ann Int Med.* 1984;100:843.

148. Pate R, Miller B, Davis J, et al. Iron status of female runners. *Int J Sports Nutr.* 1993;3:222-231.

149. Newhouse IJ, Clement DB. Iron status in athletes. *Sports Med.* 1988;5:337-352.

150. Fogelholm M. Indicators of vitamin and mineral status in athletes' blood: A review. *Int J Sports Nutr.* 1995; 5:267-284.

151. Clarkson PM. Antioxidants and physical performance. *Crit Rev Food Sci Nutr.* 1995;35:131-141.

152. Kanter MM, Nolte LA, Holloszy JO. Effects of an antioxidant vitamin mixture on lipid peroxidation at rest and postexercise. *J Appl Physiol.* 1993;74:965-969.

153. Meydani M, Evans WJ, Handelman G, et al. Protective effect of vitamin E on exercise-induced oxidative damage in young and older adults. *Am J Physiol.* 1993; 264:R992-R998.

154. Peters EM, Goetzsche, Grobbelaar B, Noakes TD. Vitamin C supplementation reduces the incidence of postrace symptoms of upper-respiratory-tract infection in ultramarathon runners. *Am J Clin Nutr.* 1993;57: 170-174.

155. Levine M, Dhariwal KR, Welch RW, et al. Determination of optimal vitamin C requirements in humans. *Am J Clin Nutr.* 1995;62 (suppl 6):1347S-1365S. Review.

156. Food and Nutrition Board. *Recommended Dietary Allowances.* 10th ed. Washington, DC: National Academy of Sciences; 1989.

157. Senay LC Jr. Temperature regulation and hypohydration: A singular view. *J Appl Physiol.* 1979;47:1-7.

158. Food and Nutrition Board, Institute of Medicine. *Fluid Replacement and Heat Stress.* Washington, DC: National Academy Press; 1994:86.

159. Food and Nutrition Board, Institute of Medicine. *Nutritional Needs in Hot Environments.* Washington, DC: National Academy Press; 1993:90-92.

160. Mahan LK, Arlin MT, eds. *Krause's Food, Nutrition, and Diet Therapy.* 8th ed. Philadelphia: Saunders; 1992:348.

161. Sawka MN, Young AJ, Latzka WA, et al. Human tolerance to heat strain during exercise: Influence of hydration. *J Appl Physiol.* 1992;73:368-375.

162. Position of the American Dietetic Association and the Canadian Dietetic Association: Nutrition for physical fitness and athletic performance for adults. *J Am Diet Assoc.* 1993;93:691-696.

163. Food and Nutrition Board, Institute of Medicine. *Nutritional Needs in Hot Environments.* Washington, DC: National Academy Press; 1993:90-92.

164. Food and Nutrition Board, Institute of Medicine. *Nutritional Needs in Hot Environments.* Washington, DC: National Academy Press; 1993:90-92.

165. Williams MH. *Nutrition for Fitness and Sport.* 3rd ed. Dubuque: Brown; 1992.

166. Ladell WSS. Water and salt (sodium chloride) intakes. In: Edholm O, Bacharach A, eds. *The Physiology of Human Survival.* New York: Academic Press; 1965.

167. Fortney SM, Nadel ER, Wenger CB, Bove JR. Effect of acute alteration of blood volume on circulatory performance in humans. *J Appl Physiol.* 1981;50:292-298.

168. Fortney SM, Nadel ER, Wenger CB, Bove JR. Effect of blood volume on sweating rate and body fluids in exercising humans. *J Appl Physiol.* 1981;51:1594-1600.

169. Fortney SM, Wenger CB, Bove JR, Nadel ER. Effect of blood volume on forearm venous and cardiac stroke volume during exercise. *J Appl Physiol.* 1983;55:884-890.

170. Nadel ER. Body fluid and electrolyte balance during exercise: Competing demands with temperature regulation. In: Hales JRS, ed. *Thermal Physiology.* New York: Raven; 1984.

171. Tipton CM. Consequences of rapid weight loss. In: Haskell W, Scala J, Whitman J, eds. *Nutrition and Athletic Performance.* Palo Alto: Bull;1982:176-199.

172. Ahlman V, Karoven M. Weight reduction by sweating in wrestlers and its effect on physical fitness. *J Sports Med Phys Fit.* 1962;7:58.

173. Costill DL, Saltin B. Factors limiting gastric emptying during rest and exercise. *J Appl Physiol.* 1974;37:679.

174. Coyle EF, Montain SJ. Benefits of fluid replacement with carbohydrate during exercise. *Med Sci Sports Exerc.* 1992;24(suppl 9):S324-S330.

175. Position of the American Dietetic Association and the Canadian Dietetic Association: Nutrition for physical fitness and athletic performance for adults. *J Am Diet Assoc.* 1993;93:691-696.

176. Food and Nutrition Board, Institute of Medicine. *Food Components to Enhance Performance.* Washington, DC: National Academy Press: 1992:49-50.

177. Ensminger AH, ed. *Foods and Nutrition Encyclopedia.* Clovis, CA: Pegus; 1983.

178. Williams MH. Nutritional ergogenics: Help or hype? *J Am Diet Assoc.* 1992;92:1213-1214.

179. Zulani U, Bonetti A, Compana M, et al. The influence of ubiquinone (CoQ10) on the metabolic response to work. *J Sports Med Phys Fit.* 1989;29:57-62.

180. Guthrie S. Prevalence of eating disorders among intercollegiate athletes: Contributing factors and preventative measures. In: Black D, ed. *Eating Disorders Among Athletes.* Reston, VA: American Alliance for Health Physical Education and Dance; 1991.

181. Weight L, Noakes T. Is running an analog of anorexia? A survey of the incidence of eating disorders in female distance runners. *Med Sci Sports Exerc.* 1987;19:213-217.

182. Burkes-Miller M, Black D. Male and female college athletes: Prevalence of anorexia nervosa and bulimia nervosa. *Athletic Train.* 1988;23:137-140.

183. Kirkley B. Bulimia: Clinical characteristics, development and etiology. *J Am Diet Assoc.* 1986;86:468-475.

APPENDIX 2–1. SAMPLE MEAL PLANS FOR TWO COMPETITIVE ATHLETES

Athlete 1: 25-year-old male, 5′9″, 145 lb (66 kg), competing in an endurance triathlon in September on the East Coast. Air temperature 55–70°F over 11 hours (7 AM–6 PM), water temperature (ocean) 69°F, high humidity, light wind.

Precompetition Day:

Training: rest day—easy 20-minute swim and stretching. Diet: 2300 kcal (35 kcal/kg), 65% carbohydrate (375 g, 7 g/kg), 15% protein (86 g, 1.3 g/kg), 20% fat (51 g). Total fluid intake = 2.5 L.

Breakfast:
1 bowl cereal with milk
Banana
1 English muffin with jam
2 C coffee with milk
8 oz juice

Lunch:
Ham and cheese sandwich with mustard
1 oz potato chips
8 oz fruit yogurt
12 oz juice

Snack:
16 oz water
1 1/2 oz pretzels
Apple

Supper:
2 C pasta with meat sauce
1 piece garlic bread
16 oz water
Popsicle

Competition Day:

2.5-mile swim, 112-mile bike, 26.2-km run. Diet: 4600 kcal (70 kcal/kg), 62% carbohydrate (700 g, 10 g/kg), 10% protein (115 g, 1.7 g/kg), 28% fat. Total fluid intake = 8 L.

Breakfast (3 hours prior to competition):
1 bagel with jam
Banana
2 C coffee with milk
8 oz juice

Snack/fluid intake (30 minutes prior to race):
32 oz Gatorade or other carbohydrate sports beverage

Snacks/fluid intake (after the swim about 1 hour into race):
(16 oz Gatorade or other carbohydrate sports beverage per hour over 7-hour bike = 3.5 L (4 large water bottles), plus 2 sports bars and 1 gel pack.
16 oz Gatorade or other carbohydrate sports beverage per hour over 3-hour run = 1.5 L.

Snack/fluid intake (30 minutes after race):
16 oz water
8 oz yogurt
12 oz juice

Supper (post race):
1/2 large cheese pizza
1 C ice cream
16 oz water

Postcompetition Day (similar to regular training day):

Training: 3 hours or varied run/bike and/or swim. Diet: 3300 kcal (50 kcal/kg), 65% carbohydrate (536 g, 8 g/kg), 15% protein (124 g, 1.8 g/kg), 20% fat (73 g).

Breakfast:
1 bowl cereal with milk
Banana
Bagel with jam
8 oz juice
1 C coffee with milk

Snack:
1 muffin
1 C coffee with milk

Lunch:
Turkey sandwich with low-fat mayonnaise
1 bag lite popcorn
8 oz fruit yogurt
12 oz juice

Snack:
1 apple
4 cookies
1 C milk

Supper:
2 C rice
6 oz. baked chicken
1 C carrots
1 C broccoli
1 Tbs margarine
12 oz juice or soda

Athlete 2: 40-year-old female, 5′2″, 108 lb (49 kg), competing in a half-marathon in the spring on the East Coast. Air temperature 45–50°F over race time (9 AM–10:45 AM), low humidity, light wind.

Precompetition Day:

Training: rest day—stretching. Diet: 1650 kcal (34 kcal/kg), 65% carbohydrate (270 g, 6 g/kg), 15% protein (60 g, 1.2 g/kg), 20% fat (36 g). Total fluid intake-2 L.

Breakfast:
English muffin with jam
8 oz juice
2 C coffee with milk

Lunch:
2 C pasta salad
pear
16 oz water

Snack:
12 wheat crackers
8 oz fruit yogurt
20 oz diet soda

Supper:
1 C skim milk
6 oz baked fish with bread crumbs
1 large baked potato with sour cream
1/2 C green beans
2 tsp margarine
2 rolls

Competition Day:

13.1 mile run. Diet: 2450 kcal (50 kcal/kg), 65% carbohydrate (398 g, 8 g/kg), 12% protein (74 g, 1.5 g/kg), 23% fat (63 g). Total fluid intake-3.5 L.

Breakfast:
English muffin with jam
1 bowl cereal with skim milk
2 Tbs raisins
8 oz juice
2 C coffee with milk

Snack/fluid intake (30 minutes prior to race):
16 oz Gatorade or other carbohydrate sports drink

Snack/fluid intake (during race)
32 oz Gatorade (1 L)

Snack/fluid intake (30 minutes postrace)
8 oz fruit yogurt
Banana
1/2 bagel
16 oz water

Supper:
2 pieces vegetable lasagna
2 rolls
Salad with 2 Tbs dressing
16 oz water

Postcompetition Day (similar to regular training day):

Training: 1 1/2 hours running and or weight training. Diet: 2000 kcal (40 kcal/kg), 65% carbohydrates (325 g, 7 g/kg), 15% protein (75 g, 1.5 g/kg), 20% fat (44 g). Total fluid intake 2 L.

Breakfast:
1 bowl cereal with skim milk
1 C strawberries
1/2 bagel with jam
8 oz juice
2 C coffee

Lunch:
Salad with 2 Tbs lite dressing, 1 oz cheese, 1/2 C beans
2 oz pita bread
2 low-fat cookies
16 oz water

Snack:
8 oz fruit yogurt
Apple
3/4 oz pretzels

Supper:
1 C skim milk
3 oz chicken stir fried in 1 Tbs oil and soy sauce
1 1/3 C rice
1/2 red pepper
1 C broccoli

Chapter 3

Roles of the Primary Care Physician, Coach, and Athlete in Rehabilitation

Primary Care Team Physician

Margot Putukian

The role of the primary care team physician in the care and rehabilitation of athletes is an exciting and challenging one. There are many individuals who contribute to the success of the athlete, including foremost the athlete himself or herself. Outside of the athlete there are parents, coaches, athletic trainers, physical therapists, strength and conditioning specialists, nutritionists, primary care physicians, and other consulting physicians. There can also be support to the athlete from school administrators and professional organizations. The challenge to the primary care team physician is to interact with many of these individuals in the common goal to provide quality medical care to the athlete.

The day is long gone that being the "team doc" meant showing up 15 minutes prior to kick-off and taking care of acute injuries, then washing up and saying good-bye until the next week. Not only do team physicians take care of more than just acute football injuries, but the extent and depth of their interaction with many athletes is much more complex. Because of this, the team physician must have a broad depth of understanding of numerous medical problems and the effect of exercise and athletic competition on these problems. The primary care team physician must have thorough train-

ing and excellent physical examination skills of the musculoskeletal system, as well as other systems of the body. Primary care sports medicine is an exciting new field that has only scratched the surface of many medical issues that pertain to exercising individuals.

RESPONSIBILITIES OF THE TEAM PHYSICIAN

There are numerous responsibilities that the team physician has to assume in order to be effective. These include medical supervision (supervision, injury prevention, evaluation of physical status, and management of medical needs), administrative functions, communication, and education of the athlete, coach, family, and sports medicine team. This education is crucial for the ongoing growth and development of sports medicine. It is important for the team physician to establish a general plan of care for the athlete and establish guidelines for the athletic trainer and physical therapist. The coordination of medical supervision and communication with the athletic trainers, paramedics, and visiting teams during competition are a critical responsibility of the team physician.

Emerging Responsibilities

In the past few decades, there has been new challenges facing those that provide medical care to athletes. There are many medical questions that must be answered. Among them are when is it safe for a wrestler with herpes to return to wrestling practice, evaluation of the the risks of competing with a viral illness, asthma, ulcerative colitis, or multiple sclerosis, and the safety of a gymnast or swimmer with anorexia nervosa. Further questions include the risk for HIV transmission during boxing, soccer, or tennis, evaluation of brain injury following concussions, and the safety of the athlete with acute infectious mononucleosis returning to soccer or golf. How these medical problems affect sports participation, and how these particular exercise activities themselves affect the disease process are found in current literature. The suggested reading list for this chapter addresses these issues.

These are some of the recent questions being asked of the sports medicine team. Not only is it important to address musculoskeletal injuries and rehabilitation, but there are many other areas of the athlete that relate to their overall health.

Musculoskeletal Focus

Musculoskeletal sports medicine is progressing with the application of orthopedic surgery, athletic training, physical therapy, and strength and conditioning, resulting in a rapidly developing competitive athlete. The usefulness of isokinetic testing, range-of-motion measurements, gait and motion analysis, and functional testing performed by members of the sports medicine team is critical in the decisions surrounding an athlete's progress and return to activity. The information provided by athletic trainers, physical therapists, and strength and conditioning specialists is often instrumental in these return to play decisions, demonstrating the importance of communication. More work lies ahead in answering sports medicine related issues that can bring an injured athlete back to activity in a safe and timely manner.

The primary care team physician's role often starts with the preparticipation physical examination. The depth of the examination will vary depending on the age and gender of the individual as well as the proposed activity. The preparticipation physical examination should screen for problems that preclude activity, such as underlying cardiovascular or neurologic abnormalities, ligamentous instability or other musculoskeletal abnormalities, organomegaly, or any acute medical illness. It should also assess for an injury that has not been properly rehabilitated, and for strength or flexibility deficits that might put an individual at increased risk for injury. In the female athlete, the preparticipation physical examination should also screen for menstrual dysfunction, prior stress fractures, and those at risk for eating disorders, together known as the female athlete triad. Finally, the preparticipation physical examination is for many young athletes an introduction to the health care system. It also gives the physician an opportunity to address concerns such as recreational and performance enhancing substance use, sexuality issues, depression and emotional issues, and other health promotional activities such as wearing seatbelts, helmets, and performing the self-breast and self-testicular exams. The preparticipation physical examination is the initial screening process that is very important. Although it may appear to be straightforward and simple, it requires considerable attention and can reveal valuable information.

It is important for the primary care team physician to integrate with participants and be the focal person to those involved in the care of the athlete. In this way, there is one "captain of the ship," which ultimately makes a consistent plan possible. Often, an athlete will become confused and ultimately lose faith in the medical team if he or she is receiving varied information and terminology from different health care providers without integration. Ideally, the primary care team physician is able to communicate and impart cooperation among all members of the health care team. It is important for the consulted health care provider to understand what his or her role is. In many situations, the primary care physician can speak directly to another health care provider, or in written form ask the provider to contact them once the athlete is evaluated so that necessary decisions can be made. In some situations, the primary care team physician may ask the consulting individual to evaluate and treat, and in others may ask for the consultant to evaluate only and hold off treatment. Finally, the same applies in terms of return to play decisions. This decision lies primarily with the team physician. In many situations, the treatment will depend on the expertise of the consulting physician or health care provider, and in that situation, the team physician can rely on the consulting expert to take over as principal decision maker. For example, if surgery is required, the orthopedic surgeon may ultimately make decisions regarding rehabilitation as well as return to play decisions. If the physical therapist or athletic trainer provides extensive care, they may be the best individual to guide and progress treatment and provide essential input to the physician regarding return to play decisions. Primary care team physicians need to use great caution in knowing their own limits, and use the expertise around them as needed for the best overall outcome for the athlete. Ultimately, it is imperative for communication to occur at every level. If communication *fails*, ultimately the medical team *fails* to provide excellent care, and in the end, the athlete loses.

Early referral to the team physician can allow for early diagnosis, further diagnostic testing, medication, and initiation of rehabilitation and referral to physical therapy if indicated. If a consulting physician, such as an orthopedic surgeon, cardiologist, or neurologist becomes involved, it is important for the team physician to get the necessary information sent to the consulting physician, and attempt to expedite the visit. It is also important to remember that the physician–patient relationship holds in this athletic setting as well, and that release of information should be discussed first with the athlete (and parents if the patient is under age 18). Maintaining this professional confidentiality extends to all those involved in the medical care of the athlete, and can create some difficulty, especially for the high-profile athlete. In addition, it is at times difficult for the physician, who at times is a personal physician and at others is the team physician. If the physician remembers to keep the athlete's care and welfare as the primary concern, this usually avoids any problems.

In this most ideal setting, the athlete excels and is able to return to the activity as safely and quickly as possible. Hopefully, athletes also learn something about the potential risk factors they had for their injury. They can work on methods of training, strengthening and conditioning, or in some other way come away with something more than they expected when they were first injured. This will improve their confidence and possibly enhance their performance in a safe and healthy manner.

Being an effective primary care team physician is a tremendous responsibility. The knowledge base required is broad, and the need to communicate with others involved in the care and performance of athletes is paramount. The application of medicine to sport as well as the effect of exercise on medical problems present issues that are exciting. Understanding the role and responsibilities of the team physician, integrating the sports medicine team, and providing quality medical care to the athlete is the challenge that faces the primary care team physician. It is a challenge well worth accepting.

SUGGESTED READING LIST

American Academy of Pediatrics Committee on Sports Medicine and Fitness. Medical conditions affecting sports participation. *Pediatrics.* 1994;94:757-760.

American Medical Society for Sports Medicine, American Academy of Sports Medicine, and American Orthopedic Society for Sports Medicine. Human immunodeficiency virus and other blood-borne pathogens in sports. *Clin J Sport Med.* 1995;5:199-204.

Andrews JR, Kupferman SP, Dillman CJ. Labral tears in throwing and racquet sports. *Clin Sports Med.* 1991;10:901-911.

Berquist TH, ed. *Imaging of Orthopedic Trauma.* 2nd ed. New York: Raven; 1992.

Cantu RC, Voy R. Second impact syndrome: A risk in any contact sport. *Phys Sports Med.* 1995;23:27-34.

Clancy WG, Ray JM, Zoltan DJ. Acute tears of the anterior cruciate ligament. Surgical versus conservative treatment. *J Bone Joint Surg.* 1988;70A:1483-1488.

Colorado Medical Society. Report of the Sports Medicine Committee: *Guidelines for the Management of Concussion in Sports,* revised. Denver: Colorado Medical Society; 1991.

Coyle EF, Montain SJ. Benefits of fluid replacement with carbohydrate during exercise. *Med Sci Sport Exerc.* 1992;24: S324-S330.

DeLee JC, Drez D. *Orthopedic Sports Medicine; Principles and Practice.* Philadelphia: Saunders; 1994.

Drinkwater B, Nilson K, Chestnut C, et al. Bone mineral content of amenorrheic and eumenorrheic athletes. *N Engl J Med.* 1984;311:277-280.

Eichner ER. Infection, immunity, and exercise. *Phys Sports Med.* 1993;21:125-135.

Eichner ER. Sickle cell trait, heroic exercise, and fatal collapse. *Phys Sports Med.* 1993;21:51-64.

Kannus P, Bergfeld J, Jarvinen M, et al. Injuries to the posterior cruciate ligament of the knee. *Sports Med.* 1991;12:110-131.

Kobayashi RH, Mellion MB. Exercise-induced asthma, anaphylaxis, and urticaria. *Sports Med Prim Care.* 1991;18:809-831.

Magnes SA, Henderson JM, Hunter SC. What conditions limit sports participation? Experience with 10,540 athletes. *Phys Sports Med.* 1992;20:143-160.

Maron B, Epstein S, Roberts W. Causes of sudden death in competitive athletes. *J Am Coll Cardiol.* 1986;7:204-214.

McKeag DB, Hough DO, Zemper ED, eds. *Primary Care Sports Medicine.* Dubuque, IA: Brown & Benchmark; 1993.

Micheli LJ, ed. Injuries in the young athlete. *Clin Sports Med.* 1988;7:513.

Puffer JC, ed. Medical problems. *Clin Sports Med.* 1992; 11:259-487.

Putukian M. The athletic woman. In Mellion MB, ed. *Office Management of Sports Injuries and Athletic Problems.* St. Louis: Hanley & Belfus; 1994.

Putukian M. The female triad: Eating disorders, amenorrhea, and osteoporosis. *Med Clin North Am.* 1994;78:345-356.

Putukian M, McKeag DM, Buschbacher RM, Braddom RL, eds. The prepartcipation physical examination. In: *Sports Medicine and Rehabilitation: A Sport-specific Approach.* St Louis: Mosby; 1994.

Rosen LW, McKeag DB, Hough D, et al. Pathogenic weight control behavior in female athletes. *Phys Sports Med.* 1986;14:79.

Shelbourne KD, Nitz P. Accelerated rehabilitation after anterior cruciate ligament reconstruction. *Am J Sports Med.* 1990; 18:292-299.

Shelbourne KD, Whitaker HJ, McCarroll JR, et al. Anterior cruciate ligament injury: Evaluation of intraarticular reconstruction of acute tears without repair. *Am J Sports Med.* 1990;18:484-489.

Silliman JF, Hawkins RJ. Classification and physical diagnosis of instability of the shoulder. *Clin Orthop.* 1993;291:7-19.

Smith DM, Lombardo JA, Robinson JB. The preparticipation evaluation. *Primary Care*. 1991;18:777-807.

Torg JS, Glasgow SG. Criteria for return to contact activities following cervical spine injury. *Clin J Sports Med*. 1991;1:12-26.

Torg JS, Sennett B, Vegso JJ, Pavlov H. Axial loading injuries to the middle cervical spine segment: An analysis and classification of twenty-five cases. *Am J Sports Med*. 1991; 19:6-20.

Twenty-sixth Bethesda Conference. Recommendations for determining eligibility for competition in athletes with cardiovascular abnormalities. *Med Sci Sports Exerc*. 1994;26 (suppl 10):S223-S283. Published erratum appears in *Med Sci Sports Exerc*. 1994;26: following table of contents; also in *J Am Coll Cardiol*. 1994;24:845-899.

Williams MH. Ergogenic and ergolytic substances. *Med Sci Sports Exerc*. 1992;24:S344-S348.

Yeager KK, Agostini R, Nattiv A, Drinkwater B. The female athlete triad: Disordered eating, amenorrhea, osteoporosis. *Med Sci Sports Exerc*. 1993;25:775.

Zehender M, Meinertz T, Keul J, Just H. ECG variants and cardiac arrhythmia in athletes: Clinical relevance and prognostic importance. *Am Heart J*. 1990;119:1378-1391.

Zeppilli P. The athlete's heart: Differentiation of training effects from organic heart disease. *Pract Cardiol*. 1988;14:61-84.

A Coach and Athlete's Perspective

Becca Main

The relationship between a coach and an athlete involves a system of separate, but associate relations. When an athlete sustains an injury a triangle forms involving the athlete, the coach, and the sports medicine staff. In some situations the injury remains unclear and sometimes contrasting opinions form. Often the simple solution to mend the wavering lines is communication. Communication in its full definition also includes compromise and acknowledgment of what is best for the athlete's future. The future of the athlete is often overlooked for the seemingly more pending question of how soon the athlete can return to competition.

Ultimately, the coach's job is to develop the athlete's skills, tactics, and sport sense so that the athlete can compete with confidence and success at his or her highest possible level. Once an injury enters the picture, the medical team begins to diagnose and dictate the guidelines for the rehabilitation of the athlete and eventually attempts to clear the athlete for performance. Sometimes, communication barriers develop even in the early stages of an athlete's injury in making the diagnosis. Upon completion of the medical staff's evaluation of an injury, and sometimes before the tests and x-rays are performed, the coach has already looked into the team's future and questions the medical staff on the athlete's return to practice and competition. Here, the athlete and the coach need to acknowledge that the medical staff has one main goal in mind, successful and complete rehabilitation of the athlete.

More often than not, an athlete who does not complete the rehabilitation protocol does so because of two factors, time and pain. Once an athlete realizes that range-of-motion exercises and treatment will take up more time in their already busy day, they tend to cut short the rehabilitation sessions and ultimately delay the process. Many athletes tell their physical therapist or athletic trainer that they will continue stretching and exercising at home, but often they do not. The time factor also will vary from athlete to athlete depending on the commitment to rehabilitation. Some athletes believe in the "leave it alone and it will heal" type of therapy, and often these types of ideas hinder the healing process in far greater ways than any outside influences. With the elite and competitively successful athlete, hard work and determination has helped them to reach the higher level and this will usually filter into the rehabilitation process. It is important to acknowledge what type of commitment the athlete seems to be giving in order to devise the protocol and time frame for return to play.

Pain level is probably what dictates the commitment to therapy sessions. Once an athlete is relieved of pain and is close to normal range of motion, they usually feel ready to graduate and move back exclusively to the playing field. This is far from the end of their therapy sessions. In order to prepare athletes mentally to compete again, the most important part of the therapy is still to come, strengthening the injured part and surrounding area. The strengthening phase can prevent injuries from occurring repeatedly and will also offer the athlete the best possible scenario to return to action. The medical team must communicate to the athletes the importance of continued treatments and strengthening exercises.

The most difficult situations that arise within the triangle of athlete, coach, and sports medicine staff are most often the less severe injuries (those that do not require a cast or surgery). Acute, more serious, injuries usually render the athlete fairly stable and the protocol is more defined. This is because the athlete usually receives prompt and thorough care. Often, it is conflicting opinions among the medical team regarding treatment for the undefined injuries that can delay the healing process. Injuries such as ankle sprains, IT band strains, shin splints, tendonitis, bruised muscles, and other less serious injuries are the most difficult to deal with as an athlete and a coach. In these undefined case scenarios, conflicting medical opinions may lead an athlete towards a more emotional response.

To define the problem areas, it is best to evaluate a successful interaction between an athlete, coach, and sports medicine staff. To be most effective as a coach and a medical team, it is important to be honest and evaluate each athlete as a separate case. This aspect is further complicated by the type of athlete who is injured in terms of role on the team, level of experience, and likelihood of an available replacement player. The coach runs these thoughts through his or her mind in the flash of a second, because most coaches will treat their athletes differently depending on the athlete's importance to the team. It is very difficult to separate these thoughts as a coach and to understand that the "benchwarmer" may ultimately become your "star." As a head coach involved in an athlete's recovery process, you have encounters with pivotal players more often than the first-year walk-on. This reasoning is based solely on the coaches need for certain players. By treating each athlete separately, the athlete will not fall into any preconceived ideas and protocols. The medical team needs to understand the coach's level of concern to return the athlete to the playing field.

The coach must be included in the rehabilitation process from the start. The more often the coach is updated, the better. In most cases, updates will come from the athletic trainers and on occasion, a physical therapist is utilized to assist the patient. This athletic trainer–physical therapist relationship is *crucial* in providing appropriate and complimentary care. In fact, consistent communication to the coach will help to heal problems that may occur later on the road to recovery. The less the coach has to look for answers, the better the coach will feel about the rehabilitation of the athlete. In successful cases, part of the rehabilitation process takes place in the presence of the coach at practice. The coach will be able to actually see the process and will feel comfort in knowing that the athlete is progressing. Whether it involves jogging, stationary bicycling, strengthening, or even the athlete watching practice, the coach sees the active progression of the athlete. Some coaches want an athlete to return to the sport only if fully recovered, so that the progress of the rest of the team is not hampered by an athlete who may only be able to perform at 50 percent of normal capacity. Coaches must understand the importance of a gradual return to action for the overall psyche of the athlete. The gradual return to play will help the athlete return to full competition potential by helping the mental progression of the player.

Athletes often struggle with the fear of reinjury, of never getting back to their original form, and of letting their coach and team down with subnormal play.

If the communication avenues are open throughout the rehabilitation process, then the time in which the athlete returns to competition will not only be efficient but can be with minimal controversy. The serious conflict will seldom be derived from the athlete's desire to compete; this is deemed a positive attribute for an athlete. Real conflict arrives when a specific time frame is demanded by the coach and athlete. Instead of utilizing a time frame as the guidelines of a protocol, an athletic trainer or physical therapist may feel it clouds the overall rehabilitation process and, unfortunately, the vision of the athlete and coach.

While being definite and precise in the calculation of the athlete's return to competition may seem the best process, leaving the doors open for the healing and strengthening of the athlete proves most advantageous in the future for the athlete. By giving the coach and athlete a large time frame for the healing process, the medical staff can monitor the rehabilitation and adjust the window accordingly. In the long run, most recoveries will occur well within the large frame of time and the medical staff appears successful in the eyes of the coach and athlete.

Many factors ultimately influence the successful and complete recovery of an injured athlete. Communication may be the most important factor to contribute to the efficient and most complete rehabilitation. As the medical team progresses with an athlete throughout the many stages of therapy, the athlete and coach need to be updated so that the triangle of communication maintains a steady constant.

Chapter 4

Physiologic Basis for Strength Training in the Prevention of and Rehabilitation from Injury

William J. Kraemer, Noel D. Duncan, and Fred S. Harman

Musculoskeletal injury or damage is a phenomena that most individuals experience at some point in their lives. Irrespective of the cause of injury, it is of critical importance to employ treatment methods that enhance the recovery of the injury to, or as close to preinjury levels as is functionally possible and protect the injured site from future damage. Numerous treatment methods aim to achieve this; however, a modality that is often dismissed but that has significant potential to prevent and rehabilitate musculoskeletal injury, is resistance or strength training.[1] Resistance exercise training increases the size and strength of bone, skeletal muscle, and connective tissue.[2-4] This type of training also modifies body shape, increases range of movement, improves posture, attenuates age-related sarcopenia, and protects vital organs. These positive adaptations will assist in minimizing the incidence of musculoskeletal injury, expedite injury rehabilitation, and reduce the possibility of future injury.

This chapter focuses on the cellular mechanisms associated with skeletal muscle damage in addition to discussing practical exercise principles that can be employed to enhance injury recovery and minimize the incidence of musculoskeletal damage.

RESISTANCE TRAINING AND INJURY

In comparison to other physical activities (football, downhill skiing, basketball), the incidence of injury resulting from resistance exercise training is negligible. The weight room injury rate in college football players is estimated at 0.13 injuries per 1000 athletic exposures or 0.35 per 100 players per season.[5] As a result, weight room injuries accounted for only 0.74 percent of the total reported time lost due to injury during the football season. Because correct technique is paramount to the success of all resistance training programs, the authors speculated that this injury rate could be reduced even further if more rigorous attention was paid to correct technical procedures in the weight room.[5] When weight training is performed with precise technical application—ensuring the completion of the exercise through the full range of motion, adequate spotting, and strict breathing techniques—even movements using heavy loads are relatively safe.[6]

Resistance training can be successfully employed to reduce the incidence of muscle injury. Individually designed resistance training programs have been shown to minimize musculoskeletal injuries in tennis players[7] and swimmers.[8] Athletes in these sports reported a lower injury rate when resistance training was incorporated into their training programs, compared to athletes who did not. These findings indicate that resistance training is a useful exercise modality for offsetting or attenuating the incidence of injury and beneficial if incorporated into training designs of similar sporting programs.

The exact mechanisms responsible for reducing muscle injury have not been identified; however, the increases in size and strength of bone, muscle, and connective tissue that occur concomitantly with resistance training are expected to contribute largely to this phenomenon. At the cellular level, resistance training increases the collagen content of skeletal muscle.[1] Collagen is the major component of the epimysium, which surrounds the entire muscle; it envelops the fascicles; and of the endomysium, which encloses the individual muscle fiber. This connective tissue is responsible for maintaining the integrity of the muscle and increasing the thickness of these sheath, increasing the strength of the framework that supports overloaded skeletal muscle. This cellular response is expected to contribute to reducing or offsetting musculoskeletal damage.

Many injuries result from the breakdown of bone and connective tissue (tendons and ligaments). Evaluation of these regions with CT scans indicate hamstring strains often occur at the myotendinous junction, which is susceptible to strain-induced muscle injury.[9] Connective tissue responds to resistance training with increases in metabolism, thickness, weight, and strength.[10,11] This form of training may be effective in reducing musculoskeletal damage at this level. In addition to aiding the prevention of injury, investigations employing animal models indicate that the recovery of damaged ligaments is also enhanced if physical activity is performed during the rehabilitation period.[10,11] Exercise training with resistance also increases the structural integrity of bony tissue and can minimize the incidence of injury at this structural level.[1] As a result of these positive adaptations, resistance training and other forms of weight-bearing exercise should be incorporated into exercise training and rehabilitation programs to offset injury and facilitate recovery.

Major skeletal muscle imbalances between agonist and antagonist muscle groups (hamstring and quadriceps) may predispose an individual to musculoskeletal injury. These imbalances can be identified and corrected with well-designed exercise training programs.[12,13] As a result, it is recommended that all athletes be physiologically screened to identify such musculoskeletal imbalances so that they can be corrected to attenuate imbalance-related injuries.[1]

Not only will muscle imbalances within a limb predispose an athlete to injury, but major imbalances between limbs can also be potentially harmful. While it is natural for one arm or leg to be stronger than the other,

individualized exercise programming involving the use of unilateral exercises can reduce major variations in strength observed. If differences in strength between limbs do exist, they should be less than 10 percent. Unilateral exercises such as the lunge, single-legged knee extensions, and curls on a machine should be employed to allow the symmetrical development of muscle. If only double arm or leg (bilateral exercises) are used, the stronger limb can compensate for the weaker limb. This is especially true on most resistance training machines.

An optimal degree of flexibility is essential to ensure adequate range of movement. Reduced flexibility around a particular joint will minimize its range of movement.[14] A tight joint may also lead to muscle imbalances around a joint, predisposing this site to injury. An optimal degree of flexibility is recommended because overstretching could lead to muscle tendon injuries, dislocations, and subluxations.

MUSCULOSKELETAL INJURY AND DAMAGE

Injury Evaluation

The aim of rehabilitation is to restore function to, or as close to preinjury levels as is functionally possible. Although the commencement point of healing is molecular, it is the evaluation of the injury that leads to the application of therapies that will enhance healing. Skilled evaluation and treatment procedures will restore strength, size, and range of movement to the damaged site and minimize scarring and pain. Incorrect evaluations and subsequent treatment may result in excessive scarring, soft tissue adhesions, and continued pain. In addition to this, any reduction in function, range of motion, muscle size and strength, and the development of abnormal and compensatory movement patterns will predispose the individual to reinjury.

Several factors are employed to assess an injury. Initially, the severity of tissue degradation will determine the status of the injury. This involves assessing the level of inflammation, whether the injury is acute or chronic (overuse, cumulative trauma, or repetitive motion disorder), and functionality. In addition, the demands that will be placed on the tissue are established (athletic versus nonathletic workloads). The speed and effectiveness of the treatment process is also dependent upon the individual's willingness to assist the body's healing process. In a survey of athletes with knee or ankle injuries, participants who scored high on the use of goal setting, positive self-talk, and mental imagery during rehabilitation exhibited faster recoveries than athletes who scored low on these factors.[15]

Tissue Homeostasis

Tissues within the human body are capable of adapting to external stimuli. The cellular responses to these stimuli fall within a continuum that is bordered by cell death and immortality (cancer) and include atrophy (a decrease in cellular structure and function) and hypertrophy (an increase in cellular structure and function). Each of these adaptive responses contains a homeostatic state that is the maintenance of the cellular structure and function within a given stimulus. In order for an adaptive state to continue, the degree of stimulus exposure must be maintained. Whenever the exposure to physiologic external stimuli exceeds the cell's capacity to adapt, injury results. If the exposure is prolonged, irreversible injury occurs, leading to cell death. Importantly, recovery of a cell from injury can be enhanced by the methods of rehabilitation.

Cellular Damage Resulting in Cell Death

Although a number of mechanisms have been proposed detailing the cascade of events that occurs at the cellular level with muscle injury, an unequivocal process of events is yet to be identified. Reports from both animal and human investigations indicate the process begins with the initial injury decreasing the level of cellular oxygen via ischemia, resulting in hypoxia. The cell's aerobic respiration is significantly compromised and ATP generation is reduced. Oubain-sensitive ATPase activity is impaired in the cell membrane, resulting in the failure of the sodium-potassium pump. An accumulation of intracellular sodium and the diffusion of potassium to the cell's exterior causes an increase in intracellular water. Edema increases the chance of acute inflammation, which initiates (by an unknown mechanism) the production of arachidonic acid, which in turn synthesizes prostaglandins. Prostaglandins activate cellular pain nerve endings and these nerve cells generate substance P, which effectively activates mast cells in the cell cytosol to produce histamines. Histamines continue the cycle, resulting in the continued influx of water, and edema is maintained.

With a reduction in the cell's energy charge and a concomitant increase in intracellular adenosine monophosphate (AMP) concentration, phosphofructokinase is stimulated to produce ATP through anaerobic glycolysis from the cell's glycogen stores. Anaerobic glycolysis results in an increase in intracellular lactic acid and inorganic phosphates, which subsequently decreases intracellular pH. As hypoxia continues, there is detachment of ribosomes from the granular endoplasmic reticulum, and the dissociation of polysomes into monosomes results. With continued membrane permeability and diminished mitochondrial function, evaginations of the membrane appear extracellularly while myelin figures are seen intracellularly. Continued hypoxia will lead to irreversible cell damage that is evidenced by severe vacuolization of the mitochondria, plasma membrane disintegration, lysosomal swelling, intracellular influx of calcium, development of calcium-rich bodies in the mitochondria, loss of essential proteins, coenzymes, and ribonucleic acids, and accelerated leakage of metabolites. The continued decline in intracellular pH appears to be the stimulating factor for the activation of acid hydrolases and enzymatic digestion of cytoplasmic and nuclear components. At this juncture, cell death is imminent.

Skeletal Muscle Soreness

Two types of muscle soreness are commonly reported, acute and delayed-onset muscle soreness (DOMS). Acute soreness is apparent during the later stages of an exercise bout and during the immediate recovery period. This results from the accumulation of end products that occur with exercise, H^+ ions or lactate. This sensation generally disappears between 2 minutes and 1 hour after cessation of exercise.

Delayed-onset muscle soreness (DOMS) is evident after unaccustomed eccentric or lengthening muscle actions (see Fig. 4–1A & B). This soreness results from structural damage at the cell level that occurs essentially in the area of the Z disc and also an inflammatory response within the muscles. Soreness from these actions typically results from walking downhill, horse riding, or downhill skiing, and appears 24 to 56 hours after the exercise bout. Armstrong and colleagues have proposed a model identifying the cellular mechanisms responsible for the delayed onset of soreness.[16] Briefly, the cascade of events is thought to follow this structured sequence of events.

1. Lengthening muscle actions or muscle stretch disrupts the structural proteins within the muscle fibers, connective tissue, and sarcolemma. This alters the permeability of the cellular membrane.
2. Intracellular calcium ion infiltration results, impairing cellular respiration.
3. Ca^{2+} activates proteolytic and phospholipytic enzymes. This results in the degradation of membrane-bound phospholipids, Z discs, troponin, and tropomysin.
4. The inflammatory response that occurs as a result of cell damage occurs concomitantly with an increase in macrophages, mast cells, histocytes, and lysosomal proteases.
5. Histamines, kinins, and K^+ accumulate in the interstitial spaces. The resulting edema and increase in temperature stimulates nerve endings, culminating in the sensation of pain (DOMS).
6. Stress proteins protect the cell from further damage and regeneration begins. The stress proteins are thought responsible for future protection of the muscle with similar lengthening actions.

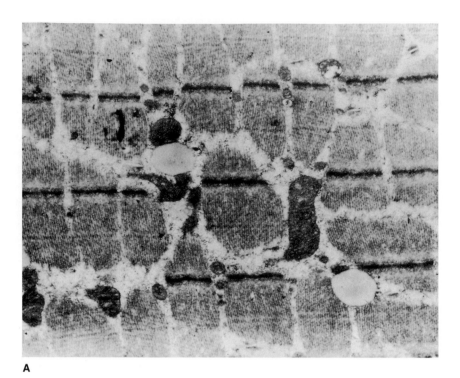

A

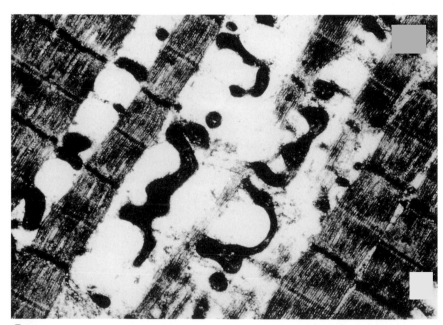

B

Figure 4–1. Ultrastructural changes in human vastus lateralis muscle that result from unaccustomed eccentric muscle actions. Pre **(A)** and post **(B)** muscle micrographs clearly display the damage that occurs to the individual sarcomere. (*Courtesy of William Kraemer, PhD [original work].*)

However, the protective mechanism is transient and will cease to have an effect if training is not continued.

Although unaccustomed eccentric muscle actions result in the damage process described, this type of muscle contraction is regularly employed by athletes to improve performance and overcome training barriers. Eccentric muscle actions permit the use of heavier weights and thus greater muscle tensions are evoked in comparison to concentric muscle contractions. This

increase in tension induces improvements in muscle strength and size. As a consequence of the damage and subsequent soreness that occurs concomitantly with eccentric exercise training, these muscle actions should be performed with a minimum of 7 to 10 days rest between exercise bouts. Typically each repetition is executed slowly (8 to 10 seconds) and loads in excess of 1 RM are used (110 to 120 percent 1 RM).

Gross indicators of skeletal muscle damage include soreness, mobility, and reduction in the level of force production. Cellular indicators of damage include the protein myoglobin (present in urine and indicative of severe crush injuries) and the enzymes creatine kinase (CK), lactate dehydrogenase (LDH), and aspartate trans-aminase. CK and LDH are the most commonly used indicators of skeletal muscle damage; however caution should be taken when using these enzymes as direct markers of muscle damage.

Cell Regeneration

Before the healing process can began, the stimuli responsible for the initial injury must be removed. Once this is achieved, the methods commonly used to aid muscle regeneration and restore functionality can be employed: cryotherapy, hydrotherapy, electrical stimulation such as electrical muscle stimulation, and massage.

The recovery process begins by minimizing the inflammatory response that occurs with tissue injury. Possibly the simplest and most effective method of achieving this, especially for acute inflammation, is cryotherapy. Ice applied to injury reduces the rate of damage by lowering the heat or energy expenditure of the injured tissue. Ice also limits the amount of secondary tissue hypoxia, inflammation, and cellular metabolism. The speed with which many of the resultant molecular and biochemical reactions occur is slowed as a consequence of the reduction in activation energy. During the repair and remodeling phase, numerous methods are employed to restore tissue functionality. Electrical stimulation, hydrotherapy, massage, and immunochemical therapies assist in bolstering the body's immune activity by increasing circulation and vascularization. The maturation phase of regeneration follows the inflammatory and then the repair and remodeling phases. During the maturation phase, resistance exercise protocols and specific activity movement patterns can be employed to enhance functionality and in some cases hypertrophy.

Once injured, skeletal muscle has the ability to regenerate and repair damaged tissue. Satellite cells are primarily responsible for this regenerative process, which is dependent upon the degree of damage to the basement membrane and the extent to which the blood vessel and nerve supply remains intact.[17] The regeneration process follows a structured sequence. As discussed, initial injury causes the disruption of the cellular structure. Mononuclear cells such as macrophages and T lymphocytes then infiltrate the tissue via the blood vessels. The basement membrane of the muscle cell acts as a guide for the myoblasts to redevelop and fuse to form new muscle fibers. The surviving satellite cells divide, mature into myoblasts, and form new myotubes within the muscle cell, and subsequent development follows the embryonic sequence.

In summary, effective treatment of an injury involves slowing and eventually stopping the rate of cellular injury during the inflammatory stage. In the second stage, the initiation and maintenance of physiologic processes occur that promote new fibroblast activity. This happens in the repair and remodeling stage. Finally, the maturation stage involves developing a matrix.

PRACTICAL REHABILITATION EXERCISE PROTOCOLS

Rehabilitation from injury involves the improvement of morphologic and performance characteristics of the neuromuscular system. In sports rehabilitation, the challenge is related to the ultimate requirement for effective and pain-free joint function and highly integrated multiple joint movement patterns. The basis for the optimal development of a strength training program is related to a needs analysis of the sport or activity. This involves a biomechanical and metabolic evaluation of the sport and a profile of the injury pattern.[18] The fundamental training principle that governs program choices is related to that of training specificity. Effective resistance training programs for both the prevention and rehabilitation of injury are based on this principle. In the case of injury rehabilitation, the exercise stimulus must effectively stimulate tissue remodeling and repair to promote adaptation and healing.

When designing a resistance exercise training program for rehabilitation purposes, the functional capabilities of an injured athlete should be assessed. Invariably, the functional capabilities of an injured athlete are lower than those of a healthy individual attempting to prevent injury (prehabilitation). Despite this, a similar set of principles of progression and program design features are utilized. The basis for the functional ability presented in normal joint function ranges from integrity of the cellular components through to the biomechanical function of joints. This requires the intact status of the biomolecular structures and physiologic function at the cellular level to the whole body's biomechanical function of the integrated patterns of joint movements in sports. With rehabilitation, it is essential that the program matches the injury and the eventual demands for function in the sport.

Developing a Basic Workout

All strength training programs begin with a basic workout design.[18] The variables that need to be considered in the development of a workout are the choice of exercise, order of exercises, number of sets, intensity of exercise, and amount of rest between sets and exercises.

To ensure continual adaptation to resistance exercise stimuli, some type of periodization cycle or program variation is employed.[19] This systematic variation of the strength training program variables (intensity of the exercise) should be applied universally. Without program variation, strength training programs will be boring and ineffective, resulting in a lack of enthusiasm and physical benefit as the individual may cease training.

1. *Choice of exercise*. Choose resistance exercises that activate the major muscle groups of the body and as discussed ensure each side of a joint is exercised (e.g., biceps and triceps of the arm). In addition, both upper (bench press) and lower body (squat) exercises should be performed. The choice of equipment is crucial. Ensure that the apparatus can be adjusted to suit body dimensions, as some machines are made for the normative male. If in doubt, use free weights as they fit any body size.

2. *Order of the exercises*. Typically the large muscle group exercises or more complex exercises are performed at the beginning of a workout. If a circuit program is employed, arm exercises should be followed by leg exercises.

3. *Number of sets*. One set of each exercise is performed at the onset of a resistance training program. Once the trained individual adapts to this, the exercise program can progress to 3 or more sets of each exercise in a program. Typically 6 sets is the upper limit performed for one exercise movement.

4. *Intensity of the exercise*. For younger (prepubescent) children, loads of 6 repetition maximum (RM) or greater are recommended. As one develops into adolescence (e.g., age 15 or 16), heavier loads can be employed in program design. Training zones are used as targets to establish exercise intensity, for example, a target load that allows only 6 to 8 or 10 to 12 repetitions. This allows specific adaptations to be achieved (e.g., greater strength with 6 to 8 RM than with a 12 to 15 RM target repetition range).

5. *Amount of rest taken between sets and exercises*. Rest periods are generally scaled according to the load and repetition range employed. At least 3 minutes rest is recommended when heavy resistances (1 to 6 RM) are employed, 2 to 3 minutes rest with moderate (7 to 10 RM) loads, and 1 to 2 minutes when lighter resistances (11 RM or greater) are used. Despite these recommendations, the individual should rest until recovered to a level where the next set can be safely and effectively performed.

Progressive Overload

Progressive resistance exercise or progressive overload refers to the need to continually increase the stress placed on the muscle as it increases its force or endurance capabilities. If the training stimulus is not increased at this point, no further gains in strength will occur.

Several methods are employed to progressively overload skeletal muscle. The resistance (amount of weight utilized) to perform a certain number of repetitions can be increased. The use of RM automatically provides progressive overload, because as the muscle's strength increases, the amount of resistance necessary to perform a true RM also increases. A 5 RM may increase from 50 to 60 lb after several weeks of training. Another method to progressively overload the muscle is by increasing the volume of training performed (the number of sets and repetitions of a particular exercise). Due to the possibility of overtraining, care must be exercised when progressively overloading the muscle. This is especially true when the progressive overload is in the form of an increased volume of training.[20] Therefore, as a general rule, large increases in the resistance or volume of training, especially for individuals with little resistance training experience, should be avoided. A reasonable guideline is not to increase the resistance for a particular number of repetitions or volume of training more than 2.5 to 5 percent at any one time.

Neural Activation

Voluntary strength is determined not only by the quantity and quality of recruited skeletal muscle mass but also by the nervous system that innervates it. Training this system will increase the synchronization and number of MUs recruited and increase the activation of contractile apparatus and skill of the movement pattern. Long-term training is also capable of decreasing autogenic inhibition (protective measure of muscle), leading to a more forceful muscle contraction.

Specificity of Resistance Training

Speed Specificity

Most coaches and athletes maintain that resistance training should be performed at the velocity encountered during the actual sporting event. For many sporting events this means a high velocity of movement. This belief is based on the concept that resistance training produces its greatest strength gains at the velocity at which the training is performed (see Fig. 4–2). There is scientific evidence that supports this view. However, an intermediate training velocity is best if the aim of the program is to increase strength at all velocities of movement.[21] Thus, for an individual interested in general strength, an intermediate training velocity is recommended. However, training at a fast velocity results in gains in strength and power at a fast velocity to a slightly greater extent than training at a slow velocity.[22] Thus, use of velocity specific training to maximize strength and power gains at a specific velocity is appropriate for athletes at some points in their training.

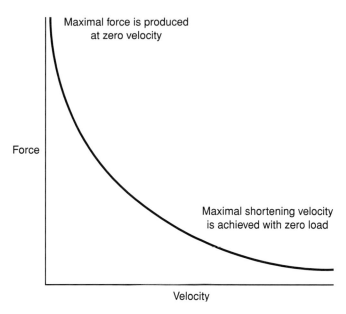

Figure 4–2. Force–velocity relationship of skeletal muscle actions displaying concentric or shortening skeletal muscle actions. When the curve meets the Y axis, the maximum isometric force exists. As the velocity of the concentric muscle action increases, the force produced decreases. (*Courtesy of William Kraemer, PhD.*)

Specificity of Muscle Action

If an individual trains isometrically, and progress is evaluated with a static muscle action, a large increase in strength may seem apparent. However, if this same individual's progress is determined using concentric or eccentric muscle actions, little or no increase in strength may be demonstrated. This is called testing specificity. This testing specificity indicates that gains in strength are specific to the type of muscle action (isometric, variable resistance, isokinetic) used in training performed. This specificity of strength gains is related to the individual learning to recruit the muscles to perform that particular type of muscle action. Therefore, a training program for a specific sport should have in it the types of muscular actions encountered in that sport. As an example, because isometric muscle actions are frequently performed while wrestling, it is beneficial to incorporate some isometric training into the resistance training program for wrestling.

Adaptations resulting from strength training are specific to the training stimulus. Improvements made while executing a contraction at a fast speed do not directly correlate with a similar muscle contractions performed at a slower speed. Lifting heavy weights must be performed at slow speeds. This recruits the glycolytic muscles fibers that are used for explosive movements (jumping, sprinting). This is not very sport specific; however, when using weights this is the only way it can be achieved. In an attempt to bridge the gap between the traditional style lifts (bench press, squats) athletes may

employ components of the Olympic lifts. For these explosive Olympic lifts to be successfully performed, speed, skill, and technique are critical (clean and jerk and the snatch). There is a large neural element involved in these lifts and the fast glycolytic muscle fibers are heavily recruited. Training should simulate the athletic movement. This may require modifying equipment, contraction speed, or starting position.

Muscle Group Specificity

Muscle group specificity simply means that each muscle group requiring strength gains must be specifically trained. If an increase in strength is desired in the flexors (biceps group) and extensors (triceps) of the elbow, exercises for both groups need to be included in the program. There must be exercises in a training program specifically chosen for each muscle group in which an increase in strength, local muscular, or hypertrophy is desired.

Energy Source Specificity

There are two anaerobic sources and one aerobic source of energy for muscle actions. The anaerobic sources of energy supply the majority of energy for high-powered, short-duration events, like sprinting 100 meters. The aerobic source of energy supplies the majority of energy for longer-duration, lower-power events, like running 5000 meters. If an increase in the ability of a muscle to perform anaerobic exercise is desired, the bouts of exercise should be of short duration and high intensity. If increases in the muscle's ability to perform aerobic exercise is desired, the training performed will be of a longer duration and lower intensity. Resistance training is usually associated with training the anaerobic energy sources. The number of sets and repetitions and the length of rest periods between sets and exercises need to be consistent with the energy source in which training adaptations are desired.

Program Variation and Periodization

Variation in the volume and intensity of training, or periodization, is extremely important for optimal gains in strength.[23-26] Slight variations in the position of the foot, hand, or other body parts that do not affect the safety of the lifter can also be valuable in producing continued gains in strength.[27] Periodization of resistance training is important for optimizing recovery and enhancing muscle force production.[19] The use of several exercises as a means to vary the conditioning stimulus of a particular muscle group is also a valuable means to assure continual increases in strength. Variation in training or periodization is needed to achieve optimal gains in strength and power. This systematic process of varying a strength training program has been called periodization of training.[19]

The purpose is to avoid overtraining, provide time for physical and mental recovery, and allow the athlete to make continued gains with a training program. Over the past 10 years, many systems of program periodization have been developed. It appears that the key to the general concept is based in the need for variation of the workout stimulus.

The challenge to any long-term training program is based in adherence to the program. Furthermore, the program must be effective. Too many of the programs that have been studied have used what might be called constant progressive resistance training programs. In other words, the individual did the same basic workout and progressed in the amount of resistance used for each exercise for a set number of repetitions. Thus, little or no variation was provided for the intensity or volume (sets × repetitions × resistance) of training nor for any other program variable. The problem is that without variation, a program becomes boring and the athlete becomes stale and does not look forward to a workout. One of the solutions to this adherence problem, which might encourage long-term adherence, is to use periodized strength training programs.

Periodized training can be achieved by altering workout variables such as the choice of exercise, order of exercise, and rest between sets and exercises. This section will focus on how the intensity and volume (sets × repetitions × resistance) might be altered for a core group of large muscle group exercises such as the squat/leg press, bench press, seated rows, military press, and lateral pull-down.

Typically, the larger muscle group exercises are periodized, but all exercises can be varied for intensity. One can vary the intensity over the week: Monday (light), Wednesday (heavy), and Friday (moderate). This goes on for a given training period (usually 8 to 12 weeks) and then competition is started or an active rest (activity but not lifting) is allowed before the training program starts a new 8- to 12 week cycle. Another method of periodization of training varies the intensity over several weeks (or cycles) of training: weeks 1 to 4 (light), weeks 5 to 8 (moderate), and weeks 9 to 12 (heavy). Usually the number of weeks used in what is called a microcycle ranges from 2 to 4. After the last cycle, or at the end of a training period, competitions are usually scheduled as the athlete is at his or her peak for that period of training. An athlete can also enter into a maintenance program where the individual lifts once or twice a week to maintain gains.

The key element of this type of training is the variation and ability to allow rest after a training or competition period. Strength can be maintained easier than it can be gained, so periods of active rest allow the athlete to stay active but not necessarily lift weights. The length of active rest is related to the amount of training the athlete has and where it is taken in the yearly cycle. Usually active rest ranges from 1 to 4 weeks in adults, with the less experienced taking the shorter 1 to 2 week breaks before a new cycle of training begins. Children and older adults may need more recovery, and each individual has to be taught to carefully assess his or her energy level. It is important that programs are individualized and used just as a guide.

Empirical evidence suggests that variation in exercises for the same muscle group causes greater increases in strength and power than no variation in exercises. This does not mean that the exercises performed must be changed every single training session, or that all exercises must be changed when one change is made. However, changes in exercises may be made every 2 to 3 weeks, or some exercises varied on an every other training session basis (two somewhat different training sessions performed alternately). As examples, the exercise included for the arms and shoulder might be the bench press and changed to the incline press or a bench press with dumbbells at 2- to 3-week intervals. These same types of changes could also be made on alternate training sessions. As an example, on Monday and Friday the bench press might be performed, and on Wednesday the incline press. Still, certain core exercises need to be maintained through the training program so that progress can be made.

EXAMPLE PROGRAM GUIDELINES

General Prepreparation Phase

Six to eight weeks are used for general strength conditioning to allow the individual to gain toleration of performing a strength training program. Teaching exercise technique should be stressed with little or no resistance. Start out at a low intensity that allows the individual to perform at least 12 to 15 repetitions with the resistance. Start with a low volume of exercise by using only 1 or 2 sets and a low number of exercises. Add exercises as the individual learns how to properly perform the exercises. The key is to introduce the concept of a strength training program. Usually large muscle group exercises are periodized and small muscle group exercises (arm curls, leg curls) are performed with a moderate intensity (8 to 10 RM). Nevertheless, all exercises can be periodized similar to the large muscle group exercises.

The number of times an athlete moves through the training cycle phases will be determined by the length of the training cycle (e.g., 1 year). It is thought that several cycles are better than one large cycle. Thus, the length of each phase is typically reduced to as low as 2-week cycles.[22,25] Typically a minimum of 6 weeks is allowed for the three cycle phases to be completed. Most programs perform 3 to 4 sessions per week when it is considered a building type program.[18]

Preparation Phase

Choose a cycle length from 2 to 4 weeks that will be used for all of the following lift cycles. This phase formally starts a training cycle as the number of exercises and initial toleration should be in place from the prior cycle. Perform 2 to 3 sets of each exercise at an intensity that allows 12 to 15 repetitions. This will create a high-volume, low-intensity stimulus. A 1- to 2-minute rest period is used between sets and exercises.

Power Phase

Using the same length cycle of 2 to 4 weeks, the individual uses a resistance that allows only 8 to 10 repetitions. The athlete performs 2 to 3 sets of each exercise with a 1.5 to 2-minute rest period between sets and - exercises. Again, technique is stressed along with progression in the resistance that can be used for the repetitions performed.

Strength Phase

Using the same length cycle of 2 to 4 weeks, the individual uses a resistance that allows only 3 to 6 repetitions. The individual performs 2 to 4 sets of each exercise with a 2- to 2.5-minute rest period between sets and exercises. Again, technique is stressed along with progression in the resistance that can be used for the repetitions performed.

High Strength Phase (optional)

Using the same length cycle of 2 to 4 weeks, the individual uses a resistance that allows only 1 to 3 repetitions. The individual performs 2 to 4 sets of each exercise with a 2- to 2.5-minute rest period between sets and exercises. Again, technique is stressed along with progression in the resistance that can be used for the repetitions performed.

Transition Phase

The athlete moves into a sport season and initiates an "in-season" program. It is also important for an individual training for fitness to use the transition phase for rest and recovery from the training cycles.

Active Rest Phase

This is a phase of the training cycle when the individual does not perform any resistance training but remains active with other activities. This phase lasts from 1 to 3 weeks depending upon the amount of training prior to this rest phase. This type of active rest phase helps fight overtraining and overuse injuries.

Nonlinear Periodized Training

1. Start with a general prepreparation phase.
2. This nonlinear method uses 8- to 12-week cycles of training where on different days the athlete utilizes a light (12 to 15 RM, 2 to 3 sets, 1 to 2 minutes rest) day; heavy (3 to 5 RM, 2 to 3 sets, 2 to 3 minutes rest) day; or a moderate (8 to 10 RM, 2 to 3 sets, 1.2 to 2 minutes rest) day.

The thought behind nonlinear periodized training is that by varying the workout within the week, adequate recovery and variation is provided for the individual. At the end of a training cycle, the athlete enters into an active rest phase of the program. One might also enter a maintenance phase using the same method of intensity variation but with a reduced number of exercises or sets to lower the volume of training.

METHODS TO ENHANCE STRENGTH

Machines or Free Weights

Right after the first resistance machine was invented, the controversy over whether resistance machines or free weights produce the greatest gains in strength and power probably started, and has continued ever since. Advocates of free weights point out that machines allow movement only in a predetermined plane and path of movement, so balancing of the resistance in all directions is not necessary. The need to balance the resistance requires the use of muscles not involved in the movement as prime movers. Prime movers in the military press are the outside of the shoulder area (deltoid) and the back of the upper arm (triceps). However, the muscles of the upper and lower back, smaller muscles around the shoulder area, and even the abdominals are involved in balancing the resistance. The involvement of these secondary, or balancing muscles, is greater with free weights than with machines. Advocates of free weights claim that the need to balance the resistance is more like a sporting event or daily life where balancing of any resistance moved is needed. Therefore, free weight training is an important part of resistance training. Conversely, machine advocates claim that the lack of a need to balance the resistance is good because it allows greater isolation of the muscles involved in the exercise as prime movers. In addition, machine advocates claim that because movement is allowed only in one plane and direction, it is easier to teach proper exercise technique. Both sides in this controversy use the same facts, but interpret them to be positive from their particular point of view. This can lead to confusion when trying to make decisions regarding equipment.

In reality, the strengths or weaknesses of machines or free weights can all be used to advantage in a resistance training program. Machines allowing movement in only one plane and direction providing isolation of a muscle group are very useful when the goal of the program is to increase strength, power, or local muscular endurance of a specific muscle group. Due to the isolation of a muscle group possible with machines, they are ideal for rehabilitation programs after an injury. Machines are also ideal for programs aimed at increasing strength, power, or local muscular endurance of a particular muscle group or joint prone to injury in a sport or in a muscle group that is the weak link in performance of a certain sporting activity. Free weight exercises, where it is necessary to balance the resistance in all directions, are a good choice where the goal of the program is to strengthen total body movements and provide coordination between various muscle groups. Thus, both machine (fixed form) and free weight (free form) exercises have a place in a well-designed resistance training program. Therefore, a well designed program will consist of both free weight and machine exercises.

Two other factors need to be addressed concerning free weights and machine exercises. Although the research is not conclusive, it appears that in adults doing free weight exercises such as squats results in greater increases in vertical jumping ability than performance of machine leg press type exercises. This is probably due to a greater mechanical similarity of squat type exercises to the jumping motion. It is, however, important to note that both squat and leg press type exercises can cause an increase in vertical jumping ability. The second factor concerns exercise technique. Due to the need for balancing the weight during the performance of free weight exercises, proper technique is more difficult to learn with free weights than machines. Thus, a greater amount of time must be planned for when teaching free weight exercise techniques.

SUMMARY

The prevention of injury is based on the ability of the musculoskeletal system to tolerate the demands of the activity. Activity itself has inherent risks of injury, and the biologic consequences of injury are related to both the mechanical and chemical stresses placed on the cells of various tissues. Resistance training designed specifically for a sport or given activity can help strengthen the underlying structures that mediate injury prevention and enhance tissue repair when injury does occur. Furthermore, the responsiveness to a resistance training program is enhanced even after longer periods of detraining when a prior long-term program has been adhered to.[28] Implementing a proper resistance training program is vital to the protection of the basic morphologic structure and function of the neuromuscular system.

Acknowledgments

This chapter was supported in part by a grant from the Robert F. and Sandra M. Leitzinger Research Fund in Sports Medicine at the Pennsylvania State University. Dr. Duncan's affiliation is with the Department of Physiology at the University of Melbourne in Australia, where he was a postdoctoral scholar in 1996–1997 in Dr. Kraemer's laboratory. Mr. Harman is a doctoral fellow in Dr. Kraemer's laboratory and the Department of Kinesiology.

REFERENCES

1. Fleck SJ, Falkel JE. Value of resistance training for the reduction of sports injuries. *Sports Med.* 1985;3:61–68.
2. Stone MH, O'Bryant H. *Weight Training: A Scientific Approach.* Minneapolis, MN: Belweather Press; 1987.
3. Stone MH. Implications for connective tissue and bone alterations resulting from resistance exercise training. *Med Sci Sports Exerc.* 1988;20:S162–S168.
4. Chandler JT, Wilson GD, Stone MH. The effect of the sqaut on knee stability. *Med Sci Sports Exerc.* 1989;21:299–303.
5. Zemper ED. Four year study of weight room injuries in a national sample of college football teams. *NSCA J.* 1990; 12:32–34.
6. Hutton WC, Adams RA. Can the lumbar spine be crushed in heavy lifting? *Spine.* 1982;7:586–590.
7. Gruchow W, Pelleiter D. An epidemiologic study of tennis elbow. *Am J Sports Med.* 1979;7:234–238.
8. Dominguez R. Shoulder pain in age group swimmers. In: Eriksson B, Furberg B, eds. *Swimming Medicine.* Baltimore: University Park Press; 1978;4.
9. Garrett WE Jr. Muscle strain injuries: Clinical and basic aspects. *Med Sci Sports Exerc.* 1990;22:436–443.
10. Tipton CM, Mathes RD, Maynard JA, Carey RA. The influence of physical activity on ligaments and tendons. *Med Sci Sports Exerc.* 1975;7:165–175.
11. Staff PH. The effect of physical activity on joints, cartilages, tendons and ligaments. *Scand J Sports Med.* 1982;29:59–63.
12. Parker MG, Ruhling RO, Holt D, et al. Descriptive analysis of qaudricep and hamstring muscle torque in high school football players. *J Orthopaed Sports Phys Ther.* 1983;5:2–6.
13. Costain R, Williams AK. Isokinetic qaudriceps and hamstring torque levels of adolescent, female soccer players. *J Orthopaed Sports Phys Ther.* 1984;5:196–200.
14. Shellock FG, Prentice WE. Warming-up and stretching for improved physical performance and prevention of sports related injuries. *Sports Med.* 1985;2:267–268.
15. Granito VJ, Hogan JB, Varnum LK. The performance enhancement group program: Integrating sport psychology and rehabilitation. *J Athletic Training.* 1995;30:328–331.
16. Armstrong RB, Warren GL, Warren JA. Mechanisms of exercise induced muscle fiber injury. *Sports Med.* 1991;12: 184–207.

17. Carlson BM, Faulkner JA. The regeneration of skeletal muscle fibers following injury: A review. *Med Sci Sports Exerc.* 1983;15:187-198.

18. Fleck SJ, Kraemer WJ. *Designing Resistance Training Programs.* 2nd ed. Champaign, IL: Human Kinetics; 1997.

19. Fleck SJ, Kraemer WJ. *Periodization Breakthrough.* New York: Advance Research Press; 1996.

20. Stone MH, O'Bryant H, Garhammer JG, et al. A theoretical model for strength training. *NSCA J.* 1982;4:36-39.

21. Kanehisa H, Miyashita M. Specificity of velocity in strength training. *Eur J Appl Physiol.* 1983;52:104-106.

22. Kanehisa H, Miyashita M. Effect of isometric and isokinetic muscle training on static strength and dynamic power. *Eur J Appl Physiol.* 1983;50:365-371.

23. Stone MH, O'Bryant H, Garhammer JG. A hypothetical model for strength training. *J Sports Med Phys Fitness.* 1981;21:342-351.

24. Matveyev L. *Fundamentals of Sports Training.* Moscow: Progress; 1981.

25. O'Bryant HS, Byrd R, Stone MH. Cycle ergometry performance and maximum leg and hip strength adaptations to two different methods of weight-training. *J Appl Sports Sci Res.* 1988;2:27-30.

26. Willoughby DS. The effects of mesocycle-length weight training programs involving periodization and partially equated volumes on upper and lower body strength. *J Strength Condition Res.* 1993;7:2-8.

27. Garhammer J. Equipment for the development of athletic strength and power. *NSCA J.* 1981;3:24-26.

28. Staron RS, Leonardi MJ, Karapondo DL, et al. Strength and skeletal muscle adaptations in heavy-resistance trained women after detraining and retraining. *J Appl Physiol.* 1991;70:631-640.

Chapter 5

Psychological Considerations in Working with Injured Athletes

David Yukelson and John Heil

Over the past 10 years, many articles have been written about the psychological processes athletes go through when injured.[1-14] Unfortunately, a dearth of literature exists regarding what athletes need from athletic trainers to facilitate the rehabilitation process.[13,15,16] Athletic trainers and sports medicine personnel often possess experiential knowledge about how athletes respond psychologically to injury, but lack specific scientific information about how best to intervene. Therefore, the purpose of this chapter is to provide an educational framework for sports medicine personnel to better understand the psychosocial intricacies that affect an athlete's response to injury.

Although many reasons for injury occurrence can be attributed to physical factors (e.g., poor equipment or playing surfaces, high-force collisions, strength and muscle imbalances, fatigue and overtraining), certain psychological factors and predisposing attitudes on the part of the athlete have also been shown to influence vulnerability to injury.[1,16-18] Along these lines, many psychological and physical factors interact to influence the risk of injury. Increased muscle tension due to anxiety can lead to muscular guarding, which puts the athlete at risk for injury because it reduces flexibility and motor coordination, and puts the muscles under a great deal of strain. Similarly, the stresses of everyday life, combined with competitive pressures, can cause attentional disruptions, tightening of the muscles, and breakdowns in concentration.[18]

Several studies have shown a relationship among personality factors, life stress, and injury occurrence.

Based on their model of stress and athletic injury, Anderson and Williams[1] proposed that individuals with high life stress, personality characteristics that provoke the stress response, and few coping resources are at increased risk for injury compared to athletes with the opposite profile. Similarly, Smith and associates[11] found high school athletes experiencing high life stress who possessed low social support and limited coping skills to be at greater risk for sustaining athletic injury. Sports medicine personnel need to be aware of the interaction of antecedent psychological variables that may affect injury, and implement appropriate intervention programs for athletes with high-risk profiles.[19]

In terms of psychological reactions to athletic injury, there are individual differences in how athletes respond physically, mentally, emotionally, and behaviorally. The degree of psychological impact an injury has on an individual is dependent on a number of mediating psychosocial factors including one's personality, self-esteem, locus of control, motivation, achievement orientation, importance of sport in the athlete's life, past history with being injured, and psychological coping skill strategies. Situational factors also come into play including the nature and severity of the injury, time of the season the injury occurs, role ambiguity, interpersonal team dynamics, and social support networks available to the athlete.[1,11,13,20] Other stress-related psychological reactions to injury include loss of identity, shattered hopes and dreams, separation, loneliness, fear of reinjury, anxiety and uncertainty, physical inactivity, unrealistic expectations regarding return to preinjury levels of performance, and diminished self-confidence.[5,9]

Accordingly, athletes respond to injury in different ways. Depending on the type of injury, personality disposition, and motivational orientation, some athletes perceive the ramifications of injury to be a disaster, while others simply take things easily in stride.[17] Aches and pains associated with minor injuries are accepted by most athletes as part of the game, and as a result subsequently are handled in routine fashion. However, lost time due to moderate or severe injury is another matter. To most competitive athletes, the latter scenario represents loss of opportunity to participate in a highly valued activity and can be perceived as a potential threat to continued success at sport. If the injury is appraised as threatening, or the athlete perceives limited control over things causing them to be stressed, various forms of emotional distress can develop. For instance, it is not uncommon for injured athletes to become irritable, impatient, frustrated, and worried or anxious about an uncertain future that lies ahead. Sometimes, the nature, frequency, and severity of psychological symptoms are such that a bonafide depression can develop. Thus, careful and consistent attention to the athlete's mental and emotional state of mind will optimize the rehabilitation process and facilitate timely intervention.

PSYCHOLOGICAL ADJUSTMENT TO INJURY

Initial attempts to understand the psychology of athletic injury drew on the work of Kubler-Ross.[21] In *On Death and Dying*, Kubler-Ross suggested that terminally ill patients move through a series of stages as they struggle to cope with feelings of loss and grief. The stages she proposed are denial, anger, bargaining, depression, and acceptance. In the denial stage, the injured athlete typically downplays the significance of the injury. After the reality of the situation sets in, anger often follows. The injured athlete may lash out at themselves or those around them. Bargaining soon follows, where the athlete tries rationalizing to avoid the reality of the situation. Distraught over the true sense of loss, depression may take over. Finally, the athlete accepts the injury for what it is and is hopeful for a successful return to competition.

This stage theory has been applied to a broad range of conditions involving loss, including athletic injury. The strength of the theory is that it provides a simple yet intuitively sensible approach to understanding the disruptive and sometimes puzzling emotions displayed without the assumption of underlying pathology. Unfortunately, research has failed to demonstrate that terminally ill patients or injured athletes consistently move in a sequential, predictable, orderly fashion through the stages described by Kubler-Ross. Rather,

emotional reactions to injury appear to be more cyclical in nature, and to vary more based on individual differences in response patterns, than stage models would seem to predict.[2,6] In addition, this model has limited value because of the obvious difference between terminally ill patients and injured athletes.

Whereas stage models fail to account for individual differences in emotional responses to injury, a number of conceptually similar cognitive-based appraisal models have recently been proposed to examine the multitude of psychosocial factors that could affect athletic injury.[2,3,13,20] The underlying tenet inherent in these models is that an individual's emotional response to athletic injury is influenced by his or her appraisal or interpretation of the injury itself and by situational factors perceived to be stressful. Thus, cognitive appraisals are thought to be influenced by the combined interaction of personal and situational factors, which in turn affect emotional and behavioral responses to injury.[2,22]

Along these lines, the affective cycle of injury is proposed as an alternative to the stage theory.[6] It accounts for the emotionally disruptive nature of injury in general, and it also recognizes the ups and downs that are typically encountered throughout the rehabilitation process. The affective cycle of injury includes three elements: distress, denial, and determined coping. Distress, which recognizes the inherently disrupting influence of injury on life-style and emotional equilibrium, includes symptoms of anxiety, depression, anger, and bargaining. The key elements to consider are the magnitude of distress, and how appropriate it is relative to the severity of injury. The second element, denial, includes feelings of shock, disbelief, and failure to accept the severity of injury. Denial can range on a continuum from mild to profound, and will vary across time and circumstances. Given the specifics of its manifestation, denial may serve either an adaptive or maladaptive purpose that can facilitate or interfere with rehabilitation. At its most fundamental level, denial is a process of selective attention. The athlete's ability to remain positive and put distressing thoughts out of his or her mind is constructive when it helps the athlete from being overwhelmed by negative thoughts and emotions. However, it becomes problematic when failure to recognize the severity of injury results in a lackadaisical attitude toward rehabilitation or failure to observe prescribed limits. The final element, determined coping, moves beyond the passive sense of acceptance. Rather, it demands the channeling of knowledge and emotional fortitude to meet the challenge of rehabilitation head on. In essence, this is what mental toughness is all about: belief, commitment, willpower, full focus, and accepting responsibility for one's actions.

A fundamental assumption of the affective cycle of injury is that emotional recovery does not move through stages in a linear process, but is a cycle that may repeat itself over days, weeks, or even many times within the course of a day.[6] It is useful to envision a macrocycle (which spans the recovery process), several minicycles (which are linked to the stages of the rehabilitation process), and microcycles that can occur at any time and reflect the ups and downs of daily life for the rehabilitating athlete. In the macrocycle of recovery, the athlete generally progresses from distress and denial to determined coping. To the extent that each distinct stage of rehabilitation represents a new challenge and requires the athlete to make a readjustment, it triggers a minicycle; but even as one element of the cycle may tend to dominate at a given period of time, it will seldom prevail 24 hours a day. The microcycle recognizes the shifts in emotional response among denial, distress, and determined coping that can occur at any time. Emotional shifts are generally linked to specific experiences or events. Setbacks during treatment and pain flare-ups are the most likely triggers of a new microcycle. However, it may also occur from something as simple as a review of the game film that shows the injury, or anything that elicits a sense of loss or threat. Let's look at a couple of case studies and see how the process unfolds.

Case Study 1

Meagan is an 18-year-old freshman enrolled in a highly competitive division 1 swimming program. She was a very successful age group swimmer, competing at the senior national level against many of the top swimmers in the country. She performed well the first part of her freshman season, but developed a worn rotator cuff around the third meet of the season. Meagan was told by the team physician to take a few weeks off or risk the possibility of surgical intervention. Throughout high school, she had chronic shoulder problems but was able to cope effectively and perform well despite constant irritation and swelling in her shoulder joint area. In college, she had a difficult time adjusting to the frustration and disappointment of being injured. Watching others improve while she couldn't train or compete had a dramatic effect on her personality and athletic identity. Feeling unmotivated, undervalued, and sorry for herself, she let some of her academic and personal responsibilities slide. Socially withdrawn and somewhat homesick, she often became irritable and moody around coaches, teammates, friends, trainers, and support staff, to the point where everyone was finding her difficult to deal with. To make matters worse, the student-trainer assigned to Meagan was young and inexperienced, and did not exude much interest or genuine concern for things going on in Meagan's life outside the rehabilitation setting. Overworked and overextended, it was not uncommon for the trainer to hand Meagan a set of shoulder strengthening exercises without much explanation, warmth, empathy, or compassion. Unfortunately, the trainer did not understand the commitment, sacrifice, dedication, and hard work Meagan invested in her swimming career. To com-

pound the situation, Meagan would often spend 2 to 3 hours a day in the training room surrounded by the same people, doing the same monotonous exercises, feeling like she was not making much progress. What could you do to help Meagan cope more effectively with the stress she is experiencing?

Case Study 2

Jim is a junior all-conference linebacker who tore his ACL the next-to-last game of the season. Initially, the injury brought on a plethora of emotions (fear, anger, frustration, anxiety, apprehension), irrational thoughts (perceiving himself to be a real loser, wondering why bad things always happen to him), and the potential realization of lost dreams (missing out on this year's bowl game, anxiety and uncertainty regarding whether or not he is ever going to be able to play again). Once Jim accepted the injury for what it was, he made a commitment to his trainer, Dan, that he would do whatever was necessary to get back on the field healthy again and make his final year a great one. Jim and Dan had a very good relationship already established, and together they talked about anticipated psychosocial stressors that could affect Jim's motivation and focus (e.g., having to get around campus on crutches, feelings of social isolation from the team, keeping a healthy and balanced life style). With the help of a sports psychologist, they developed a comprehensive goal setting plan for rehabilitation, along with psychological coping skill strategies for various phases of the rehabilitation process. If you were in charge of Jim's rehabilitation program, what kinds of psychological strategies and techniques would you employ to keep him physically, mentally, and emotionally focused throughout the rehabilitation process?

Meagan appears to be suffering from a subclinical depression with symptoms of apathy, irritability, moodiness, helplessness, and hopelessness. It is probably these depressive symptoms that underlie her failure to meet her responsibilities. Unfortunately for Meagan, this sets up a vicious cycle whereby failure to follow through on responsibilities undermines not only the recovery process, but also her potential success as a college student. The longer she is depressed, the worse her pain becomes. Attempts to alleviate pain with tried and tested methods meet with little success. In the process, Meagan is coming to be identified as a nuisance. Because Meagan is new to her team and to the sports medicine providers, they may fail to see that her behavior is a maladaptive reaction to injury. Alternately, they assume the behavior that they are seeing is typical for her in general. Those who knew Meagan in high school would likely be surprised by this turn of events. She was probably respected and admired by others for her success over the adversity that her shoulder pain presented at the high school level. Meagan appears to be unmotivated and feels undervalued. If something is not done soon, Meagan is likely to develop a bonafide clinical depressive disorder. Her career in swimming is clearly at risk.

In marked contrast, Jim is well known to the treatment providers. They were there with him during his period of acute distress, which was understandable given the circumstances of his injury and potential impact on his career. The loss associated with Jim's injury, his relatively straightforward psychological presentation, and knowledge of him as a solid individual makes it easier to understand his distress and feel compassion for him. Jim's decision to take control of his life and his demonstration of determined coping are likely to rally others to support his effort. Jim is responding to adversity in a way that we all respect and admire. This, and the support that has come about as a consequence, has created a positive cycle of response. As a consequence, Jim's prognosis for doing the very best that he can is quite good. The involvement of the athletic trainer and sports psychologist have helped Jim to create a plan that is not just optimistic, but realistic. He does not assume that everything will be okay, but anticipates problems and makes preparation for dealing with these. However, it must be remembered that Jim has demonstrated vulnerability to depression, and this may be elicited in the case of a treatment setback or other playing mishap. However, with timely intervention and professional guidance, this is likely to be a minor interruption, with Jim probably returning on course for success.

ROLE OF THE ATHLETIC TRAINER IN THE PSYCHOLOGY OF RECOVERY

Athletic trainers are in an ideal position to influence the psyche of injured athletes. In a survey of athletic trainers designed to identify characteristics of athletes who coped most and least successfully with their injuries, Wiese and associates[16] found interpersonal communication skills, understanding of individual motivation and self-thoughts, goal setting, and positive reinforcement to be important factors in facilitating an athlete's ability to cope with injury rehabilitation. In a similar study, athletic trainers noted successful versus unsuccessful coping athletes were more compliant with treatment and rehabilitation programs, had a more positive attitude toward injury and life, asked questions and sought knowledge about injury and rehabilitation, and appeared to be more motivated and dedicated in their quest to return to their sport.[15] Likewise, Ievleva and Orlick[7] found fast healers to use more goal-setting strategies, positive self-talk, and healing imagery techniques than did slow healers. Finally, U.S. olympic skiers note the importance of various interpersonal resources as being important factors facilitating their recovery from injury.[5] In particular, having injured models for references,

rehabbing with others, and social support from significant others (coaches, teammates, family, and friends) were rated as being important.

There are many factors that affect adherence to rehabilitation programs. Athletes as well as athletic trainers share the responsibility of promoting adherence to the rehabilitation process. Motivational orientations, attitude, outlook, coping skill strategies to deal with stress, and efficacious beliefs are factors that lie within the individual. However, one of the most important factors to consider is the trainer's relationship with the athlete. Communication, trust, and mutual respect are essential ingredients for developing rapport and establishing effective working relationships.[23] It also helps for sports medicine personnel to be genuinely concerned about the personal welfare of the athlete, and spend more time getting to know the athlete as a unique individual, beyond his or her injuries or physical complaints.[9]

Along these lines, research indicates athletes would like sports medicine personnel to have good listening skills, show compassion and empathy, be able to provide education and clear information about injuries and rehabilitation procedures, use appropriate motivational techniques that recognize individual differences in athlete's needs and interests, provide support when needed, and have desirable personal characteristics that facilitate positive interactions.[5,9,13,16,24] Although many athletic trainers report a need for educational training in the areas of counseling and sports psychology,[15,16,25] they along with other sports medicine personnel are in a wonderful position to empower the athlete with skills that will facilitate compliance to the rehabilitation process and motivation for optimal recovery.

PSYCHOLOGICAL TRIAGE

Because of the stressful nature of injury, more severe psychological difficulties can arise. Premorbid conditions such as alcohol or drug abuse or adjustment difficulties can also complicate recovery from injury. The sports medicine injury checklist as developed by Heil[6] is a tool to guide the sports medicine professional in the triage of the injured athlete (see Table 5-1). It is divided into two parts: an acute phase component, which is relatively brief; and a chronic phrase component, which is subdivided into current factors and history sections. This checklist is designed as a guide to inquiry and evaluation. Consequently, there is no formal weighting of the checklist items. When followed, it ensures that a comprehensive assessment has been completed. Ultimately, the goal of psychological triage is to assess the athlete's motivation, vulnerability to the sequel of injury, and ability to understand and cope with the demands of rehabilitation.

TABLE 5–1. SPORTS MEDICINE INJURY CHECKLIST

Acute Phase

_____ Failure of pain to respond to routine management strategies

_____ Failure of athlete to comply with recommended rehabilitation program

_____ Rehabilitation setbacks

_____ Emotional distress (depression, irritability, confusion, guilt, withdrawal)

_____ Irrational fear or anxiety in specific situations in the otherwise well-adjusted athlete (may be seen as avoidance of feared situation)

_____ Overly optimistic attitude toward injury and recovery

_____ Persistent fatigue

_____ Sleep problems

_____ Gross overestimate or underestimate of rehabilitation progress by athlete

Chronic Phase

Current factors

_____ Persistence of pain beyond natural healing

_____ "Odd" descriptions of pain

_____ Inconsistency in "painful" behavior or reports of pain

_____ Failed attempt(s) at return to play

_____ Performance problems following return to play

_____ Inability to identify realistic goals for recovery

_____ Recent stressful changes in sport situation

_____ Stressful life circumstances (within the last year)

_____ Depression (including changes in sleep, appetite, energy, and libido)

_____ Strained relationships with coaches, teammates, or friends

_____ Personality conflicts between treatment providers and athlete

_____ Poor compliance with scheduled visits and medication use

_____ Additional medical treatment sought by athlete without consulting current treatment providers (including emergency room visits)

_____ Iatrogenic problems

_____ Repeated requests for pain (especially psychoactive) medication

_____ Evidence of illicit drug use (recreational or ergogenic)

History

_____ Multiple surgeries at pain site

_____ Chronic pain in the same or another physiologic system (may be resolved)

_____ Family members with chronic pain

_____ Problematic psychosocial history (behavior problems in school; vocational, marital, or legal problems; history of physical or sexual abuse)

_____ Problematic psychological history (repeated or prolonged psychological adjustment problems; alcohol/drug problems; eating disorders)

From Heil J,[6] with permission.

The acute phase component includes nine items that can be assessed by observation. The current factor section of the chronic phase component assesses a wide range of behaviors. Of these, some are relatively easily observed while others will require a more systematic approach to assessment. The athletic trainer will need to take the time to speak with the athlete at length and to seek feedback from the coaching staff. The history section of the chronic phase component includes five items that encompass an in-depth look at the athlete's personal history. Much of this information is usually available through existing medical records. However, it is likely that direct and sometimes probing questions need to be asked. There are times when the whole story is not told. Because of the sensitive nature of these questions, it is important to proceed cautiously and with respect for the athlete's privacy. To the extent that this interchange between athletic trainer and athlete conveys a sense of concern, it will be well received by the athlete.

The checklist can be used in its entirety or in a piece-by-piece manner as problems with injury become chronic. The initial acute phase component may be used alone in the immediate postinjury period to assess risk for problems with rehabilitation. One may proceed to the chronic phase component when the athlete fails to recover from an injury within the usual time frame or experiences repeated setbacks in treatment. The elements of the history section of the checklist should be investigated in the case of entrenched injury syndromes. In summary, the questionnaire is designed to help the athletic trainer look beyond what is immediately apparent and ensure a thorough and systematic psychological evaluation.

Case Study Update: Application of Sports Medicine Injury Checklist

Given the depth and complexity of the problems faced by both Meagan and Jim, the use of the sports medicine injury checklist is appropriate. Additional information gained will help shape the athletic trainer's impression of the athlete and guide treatment planning. As you work through the checklist for Meagan, it literally begins to light up with hits. However, most interesting is what is found in the history section of the chronic phase component. You find that Meagan suffered chronic asthma as a child, which she eventually overcame through her swimming. You also discover that her mother suffers chronic pain that has led to repeated hospitalizations over time. At about puberty, Meagan went through a brief period of psychological counseling for adjustment problems that appear to have begun at a time when Megan's mother was hospitalized. In the process, you also discover that her mother has recently completed a hospital stay. You then realize that things have never been easy for Meagan. One way or another, she has always struggled with adversity. While on one hand this tends to build good coping skills, on the other, it leaves the individual vulnerable to that "not again" feeling. Understanding stressors Meagan has had to deal with in her life helps build compassion. In the context of her freshman transition, you realize that this is a significant stressor for her. With a minimal support network, she has no one to lean on. It is readily apparent that work with Meagan is going to be labor intensive and of extended duration.

Because you know Jim well and have had extended conversations with him, you question whether the checklist will be useful but elect to use it anyway. As expected, not many items are found. However, you are surprised to discover that Jim has been having persistent sleep problems and is feeling increasingly fatigued. He seems to look fine, but describes himself as crashing after rehabilitation. The combination of pain and restlessness he experiences leads to problems with sleep. He is attempting to compensate for this by occasional naps during the day, but this in turn is interfering with his study schedule. In Jim's efforts to project a positive attitude, he declined to report just how great a struggle he was experiencing. He is not being evasive, but simply did not see the relevance of this to recovery from injury. This discovery helps you realize that you are on track in working to establish underlying realistic goals for Jim's recovery. At the same time, you realize that he is likely to need help with pacing his effort over the course of rehabilitation. You decide to supplement the existing treatment plan with a sleep management program and brief overview of time management skills.

PAIN MANAGEMENT

Many of the problems that occur during rehabilitation can be traced to problems with pain management. In health and in injury, pain is an integral part of the athlete's experience. Pain must be understood not only as a signal of tissue damage, but also in terms of the personal meaning it has to the athlete. The athlete must deal with routine performance pain, the nuisance of muscle soreness and other feelings of discomfort, the intense pain of sudden severe injury, the grind of rehabilitation, and the uncertainty of chronic injury.

In coping with pain, the mind and body interact in complex ways.[26] Pain begins as an electrochemical signal that proceeds to the spinal cord and then the brain. This gives rise to psychological awareness (perception). From this, follows a series of brain processes that attempt to provide meaning to pain. For example, pain may be identified as routine or alternately, as a warning that injury is in the making. The meaning assigned to pain ultimately serves as a guide to action.

There are individual differences in how people respond to pain. Through proper education, sports medicine personnel must teach athletes to differentiate routine injury pain from dangerous injury pain. Consider an athlete who has the perception of a burning pain in her leg as she completes a set of resistance training exercises

prescribed as part of her rehabilitation. If she determines that the meaning of this pain is routine, she is likely to continue with her rehabilitation, and to feel good about the effort expended. Now consider another variation of the situation just described. What if the athlete interprets pain as a signal of reinjury? The athlete is likely to avoid the task altogether, or if she continues the exercise, she is likely to do so in a way that is hesitant or fearful.

The complexity of pain is reflected in the gate control theory of Melzack and Wall.[27] They observed that the spinal cord functions as an electrochemical switching station where pain and other sensory inputs are mixed and modified. Special descending tracks that move from the brain downward appear to exert a moderating influence on pain, essentially turning it up or down, in much the same way a rheostat on a light switch modifies an electrical signal and hence, the brightness of light. The gate control theory has been used to explain the remarkable feats of pain tolerance often demonstrated in sport and the therapeutic benefits of heat, cold, ultrasound, and acupuncture. Over 30 years later, Melzack and Wall's gate control theory continues to withstand the test of time as additional research continues to add shades of meaning to this theory.

When pain is prolonged, psychological factors come to play a progressively more prominent role. As a result, pain becomes increasingly situation-specific and is triggered by situational circumstances that elicit psychological reactions such as fear, anxiety, mistrust, or lack of confidence. When the athletic trainer and the athlete's perspectives on pain diverge, problems are in the making. If the athletic trainer observes inconsistency in pain and behavior, the athlete's credibility may be called into question and suspicions of malingering may be raised. Simultaneously, athletes may feel that their complaints of pain are not being taken seriously, thereby undermining trust and confidence in their treatment providers. The best remedy to this potential set of problems is clear and consistent communication about pain, clarification of its status as benign or as a signal of danger, and careful attention to the meaning that pain holds for the athlete. Consequently, athletes need to be empowered with the right kind of information to help them take responsibility for their own health care.

PSYCHOLOGICAL TECHNIQUES TO FACILITATE RECOVERY

Mental training techniques are a wonderful tool to help athletes cope with the demands and rigors of rehabilitation. The same skills that help athletes succeed on the playing fields (goal setting, accountability and commitment to excellence, relaxation and visualization, concentration and confidence, emotional self-control and positive self-talk, developing mental plans for success, and coping skill strategies for dealing with adversity) are transferable life skills that carry over into other domains like injury rehabilitation.[9,13,14,17,28,29]

Based on examination of specific cognitive, behavioral, and affective responses to athletic injury, a number of psychological skills and strategies can be suggested. First and foremost, it is important to develop trust and rapport with the injured athlete. Hence, a premium is placed on effective communication skills, particularly active listening. Good communication involves mutual sharing and mutual understanding.[23] You must take the time to get to know the athlete, and for the athlete to develop a personal relationship with you. I recognize this is difficult to do if you are seeing 20 to 30 patients a day; however, it will pay dividends in the long run. For instance, many intercollegiate athletes have reported to me the therapeutic benefits of having a personal relationship already established with their trainer, someone to talk to about the frustrations associated with injury, someone who understands the commitment, sacrifice, many hours invested to get to where the athlete is currently at now. The trainer needs to know when to push and when to back off, which can only be accomplished by knowing something about the individual ahead of time. Consequently, the communication skills of active listening, clarifying, paraphrasing, nonjudgmental empathy, and reassurance builds trust, hope, and respect.

Second, it is important to help athletes develop a plan to deal with the injury effectively so they know what to expect. Empower the athlete with knowledge about the nature of the injury itself and what the recovery process is all about. Pictures, anatomic diagrams, and CD-ROMs are helpful educational learning tools that can facilitate visualization scenarios. Remember to speak in language the athlete can understand. Reinforce the commitment that is required and the expectations you have. Jim's trainer Dan is very well organized, plans things out, and discusses what to expect each day of rehab, which in turn builds trust in Jim. Thus, a plan provides direction and helps the athlete understand what is going to happen along the way. It gives the injured athlete a mental picture of what to expect, a schemata from which to develop goals and expectations, a framework from which to evaluate progress that has been made.

The third consideration is attitude and outlook. Psychological outlook on how athletes feel about themselves at any particular point in time can impact what they do in rehab. As noted in Meagan's case study, intercollegiate student-athletes have a tremendous amount of academic and interpersonal stress to deal with, which can undermine identity, confidence, and self-esteem. The extent to which sports medicine professionals can help the athlete feel positive, optimistic, and in control of the rehabilitation process will greatly affect the sense of determined coping.

Likewise, the trainer's attitude and outlook can affect motivation and desire to get better. Athletic trainers and sports medicine practitioners need to be aware of the various psychosocial stressors that can affect their own motivation and concentration (handling high patient loads and multiple demands effectively, dealing with patient idiosyncrasies, dealing with multiple personalities of doctors and other support staff, having a life for yourself outside the health care facility), which in turn affects their self-esteem and quality of care provided. Hence, you have to take care of yourself before you can give to others. Consequently, the practitioner needs to keep things in perspective, and be highly motivated, enthusiastic, and committed to helping the injured athlete get better.

A fourth area to address is that of goal setting. Goals provide direction and purpose. They focus attention and action on the task at hand, help mobilize intensity of effort and persistence by giving the individual something to shoot for, and facilitate strategy development and subsequent action plans for achievement.[30] Beginning with the end in mind, the injured athlete should set short-term goals in relation to long-term objectives. Goals should be difficult enough to challenge, yet realistic and attainable. The sports medicine practitioner can facilitate the process by finding creative ways of providing feedback to the injured athlete. For instance, for a postsurgical ACL patient, the practitioner may want to see an increase in knee flexion of 10 degrees this week. Subsequently, there could be daily goals, weekly goals, leading to monthly goals where the trainer is looking for definite changes in range of motion, proprioception exercises, strength, or endurance. The key is to have the athlete set short-terms goals that are specific and measurable so the athlete feels like they are making appropriate progress toward the end result.

Two very important psychological skills for rehabilitation are relaxation and healing-based visualization techniques. Relaxation training can be taught in a number of different ways (e.g., autogenic training, progressive muscle relaxation, diaphragmatic breathing, biofeedback training), and a number of authors have described imagery methods applicable to helping injured athletes.[17,28,31,32] Visualization can be used to create the proper attitude and mindset for recovery, or as a tool for coping with adversity or overcoming counterproductive thinking. With proper education on the anatomy of injury and subsequent healing processes, it can be used as part of rehabilitation imagery or as a performance enhancement tool for return to competition.

Likewise, it is important to teach athletes how to cope with setbacks and deal with their emotions effectively. Elite competitive athletes sacrifice so much to get to where they are that when something like severe injury occurs, often everything seems to fall apart. Patience is a wonderful virtue and injured athletes need to learn how to keep everything in proper perspective. This is where positive self-talk and an optimistic outlook come into play. It takes great willpower and volition to *choose* to think confidently, even when adversity surrounds you. Consequently, sports medicine practitioners (with the aid of a sport psychologist) can teach athletes how to reframe negative, self-defeating thoughts into something more constructive and task oriented. For instance, rather than dwelling on negative things out of Meagan's control (e.g., watching others improve while she couldn't train), she should focus her mind and energy on short-term rehabilitation goals that affirm the progress she is making. Self-monitoring techniques that bring awareness and attention to faulty internal dialogue are the first step in gaining control of self-defeating thoughts and attitudes.

In addition to resilient coping skill strategies, an important intervention strategy that has great relevance for injured athletes is that of peer helping and social support. Common psychological reactions to athletic injury are feelings of isolation and withdrawal and perceptions within injured athletes that they are no longer valued or an important part of the team. By reaching out and providing genuine support and encouragement, peers or other injured athletes can be a source of emotional, informational, or tangible support during recovery from injury.[33]

REFERRAL AND COORDINATION OF CARE

Because athletic trainers are the primary points of contact for the injured athlete, they most directly influence the accessibility of psychology to the injured athlete. Once the athletic trainer decides that psychological intervention is indicated, careful consideration of the process of referral is necessary. An initial unspoken hurdle to overcome is the lack of understanding of what psychologists do, and what for some may be the stigma of psychological referral. Some athletes may interpret this as suggesting that they are a head case or that they are imagining or otherwise faking their injury. As a consequence, referral is best thought of as a process that includes preparation, referral, and follow-up.

Preparation of the athlete begins with clear statements of the potential benefits of referral. It is important to emphasize the stressful nature of injury and the performance benefits of psychology. A brief description of what is involved in working with the psychologist can be provided next. For the athlete who has made a commitment to see a psychologist, the single most effective way to assure follow-through is to schedule the appointment

at the time the athlete commits to psychological intervention. A follow-up meeting with the athlete after initial psychological consultation helps reassure the athlete and facilitates coordination of care. Referral is most effective when done in a way that not only assures the athlete of continuing concern and support, but also implies an understanding and endorsement of psychological intervention.

How vigorously referral should be recommended will be influenced by the severity and urgency of the problem. In cases of acute psychological distress, prompt referral is essential. In less pressing situations or where the athlete elects to defer intervention, the athletic trainer may suggest that the athlete attempt some coping measure and that if the situation does not improve, referral will again be considered. Do not hesitate to reintroduce the idea of referral. The athlete who is mentally prepared and receptive to treatment will experience the greatest benefits.

Case Study Update

Let's consider what is potentially involved in making referral work for Meagan and Jim. Because Meagan appears somewhat fragile and there are strained relations between her and the athletic training staff, a cautious and sensitive approach is essential. You begin by sharing with Meagan your sense of compassion for the difficult situation in which she finds herself. At the same time, you convey your respect for her ability to overcome adversity in the past. Your suggestion to Meagan that she consider working with you and a psychologist is followed by comments on how helpful you have found this to be with other athletes. In your conversation with her, you emphasize its benefits not only in injury management, but also as a practical skill for developing the mental game. Because Meagan is initially reluctant, you ask her to think it over and suggest that you will discuss it with her at another time. You close your conversation by emphasizing that you want to make sure that everything possible is done to help her. The next time you see Meagan, she appears more at ease and opens up to you about her problems. Then you ask her if she would like to follow up with the psychologist. When she agrees, you offer to give the psychologist a call to set up the appointment. You then reassure Meagan by letting her know that if she is uncomfortable with the psychologist or at any time feels any reservations, to be sure to let you know.

For Jim, no formal referral is necessary. You just suggest that he discuss the concerns that you and he have identified with fatigue and sleep the next time he sees the sports psychologist. You reflect for a moment on how Jim developed such a comfortable working relationship with the psychologist and realized it evolved as a natural extension of the performance enhancement work the sports psychologist had done with the football team. You may even consider having Jim talk with Meagan. As an upper classman with star status who has direct experience with both injury and sports psychology interventions, he is an excellent model. His comments would likely help Meagan keep the intent behind the referral in the proper perspective and help reinforce that people really do care about her. The sports psychologist is an integral member of the sports medicine team; referral is relatively simple, timely, and efficient.

SUMMARY

Injury can be one of the most debilitating obstacles an athlete can face. Although there are individual differences in how athletes respond, many have a difficult time coping with psychosocial stressors associated with injury. Consequently, the purpose of the present chapter is to provide the sports medicine practitioner with various sports psychology guidelines in hope that each patient is treated as a unique individual, not just another entry on the daily treatment log. Models of psychological adjustment have been presented, along with suggested interventions sports medicine practitioners can adopt to facilitate successful recovery. It is important to get the injured athlete actively involved in the rehabilitation process, and to educate, motivate, communicate, and inspire athletes to take responsibility for their own health care. Along these lines, athletes should be encouraged to approach rehabilitation the same way they do their athletic competitions: with desire, dedication, commitment, planning, confidence, belief, and trust. Likewise, athletes should be encouraged to set goals for themselves, and develop plans to deal with potential setbacks if they arise in an emotionally constructive way. Finally, it is important to recognize the role psychosocial stressors play on the perceptions, emotions, and behaviors of injured athletes, and to encourage determined coping skills in response to these stressors.

REFERENCES

1. Anderson MB, Williams JM. A model of stress and athletic injury: Prediction and prevention. *J Sport Exerc Psychol.* 1988;10:294–306.
2. Brewer BW. Review and critique of models of psychological adjustment to athletic injury. *J Appl Sport Psychol.* 1994;6:87–100.
3. Brewer BW, Linder DE, Phelps CM. Situational correlates of emotional adjustment to athletic injury. *Clin J Sports Med.* 1995;5:241–245.
4. Brewer BW, Van Raalte JL, Linder DE. Role of the sport psychologist in treating injured athletes: A survey of sports medicine providers. *J Appl Sport Psychol.* 1991;3:183–190.
5. Gould D, Udry E, Bridges D, Beck L. The psychology of ski racing injury rehabilitation: Final report. Paper presented as part of *U.S. Olympic Committee Sports Science and Technology Grant Project*, 1996.
6. Heil J. *Psychology of Sport Injury.* Champaign, IL: Human Kinetics; 1993.
7. Ievleva L, Orlick T. Mental links to enhanced healing: An exploratory study. *Sport Psychol.* 1991;5:25–40.
8. Pargman D. *Psychological Bases of Sport Injuries.* Morgantown, WV: Fitness Information Technology; 1993.
9. Petitpas A, Danish SJ. Caring for injured athletes. In: Murphy SM, ed. *Sport Psychology Interventions.* Champaign, IL: Human Kinetics; 1995.
10. Smith AM, Scott SG, O'Fallon W, Young M. Emotional responses of athletes to injury. *Mayo Clin Proc.* 1990;65:38–50.
11. Smith RE, Smoll FL, Ptacek JT. Conjunctive moderator variables in vulnerability and resiliency research: Life stress, social support, coping skills, and adolescent sport injuries. *J Personal Social Psychol.* 1990;55:360–370.
12. Wiese DM, Weiss MR. Psychological rehabilitation and physical injury: Implications for the sports medicine team. *Sport Psychol.* 1987;1:318–330.
13. Wiese-Bjornstal DM, Smith AM, LaMott EE. A model of psychologic response to athletic injury and rehabilitation. *Athlet Train Sports Health Care Perspect.* 1995;1:17–30.
14. Yukelson D, Murphy S. Psychological considerations in injury prevention. In: Renstrom P, ed. *Sports Injuries: Basic Principles of Prevention and Care.* Cambridge, MA: Blackwell; 1993.
15. Larson GA, Starkey C, Zaichkowsky LD. Psychological aspects of athletic injuries as perceived by athletic trainers. *Sport Psychol.* 1996;10:37–47.
16. Wiese DM, Weiss MR, Yukelson DP. Sport psychology in the training room: A survey of athletic trainers. *Sport Psychol.* 1991;5:25–40.
17. Rotella RJ, Heyman SR, Williams JM. Stress, injury, and the psychological rehabilitation of athletes. In: Williams J, ed. *Applied Sport Psychology: Personal Growth for Peak Performance.* 3rd ed. Mountain View, CA: Mayfield; 1997.
18. Williams JM, Tonyman P, Anderson MB. The effects of stressors and coping resources on anxiety and peripheral narrowing. *J Appl Sport Psychol.* 1991;3:126–141.
19. Williams JM, Roepke N. Psychology of injury and injury rehabilitation. In: Singer R, Murphey M, Tennant L, eds. *Handbook of Research in Sport Psychology.* New York: Macmillan; 1993.
20. Udry E. Coping and social support among injured athletes following surgery. *J Sport Exerc Psychol.* 1997;19:71–90.
21. Kubler-Ross E. *On Death and Dying.* New York: Macmillan; 1969.
22. Wagman D, Khelifa M. Psychological issues in sport injury rehabilitation: Current knowledge and practice. *J Athlet Train.* 1996;31:257–261.
23. Yukelson D. Communicating effectively. In: Williams J, ed. *Applied Sport Psychology: Personal Growth for Peak Performance.* 3rd ed. Mountain View, CA: Mayfield; 1997.
24. Fisher AC, Hoisington L. Injured athletes' attitudes and judgements toward rehabilitation adherence. *J Athlet Train.* 1993;28:48–53.

25. Moulton MA, Molstad S, Turnerr A. The role of athletic trainers in counseling college athletes. *J Athlet Train.* 1997;32:148-150.

26. Brewer BW, Van Raalte JL, Linder DE. Effects of pain on motor performance. *J Sport Exerc Psychol.* 1990; 12:353-365.

27. Melzack R, Wall PD. Pain mechanisms: A new theory. *Science.* 1965;150:971-979.

28. Ievleva L, Orlick T. Mental paths to enhanced recovery from sports injury. In Pargman D, ed. *Psychological Bases of Sport Injuries.* Morgantown, WV: Fitness Information Technology; 1993.

29. Weinberg RS, Gould D. *Foundations of Sport and Exercise Psychology.* Champaign, IL: Human Kinetics; 1995.

30. Gould D. Goal setting for peak performance. In: Williams J, ed. *Applied Sport Psychology: Personal Growth for Peak Performance.* 3rd ed. Mountain View, CA: Mayfield; 1997.

31. Simonton OC, Mathews-Simonton S, Creighton J. *Getting Well Again.* New York: St. Martin's; 1978.

32. Yukelson D. Psychology of sports and the injured athlete. In: Bernhardt DB, ed. *Sports Physical Therapy: Clinics in Physical Therapy.* New York: Churchill Livingstone; 1986.

33. Hardy C, Crace K. Dimensions of social support in dealing with sport injuries. In: Pargman D, ed. *Psychological Bases of Sport Injuries.* Morgantown, WV: Fitness Information Technology; 1993.

Chapter 6

The Cervical Spine

Wayne Stokes and Craig Denager

Treatment of cervical injuries requires a broad understanding of the soft-tissue structures, biomechanics, functional anatomy, and pathology to formulate a rehabilitation program. The history, physical examination, awareness of multiple diagnoses, and varied pain patterns can enable the therapist and physician to work in conjunction to achieve rewarding outcomes for patients. X-rays, MRIs, electrodiagnoses, and nerve blocks can supplement the diagnostic and treatment program.

It is important to recognize that multiple diagnoses may exist in the same patient, and that the prominence of each may shift in a recognizable pattern. Clinicians must continue to reevaluate and communicate to achieve pain-free range of motion, enhanced function, and early return to sport activity in patients.

ANATOMY AND BIOMECHANICS

The cervical spine is traditionally recognized to protect neural structures and provide support of the head. Its structural rigidity provides attachments for ligament and muscle and subsequently subserve mechanical motion. The cervical spine is unique and principles derived from the lumbar spine cannot always be directly applied to the cervical spine.

The cervical region is composed of seven vertebra with eight cervical roots and maintains a lordotic curve. The C1 to C2 atlantoaxial complex provides up to 50 percent of cervical rotation of the 80 degrees available (see Fig. 6–1A).[1]

The atlas consists of a bony ring with two lateral masses and no vertebral body. It articulates with the odontoid process of the axis on the atlas's posterior portion of the anterior arch. The odontoid limits movement backward of the axis. The transverse ligament of the axis functions as a restraint ligament posterior to the odontoid (see Fig. 6–1B).[2]

A synovial joint is formed between the facet of the posterior portion of the odontoid and the anterior portion of the transverse ligament. Rupture of the transverse alar ligament results in forward subluxation of C1 on C2 and subsequent spinal cord compression (see Fig. 6–1C). The superior articular process of the atlas rides on top of the lateral mass and articulates with condyles of the skull. This is the atlantooccipital joint (AO), and its shape helps stipulate the amount of motion present at the AO joint, which is primarily nodding.[3]

The AO joints are synovial joints with capsullary attachments that act as stabilizing restraints under tension and result in the head and atlas moving as one in rotation around the axis.[4] From the inferior surface of C2 through C7, the cervical vertebrae are termed typical. The vertebral body is smaller in relation to the posterior arch compared to the lumbar segment.[5]

The transverse process of C1 through C7 contain the foramen transversarium. The vertebral artery runs through this foramen from C1 through C6 (see Fig. 6–2). The uncovertebral joints, or joints of Luschka, are clefts that appear in the annulus fibrosis of the cervical intervertebral disk in later childhood at the location of the uncus.[6] The uncovertebral joint may provide protection to the cervical disk from prolapse. Degenerative changes and osteophytic bars can impinge upon the cervical spinal canal as well as the soft-tissue structures of the lateral foramen.[7]

These changes are quite concerning clinically when found on x-ray and on CT scan. The fissures that result in the formation of the uncovertebral joint increase the fibrocartilage content of the cervical disk compared to the

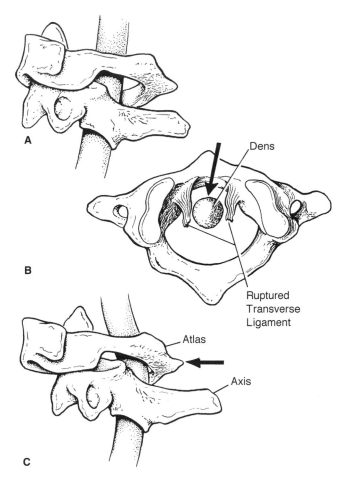

Figure 6–1. Rupture of the transverse ligament leads to forward subluxation of the axis. **A.** Normal anatomic relationship of the atlas, axis, and spinal cord. **B.** Overhead view showing rupture of the transverse ligament and loss of contact of the anterior arch of C1 and odontoid. **C.** Forward subluxation of C1 on C2 secondary to rupture of the transverse ligament. Note how the spinal cord can be compressed. (*From Schultz RJ. The Language of Fractures. Baltimore: Williams & Wilkins; 1972:183. With permission.*)

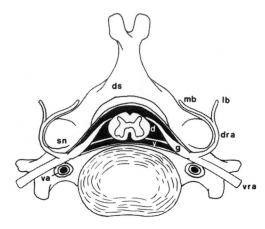

Figure 6–2. A top view of the course and relations of typical cervical nerve roots. (ds, dural sac; d, dorsal root; g, ganglion; v, ventral root; sn, spinal nerve; dra, dorsal ramuns; vra, ventral ramus; mb, medial branch; lb, lateral branch; va, vertebral artery.) (*From White AH, Schofferman JA. Spine Care. St. Louis: Mosby-Year Book; 1995; 2:830. With permission.*)

lumbar disk and may help explain the decreased frequency of cervical disk herniation.[8] The width and thickness of the posterior longitudinal ligament and decreased loads across the cervical spine may contribute to this phenomenon as well.[9] The cervical intervertebral disk and the zygapophyseal joints each distribute approximately half of the vertebral load.[10] This stands in contrast to the lumbar disk, which may transmit up to 85 percent of the axial load.[11]

The zygapophyseal joints (Z-joints) are formed by the inferior articular process of the higher vertebra and the superior articular process of the vertebra below. The Z-joint, or facet, is covered by an innervated fibrous capsule and the articular process itself is covered by smooth articular cartilage subject to high forces and degenerative changes. There are intra-articular inclusions of fibroadipose tissue most notably in the poles of the facet joints and a synovial membrane lines the capsule.[12]

The orientation of the facet joints of C3 through C7 allow for extension, flexion, and some rotation. They face backward and upward at an angle of approximately 45 degrees from the horizontal. This is in contrast to the lumbar facet joints, which allow only a small amount of axial rotation (see Figs. 6-3 and 6-4).[13] The end range of motion of the flexed cervical spine is felt to be more dependent on increased tension in the soft tissues of the neck as the comparison to bony facet compression forces preventing further flexion in the lumbar spine.[14] Extension of the neck decreases lateral foraminal size in the cervical spine. The spinal ligaments include the anterior longitudinal ligament along the anterior vertebral body, which may limit hyperextension. The posterior ligament in the cervical spine is an extension of the tectoria membrane and is located on the posterior aspect of the vertebral body, anterior to the spinal cord. It may protect against disk herniation by impinging upon the thecal sac. The ligament of flavum lies ventral to the facet joints. The capsule of the facet joints provide stability when the cervical spine is flexed.

The muscles of the cervical region include the suboccipital, multifidus, erector spinae, semispinalis, and splenius. In addition, the scalenes, trapezius, and levator scapulae play a significant role in the cervical spine. Injury to the soft-tissue structures contributes significantly to pain and dysfunction (see Fig. 6–5).

The suboccipital muscles control the nodding motion at the AO joint and rotation at the atlas axial joint. The semispinalis capitis, semispinalis cervicis, and longissimus capitis extend and rotate the head. The semispinalis capitis originates from the upper thoracic and cervical transverse process and inserts into the occipital base. It is a large muscle involved in head extension and may

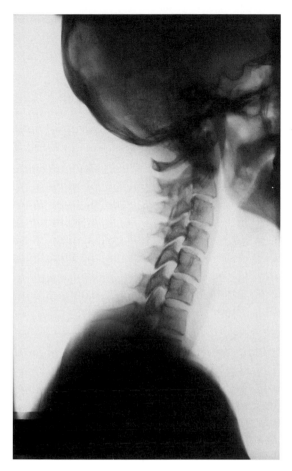

Figure 6–3. Lateral radiograph of the cervical spine.

play a significant role as a rein during flexion. The splenius extends the head and neck and the splenius capitis assists in rotation of the head in conjunction with the opposite sternocleidomastoid. The eructs spinae, which crosses multiple levels, is generally felt to assist in extension. The specific function of the multifidi in rotation has been debated. The unisegmental muscles of the spine may serve proprioceptive function because they contain the third highest density of muscle spindles, behind those of the eye and the hand (see Fig. 6-6).[15]

The levator scapulae attaches at the superior angle of the scapula and the first four cervical transverse processes and assists in elevation and downward rotation of the glenohumeral joint. Its relationship to neck pain and poor posture cannot be overlooked (see Fig. 6-7). The scalene muscles contribute significantly to myofascial pain patterns and neurovascular entrapment. The anterior and medial scalene attach to the first rib and the posterior scalene to the second rib. They assist in lateral motion, cervical spine stabilization, and respiration. The scalenes attach proximally at the transverse processes of the cervical vertebra, on the cervical nerves and roots. The paired cervical-spinal nerves that exit the cervical cord consist of motor fibers in the ventral root and sensory fibers going into the spinal cord in the dorsal root (see Fig. 6-8). The cervical spine nerves exit above the named vertebra, except for the C8 spinal nerve, which exits below the seventh cervical vertebra. The ventral and dorsal roots combine to leave the intervertebral foramen as a mixed spinal nerve root. When the

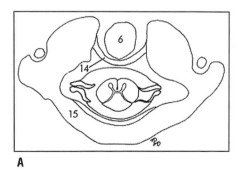

A

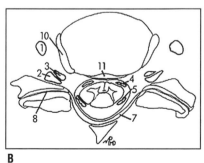

B

Figure 6–4. Schematic representations of the normal cervical spine at **(A)** C2 and **(B)** just above the inferior endplate of C4 (at the C4 to C5 intervertebral disk). (1, vertebral body; 2, dorsal root ganglion; 3 and 4, ventral roots; 5, dorsal root; 6, odontoid process; 7, ligamentum flavum; 8, facet joint; 9, neural foramen; 10, Luschka process; 11, posterior longitudinal ligament; 12, superior articulating process; 13, inferior articulating process; 14, transverse ligament; 15, lamina.) *(From Firooznia HF, Golimbu C, Raffi M, et al. MRI and CT of the Musculoskeletal System. St. Louis: Mosby-Year Book; 1992. With permission.)*

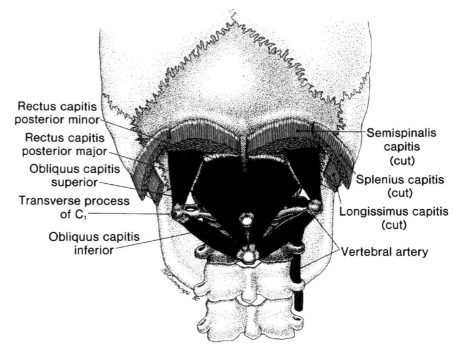

Figure 6–5. Attachments of the suboccipital muscles. The most lateral three of these four muscles define the suboccipital triangle. The triangle surrounds the transverse portion of the vertebral artery and should be avoided when injecting trigger points in the posterior neck muscles. *(From Travell JG, Simons DG. Myofascial Pain and Dysfunction: The Trigger Point Manual. Baltimore: Williams & Wilkins; 1983;1:323. With permission.)*

spinal root leaves the foramen, the dural sleeve terminates. The epineurium surrounds the nerve fibers.[16]

The ventral rami form the brachial plexus via C5 through T8, and C1 through C4 primarily supply much of the neck muscles (see Fig. 6-9). The sympathetic trunks are present along the entire spinal cord and their relationship to propagating chronic neck pain is imprecisely understood.

Nociceptive pain fibers and proprioceptive fibers are increasingly being documented in most segments of

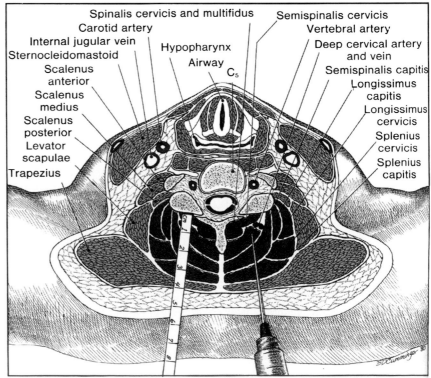

Figure 6–6. Cross-section of the neck through the C5 vertebra, which corresponds to the level of trigger point 1. The bony parts of the vertebra are stippled black and are outlined by a dark line surrounding black stipples. The rule shows that the 5-cm needle cannot penetrate the full depth of the posterior cervical muscles without compression of the skin. The vertebral artery is surrounded by the vertebral transverse processes. It travels anterior to and along the lateral border of the posterior cervical muscles. *(From Travell JG, Simons DG. Myofascial Pain and Dysfunction: The Trigger Point Manual. Baltimore: Williams & Wilkins; 1983;1:316. With permission.)*

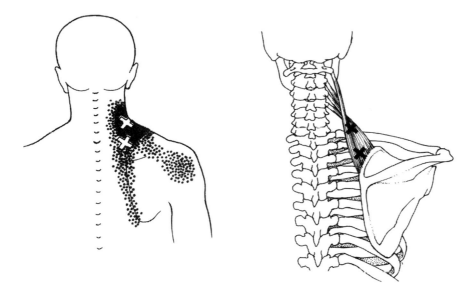

Figure 6–7. Consolidation referred pain pattern of the two trigger point locations (Xs) for the right levator scapulae muscle. The essential pain pattern is solid black and the spillover pattern is stippled. *(From Travell JG, Simons DG. Myosfascial Pain and Dysfunction: The Trigger Point Manual. Baltimore: Williams & Wilkins; 1983;1:335. With permission.)*

the spine. Abnormally sustained firing patterns of these fibers after injuries have healed may help explain the chronicity of cervical neck pain. Pain can be associated with mechanical pressure on nerve roots via herniated nucleus pulposus or osteophytic obstruction in the foramina, resulting in impairment of venous return of the nerve root. This may result in intraneural fibrosis, edema, and perineural fibrosis.[17] Neural peptides and inflammatory peptides, phospholipase A2, substance B, leukotrienes, bradykinins, and prostaglandins are increasingly being documented in the spinal canal after

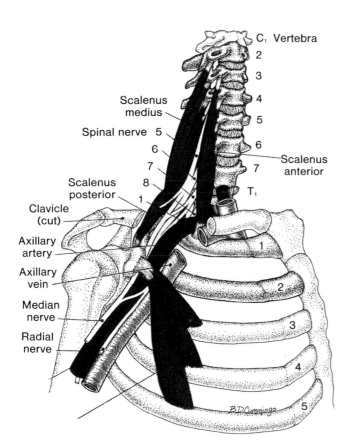

Figure 6–8. Thoracic outlet entrapment by the scalene muscles. The neuromuscular bundle is spread out to show the relations of its component parts. A portion of the clavicle has been removed. The brachial plexus and the axillary artery emerge above the first rib and behind the clavicle between the scalenus anterior and scalenus medius muscles. The spinal nerves are numbered on the left, the vertebrae on the right, and the vertebral nerves on the right. The T1 nerve lies dorsal to and beneath the subclavian artery. *(From Travell JG, Simons DG. Myofascial Pain and Dysfunction: The Trigger Point Manual. Baltimore: Williams & Wilkins; 1983;1:356. With permission.)*

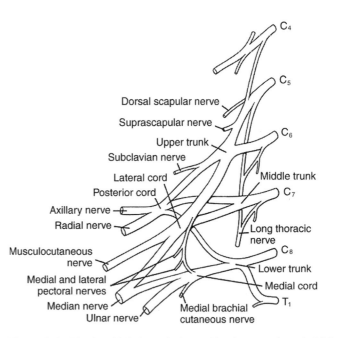

Figure 6–9. The brachial plexus is formed by the ventral rami of C5 through T1. *(From Seeley RR, Stephen TD, Tate P. Anatomy and Physiology. St. Louis: Mosby; 1989:9. With permission.)*

disk herniation. These chemical neural peptides may sensitize the dorsal root ganglion and pain receptors in the spinal cord and may sensitize nociceptive fibers.[18] Abatement of symptoms, including upper extremity paresthesias, radicular patterns, and motor weakness, early in the course of what appears to be a cervical radiculopathy may represent resolution of neural peptide mediated pain sensitization, or nerve dysfunction.

TREATMENT OF NECK AND CERVICAL SPINE PAIN

Rehabilitation of the neck and cervical spine is often challenging. A careful history and thorough physical exam will provide direction for a plan of care. The focus of this discussion is on the evaluation and rehabilitation of patients with cervical pain and dysfunction who present to a physician or an outpatient physical therapy center. The discussion will address four common conditions: disk lesions and foraminal encroachment, muscle strain, facet syndrome, and myofascial pain. This section will not address the recognition and management of fractures, dislocations, fractures with dislocations or injury to the spinal cord. The potential for these injuries must be recognized at the site of the event so that the patient can be properly transported and cared for. Rehabilitation of the cervical spine injured patient is beyond the scope of this chapter.

Evaluation

History
Patients present with a wealth of information that assists the physician and physical therapist in evaluation and treatment. Factors such as age, medical history, social history, occupation, history of sports participation, pain pattern, and onset of symptoms should be considered in forming a diagnosis and plan of care. An older patient with a history of neck pain of insidious onset presenting with radicular symptoms is more likely to be suffering from disk or bony changes, resulting in pressure on a spinal nerve. A younger patient presenting without a history of trauma, who reports an insidious onset of symptoms, demonstrates poor posture, and experiences high stress levels in their daily lives, is more likely to demonstrate a myofascial pain pattern. These myofascial pain patterns and the associated trigger points may represent a primary muscle dysfunction. However, injury to any portion of the vertebral motion segment including the disk, nerve soft structure, or facet capsular complex, may initiate or exacerbate myofascial pain patterns.

Brachialplexopathy must be considered in some patients, such as soccer players and football players, who present with cervical pain, upper extremity parathesias,

and motor deficits. Trauma that results in a whiplash mechanism will result in muscular strain. In collision sports such as football, facets syndromes can be coupled with muscle strains. These high-speed injuries can also result in ligamentous sprains, instability, and bony changes. Radiologic studies are essential in the complete evaluation of these injuries. This type of patient may also have an underlying bone or ligament injury that must be identified and treated.

Neck pain often persists beyond the expected time frame for healing of soft tissues, resulting in a myofascial pain pattern. Injury to any portion of the vertebral motion segment, including the disk, nerve, facet capsular complex, or fascia may also lead to the development of a myofascial pain pattern. These patients will relate a history of cervical strain or injury that initially caused pain that was centrally located with a subsequent achy, peripheral pain pattern. Finally, there are patients who present with painful, stiff necks that they relate to events such as a sudden turn or twist or "sleeping on it wrong." Often, the pain is very well localized, suggesting impingement within a facet.

The findings of the patient's history help clinicians identify the cause of symptoms, structure the physical examination, and identify appropriate radiologic and electrodiagnostic studies. In patients presenting with cervical pain and upper extremity parathesias, anterior-posterior, lateral, and oblique view X-rays can be supplemented with magnetic resonance imaging (MRI) or computed tomography (CT) to identify thecal sack encroachment, spinal nerve compression or displacement, and rule out more serious pathology (see Fig. 6–10). CT scanning is quite valuable in identifying fractures not seen on plain X-ray. It is felt that MRI is best utilized to evaluate soft-tissue structures. In patients with suspected cervical radiculopathy or brachialplexopathy, electromyography (EMG) is the test that will demonstrate physiologic changes in the nerve secondary to injury, identify the location of the injury, demonstrate the acuity of the injury, or demonstrate axonal damage. The physical exam and any diagnostic testing is directed at confirming or refuting the conclusions reached, rather than a blind search. During the history, patients may also report self-treatments such as stretching and posturing, which alleviate their symptoms. The importance of active listening cannot be overstated when examining patients with neck pain.

Physical Exam
The physical exam of the neck and cervical spine is similar to that of other orthopaedic conditions. The clinician should observe the patient movement patterns as they walk, sit, and remove coats and other clothing. Muscle atrophy and spinal alignment should be noted. Standing

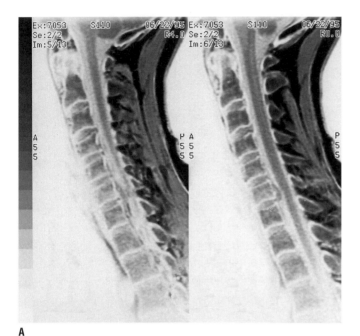

A

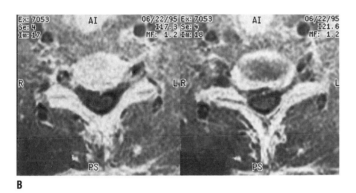

B

Figure 6–10. A, B. MRIs of cervical disk herniated nucleus pulposus (HNP).

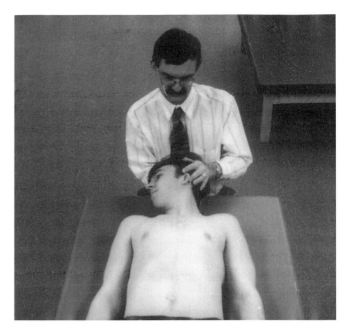

Figure 6–11. Manual cervical rotation.

while extending and side-bending the cervical spine, called Spurling's maneuver, may reproduce the patient's pattern of pain or parathesias. This maneuver narrows the intervertebral foramen and will further entrap a compromised nerve root. If this maneuver reproduces pain that is well localized to one vertebral segment, a facet syndrome may be the source of the patient's symp-

and sitting posture must also be evaluated. Poor posture and abnormal movement during daily activities can alter forces placed on the cervical spine. These stresses result in overuse of the extensor muscles that can perpetuate cervical pain patterns.

The clinician should assess the patient's willingness and ability to move the neck through all motions. Full, active, pain-free movement of the cervical spine should be the primary goal in most treatment programs (see Fig. 6-11). Rotation at the occipital-atlanto articulation can be assessed passively, as can segmental movements throughout the cervical spine. Side-gliding of the head in varying degrees of cervical flexion allow the clinicians to identify the source of motion restriction (see Fig. 6-12). Pain and motion restrictions are noted for active and passive movements. Manual compression

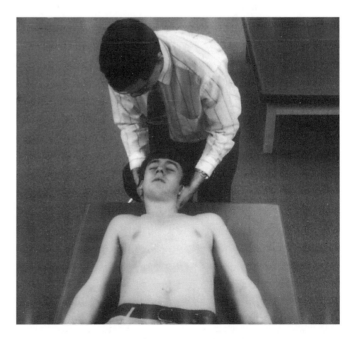

Figure 6–12. Manual side gliding.

toms. Distraction of the cervical spine may relieve symptoms of spinal nerve compression or facet dysfunction. An important finding is the relief of radicular symptoms with distraction that has been reported by patients. When distraction provides relief, distraction techniques can relieve suffering. This enables patients to alleviate or reduce their pain throughout the day. Psychologically, this empowers them in their ability to manage their condition. Manually resisted isometric contractions will identify weakness in the cervical musculature and elicit pain in cases of muscle strain. Palpation can help identify the site of a lesion, assess the degree of muscle spasm, and identify trigger points. The clinician should not interpret muscle spasm as confirmatory evidence of strain, as pain in the cervical region results in protective guarding and spasm. Incorporating a self stretching program is essential in the rehabilitation process (see Fig. 6–13).

Active range of motion of the upper extremities should also be measured. If motion is limited, passive range of motion must also be assessed. A neurologic exam assessing upper extremity strength, sensation, including response to pin prick and light touch, deep tendon reflexes, and proprioception yields valuable information regarding neurologic involvement. Loss of sensation or function in the upper extremities is a significant finding. In cases of disk injury or foraminal stenosis, surgery may be indicated if peripheral symptoms are severe or progressing. The relationship between cervical pathology and shoulder dysfunction must also be kept in mind. A C6 or C7 radiculopathy may result in abnormal function of the scapular stabilizers and rotator cuff. Impairment of the scapular stabilizers alters glenoid positioning, which can lead to the shoulder impingement syndrome and symptoms of instability.

In patients with nerve injury secondary to herniated disk injuries and stenosis, peripheral parathesias and radicular patterns may dominate the patient's oral history. Associated findings such as reflex changes, sensory abnormalities in a dermatomal pattern, and weakness in a myotomal distribution, suggest a diagnosis of radiculopathy. EMG and MRI further delineate the diagnosis. Also, other conditions such as thoracic outlet syndrome, entrapment of the ulnar nerve in the ulnar groove, or the median nerve in the carpal tunnel must be considered in patients with radicular symptoms in the upper extremity.

Myofascial trigger points have well-documented, reproducible referral patterns. Cervical facet referral patterns have also been documented in the posterior neck, scapular region, and upper extremity, but in a less precise and more overlapping manner. Thus, multiple pain and referral patterns may exist in one patient. These pain

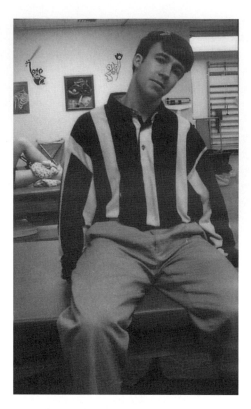

Figure 6–13. Cervical self-stretch.

patterns evolve over time. The hallmark of myofascial pain is the existence of exquisitely tender trigger points in the cervical, occipital, and periscapular regions. Patients with myofascial pain patterns frequently complain of headaches and neck pain that worsen throughout the day. Pain to palpation in the suboccipital, cervical, and scapular muscles may represent trigger points with relatively defined referral patterns that assist in making a diagnosis of myofascial pain.

Impingement at a cervical facet usually presents with well-localized tenderness and spasm of the cervical paraspinal muscles. It results in a restriction of sidegliding at the level of involvement. Examination of upper extremity function is rarely remarkable. The clinical examination correlates of facet syndrome are not fully understood. Altered mobility, restricted translation and side-gliding of the facet provide subtle clues, especially in patients with traumatic onset, an MRI without evidence of disk injury, and an absence of trigger points.

Patients with muscle strain will present with a history of a traumatic episode and often are reluctant to move their head and neck. Spasm and tenderness are evident. Patients with strains rarely complain of radicular symptoms. The clinician should rule out instability due to injury to the bony and ligamentous elements of the spine before assessing active and passive movements of the head and neck. The violent forces needed to cause strain injury are sufficient to injure these tissues. In fact, many patients referred for cervical strain injuries without evidence of instability probably have some involvement of surrounding connective tissues. In our view, the absence of trauma precludes the diagnosis of cervical strain in most cases. If one appreciates the forces required to injure muscle, pain of insidious onset is not consistent with the diagnosis. Many patients diagnosed with cervical strain are suffering from pain stemming from a facet or disk. All cervical pain can result in guarding and muscle spasm; thus spasm is insufficient evidence to confirm the existence of a muscle strain.

Treatment

Each of the conditions requires a different approach to treatment and responds at different rates. Muscular strains heal slowly as the body works through an acute inflammatory response to remove damaged tissue, a repair phase, and finally, tissue remodeling. In the acute phase, treatment should be directed at pain control and protection from further injury. Ice or moist heat and transcutaneous electrical nerve stimulation TENS may be used depending on how recently the injury occurred, the degree of pain and spasm, and the patient's preference. Analgesic and nonsteroidal antiflammatory medications can be quite helpful in the acute phase. As the symptoms of acute inflammation resolve, patients should be guided through a progression of exercises to restore range of motion, build endurance and strength in *the postural* muscles, improve postural awareness, and a return to all occupational and recreational pursuits.

Range of motion can be improved through muscle energy and proprioceptive neuromuscular facilitation (PNF) techniques as well as passive and active stretching. Soft-tissue restrictions, including ligamentous contracture and shortened muscles, respond well to these techniques. PNF contract and relax stretches work particularly well when treating spasm in the cervical musculature. The clinician should also assess and treat limitations stemming from abnormal arthrokinematics of facets. Painful, forced, stretching must be avoided. Pain will result in spasm and guarding and activation of the pain and spasm cycle.

Isometrically resisted cervical flexion, extension, side-bending, and rotation can be used to facilitate the restoration of strength. It has been our experience that patients complain that their cervical musculature fatigues easily after injury, while strength returns rapidly when pain resolves. Frequent, high-repetition bouts of exercise are more valuable than one intense bout. Enhancing postural awareness and general upper body conditioning can be as important as strengthening and stretching specific muscle groups.

Patients should gradually discontinue the use of cervical collars as their muscular endurance and postural awareness improves. Patients may return to work and recreational activities as symptoms permit. A patient with a sedentary job will likely be able to return to work sooner than someone employed in a job requiring a lot of physical effort. Likewise, returning to recreational pursuits such as swimming, hiking, or cycling will be tolerated sooner than sports such as wrestling, football, or gymnastics. The physician, therapist, and athletic trainer should work with the patient to individualize functional programs to meet the needs of each patient.

Some patients delay treatment following cervical strain. They usually present complaining of loss of motion and pain. In these patients, soft-tissue restrictions including ligamentous contracture and shortened muscles will respond to active and passive stretching. Restricted motion in the articular facet responds best to joint mobilization. The restricted motion may have multiple causes. The clinician must evaluate and address soft-tissue and facet involvement.

Facet dysfunction differs from muscle strain in presentation as well as treatment. Motion is usually restricted in side-bend and rotation to one side. Side-gliding at each cervical level will identify the site of dysfunction. There is usually not a history of trauma, but the onset may be acute; occurring with rapid rotation or side-bending. Muscle spasm is almost always present. Successful treatment depends on management of pain and spasm. Moist heat, TENS, gentle massage, and oral medications can be very helpful in the first few days of a painful facet dysfunction. Cervical mobilization and muscle energy techniques can then be used to restore facet arthrokinematics. Considerable relief is frequently achieved during the initial visit. Pain-free, unrestricted function is generally achieved within 2 weeks.

Occasionally, a patient will not respond to treatment or present with a more protracted history of pain and dysfunction. Unfortunately, facet dysfunction and irritation is not correlated to radiographic x-ray, CT scan, or MRI changes. The pain generators in the facet-joint, including the capsule, capsular joint inclusions, synovial lining, and subchondral bone, are not readily apparent on radiologic studies. Fluoroscopy-guided facet injections or procedures that anesthetize the medial branch of the dorsal rami that subserve the facet joint may block perpetuated nociceptive afferent input and alleviate symptoms. This procedure is diagnostic and therapeutic. Chronic facet irritation may result from degenerative changes in the cervical spine. The treatment approach described can assist these patients. Cervical traction may also provide relief of pain and increase range of motion (see Fig. 6–14). Unfortunately, symptoms often recur.

Conservative care of foraminal encroachment in the cervical spine due to bony changes, degenerative changes in the cervical disk, and acute cervical disk injuries can be frustrating for the patient and clinician. These patients usually present with complaints of radicular symptoms and burning pain in the neck and shoulders. Younger patients with acute lesions frequently do recover completely without surgical intervention. However, recovery can be slow and trying for the patient. Significant degenerative changes, resulting in radicular symptoms, often require surgical management to relieve pressure on the spinal nerves. Decisions on surgical intervention are often preceded by epidural blocks utilizing small amounts of anesthetic and anti-inflammatory corticosteroid preparations. The steroid preparation can counteract the sensitization of the nerve root and pain caused by the chemical mediators and neuropeptides. The anesthetic can interrupt the pain and spasm cycle and subsequently decrease stress across the cervical spine, providing considerable relief.

In all cases, the physician and physical therapist must address neck pain and muscle spasm. Therapeutic modalities may also benefit these patients. Frequently, patients identify positions that relieve symptoms. Flexion, rotation, side-bending, and distraction of the spine may decrease spinal nerve irritation and thus radicular symptoms. If radicular symptoms can be managed, the treatment approach is similar to that for cervical muscle strains. The emphasis of treatment should be dynamic control of the cervical spine to reduce radicular symptoms. Improved postural awareness and muscular endurance may alleviate some symptoms. The physician, physical therapist, and patient should work together to develop a progressive rehabilitation program. The goals should encompass daily cervical function, including driving where quick head movement and near normal cervical motion is required to back up, maneuver in traffic, and read signs. Patients with significant MRI changes, motor weakness, and pain, who fail to respond to conservative care, could benefit from surgery to decompress the spinal nerve. Postoperative therapy is similar to the preoperative course. Cervical range of motion is generally limited. When the tissues heal sufficiently, gentle active range-of-motion exercises and stretching should be encouraged. The clinician should also assess the arthrokinematics of the cervical facets. Gentle joint mobilization (grades II and III) can result in rapid improvement in range of motion. The clinician should also stress postural control and awareness as the patient builds endurance in the postural stabilizers and begins to decrease the use of a cervical collar, postoperatively.

Damage to the cervical intervertebral disks may result in localized discomfort, intermittent radicular symptoms, or constant, incapacitating radicular symptoms. Diagnosis is often difficult because other conditions such as thoracic outlet syndrome, entrapment of the axillary nerve and posterior humeral circumflex artery in the quadrangular space, ulnar nerve entrapment, cubital tunnel syndrome, and carpal tunnel syndrome can present with similar symptoms. TENS, heat or cold, and manual or mechanical traction may be useful in managing acute or more long-standing symptoms. Following acute injury, efforts are directed at managing the patient's symptoms and protecting the injured tissue. As symptoms abate, the course of rehabilitation is similar to that described in this chapter for foraminal encroachment. However, some patients do not respond to conservative care and continue to experience radicular symptoms. The decision on when surgical intervention is indicated is made by the surgeon and the patient.

Persistent pain in the neck, upper back, and shoulders is often best described as myofascial. Because there is no single cause of myofascial pain, there is no single treatment approach. Often the clinician must address stretching, postural awareness, stress reduction, and general overall conditioning. The hallmark finding in patients suffering from myofascial pain is the presence of

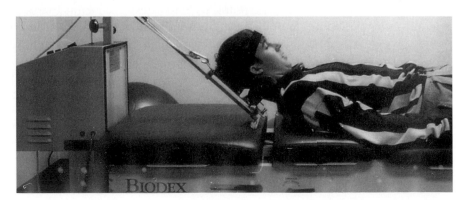

Figure 6–14. Cervical traction.

areas of localized tenderness called trigger points and decreased ROM.

Trigger points are hypersensitive to all forms of energy—mechanical, electrical, thermal, and acoustic. The clinician may direct initial treatments toward desensitization of trigger points and the initiation of pain-free exercise in a home exercise program. Stimulation of trigger points with brief (30 to 40 seconds), intense (noxious) stimulation is effective in desensitizing the trigger points and relieving pain. Long-phase duration (200 plus microseconds), low-frequency (2 to 5 pulses per second) TENS application is effective in trigger point treatment for many patients. A probe, approximately the size of the tip of a little finger, is used to maximize current density over the trigger point. In absence of these parameters, conventional TENS applied with small electrodes over the most sensitive points combined with moist heat may be effective. This treatment can be followed with acupressure and massage. In patients who are extremely sensitive, ultrasound over the trigger point for 30 to 40 seconds will elicit a burning, needling sensation similar to that achieved with long-phase duration, low-frequency TENS. Flouromethane spray and injection of trigger points with a local anesthetic can provide relief (see Fig. 6–15). This approach can also help confirm the diagnosis of myofascial pain and increase ROM. When combined with contract and relax stretching and active range-of-motion exercises, cervical motion can be greatly increased.

Myofascial release techniques are also effective in managing persistent neck pain of soft-tissue origin. Indirect release techniques, such as a suboccipital release, relieve stress on tense tissues and break the cycle of pain, tension, and spasm. Direct techniques are used to stretch tight fascial tissues. Abnormal joint mechanics may promote myofacial trigger points; conversely, muscle pain and dysfunction may lead to abnormal joint mechanics. Joint mobilization should be done to address restrictions in the articular facets. By treating soft tissue as well as joint restriction, the clinician promotes a better therapeutic outcome.

When trigger point therapy and myofascial release techniques are effective, the results are usually noted immediately with pain relief. In patients who respond, subsequent treatments can result in longer and longer periods of pain relief. A home program incorporating stretching and general upper extremity conditioning is invaluable in preventing recurrence of pain. Use of a TENS at home may also be effective in providing the patient with control of their symptoms. Many people "hold their stress" in their neck and shoulders. In fact, many have forgotten what it feels like to relax these muscles and do not realize how stress effects them.

Many activities of our society, including driving and working on a computer keyboard, contribute to a posture where the head is forward and the shoulders are rounded. Improved postural awareness and daily attention to a few simple exercises such as scapular retraction and chin tucks can have a dramatic impact within a few weeks. However, patients must be reminded that muscle reconditioning takes time. Improvement in flexibility and muscular endurance result from daily attention over a period of time. Moreover, when gains are made, they must be maintained through a regular exercise regimen.

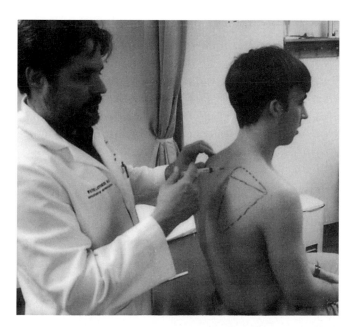

Figure 6–15. Injection into a trigger point.

SUMMARY

Treating patients with neck and upper back pain requires a thorough review of the patient's history and physical exam. Multiple anatomical sites may be injured and can be potentially the cause of an individual's pain. This results in complaints of neck pain and evidence of guarding muscle spasm and dysfunction. Careful evaluation is often the key to successful treatment. The physician, physical therapist, and athletic trainer have a number of treatment options available and work to match the problem with the most effective plan of care. Initial emphasis should be on decreasing pain and spasm, as well as improving motion. This should be followed by stretching and strengthening. Analysis of an individual's demands throughout the day is needed to establish a rehabilitation program. A failure to respond to treatment warrants a complete review of the patient's complaint and the plan of care.

Imaging and radiographic findings play a part in the development of the treatment and rehabilitation plan.

Hopefully, this chapter will assist the clinician in the evaluating and treating patients with neck pain and dysfunction but no evidence of spinal instability or spinal cord injury. Neck pain is a common complaint among patients. However, the causes of neck pain are not fully understood, making the treatment of neck pain a challenge.

REFERENCES

1. Heulke D, Nusholtz G. Cervical spine biomechanics: A review of the literature. *J Orthop Res.* 1986;4:232–245.
2. Dvorak J, Panjabi MM. Functional anatomy of the alar ligaments. *Spine.* 1987;12:183.
3. White AA, Panjabi MM. The clinical biomechanics of the occipitoatlantis-axial complex. *Clin Orthop.* 1978;9:867.
4. Bogduk N. Anatomy of the spine. In: White AH, Schofferman JA, eds. *Spine Care.* St. Louis: Mosby; 1995;2:822.
5. Greenman PE. *Principles of Manual Medicine.* Baltimore: Williams & Wilkins; 1989:50.
6. Hayashi K, Yakubi T. Origins of the uncus and of Luschka's joint in the cervical spine. *J Bone Joint Surg.* 1985;67:788.
7. Twomey LT, Taylor JR. Development and growth of the cervical and lumbar spine. In: White AH, Schofferman JA, eds. *Spine Care.* St. Louis: Mosby; 1995;2:794.
8. Twomey LT, Taylor JR. Development and growth of the cervical and lumbar spine. In: White AH, Schofferman JA, eds. *Spine Care.* St. Louis: Mosby; 1995;2:794.
9. Bland JH, Boushey DR. Anatomy and physiology of the cervical spine. *Semin Arthritis Rheum.* 1990;20:1.
10. Pal GP, Sherk HH. The vertical stability of the cervical spine. *Spine.* 1988;13:447.
11. Miller, JAA, Haderspeck KA, Schultz AB. Posterior element loads in lumbar motion segments. *Spine.* 1983;8:331.
12. Bogduk N. Anatomy of the spine. In: White AH, Schofferman JA, eds. *Spine Care.* St. Louis: Mosby; 1995;2:12.
13. Greenman PE. *Principles of Manual Medicine.* Baltimore: Williams & Wilkins; 1989:126.
14. Twomey LT, Taylor JR. *Physical Therapy of the Low Back.* New York: Churchill-Livingstone; 1987.
15. Bogduk N, Twomey LT. *Clinical Anatomy of the Lumbar Spine.* 2nd ed. Melbourne: Churchill-Livingstone; 1991.
16. Sunderland S. *Nerves and Nerve Injuries.* 2nd ed. New York: Churchill-Livingstone; 1978.
17. Parke W. The significance of venous return impairment in ischemic radiculopathy and myelopathy. *Orthop Clin North Am.* 1991;22:213.
18. Weinstein J. Neurogenic and non neurogenic pain and inflammatory mediators. *Orthop Clin North Am.* 1991;22:235.

Chapter 7

The Thoracic Spine

Differential Diagnosis for Thoracic Pain

Jacob Heydemann

There are many possibilities to consider when the athlete presents with thoracic pain. Pain in the thoracic spine, as in many other places of the body, is commonly a muscular pain due to overuse or straining. It can be related to specific events or activities in which the athlete participated. Throwing, twisting, rotational-type activities such as golf, tennis, or throwing-type sports may cause a straining or pulling of the muscles of the chest wall or the thoracic paraspinous muscles. Lifting-type sports may also cause transient muscular pain. These pains are often acute in onset, short lived, responding to a period of modification of activity, ice, massage, and anti-inflammatories.

Pain in the thoracic portion of the body may also be associated with a specific traumatic event such as direct blow, fall, or violent impact. These types of injuries may be associated with contusions or fractures of the bony structures of this region. Fractures may occur in the spine, ribs, or scapula. Fractures of the spine may be associated with neurologic involvement. Fractures of the ribs may be associated with injuries to the chest wall or pleura, or the chest cavity, lungs, heart, or vascular structures of the aorta and subclavian region. Lower rib fractures may be associated with visceral trauma to the spleen or liver. Fractures of the scapula may be associated with chest wall trauma or neurologic or vascular insult.

Pain associated with lifting, torsional or twisting activities may also cause a thoracic disk herniation. Rarely are they associated with falls; they may be associated with a preexisting spinal abnormality of Scheuermann's disease or progressive wedging of the vertebral bodies. This type of pain is quite variable in presentation.

Pain may also be secondary to an infection or tumor. This pain develops for no apparent cause and is of a progressive, unrelenting nature that does not respond to modification of activity. The pain may present not only as daytime pain but as nighttime pain. This type of pain would raise a suspicion of an infection that could be intraspinal, intrathoracic, or intra-abdominal. It may also raise the suspicion of a tumor. Benign or malignant, tumors may occur in the thoracic region either as primary or metastatic. These tumors may present in the thoracic region within the spinal canal, spinal column, thorax, or abdomen.

Pain may also arise from a vascular origin. This pain may be associated with an aneurysm of the aorta or of the subclavian vessels. It may be of a neurogenic origin such as injury to the long thoracic nerve. Injury to the spinal segmental nerves may cause rib cage pain or may be a viral infection of the rib cage segmental nerves, such as shingles, which can be associated with severe pain, burning, and itching. Visceral pain from the abdominal cavity irritating the phrenic nerve of the diaphragm can be felt in the shoulder area.

In summary, one must always look for a history of trauma or injury. One should always try to localize the pain to a specific area. With specific traumatic injuries such as fractures, one must rule out injury to associated structures of the lung, abdomen, vasculature, and nerves. If a specific event cannot be defined and the pain is unrelenting, progressive, and associated with night-time pain, one must consider tumors and infection in a differential diagnosis.

TRAUMA

The majority of injuries to the thorax are sprains, strains, contusions, or deep bruising. The player is knocked to the ground and has the wind knocked out. This is a forceful expiration secondary to an acute upward migration of the diaphragm. The player will temporarily feel short of breath and have difficulty insufflating from the associated pain from the blow. The athlete often responds to a brief period of rest. Strains and sprains are more commonly associated with lifting, twisting, and rotational-type injuries. The muscle is suddenly contracted or stretched with such force as to cause a partial tearing of these structures. Most commonly, this is seen in lifting-type sports, but may also be seen in activities such as golf, baseball, throwing sports, and volleyball.

Common types of blunt trauma include blast injuries, which can produce cardiac and pulmonary contusion, and rupture of the tracheal bronchial tree and the diaphragm. Crushing injuries are often associated with disruption of the chest wall, diaphragm, or tracheal bronchial tree. Deceleration injuries are found to occur to the chest wall, lung, myocardium, bronchi, and aorta. Hypertension injuries occasionally disrupt the intrathoracic portion of the thoracic duct. Flexion injuries produce overlapping transverse sternal fractures. Penetrating chest injuries can be produced by either knife or missile. They may be associated with pulmonary and vascular complications. Wounds at the base of the neck and upper part of the thorax may involve the trachea, larynx, great vessels, thoracic duct, esophagus or lungs. Wounds in the midthorax may damage the heart, aorta, or lungs. Penetrating injuries in the lower chest may involve the lungs, diaphragm, spleen, liver, stomach, or colon. One must carefully assess the entrance and exit sites and note the respiratory pattern of the patient, skin color, and degree of distress. When chest wall instability is present, this must be partially stabilized either by pressure dressing or sandbags, or if

available, positive pressure assisted ventilation. When there is a sucking wound, it must be occluded by a dressing such as petroleum jelly on gauze. Large air and fluid collections must be evacuated with a chest tube. Most thoracic trauma is accompanied by some degree of chest wall damage, ranging from localized contusion to extensive flail disruption. Contusions may be associated with localized pain, interference with respiration, and coughing. Contusions should be treated as simple rib fractures with symptomatic management. They usually resolve within 1 to 2 weeks. Simple rib fractures are usually caused by a direct blow to the chest wall. Pain is of sudden origin and aggravated by sudden motion. The fracture site is always tender. Crepitation may be palpated. Anterior, posterior, or lateral compression of the chest wall may elicit pain that can be localized to a specific rib area. Treatment of simple rib fractures is symptomatic. The physician must determine whether there has been an associated intrapleural collection of blood or air, and whether or not this is large enough to require evacuation with a chest tube. Flail-type chest injuries typically result from fractures of at least three consecutive ribs each in two or more places. Posterolateral lateral flail chest is the most common site. This is due to a momentary driving of the scapula into the chest. These injuries can be associated with severe chest wall contusion, interruption of the intercostal vessels and nerves, as well as bleeding. Contusion and laceration of the lung may occur, producing a hemopneumothorax. The patient will exhibit painful, rapid, shallow, grunting respiration. The flail segment is visible and palpable as it moves paradoxically with respiratory effort. In other words, as the patient breathes in, the chest wall will move out, and vice versa. These patients require ventilatory assistance and intubation with positive pressure ventilation.

The rib fractures in the lower ribs may also be associated with injury to the visceral structures of the abdomen. Structures at greatest risk are the liver, spleen, and kidneys. One must look for associated rigidity of the abdomen, tightness of the abdominal muscle, pain with pressure to the abdomen, diffuse tenderness about the abdomen, and flank tenderness in the lower back. This may or may not be associated with swelling or bruising. One must also check the urine for anuria (the lack of urine production) or hematuria (blood in the urine). Injuries to the visceral structures may cause acute changes such as abdominal rigidity, hypovolemia, hypotension, and tachycardia; but may also be associated with slow leaks that can take some time to present following the trauma to these visceral structures. Several days may pass during which the patient develops progressive abdominal pain, blood pressure changes, hypotension, and progressive anemia. These visceral injuries can be life threatening; either acutely or subacutely. Penetrating injuries of the chest produce two problems. The first is a potentially open wound in the chest wall. The second is a perforation or laceration of the intrathoracic or intra-abdominal organs or both. The classic sucking wound of the thorax consists of a chest wall defect with missed air on inspiration, but acts as a flat valve to prevent expulsion or expiration. This leads to a tension pneumothorax that must be treated with evacuation of the air.

In the chest cavity area, one must be aware of specific signs and symptoms associated with a tension pneumothorax or hemothorax. There will be acute respiratory changes, and rapid breathing may be noted. The patient may have difficulty breathing; short, shallow breaths may be all the athlete is capable of. There may be associated chest wall asymmetry. Because of this, the patient may become cyanotic. One may note a tracheal deviation with a tension pneumothorax where the windpipe has been pulled off to the side on the expanded lung. There may be associated air in the soft tissues or subcutaneous emphysema. With this particular disorder, the skin and soft tissues will have a crackly-type feel. This is due to the injection of air into the soft tissues. If there is a penetrating injury, air may be sucked into the chest cavity, collapsing the lung as the vacuum effect of the chest cavity is lost. In such instances, there are absent or diminished breath sounds on that side. Associated with a tension pneumothorax is a distention of the neck veins as well. Treatment is emergent. One must maintain or reestablish an airway and ventilate the patient. Ventilation may require an emergency intubation or assistive mechanical ventilation. For a tension pneumothorax, a large-bore needle must be placed into the second intercostal space along the midclavicular line to relieve the pressure within the lung cavity on the collapsed side. Once the patient has been stabilized, further study including chest x-ray and possibly chest tube placement can be done. The sucking wound to the chest wall should be occluded with a dressing of petroleum gauze and elastoplast to prevent further air entry while the pneumothorax is evacuated with a chest tube.

Spinal fractures in the thoracic spine are generally stable as the rib cage provides stability to the spinal column. This is true up until the thoracolumbar junction, which is an area of increased propensity for unstable injuries. Multiple types of fractures may occur to the spinal column. In the immature spine, vertebral end plate fractures may occur. These fractures are seen as small bone fragments attached to the ring apophysis of the vertebra that may become displaced with this fragment of bone. This is an epiphyseal or growth-plate type fracture. It may act like a herniated disk and present with radicular-type symptoms. These fractures are more common in the lumbar spine than in the thoracic spine. Major column fractures more commonly occur at the thoracolumbar junction, because of the greater risk of instability at this area. Denis divided the spinal column into three segments. The anterior is made of the anterior vertebral body, the anterior annulus fibrosis, and the anterior longitudinal ligament. The middle column is made of the posterior vertebral body, posterior annular fibrosis, and the posterior longitudinal ligament (see Fig. 7-1). The posterior column is made of the posterior laminar arch, supraspinous ligament, interspinous ligament, posterior lateral capsule, and ligamentum flavum.

Several fracture types can occur based on this division of spinal columns. The compression-type fracture is secondary to failure of the anterior column (see Fig. 7-2A). These are mostly stable fractures. Unless the fracture is greater than 50 percent of vertebral body height, it can be treated with an external brace. When the fracture is greater than 50 percent of the vertebral body height, the posterior longitudinal ligament fails and a posterior spinal fusion is indicated with instrumentation for spinal stabilization.

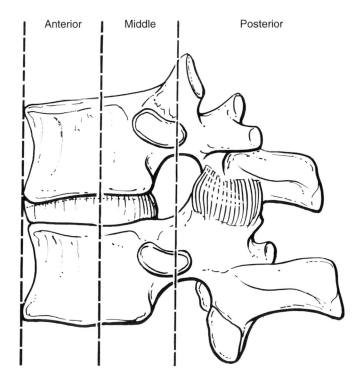

Figure 7–1. The three segments of the spinal column: anterior, middle, posterior.

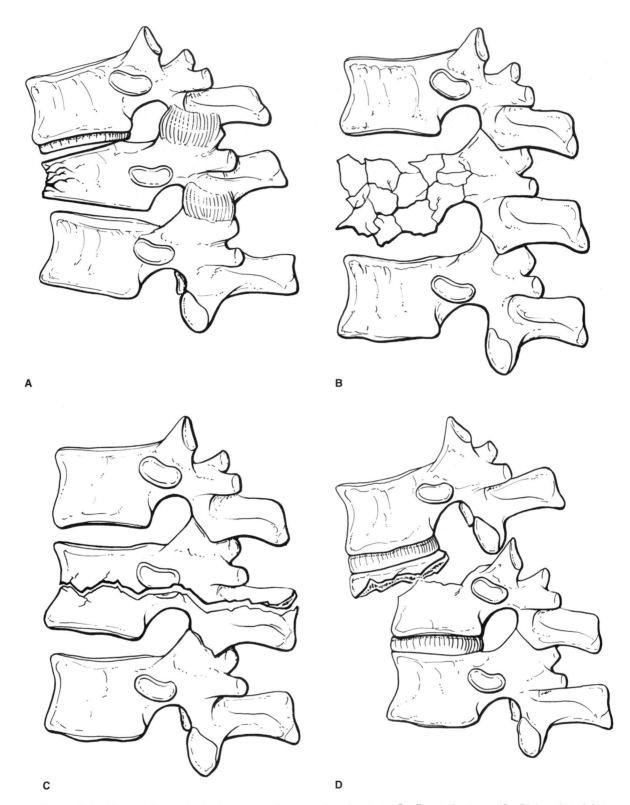

Figure 7–2. Types of spinal fractures. **A**. Compression fracture. **B**. Burst fracture. **C**. Dislocation injury. **D**. Fracture-dislocation.

A burst fracture is a failure of the spine under compression of the anterior and middle column (see Fig. 7–2B). Usually, this involves the lower thoracic, thoracolumbar junction as well as the lumbar portion of the spine. There may be mechanical instability or neurologic instability. This means that the spine itself may be unstable, but the patient is neurologically intact, or the patient may have neurologic compromise even though the spinal column does not appear to be significantly displaced into the spinal canal. A CT scan is needed to help define the degree of spinal canal compression. If the degree of compression of the vertebra is less than 60 percent collapse, either a posterior or an anterior fusion is indicated. If the fracture is greater than 60 percent collapse, an anterior surgical procedure with a buttress grafting is indicated.

The third type of fracture is the seat belt flexion distraction injury (see Fig. 7–2C). There are three types. These are commonly referred to as "chance" type fractures. In type 1, the fracture travels through the vertebral body and then through the spinous process. In type 2, the fracture travels through the vertebral body and between the spinous processes. And in type 3, the fracture travels through the vertebral body and asymmetrically through the posterior elements of the vertebra. An MRI is necessary to rule out disk displacement and to assess the approach for surgical stabilization.

If all three columns fail in compression with rotation, a fracture-dislocation may occur (see Fig. 7–2D). These are always unstable injuries and always require surgery. They most commonly occur at the thoracolumbar junction (see Fig. 7–3A,B).

Instability can be defined in three degrees. First-degree instability is mechanical. This is where there is a fracture of the vertebral body without neurologic compromise and there is risk of a progressive kyphosis (or rounding of the back). Second degree instability is neurologic and commonly seen with a collapsing burst fracture where a fragment protrudes into the spinal canal. Finally, there is a mechanical and neurologic instability. This type of instability is associated with the unstable

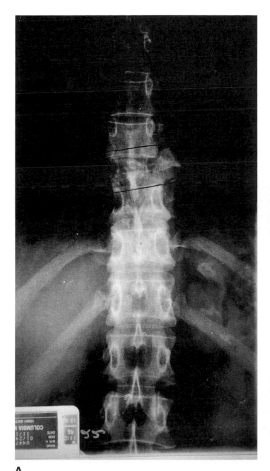

A

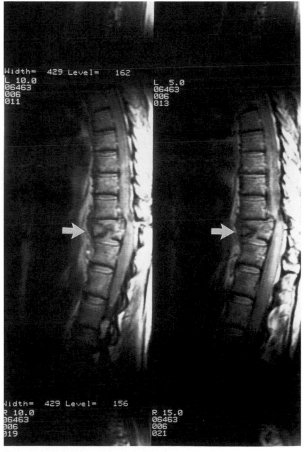

B

Figure 7–3. A, B. Fracture-dislocation.

burst fracture or the fracture with dislocation. This is most commonly a three column injury—anterior, middle, and posterior. Instability requires surgical stabilization.

Minor fractures may also occur. These are fractures of the transverse process that are associated with direct blow type trauma. Violent muscle contraction can also be associated with transverse process fractures. Track spinous process fractures are most commonly associated with a direct blow. Articular process fractures are also associated with a direct blow. These types of fractures are all considered stable. But another type of minor fracture, a fracture of the pars interarticularis, may or may not be stable. These fractures are commonly seen with the gymnast who does extension type backflips, the cheerleader who does similar stunts, and the interior lineman who does extension blocking. Pars interarticularis fractures may be associated with more significant trauma such as motor vehicle accidents. These associated traumatic injuries need to be ruled out with a CT scan. Treatment of pars interarticularis fractures, when identified either radiographically or with bone scan, is treated with a thoraco-lumbosacral orthosis (TLSO) until the symptoms have abated. Rarely, isolated or limited fusion is indicated. This is more common if the pars interarticularis defect is associated with a progressive spondylolisthesis than as an isolated injury.

All fractures of the spine need accurate neurologic assessment. Any suspicion of a fracture should be referred immediately for medical attention. In the thoracic spine, the physician needs to carefully examine not only the segmental distribution through the chest and upper abdomen, but also the lower extremities for possible nerve root involvement. If paralysis does occur, it may be transient or persistent. Transient paralysis is associated with spinal cord shock. Generally, spinal shock will resolve within 48 hours. The bulbocavernosus reflex is considered the critical determinant of the resolution of spinal shock. When the bulbocavernosus reflex returns or 48 hours passes, the period of spinal shock is felt to have resolved.

Common signs and symptoms of fractures of the spinal column are consistent with any fracture. An examiner would expect to see acute, localizing pain. There may be associated swelling due to hematoma or deformity of the spine if there has been an unstable injury. One may be able to palpate an acute angulatory or kyphotic, gibbous deformity, displacement of the spine, or widening of the interspinous space.

Treatment of spinal fractures, if stable, requires immobilization for pain management. If the fractures are associated with an unstable injury, then immobilization requires rigid fixation. For transporting these individuals, a spine board and sandbags are necessary. Because these injuries are often associated with significant trauma, medical stabilization of airway, breathing, and circulation must be carried out as well.

The last group of fractures for this region is the scapular fractures. Scapular fractures are unusual in their occurrence composing 1 percent of total body fractures. Fifty percent of these fractures involve the scapular spine and body, 25 percent the glenoid, 10 percent the acromion, and 7 percent the coracoid. Scapular fractures are usually high-energy injuries. Therefore, greater than 80 percent of scapular fractures are associated with other trauma. Associated signs and symptoms of scapular fractures are a point tenderness to the area of the scapula, decreased shoulder motion, swelling to the area, and bruising. Associated chest trauma, fractured ribs, pneumothorax, and vascular injuries to the major vessels such as the subclavian artery and vein must be ruled out. Treatment of scapula fractures most commonly requires immobilization as the majority are nondisplaced. Symptomatic treatment for pain management is appropriate. Fractures that are displaced, especially those involving the articular region of the glenoid, do require surgical management.

The last major trauma injury to the thoracic portion of the body is a very rare scapulothoracic dissociation or dislocation. The etiology of this injury is that of a severe, direct blow laterally that displaces the scapula with associated traction to the upper extremity. The scapula tears away from the posterior chest wall. This injury may commonly be associated with fractures to the area and there may be injury to the subclavian vessels or axillary vessels, as in the displaced scapular fractures. The associated signs and symptoms of this region are a history of violent trauma and massive swelling. There will be significant lateral displacement of the scapula and most commonly, a pulseless extremity. There may be complete or partial brachial plexus palsy. Treatment involves stabilizing the fractures, immobilizing the arm, and evaluating the neurovascular insult and treating it as needed. Surgery is often necessary and is dependent upon the degree of neurovascular involvement of the glenohumeral joint, as is amputation of the arm above the elbow, depending upon the degree of neurovascular involvement.

Traumatic pain can also be associated with neurogenic origin. Thoracic disk herniation is associated with a traumatic event 25 to 50 percent of the time. These events are generally torsional or twisting injuries and are rarely associated with falls. Presentation of a herniated disk in the thoracic spine is that of pain, which can be quite variable from constant to intermittent and dull to sharp. It can be associated with axial unilateral or bilateral radiculopathy or pain that is circumferential around the chest. It can be aggravated by a cough, sneeze, or increase in exertion. There may be associated groin, chest, or abdominal pain depending on the level of the herniation. There may be associated neck pain, upper extremity involvement, and Horner syndrome. Horner syndrome is drooping of the eye with a small pupil and decreased sweating on the injured side of the face. This would be seen with a herniated disk when the lesion is in the area of T1 and T2. There may be associated numbness, paresthesias, dysesthesias, motor weakness, and possibly bladder dysfunction. The levels of these findings will be dependent upon the level of the herniation in the thoracic spine. Treatment of a herniated disk in the thoracic spine depends on whether or not there is associated myclopathy. Without myelopathy the treatment is nonsurgical; rest, anti-inflammatories, and possibly a brace. Physical therapy with postural training, hyperextension, strengthening, back school, and cardiovascular conditioning are also appropriate. When there is associated myelopathy, then management is surgical.

Scheuermann's disease is another cause of back pain (see Fig. 7-4). This is a wedging of three or more thoracic vertebra in a row of greater than 10 degrees each. This is most commonly seen in adolescence. It may progress and lead to a significant functional and cosmetic deformity. Early intervention includes a course of bracing, or if the curve becomes excessive or is unresponsive to bracing, surgical intervention is indicated. Scheuermann's disease may be associated with a thoracic herniated disk.

Other possible causes for neurogenic back pain are injury to the long thoracic nerve. A palsy of the long thoracic nerve will lead to shoulder pain, winging of the scapula, and difficulty lifting the arm. The long thoracic nerve is unprotected at the inferior margin of the scapula. Nerve palsy is associated with either nerve compression with anterior scapular motion or nerve traction associated with posterior scapular movement. Treatment of the long thoracic nerve palsy is often expectant. These lesions often resolve on their own without any intervention. When the palsy is persistent, and the winging is significant, a muscle transfer may be indicated.

INFECTION

When back pain cannot be associated with a traumatic event, the possibility of an infectious etiology or a malignancy must be considered. Infections may occur anywhere in the spine and appear either as a diskitis or

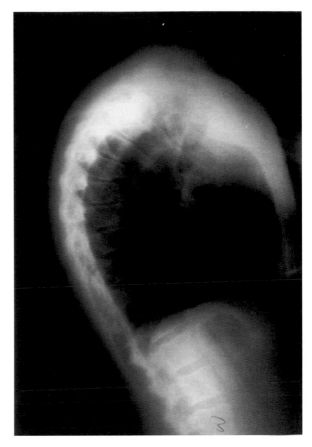

Figure 7–4. Scheuermann's disease.

an osteomyelitis. Signs and symptoms of osteomyelitis and diskitis are very similar, such as back pain that can be relentless, most commonly as night pain, as well as day pain. There may be associated fever. There is a higher incidence of osteomyelitis in paraplegics and in IV drug abusers. Laboratory studies will show an elevated sedimentation rate and C-reactive protein. Blood cultures may or may not be positive. Diagnosis depends on needle aspiration or needle biopsy of the vertebral body. X-ray changes may be present. Soft-tissue swelling may be noted as well as bony changes. An MRI is often helpful in the evaluation of these infections. Treatment of an osteomyelitis is 6 weeks of IV antibiotics, bracing, and careful neurologic assessment. If neurologic compromise occurs or there is failure of response to the IV antibiotics, surgery is indicated.

A diskitis may present with localizing pain and tenderness, back spasm, fever, neurologic deficits, tension signs, back pain, radicular pain, and spinal deformity. It may also present as an abdominal pain. A C-reactive protein, sedimentation rate, and cultures of the blood and

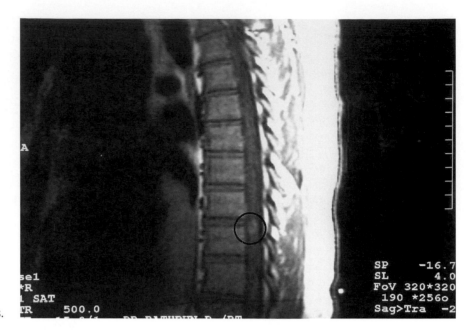

Figure 7–5. Epidural abscess.

urine are indicated. An MRI is often helpful in diagnosing a diskitis. Treatment is IV antibiotics, bracing, and rest. Surgery is indicated only when there is a failure to respond.

Epidural abscesses may also occur in and around the spine (see Fig. 7-5). This is associated with acute spinal pain, fever, and neurologic changes. Laboratory evaluations will show an elevated sedimentation rate and an elevated WBC count. Blood cultures are indicated. X-rays will show soft tissue swelling around the spine. CT myelogram is indicated. Treatment is IV antibiotics and surgery if there is neurologic involvement or failure to respond to antibiotic therapy.

TUMORS

Lastly, tumors must always be considered in the differential diagnosis. Tumors may occur in the soft tissues or bone structures (see Fig. 7-6), within the spinal column (see Fig. 7-7), nerves (see Fig. 7-8), from visceral origin, abdomen, or within the lung or chest wall cavity. They may be primary tumors or metastatic lesions and they may be a direct cause of pain due to expansion within the direct spinal structures or they may be associated with referred pain of visceral origin in the abdomen. This pain will be relentless and will not respond to alteration of activity. The pain will be progressive with associated weakness, weight loss, and

fatigue. There may or may not be associated bone tenderness or deformity depending on the origin. There may or may not be neurologic changes depending on the site of the tumor. When there are x-ray changes of spinal tumors on repeated radiographs, the lesions are often destructive. They may be expansile or they may cause vertebral collapse, such as in leukemia. Appropriate radiographic studies are indicated followed by biopsy and treatment as warranted by the nature of the tumor.

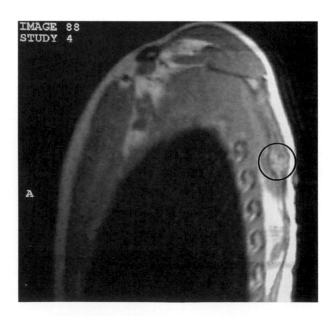

Figure 7–6. Scapular osteochondroma.

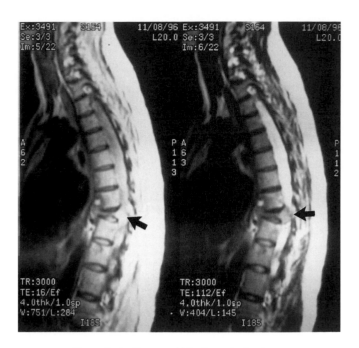

Figure 7–7. Tumor within the spinal column.

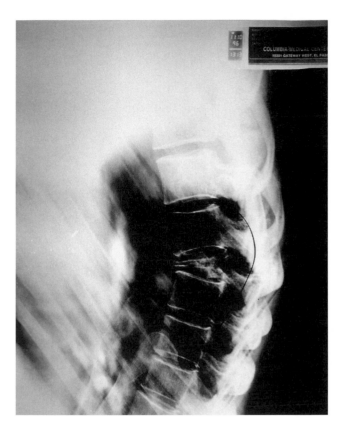

Figure 7–8. Tumor within the spinal nerves.

SELECTED READINGS

Fractures

Bohlman HH. Treatment of Fractures and Dislocations of the Thoracic and Lumbar Spine. *J Bone Joint Surg.* 1985; 67A: 165-169.

Denis F. The three column spine and its significance in the classification of acute thoracolumbar spinal injuries. *Spine.* 1983;8:817-831.

Thoracic Disk Herniation

Brown CW, Deffen PA Jr, Ahmabjian J, et al. The natural history of thoracic disc herniation. *Spine.* 1992;17(suppl 6):S97-S102.

Spinal Injections

Currier BL, Eismont FJ. Injections of the spine. In: Rothman RH, Simeone FA, eds. *The Spine.* 3rd ed. Philadelphia: Saunders; 1992.

Vincent KA, Benson DR. Differential diagnosis and conservative treatment of infectious diseases. In: Frymoyer JW, ed. *The Adult Spine: Principles and Practice.* New York: Raven; 1991; 1.

Tumors

Gubta RK, Alansari AG. Value of image guided needle aspiration in the assessment of thoracolumbar and sacrococcygeal masses. *ACTA Cytologica.* 1996 March-April 40(2): 215-221.

Thoracic Trauma

Head JM. Thoracic emergencies. In: Wilkens EW Jr, ed. *MGH Textbook of Emergency Medicine.* Baltimore; Williams & Wilkins; 1978.

Dislocation

Rockwood CA. Subluxations and dislocations about the shoulder. In: Rockwood CA Jr, Green DP, eds. *Fracture in Adults.* 2nd ed. Philadelphia: Lippincott; 1984.

Management of Thoracic Dysfunction

Louie Zuniga

This section includes a brief description of the anatomy and kinesiology of the thoracic spine. Although extensive literature exists for the cervical and lumbar spines, information regarding the thoracic spine is relatively sparse. The region anchors the movement of the shoulder as well as the muscles of respiration. Early studies by Lovett and later Fryette attempted to produce models for identification of movement coupling the multiple articulations between the vertebrae and ribs. Later, Panjabi, White, and associates studied movement and stability within the thoracic spine and its articulations with the costovertebral joint. The coupled movements allow for the kinesiologic chain of events between the hips and shoulders in the throwing motion or the overhead hit in a tennis swing (see Fig. 7-9). It is the base upon which rotation between the still head and leading hips occurs in the powerful golf swing. It anchors the scapula for the precise backhand in tennis or sustained and repeated overhead postures for the volleyball setter and hitter.

This chapter will link the mechanics of the movements to potential dysfunction and provide solutions through the use of manual treatment approaches and exercise. This section is not intended to be an extensive explanation of the osseous or soft-tissue structure of the thoracic spine.

ANATOMY

The thoracic spine consists of 12 vertebrae divided into three sections. The middle four are considered typical, the top and bottom four are considered atypical. Typical thoracic vertebrae have a heart-shaped body when viewed from above and an almost always round vertebral canal. T1 looks more like a cervical vertebra, has almost horizontal transverse processes, and possesses a full facet on the superior edge to accommodate the first rib. Each vertebra in the thoracic spine possesses at least one facet on its body to accommodate a rib. T1 to T10 have articular facets on their transverse processes to provide attachment for the first ten ribs. The relative size of the body of the thoracic spine increases as the spine moves caudal to accommodate for increasing weight-bearing requirements through the spine (see Fig. 7-10).

The orientation of the facets or zygapophyseal joints is in a coronal plane in the thoracic spine. In the uppermost portion of the thoracic spine between C7 and T1, the facets tend to resemble the cervical spine; moving in a more coronal orientation through the midthoracic spine to become sagittal at T12 and L1 (see Fig. 7-11).

Each vertebra is separated by an intervertebral disk. The disks in the thoracic spine are thinner relative to the lumbar spine owing to the thoracic spine's relative lack of motion. Each vertebral body is attached to the anterior longitudinal ligament as well as the posterior longitudinal ligament. The anterior longitudinal ligament along with the structural attachments between the sternum and the ribs prevents excessive hyperextension. Studies indicate that there is only a small amount of extension that occurs in an individual spinal unit made up of two thoracic vertebrae and their intervertebral disk. Posteriorly, the posterior longitudinal ligament attaches to the body of the vertebra as well as the intervertebral disk. This attachment tethers the spinal elements, and along with the muscular attachments, prevents excessive forward flexion of the spine.

The evaluation and treatment model discussed in this chapter requires a definition of terms used in the biomechanical model of movement of the thoracic spine. From the study of kinesiology, we borrow the terms kinematics, meaning movement, and kinetic, meaning forces. The terms osteo, meaning bone, and arthro, meaning joint, from Greek roots are combined with the kinesologic terms to give rise to arthrokinematics and osteokinematics. When we refer to these motions, we should define the axis upon which they occur. Arthrokinematics refers to the movement within a joint without regard to the osteokinematics of the bone. For example, the spine may bend forward (see Fig. 7-12) (osteokinematic motion) while the vertebra flex forward, glide anteriorly, distract posteriorly, and compress anteriorly (the arthrokinematic description). The arthro-

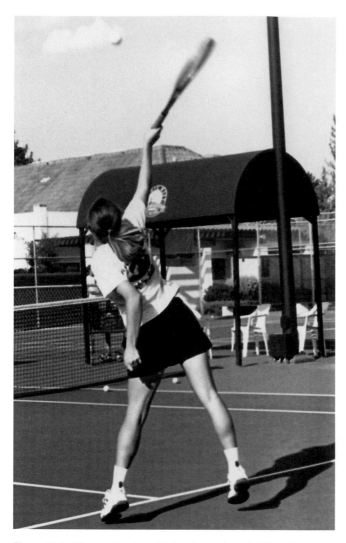

Figure 7–9. The overhead shot in tennis requires stability of the muscles of the thoracic spine to generate power in the anterior shoulder.

kinematic description should be accompanied by the axis upon which the motion occurs. This arthrokinematic description is the basis from which coupled motion is derived. Coupled motion can be described as the combination of arthrokinematic motions that combine to form movement in an osteokinematic plane. Coupled motion is the basis for the design of the forces applied for the treatment of dysfunction within the facets of the thoracic spine as well as in the costovertebral dysfunction. An often-used example of coupled motion is a wood screw driven into a board. The rotation is said to be coupled with the translation as the screw moves into or out of the board.

The zygapophyseal joints of the thoracic spine are curved both in the sagittal and transverse planes. They are considered plane joints with surfaces covered with hyaline cartilage. Each surface "cups" the other to allow

for multiple degrees of freedom of motion. Each joint is encapsulated with a loose connective tissue capsule lined with synovial membrane. The capsule is attached to the margins of the individual facets. Motion occurs in very small amounts toward flexion and a much lesser extent towards extension at the zygopophyseal joints. Side bending of the thoracic spine is minimal due to the influence of the ribcage and the ileum, but rotation is available to a large extent in this area of the spine. The amount of motion in each direction varies between individuals, but in general, the relative amount of availability of motion is determined by the structure and orientation of the individual facets. The motion, forward bending of the spine, includes flexion of the thoracic vertebra. This flexion about the x-axis is coupled with a translation inferiorly along the z-axis and slight distraction posteriorly along the y-axis (see Fig. 7–13). It is also known clinically that with flexion of the thoracic vertebra there is associated anterior rotation of the ribs. This anterior rotation is accomplished through a combination of forces exerted upon the ribs by the inferior articular process of the superior thoracic vertebra and the superior articular process of the inferior thoracic vertebra. Both combine by "pulling" and "pushing" to produce a gentle curve and the orientation to support the rotational movement of the rib about a paracoronal axis.

Stability within this portion of the spine in flexion is based on the posterior elements including the intervertebral disk, the posterior longitudinal ligament, and the costovertebral joint. Panjabi, Hausfeld, and White studied failure in both flexion and in extension. They defined the failure as complete separation of the superior from the inferior vertebra or movement of more than 10 mm in translation or 45 degrees of sagittal rotation. Flexion in the thoracic spine occurs about rotation of the x-axis with a slight anterior translation along the z-axis and a distraction along the y-axis. Movement was noted after transection of a particular element and the contribution of each structure to the stability of the spine was noted. Results of the study showed that stability was maintained until the costovertebral joint was transected. It was determined that the costovertebral joint was a key element in the stability of the thoracic spine in forward flexion.

Extension occurs within the thoracic spine as the vertebra posteriorly rotates about the x-axis and translates slightly posterior along the z-axis. There is slight compression about the y-axis as the spine bends backwards (see Fig. 7–14). The ribs are thought to follow this motion producing a posterior rotation about a paracoronal axis. As the inferior articular process of the superior vertebra moves down and back in sagittal rotation about the x-axis, the head of the rib is pushed toward posterior rotation. The stability in extension is drawn from the anterior longitudinal ligament, the anterior one half of the

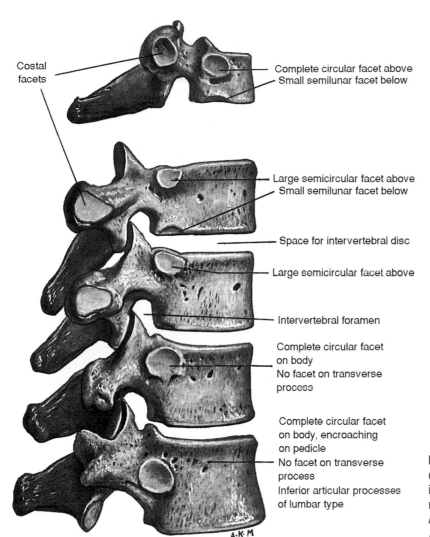

Costal facets

Complete circular facet above
Small semilunar facet below

Large semicircular facet above
Small semilunar facet below

Space for intervertebral disc

Large semicircular facet above

Intervertebral foramen

Complete circular facet
on body
No facet on transverse
process

Complete circular facet
on body, encroaching
on pedicle
No facet on transverse
process
Inferior articular processes
of lumbar type

A·K·M

Figure 7–10. Lateral view of the thoracic spine. The size of the body and the orientation of the spinous processes illustrates the change between the first and twelfth thoracic vertebrae. *(From Williams PL, Warwick R. Gray's Anatomy. 36th British ed. Edinburgh: Churchill Livingstone, 1980:565. With permission.)*

disk as well as the costovertebral joints and the posterior longitudinal ligament. In Panjabi's study, the functional spinal units remain stable until the posterior longitudinal ligament was released.

Rotation within the thoracic spine is said to be closely coupled with side bending to the same side. What is seen clinically is that when rotation occurs about the y-axis, there is a coupling of rotation about the z-axis to the same side and a translation along the x-axis to the opposite side (see Fig. 7–15). The ribs are said to behave in the following fashion. The trunk is rotated to the left, and what follows is left rotation of the superior vertebra which translates to the right. The right rib is said to be pulled forward at the costovertebral joint and anterior rotation is introduced while the left rib is pressed back into posterior rotation. The translation of the superior vertebra to the right is said to push the right rib anteriorly and laterally and eventually cause tension in the costotransverse ligaments. The left rib is said to be pulled medially

and posteriorly eventually causing tension at the costotransverse ligaments on the left side. When the ligaments become tensed, further motion can occur from the coupling of left side bending of the superior vertebra accomplished by an upward glide on the right side of the superior vertebra at the facet accompanied by a downward glide of the inferior facet on the right side. The final coupling produces the side bending left rotation that is presented clinically.

The coupling between side bending and rotation was first studied by Lovett while identifying problems with scoliotic curves. In his studies, he found that when the spine was side bent to one side, a coupling of rotation occurred to the opposite side. However, if the spine was placed in an extended position and side bent, the coupling occurred to the same or ipsilateral side. Lovett felt that the spinal element that controlled the motion was the zygapophyseal joint based on the idea of the joints being loaded in full extension. Later, Fryette, in a

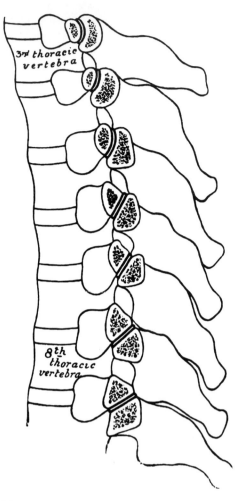

Figure 7–11. Lateral view illustrating the orientation of the vertebral facets in the thoracic spine. Note the change in orientation between the third and eighth vertebrae owing to the increase in weight bearing in transition into the lumbar spine. *(From Williams PL, Warwick R. Gray's Anatomy. 36th British ed. Edinburgh: Churchill Livingstone, 1980: 451. With permission.)*

much-quoted study, confirmed the observations made by Lovett, but found that in addition to coupling of motion to the ipsilateral side in extension, there is coupling to the ipsilateral side in the extreme flexed position as well. He later proposed the concepts that are now known as Fryette's laws of spinal motion from his observations.

1. When the spine is in a neutral position and the facets are not engaged, side bending and rotation occur to opposite sides. That is, side bending left would occur with rotation to the right.
2. When the facets are loaded in extension or flexion, the spine is said to be in nonneutral mechanics and the coupling of motion occurs to the same side—that is, side bending left, rotation left; or vice versa.
3. Spinal motion occurring in any particular plane will limit motion in the other two planes.

The muscular attachments and their influence on the thoracic spine can be divided into functional layers. The deep layers of muscles are those short band-like muscles known as the interspinalis and intertransversalis. These, although important for postural maintenance, are more completely described in a detailed anatomy text. The next layer of muscles is collectively considered the erector spinae, originates within the thoracolumbar fascia, and has been described in three parts. The muscles can be divided by medial, intermediate, and lateral fibers. The muscles within the erector spinae can be palpated between the transverse processes as well as between the spinous process throughout the thoracic spine (see color insert). In the pathologic spine, this area of palpation will reveal rolled tensed muscles that are tender to palpation and responsive to strumming by reproduction of symptoms in a local or referred area. The most superficial layer of muscles commonly associated with the thoracic spine is the large three-part trapezius muscle, the rhomboids, and the levator scapula. This most superficial group of muscles plays a prominent role in the stability of the scapular element of the thoracic spine in throwing and in overhead activities, as well as maintenance of the head posture for sports and activities of daily living.

THE CERVICOTHORACIC JUNCTION

The area between the cervical and thoracic spine is seen clinically as a region that produces considerable pain and is often associated with symptoms generated from other areas. One common dysfunction in this area is the thoracic outlet syndrome.

This may involve the muscular or fascial compression of vascular and neurologic branches as they exit the spine and descend laterally to the upper extremity, or it may involve the structural restriction from the first rib. Clinically, what is seen is often a painful region in the upper back with associated stiffness in the upper trapezius on that side. The scalenes are usually reactive to palpation and, very often, neck range of motion is limited. Pain may radiate down the arm and can be confused with carpal tunnel or epicondylar pain. The area around the first and second rib both posterior in the upper thoracic spine and anterior in the chest wall may be quite tender to palpation.

The examination process for this problem should include at least two clinical tests. The first is a classic Adson's maneuver in which the radial pulse is palpated with the arm in extension, abduction, and external rotation (see Fig. 7-16). The patient is asked to turn the head away from the arm and the observance of change in the pulse is palpated by the examiner. Some have described this test as a predominantly vascular exercise for

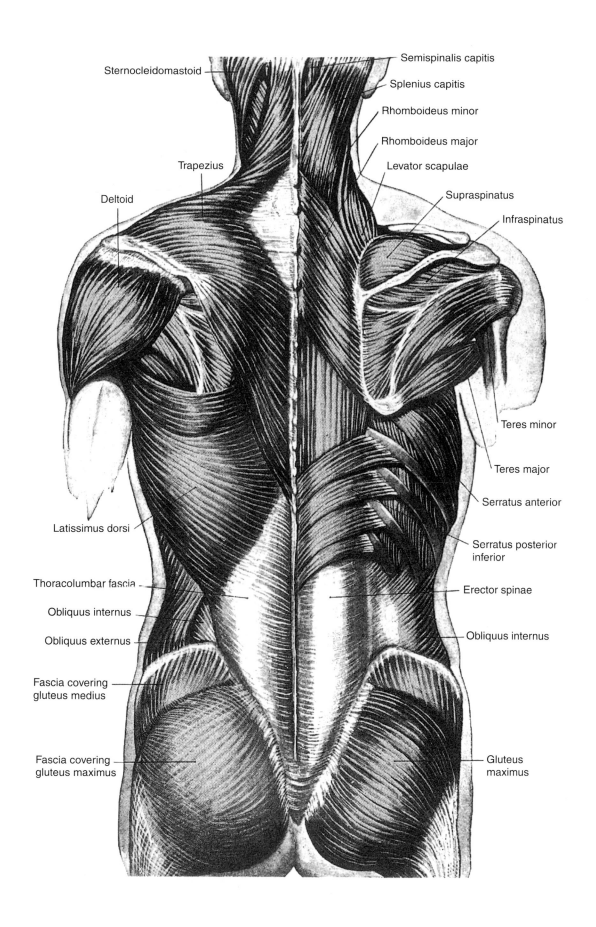

Sternocleidomastoid

Trapezius

Deltoid

Latissimus dorsi

Thoracolumbar fascia

Obliquus internus

Obliquus externus

Fascia covering
gluteus medius

Fascia covering
gluteus maximus

Semispinalis capitis

Splenius capitis

Rhomboideus minor

Rhomboideus major

Levator scapulae

Supraspinatus

Infraspinatus

Teres minor

Teres major

Serratus anterior

Serratus posterior
inferior

Erector spinae

Obliquus internus

Gluteus
maximus

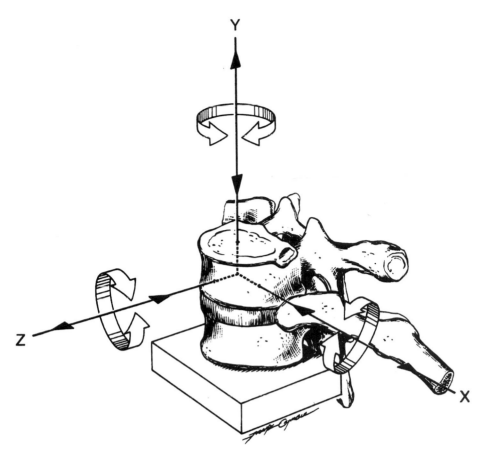

Figure 7–12. An illustration showing the planes of motion of the thoracic spine about the x, y, and z axes. The motion is coupled between these axes to produce normal spinal motion. *(From Lee D. Manual Therapy for the Thorax. Delta, BC: DOPC; 1994:24. With permission.)*

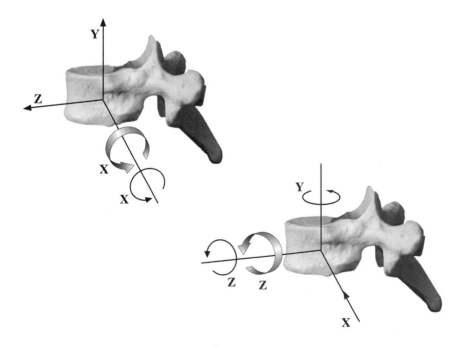

Figure 7–13. Arthrokinematic motion of the thoracic spine in forward bending about the x, y, and z axes. *(From Lee D. Manual Therapy for the Thorax. Delta, BC: DOPC; 1994:25. With permission.)*

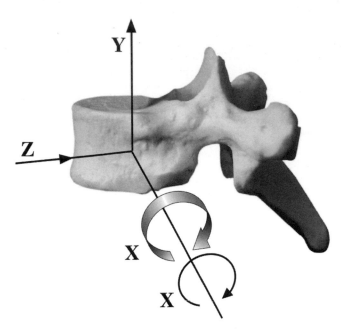

Figure 7–14. Model illustrating backward bending of the thoracic spine with arthrokinematic motion about the x, y, and z axes. *(From Lee D. Manual Therapy for the Thorax. Delta, BC: DOPC; 1994:32. With permission.)*

diagnosis of the thoracic outlet dysfunction. Another maneuver more mechanical in nature that has been shown to be quite effective in identification of the first rib component of the thoracic outlet syndrome is described as a CRLF, an acronym standing for cervical rotation lateral flexion. To complete this maneuver, the head is rotated toward the suspected side of dysfunc-

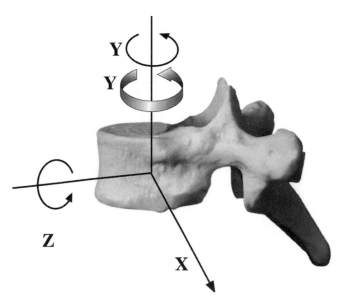

Figure 7–15. Rotation coupled with side bending within the thoracic spine.

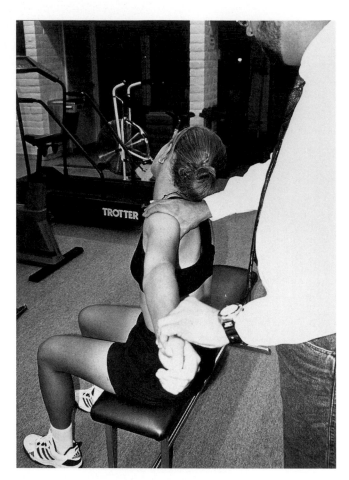

Figure 7–16. Classic Adson's maneuver to assess the influence on the outlet on upper extremity pain.

tion (see Fig. 7–17). The head is then bent toward the chest in a gentle fashion. The sense of freedom is observed as the head is bent towards the chest. A similar maneuver is performed to the opposite side away from the side of dysfunction with the same sense of freedom palpated. A positive sign is confirmed by the presence of a firm or blocked end feel when the ear is moved towards the chest when rotated away from the side of the complaint. A positive sign is an indication of a first rib dysfunction compressing the neurovascular bundle and causing the pain or perhaps the presence of a cervical rib in the patient.

The motion involving the golf swing lends itself to potential dysfunction in the cervicothoracic junction. Generally, the chin is held down with the eye on the ball. An overzealous swing around a firm placement of the chin can produce the forces to allow for the anterolateral direction of motion leading to pain and dysfunction in the thoracic outlet. In this example, the right-handed player may complain of pain in the left shoulder and arm, scapular pain on the left that may extend down through the midthoracic spine. Painful rota-

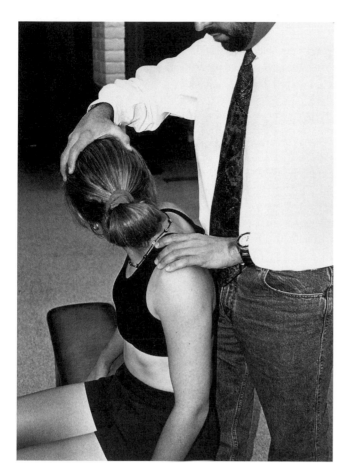

Figure 7–17. The cervical rotation lateral flexion (CRLF) maneuver to assess the influence of the first rib as associated with thoracic outlet dysfunction. This figure illustrates a test for the left first rib dysfunction.

tion of the neck to the left and painful and stiff side bending to the left is also a common complaint. The anterior margin of the first and perhaps second rib may be quite tender to palpation at the angle of Louis of the sternum. Functionally, this type of dysfunction will generally include trauma to the first rib as well as a first or second thoracic dysfunction involving rotation and side bending. Depending on the length of time from the trauma to the examination, the patient may demonstrate patterns of weakness in the shoulder girdle and about the middle or lower trapezius, rhomboids, and serratus posterior and anterior. Patterns of weakness and tightness are common in this area.

The treatment approach for the thoracic outlet syndrome is based on evaluative findings. If the problem is identified early, then muscle wasting, weakness, and inhibition are less likely, but the painful condition may still remain and a comprehensive approach must be used to solve the athlete's problem. Systematically, looking at myofascial restrictions, joint dysfunction, and muscle imbalance is most useful in the management of these cases. The patient

may be treated seated or supine. From behind, a rolling maneuver is performed across the neck. This may be coordinated with breathing until relaxation and symmetry is felt in the upper trapezius. From the same position, applying a firm contact with the lateral phalanx of the index finger to the superior border of the first rib near its attachment to T1 is demonstrated in Figure 7-18. The direction of contact is medial and posterior in a fashion as to roll the rib back towards its attachment on the T1 facet. The head is slightly flexed and side bent to the side of the dysfunction to the point where slight motion is felt by the examiner at the finger contact of the first rib. The head is rotated slightly away from the side of dysfunction until slight motion is felt at the base of the neck underneath the finger. The patient is then asked to bend the head away from the side being treated using only a small amount of pressure. The scalenes on the treatment side are reciprocally inhibited by the contraction of the opposite side. The finger contact maintains pressure on the medial aspect of the first rib. Two or three repetitions are repeated and usually sufficient for reduction of the first rib dysfunction.

The muscle imbalances including facilitation and inhibition are more apparent when the problem has become chronic. If the chronic problem is suspected, then the presence of muscle imbalance is very likely and should be assessed. The general rule is to stretch the antagonist prior to strengthening the agonist. In this case, often the scalenes along with the upper trapezius, as well as the pectoralis, may be very tight on the affected side. These muscle groups generally should be stretched prior to the strengthening exercises performed for the middle and lower trapezius and serratus anterior that are generally inhibited. Strengthening may begin almost immediately, provided that stretching is done first.

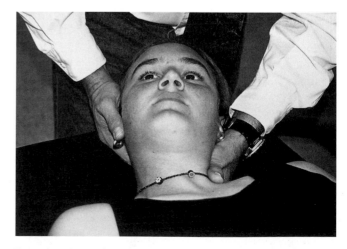

Figure 7–18. Treatment for the first rib dysfunction. The left first rib is treated with a muscle energy technique designed to reduce the influence of the first rib on the thoracic outlet dysfunction.

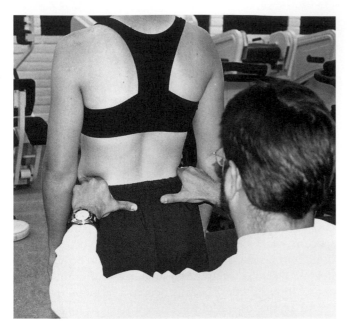

Figure 7–19. Evaluation of posture influences on thoracic dysfunction. Views of contours and relative heights are advocated to assess extrinsic influence affecting the thoracic spine.

MANAGEMENT OF THORACIC DYSFUNCTION

Manual therapy in the thoracic spine is a very useful tool in the management of pain of the injured athlete. The model for treatment involves the use of palpatory skills, understanding of anatomy and biomechanics, and patience on the part of the provider. The techniques require repetition and practice but once capable hands are realized, the results will satisfy the provider that the time and effort was well spent. The examination of the thoracic spine is performed with the operator behind the patient. Initially, the patient is observed for areas of fullness or flatness. Winging of the scapula is observed and noted. The patient is asked to raise the arms both forward and to the sides and attention is paid to the scapulothoracic rhythm that takes place. The athlete bends forward and changes and the contours are noted for scoliotic curves. A general screening exam is advocated to allow the examiner to narrow the field of focus to a specific region (see Fig. 7-19). Dysfunctions within the thoracic spine may be considered either intrinsic or

TABLE 7–1. INTRINSIC THORACIC DYSFUNCTIONS

Facet syndrome
Costovertebral joint dysfunction
Myofascial trigger point pain
Fracture dislocation
Primary pathology
Thoracic outlet syndrome

TABLE 7–2. EXTRINSIC THORACIC DYSFUNCTION

Anterior shoulder instability
Quadratus laborum and pelvic dysfunction
Short leg syndrome or hemipelvis
Ideopathic scoliosis
Cervical dysfunction

extrinsic. The intrinsic dysfunctions originate within the skeletal, muscular, or fascial systems of the thoracic spine. These may include those items in Table 7-1. The extrinsic thoracic dysfunctions are those whose origins come from structures outside of the thoracic spine and are listed in Table 7-2.

The screening exam is useful to raise the level of suspicion of the examiner to a particular element of the patient's complaint and identify whether the problem may be intrinsic or extrinsic in nature.

Case Study

Examine the case of the young athlete with a short leg or hemipelvis who has a compensatory scoliotic curve. During his throwing motion, due to the forceful eccentric loading on the trapezius and rhomboid, he develops mid to upper thoracic pain. The detailed exam may reveal the presence of the trigger points and perhaps even facet or costovertebral joint dysfunction, but will completely ignore the short leg and compensatory curve as its consequence. It may not be overstressed that the exam must consider an overall view of the athlete's premorbid condition to assist in the determination of the proper course of treatment and the order in which to proceed. The school athlete offers a unique opportunity to document and observe premorbid conditions if an adequate preparticipation screening is included in the physical.

Palpation is a critical element of the musculoskeletal treatment approach and certainly requires the most practice and patience to master. In this exam, the iliac crests are palpated for height and symmetry. The lower ribs and quadratus lumborum may be associated with the painful lower thoracic spine, so both of these areas are briefly assessed. The acromioclavicular joint is palpated for height and symmetry, as well as the position of the head related to the midline. Next, the muscles of the erector spinal group are palpated. Three divisions exist in the erector spinae group and are separated by an intermuscular septi. The intermediate division is the one most useful diagnostically in this model and is felt just lateral to the spinous process in a "gutter" overlying the lamina of the vertebra with its most lateral border the transverse process. It is this group of muscles that when palpated yields information regarding the level of the dysfunction that requires attention. The position of the transverse process relative to the opposite side and to the levels above and below offer the information that will direct the forces used in the treatment approach. A previous description of the coupling that occurs in the thoracic spine indicated that when the spine is bent to one side in a neutral posture, rotation will occur to the opposite side. It also described that when either flexion or extension occurred, the rotation occurred in the same direction when side bent. Using these basic rules, the motion segment is examined in three positions—neutral, extended, and flexed. The transverse processes are contacted to provide a landmark for reference (see Fig. 7–20). For this discussion, the figure will illustrate the right transverse process at T5 posterior relative to the left when the patient extends the spine backward. When he flexes forward, the level of T5 is about equal on the right compared to the left. Palpation along the "gutter" at the T5 level is reactive to palpation on either side. Since the coupling of spinal motion in extension is to the same side, the segment is said to be side bent and rotated to the same side. Following this example, the expectation for symmetry biomechanically is for both facets to close when the spine is extended. Since the left facet is forward relative to the right, that segment is said to be rotated to the right and side bent to the right; thus the left

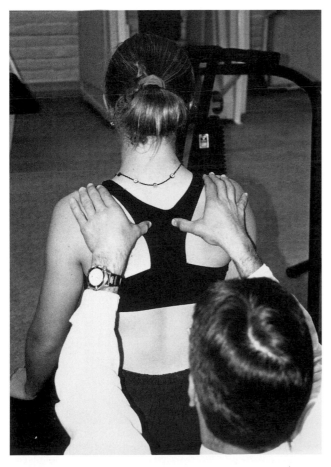

Figure 7–20. Palpation of the transverse process to determine the positional diagnosis for treatment planning.

facet will not close. The motion segment is described as flexed, rotated, right side bent right.

This particular positional diagnosis is useful in communication with treatment team members as well as medical reports. It gives the provider a positional description of the restriction and the direction to which forces should be applied to restore motion in that segment.

The treatment model described to treat these restrictions consists of the use of position with the application of gentle forces to facilitate movement. The use of high velocity and force is discouraged in this discussion. Those thrusting maneuvers often seen on sidelines possess a degree of risk that should not be dealt with casually. Although effective, high-velocity, low-amplitude manipulation or adjustments should be performed by individuals who have attained a level of skill deemed sufficient to perform these maneuvers. The potential for subluxed ribs, ruptured capsular or articular ligaments, and even death exists if performed to the cervical spine. This should always be on the mind of the operator when attempting a technique that requires force and speed. The approach described in this chapter incorporates the use of palpatory skills and knowledge of the biomechanics of coupling and anatomy to apply gentle corrective forces to improve movement and decrease pain. The forces do not move joints, but rather act on a neurophysiologic level to ease pain and facilitate movement.

Case Study

An 18-year-old high school volleyball player reports an injury during a game while blocking a shot. She feels a twinge in her neck and left shoulder in the scapular region. Upon examination 4 days later, three possibilities are considered. First, a cervical dysfunction due to the reports of pain at the base of the skull "running down into the back of the shoulder blade." Second, an anterior shoulder strain due to her reports of actual shoulder pain deep and aching with stiffness when she attempts to elevate the arm. Finally, middle to upper thoracic dysfunction is considered from point tenderness in this region. A screening examination reveals that the neck bends forward and is uncomfortable but painful backward. She can flex her arms both to 180 degrees pain free, but elevation produces pain at the T4 and 5 level along the scapular border. Palpation down the "gutter" found between the spinous and transverse process reveals reactive tissue at about the T4 and 5 level with less tenderness above. Palpation of the transverse process reveals that when she sits up tall (neutral), the right T5 transverse process is slightly posterior when compared to the left side. Asked to slump and the relative difference is more apparent. Reversal of the curve, sitting tall and bending back, allows the two sides to come to about equal. This describes the dysfunction in which the right facet will not open or the segment is said to be extended. The expectation is for the transverse processes to follow symmetrically forward when the patient slumps. The fact that the right facet stays relatively posterior compared to the left indicates its lack of ability to close and indicates an extended position. This segment is said to be extended, side bend right, and rotated to the right. The

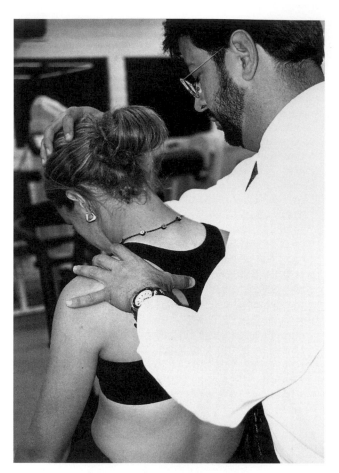

Figure 7–21. Treatment technique for a positional restriction in which the right T5 process is relatively posteror when the athlete is asked to flex the spine. The technique uses position and gentle force to improve motion and decease pain.

course of treatment would include moving that segment through its normal range of motion into flexion, side bending left, and rotation left with gentle positioning and the use of light forces.

Figure 7–21 illustrates the seated treatment position of the extended, side bent right, rotated right dysfunction. The athlete is seated on the side of the table with the operator standing behind. The left hand is placed over the shoulder with the thumb at the transverse process of T5. A gentle translatory force is applied with the thumb against the spinous process to influence left side bending and left rotation. The athlete's head is held with the right forearm and hand as she slumps backward into the operator's chest only slightly, producing tension up through the hips to the level of T5. The head is cautiously bent forward until tension comes from above and reaches the level of the thumb. She is then allowed to slightly bend the head to the left until tension is felt at the operator's thumb. Rotation is then introduced to the left, once again palpating for tension at the level of T5. The athlete is then asked to bend her head slightly to the right against constant and unyielding resistance. When completely relaxed, the left

thumb may translate to the right up to the point of resistance. Three or four 5-second efforts will generally provide sufficient treatment to alleviate the dysfunction in this area. She is then asked to sit upright and is retested.

Had the athlete been in flexion rather than extension, that is, the inability for the left facet to close, a similar technique would have been utilized. The palpatory findings in this example would include reactive tissue at about the level of T5 similar to that found with the flexion restriction. When the athlete was asked to slump, both transverse processes would have looked approximately equal. When asked to extend and bend slightly backward, the transverse process on the right would have been more posterior to that of the left. This scenario would indicate an inability for the left facet to close and therefore a flexion restriction coupled with side bending right and rotation right. That segment would be said to have been flexed, side bend right, and rotated right. In this instance, she would be asked to sit upright on the table (see Fig. 7–22). The operator's left hand would be placed over the left shoulder with the thumb at the T5 transverse process. The right forearm and hand are placed on the patient's

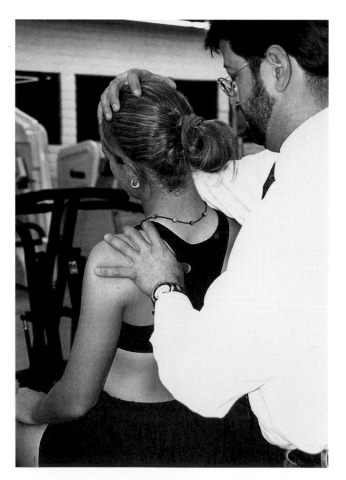

Figure 7–22. Treatment technique for a positional restriction in which the left T5 process is relatively anterior when the athlete is asked to extend the spine. The technique uses position and gentle force to improve motion and decrease pain.

right shoulder and head. The thumb of the left hand of the operator acts as a guide as the athlete is asked to push her stomach forward until the first motion is detected under the left thumb. The head is then gently translated back until motion is felt at the thumb. The head is not extended, since this may cause pain and damage to structures within the cervical spine. A gentle side bend left and rotation left are achieved with a tilt and turn of the head until first motion is felt. The activating force by the athlete is a gentle tilt to the right followed by a complete relaxation. A similar translation at T5 with the thumb will influence the coupling of side bending left and rotation left. Three or four repetitions followed by complete relaxation, then translation, are generally sufficient to treat the restricted segment.

Treatment within the thoracic spine is often an important component in the management of shoulder pain and dysfunction. The inclusion of thoracic training exercise and, very often, mobilization of the thoracic spine with anterior shoulder dysfunction rehabilitation is now standard in most protocols. Clinically, the region between about T4 and T6 seems to be most often associated with either the primary cervical dysfunction or the anterior shoulder dysfunction. It has been said that this region provides the functional axis for extension of the head as well as elevation of the arms. It is no wonder that clinically, this region is a major contributor to pain and dysfunction, especially in a chronic condition. Treatment of this area should be viewed from a variety of perspectives to be most effective. The structural element should be addressed with the use of joint mobilization techniques. Painful patterns should be identified and myofascial components to the pain addressed. Muscular imbalances should be considered with the presence of inhibited and facilitated muscular patterns addressed. Last, the appropriate exercise should be included based on the treatment provided and the deficiencies noted.

Exercise for rehabilitation of the thoracic spine includes stretching of the articular structures, postural reeducation of deep muscles, and classic general strengthening exercises for the superficial layers of muscle. The evaluation process assists in making the determination as to which areas to focus on with the specific exercise protocol. Patterns of muscular imbalance are often overlooked as an area of thoracic pain and dysfunction. Often tight muscles such as the pectoralis major, pectoralis minor, scalenes, upper trapezius, and levator scapula will inhibit strengthening of muscles important in shoulder and thoracic rehabilitation such as the middle trapezius, lower trapezius, serratus anterior, and rhomboids. Exclusive use of classic weight training programs administered to the muscle groups that are inhibited by these tight structures will provide less than optimal results and may often exacerbate pain syndromes. Stretching of the antagonist is advocated prior to the strengthening of the agonist.

Evaluation of the muscle imbalance can begin with the seated examination. The examiner can look at head and neck range of motion to determine tightness of the upper trapezius and levator scapula. The scalenes can also be assessed in the upright seated position. With the athlete laid supine, the arms can be flexed with a tight pelvic tilt and the latissimus dorsi can be assessed for its length. Abduction can be performed with the athlete supine. In this exercise, the athlete is asked to abduct the arms and maintain contact of the shoulders on the table (see Fig. 7–23). A tight pectoralis will inhibit the ability of the athlete to maintain contact as the athlete moves toward full abduction. Manual stretching can be done to improve the length of the tight muscles. However, it's essential to provide the athlete with a self-administered exercise program. The following series of exercises are used for both stretching tight structures and strengthening weak and inhibited structures. A number of authors including Janda, Bookhout, and Sharmann have de-

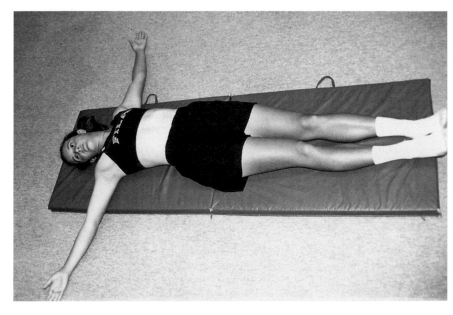

Figure 7–23. Assessment of a tight anterior shoulder that may influence the strength of the middle and lower trapezius muscles. This position is also used for strengthening of the inhibited middle and lower trapezius muscles.

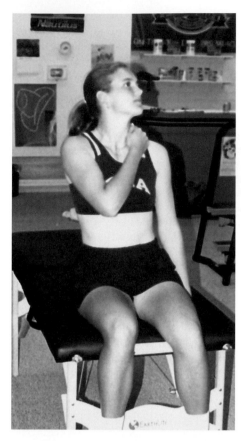

Figure 7–24. Scalene stretch seated for tight left scalene musculature. The athlete looks up to the corner, then pulls down and away with the opposite hand.

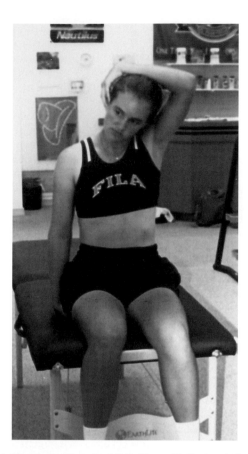

Figure 7–25. Upper trapezius stretching with the head tilted to the left and turned to the right, then supported with the left arm. The trunk rather than the head is bent to the left for comfort.

tailed exercises in more specialized publications. The reader is encouraged to look at these publications for more detail in this area. Figure 7-24 illustrates the athlete performing the stretch for the scalene muscles. These are included in this chapter because of their anterior attachment to the thorax. Tight scalenes are common contributors to persistent and chronic flexed cervical dysfunction. The tight scalenes are often found in the thoracic outlet syndrome dysfunction previously described. In order to stretch the left scalenes, the athlete is seated on the table. The left hand is placed underneath the left thigh and the athlete is asked to sit tall. The right hand is then draped over the clavicle and the first rib region. The athlete is asked to slowly extend the head, side bend to the right, and rotate to the left, feeling a general stretch in the left scalenes. Because of the presence of the carotid artery and the slight extension of the head, this exercise should be approached with caution. The amount of traction placed on the neck by the right hand should be closely monitored.

Stretching of the upper trapezius can be done in a similar seated position (see Fig. 7-25). To stretch this muscle, the right hand is placed underneath the right thigh as was done for the scalenes. Very much like the testing position, the head is slightly flexed and brought to the left side bending with rotation to the right. The right scapula is

contracted medially or downward to produce an active stretch. The trunk is leaned away from the right hand. A similar position is described for stretching of the right levator scapula. For this exercise position, the right hand is placed underneath the thigh. The head is slightly flexed, side bent to the left and rotated to the left. The head position is supported with the left hand. Pulling on the head in this position can produce neck or upper thoracic pain so bending the trunk or contracting the right lower trapezius through the scapula is a better approach to stretching these structures (see Fig. 7-26). Stretching of the pectoralis major can be accomplished by asking the athlete to initially face the wall and stand about 12 inches away. The athlete places the left palm on the wall at about 80 degrees of abduction. The right hand is placed on the wall and serves as a guide toward rotation. The pelvis and feet are rotated towards the right, immediately producing a stretch on the left pectoralis group. The right arm is pressed towards the wall in order to facilitate rotation to the right and increase the stretch to the pectoralis group. The left lower thoracic musculature including the trapezius should be recruited during this exercise to facilitate further stretching of the pectoralis group.

A common error in this exercise is to allow the left shoulder to elevate during the stretch. Stretching of the

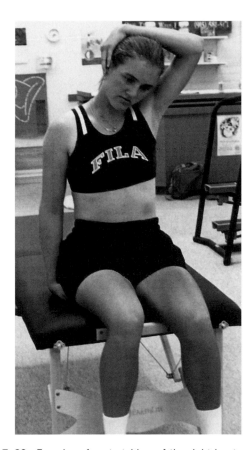

Figure 7–26. Exercises for stretching of the right levator scapula. The right hand is placed under the thigh with the head rotated and side bent to the left and supported by the left arm. The athlete leans the trunk to the left, or may contract the muscles of the lower trapezius on the right side to produce the desired stretch.

latissimus dorsi is accomplished with the athlete in a kneeling position. A table or bench about 3 feet high is placed in front of the athlete, and the elbows are placed on the bench. The shoulder blades are allowed to fall outward with the elbows held in closely toward the head, palm facing palm (see Fig. 7–27). The athlete is then asked to sit back towards the heels maintaining a straight back. A posterior pelvic tilt can be initiated to further increase the stretch on the latissimus dorsi through the lumbodorsal fascia. Stretching of the pectoralis minor can be accomplished by the elevation of the arm to approximately 120 degrees. This angle of abduction produces an advantageous angle for introduction of a stretch directly to the pectoralis minor. The exercise is easily performed using a door frame or exercise apparatus. The stretch includes holding the door frame or apparatus and moving the chest forward producing a stretch at the chest wall and stretching the pectoralis minor. This stretch may also be accomplished manually with the athlete laying supine on a treatment table with the arm abducted to 120 degrees. The hips and the knees are bent, then rotated to the right in this example. This rotation allows the torso to stretch the pectoralis minor at its origin.

Stretching of the articular structures is advocated with the thoracic dysfunction. The thoracic spine facet motions that should be emphasized are flexion, side bending, and rotation. Exercise to facilitate these articular motions is as follows. From the position of a "cat" stretch with the athlete on all fours (see Fig. 7–28), the athlete is asked to arch the back upward with the neck flexed downward to produce flexion of the thoracic spine. The hand position may be changed in order to alter the apex of the curve to the lower or upper thoracic spine. By bringing the hands closer to the knees, the apex of the curve is focused in the

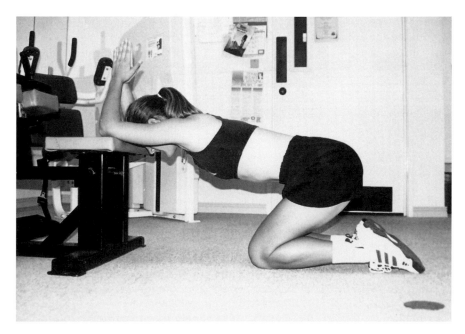

Figure 7–27. Stretching of the latissimus dorsi. The athlete is encouraged to keep the back straight while sitting back on the heels. A posterior pelvic tilt will improve the effectiveness of the stretch at its extremes.

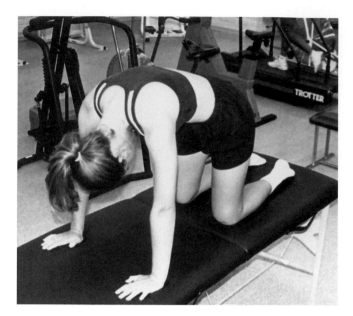

Figure 7–28. The "cat" stretch in which the athlete emphasizes flexion of the thoracic spine. This exercise may be used as an adjunct to treatment for an extension restriction with the thoracic spine. A reversal of the curve in this same position may be used to emphasize extension of the spine.

lower thoracic spine. By moving the hands further toward the head, the apex of the curve can be focused on the upper thoracic spine. When the extension dysfunction is identified during the examination and evaluation process, this exercise can be utilized to maintain a correction for an extended rotated and side bent dysfunction. The spine can also be extended in the very same position by lifting the head and allowing the spine to fall between the shoulder blades. The apex of the curve can be altered for stretching a specific area in the lower, middle, or upper thoracic spine by positioning the hands either more toward the knees or toward the head. The determination of where the apex should occur is based on the findings during the screening and evaluation of the thoracic spine. Stretching of the articular structures for side bending can be accomplished in a seated position by dropping one arm to the side and reaching to the floor while simultaneously reaching skyward with the opposite arm. Slight lateral flexion completes the stretch. Stretching of the structures for articular rotation in the thoracic spine can be accomplished with the athlete seated with the back supported. A rotation and a reach with the contralateral arm produces a middle to upper thoracic rotary stretch.

In order to determine a muscle retraining format the examiner must first evaluate which muscles are weak or inhibited. The term "inhibited" is preferred here, because the tight antagonist may be perpetuating the weakness or inhibition of the agonistic mover. An example of this relationship can often occur with a tight scalene, pectoralis minor, and latissimus dorsi. This tight relationship can inhibit the contraction of the middle and lower trapezius muscles as well as the rhomboids in scapular retraction.

Muscle testing for the trapezius can be performed prone. The fibers tested depend on the position of the arm during the test. In order to assess the strength of the middle and upper fibers, the athlete is laid prone with the head resting midline with the forehead and chin supported. The arms are internally rotated and laid alongside the trunk with the shoulders relaxed. The athlete is asked to lift the arm a few degrees upward and pull the shoulder blade medially. Resistance can be applied to medial border of the scapula to assess the amount of strength available. Both sides should be assessed and if there is weakness it should be noted for retraining. The lower fibers can be assessed with the athlete prone, forehead and chin supported. The arm is brought into a fully flexed position with the shoulder internally rotated. The athlete's arm is supported at the elbow and the athlete is asked to raise the arm off the table. Care should be taken not to allow excessive extension of the spine and force should be applied to the inferior lateral angle of the scapula. One side should be assessed against the other to form an opinion as to the degree of weakness present. The levator scapula and middle trapezius act in synergy to produce elevation of the shoulder. With the athlete in a tall sitting position, the athlete elevates both shoulders towards the ears. The evaluator applies pressure downward in order to assess the strength of the levator and middle trapezius.

The serratus anterior is the prime mover for abduction of the scapula assisting in superior rotation as well. Accurate assessment of the strength of this muscle is vitally important in shoulder rehabilitation and dysfunction of the upper and middle thoracic spine. Weakness of this muscle produces the classic scapula alata or winging of the scapula. To assess the strength of this muscle, the athlete is asked to face the wall with the finger tips in contact at about shoulder height. The athlete is then allowed to bend the elbows and flex towards the wall (see Fig. 7-29). Both scapulas must be observed for winging or asymmetry that may occur. Often, the amount of weakness in the serratus anterior is occult. Therefore, a number of testing positions for this muscle are advocated. With the athlete seated, he or she is then asked to raise the arm horizontally forward with the elbow bent. The examiner controls the athlete on the lateral side of the thorax just under the inferior angle of the scapula. The athlete is asked to push forward with the elbow producing a contraction of the serratus anterior towards abduction and rotation. Rotation is palpated by the finger contact at the inferior angle and abduction is observed as the scapula moves forward and outward. A third position is advocated in which the athlete lays supine on the table with the arm flexed to 90 degrees. The athlete is asked to raise the arm forward and upward, thereby contracting the serratus anterior. Resistance may be offered through the arm with an axillary force through the arm to assess more carefully the available strength of the serratus anterior.

Once the identification of weakness has been made, retraining must occur. After the antagonist and the articular structures have been mobilized a retraining sequence for the thoracic spine should be implemented. In order to

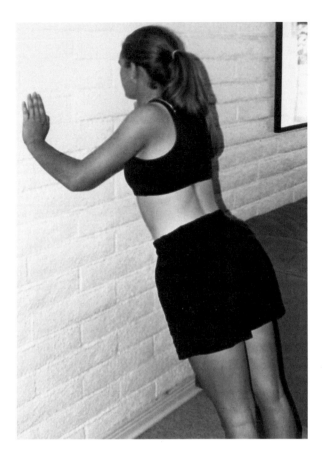

Figure 7–29. Testing position for the serratus anterior to determine the scapula alta. This position may also be used as a training position for strengthening of the serratus during the rehabilitation process.

strengthen scapular depression in the lower trapezius, the athlete is asked to kneel with the arms extended resting on a bench (see Fig. 7–30). This same position may be used for stretching of the latissimus dorsi with either the elbows bent or the arms straight. The weak arm is then raised off the bed about 2 inches. Attention is paid at this point to prevent extension of the lumbar spine and lower thoracic spine. Activation of the abdominals often inhibits the tendency to extend the lower back and lower thoracic spine. The athlete is then asked to actively contract the lower trapezius and bring the scapula into depression and

adduction. An alternative position was described by Lewit for retraining of the lower trapezius. In this position, the athlete is asked to bend the knees and lean all the way back on the heels. The hands are brought above the head and placed palm over hand with the affected side on top of the unaffected hand. The athlete is then asked to draw the shoulder blades into adduction and depression. Both of these positions tend to simultaneously stretch the antagonistic latissimus dorsi and anterior shoulder musculature while strengthening the middle and lower trapezius musculature.

Retraining of the middle trapezius and levator may be accomplished with an exercise in which the athlete is asked to lay supine with the palms facing upward. The athlete is then asked to slowly abduct the arms while maintaining contact with the treatment plinth or mat. At the point where the arm begins to lose contact, the athlete is asked to actively contract the trapezius toward scapular retraction. From this exercise, we find that once again the anterior structures are being stretched simultaneously to active contraction of the middle trapezius towards the scapular retraction; thus retraining the agonist while stretching of the antagonist is accomplished. The range of motion is not continued past that point until the athlete can maintain contact with the treatment plinth as they move upward toward full abduction. In order to perform this exercise, the pectoralis and anterior capsule must have been stretched prior to initiation. The serratus anterior will be strengthened in a sequential fashion depending on the degree of weakness. If there is significant weakness found in the serratus anterior, a prone press-up in which the athlete is asked simply to press up through the hands and arch the back may be performed. The athlete may then perform hands and knees push-ups and include complete scapular protraction at the end of the range. The athlete is instructed in this position to completely protract the scapula and depress the shoulder blades bilaterally as the end of the range is achieved. A wall press-up can be added to further achieve a complete scapular protraction with the head flexed in a downward position (see Fig. 7–31). In this position, the athlete is asked to tuck the pelvis completely and attempt to maintain a protracted position for 5 to 10 seconds. The next step in the sequence calls for an incline push-up on a 4-foot-high platform progressing down to the floor. Each

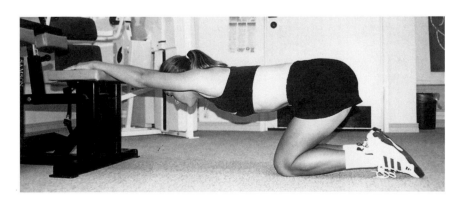

Figure 7–30. Strengthening the position for lower thoracic spine and lower trapezius musculature. Care should be taken not to overextend the upper back during the performance of this exercise.

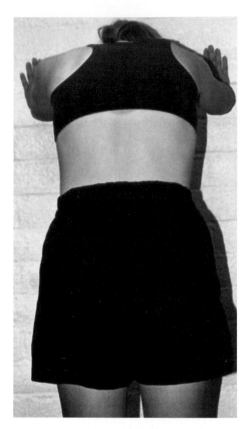

Figure 7–31. Retraining the serratus anterior standing against a wall. The athlete is asked to completely protract the shoulders at the end of the range and to press the shoulder blades downward.

muscle that requires strengthening will have an antagonist that should have previously been lengthened with stretching activities. This cross-pattern of muscle imbalance is more completely described by Janda and others. Numerous authors have recognized the presence and patterns of muscle imbalance that have been described. However, at times the approach in terms of sequence and application of exercise differs between authors such as Janda and Sharmann.

The rehabilitation and treatment of the thoracic spine should include a complete history, screening examination, and a segmental examination with identification of specific joint restrictions, followed by an assessment of muscle imbalance to apply a correct program of treatment. The sequence of treatment as is indicated in Table 7–3 in-

TABLE 7–3. SEQUENCE OF TREATMENT

1. Joint dysfunction management with manual therapy
2. Stretching of tightened articular structures with self-mobilization
3. Stretching of shortened antagonists
4. Strengthening of inhibited or weak agonists
5. General and traditional strengthening exercises

cludes the identification and treatment of a specific joint dysfunction, generally using a manual technique. Second, addressing the articular restriction with a self- or auto-mobilization technique in which the patient participates actively. The third phase includes stretching of the tight antagonistic or shortened antagonistic musculature and articular structures, followed by strengthening of the inhibited or weak agonistic musculature. Finally, a general strengthening program, as is most commonly utilized in most gymnasiums and training facilities, to include a full weight and strength program.

SELECTED READINGS

Anatomy and Kinesiology

Bourdillon JF. *Spinal Manipulation*. 5th ed. London: Butterworth-Heinmann; 1992.

Grossman MR, Sharmann SA, Rose S. Review of length associated changes in muscle. Experimental evidence and clinical applications. *Phys Ther*. 1982;62:1799–1808.

Janda V. *Muscle Function Testing*. London: Butterworth; 1983.

Lee D. Biomechanics of the thorax. 3:A, Clinical model of in-vivo function. *J Manual Manipulative Ther*. 1993;1:13–21.

Lovett RW. The study of the mechanics of the spine. *Am J Anatomy*. 1902;2:457–462.

Panjabi MM, Brand RA, White AA. Mechanical properties of the human thoracic spine. *J Bone Joint Surgery*. 1976;58A:642–652.

Panjabi MM, Hausfeld JN, White AA. A biomechanical study of the ligamentous stability of the thoracic spine in man. *Acta Orthop Scand*. 1981;552:315–326.

Panjabi MM, Takata K, Goel V, et al. Thoracic human vertebrae: Quantitative three-dimensional anatomy. *Spine*. 1991;16:888–901.

Williams PL, Warwick R, eds. *Gray's Anatomy*. 36th British ed. Edinburgh: Churchhill Livingstone; 1980.

Chapter 8

The Lumbar Spine, Ilium, and Sacrum

The Lower Back in Sports

Craig C. Young, Lee H. Riley III, and John G. Lachacz

Low back pain occurs commonly in both athletes and nonathletes with estimates of 60 to 90 percent lifetime prevalence and a 5 to 35 percent annual incidence.[1-6] Low back pain is the leading cause of disability for Americans under the age of 45 and the third leading cause of disability for Americans of all ages.[7-10] Despite the fact that only 5 percent of low back pain sufferers seek medical evaluation,[11] low back pain was the fifth most common reason for visiting a physician's office in 1990, accounting for almost 15 million office visits, 56 percent of which were to primary care physicians.[12] Even a study of school children has found a high (74 percent) prevalence of back pain.[13] Athletes, eager to return to full participation in their sporting activities, are usually highly motivated to participate in treatment for low back pain.[14] The development of an individualized treatment and rehabilitation plan for each athlete's specific problem is paramount.

ANATOMY

The lower back provides support, stabilization, and movement of the trunk. The musculature, ligaments, and vertebrae of the lower back also serve to protect the spinal cord. Weight supported by the spine increases proportionally from the cervical to the lumbar regions. Mechanically greater leverage is exerted in the lumbar spine. These two factors place the lumbar spine under great stress, which accounts for the common injury to this region of the body. Many sports, including golf, football, and ballet, involve fast movements, which place the trunk in a flexed and rotated manner.

Bones

Adults usually have 33 vertebrae consisting of 7 cervical vertebrae, 12 thoracic vertebrae, 5 lumbar vertebrae, 5 fused vertebrae forming the sacrum, and 3 or 4 rudimentary vertebrae forming the coccyx (see Fig. 8-1). The lumbar vertebrae are larger and heavier than the cervical or thoracic vertebrae. Their bodies are wider transversely than their depth anteroposteriorly. The lamina are bridged posteriorly by the ligamentum flavum, which is rich in elastin, an elastic tissue that stretches during back flexion and remains taut during extension. The curve of the lumbar spine is relatively gradual, whereas the curve at the lumbosacral junction is much sharper. While the sharper curve allows for increased mobility, it also subjects the region to greater leverage, and thus places it at increased risk of injury. This curve is especially sharp in women.

Joints

Each vertebral motion segment has three joints. The posterolateral, zygapophyseal joints are synovial joints

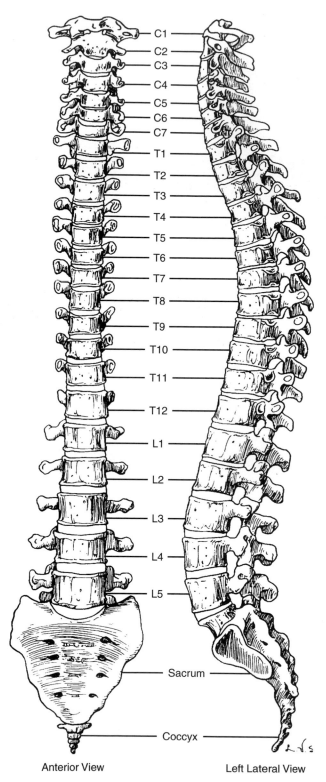

C1
C2
C3
C4
C5
C6
C7
T1
T2
T3
T4
T5
T6
T7
T8
T9
T10
T11
T12
L1
L2
L3
L4
L5
Sacrum
Coccyx

Anterior View   Left Lateral View

Figure 8–1. The vertebral column. *(From Chusid JG.* Correlative Neuroanatomy and Functional Neurology. *19th ed. Stamford, CT: Lange; 1985.)*

formed by the articulation of the superior articular processes with the inferior articular processes of the vertebrae above. In the upper spine, the zygapophyseal joints are oriented in the sagittal plane; however, a transition takes place at the thoracolumbar junction where the joints gradually become more coronally angled. The inferior articular processes of the 5th vertebra are relatively coronally placed so that they hook over the superior articular processes of the sacrum, thus mechanically assisting stabilization of the 5th vertebra on the sacrum. The articular capsules of the zygapophyseal joints are relatively lax and provide very little joint stability.

The intervertebral disks are fibrocartilaginous joints located anteriorly between adjacent vertebrae. They consist of a gelatinous nucleus pulposus surrounded by a fibrocartilaginous annulus fibrosis. The disk is reinforced anteriorly and posteriorly by the longitudinal ligaments. The anterior longitudinal ligament is a strong band that serves to limit extension of the vertebral column. The posterior longitudinal ligament is a similarly strong band that serves to limit flexion of the vertebral column. Both the anterior and the posterior longitudinal ligaments are thickest centrally and thinnest laterally.

The near sagittal orientation of the articular process facets allows good extension and flexion in the lumbar spine. Lateral bending motion is also relatively free with the inferior facets of the vertebrae sliding down on one side and up on the other. However, rotational movements in the lumbar region are very limited since the articular processes quickly lock together.

Disks

The intervertebral disks absorb shock, distribute load, allow motion, and provide joint stability between vertebral bodies. They are numbered according to the vertebra below which they lie. The disks are approximately one-third the height of the vertebral body in the lumbar spine region. They are composed of two parts, the fibrous outer portion, the annulus fibrosus, and the semigelatinous inner portion, the nucleus pulposus.

The annulus fibrosus is made up of concentric layers of obliquely running fibers that absorb compressive forces. Its functions are to withstand torsional tension of the vertebral column and horizontal pressure from the nucleus pulposus.

The nucleus pulposus lies somewhat posterior to the center of the vertebral body, and thus the annulus fibrosus is thinnest posterior to the nucleus pulposus. The normal water content of the nucleus pulposus is 70 to 88 percent. Because of its gelatinous nature, the nucleus pulposus changes shape easily and dissipates vertical forces applied to the spinal column. The functions of the nucleus pulposus are to distribute the load through the vertebral column and to absorb vertical stresses.

Large pressures can be generated in the nucleus pulposus. Studies have shown that pressure at the L3 in a 70-kg individual is about 100 kg when standing and 140 kg when sitting.[15,16] When lifting a 50-kg weight, the load on the L3 disk increases to 210 kg if the lifting is done with the back straight and the knees bent and to 340 kg if the back is bent and the knees are straight (see Fig. 8-2).[16] The tremendous stresses placed across the disks emphasizes the importance of correct lifting form, that is, lifting with a straight back and using the thigh and leg muscles instead of the back muscles.

The nucleus pulposus has no direct innervation. However, the adjacent posterior longitudinal ligaments and the posterior surface of the annulus fibrosis are rich in sensory fibers and may contribute to the pain felt by patients with discogenic pain.[17] Compression of the sensory fibers in dural sleeves and roots of a spinal nerve may contribute to the radiating pain felt by some patients.[18]

The blood supply of the intervertebral disk after birth is primarily by diffusion from the adjacent vertebral end plates. However, the foramina, through which fetal vessels traversed the cartilaginous end plates, may remain patent and are a potential site for intervertebral herniation of the nucleus pulposus.

Muscles

The muscles of the back can be divided into two general layers: the superficial layer (see Fig. 8-3) and the deep

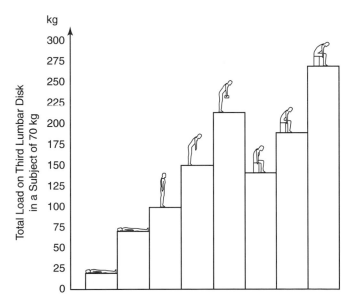

Figure 8–2. Total load on the third lumbar disk in different positions in a 70-kg subject. Positions shown are (1) reclining supine; (2) reclining lateral decubitus; (3) standing upright; (4) standing with 20 degrees of forward leaning; (5) standing as in 4 with 20-kg load in arms; (6) sitting upright, arms and back unsupported; (7) sitting with 20 degrees of forward leaning; and (8) sitting as in 7 with 20-kg load in arms. *(From Nachemson A. The load in lumbar disc in different positions of the body.* Acta Orthop Scand. *1965;36:426. With permission.)*

layer (see Fig. 8-4). The superficial layer, an extension of the shoulder girdle muscles in the lower back, is composed of the latissimus dorsi. The deep layer is composed of numerous converging and diverging fascicles that are arbitrarily grouped together by length and direction.[19] The erector spinae is the largest muscle group in the back. These muscles are primary extensors of the back. Lying beneath the erector spinae are the transversospinalis muscles. These muscles slant inward and upward and are extensors and lateral flexors of the lumbar spine. The segmental muscles are represented by the interspinales between the spinous processes and the medial and lateral intertransversarii between the transverse processes. With the exception of a few small anterolateral muscles, these back muscles are innervated by the dorsal ramus of the spinal nerve at the level superior to the origin of the muscle.

In contrast to the discrete function of limb muscles, the complex, overlapping back muscles act in various combinations to initiate and complete motions. In many instances, after the initiation of a motion by the agonist, gravity acts as the primary force with the back muscles eccentrically contracting to control the motion. The muscles involved in the motions of the lower spine are listed in Table 8-1.

Spinal Cord and Nerve Roots

The spinal cord ends near the lower edge of L1 as the conus medullaris. Below this level is the cauda equina, which descends from the L2 level to the S2 level. The typical posterolateral protruding disk usually compresses the nerve that exits through the foramen, below the level of the disk, instead of the laterally exiting nerve root at the intervertebral foramen at the same level (see Fig. 8-5). Thus, the protruding disk usually exits the nerve numbered one greater than itself (e.g., a protruding L4 disk typically affects the L5 nerve).

GENERAL HISTORY

Although the precise cause of low back pain cannot be clearly delineated in many cases, the patient history and physical examination are the first, critical steps in identifying the small subgroup of individuals with pathology that requires diagnostic testing or surgical intervention. Attention to detail in this part of the process leads to a thoughtful, directed, thorough, cost- and time-effective evaluation. Despite the importance of these early steps, they are often compromised by the busy clinician who either delegates the task to others or relies more heavily on later diagnostic studies to fill in the gaps. The interview process itself can yield a wealth of more nuanced information not readily apparent in the presenting complaint about the patient's

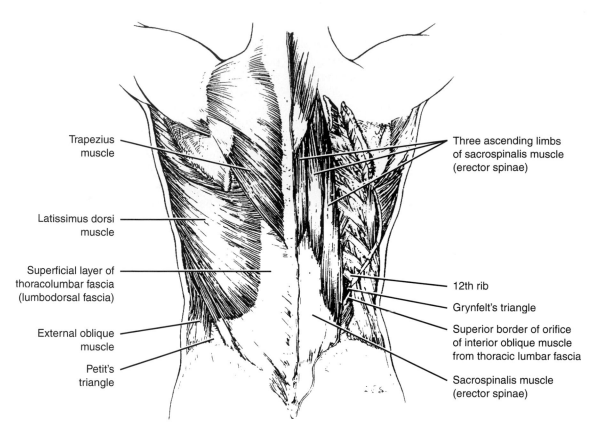

Trapezius muscle

Latissimus dorsi muscle

Superficial layer of thoracolumbar fascia (lumbodorsal fascia)

External oblique muscle

Petit's triangle

Three ascending limbs of sacrospinalis muscle (erector spinae)

12th rib

Grynfelt's triangle

Superior border of orifice of interior oblique muscle from thoracic lumbar fascia

Sacrospinalis muscle (erector spinae)

Figure 8–3. The superficial muscles of the posterolateral abdominal wall. *(From Linder HH. Clinical Anatomy 1989. Norwalk, CT: Appleton & Lange; 1989.)*

concerns, limitations, expectations, and attitudes that can have a critical impact on the overall outcome. The high false-positive rate of advanced imaging studies such as magnetic resonance imaging (MRI) and computed tomography (CT) further underscores the need to use these studies only to confirm clinical suspicions based on a complete history and physical examination.[20-22] It also avoids the folly of performing operations based on radiographic findings alone. This section reviews the areas that must be explored during the process of obtaining a patient's history of the lumbar spine injury and during the physical exam.

Pain

Pain is a common presenting complaint. The history should focus on the onset, location, character, and associated factors related to the primary complaint of pain. The interviewer should determine whether the pain occurred acutely or insidiously and where the pain is located: midline, paraspinous muscle region, buttocks, legs, or radicular. Ask patients specifically about the distribution of pain, tingling, and numbness. Referred pain should not be confused with radicular symptoms that occur in specific dermatomal patterns of motor weakness, reflex, and sensory changes. Sclerotomal pain can

extend into the buttock, hips, groin, or distal thigh in a nonspecific pattern that needs to be distinguished from the dermatomal pattern of radicular pain. Elicit whether the onset of pain was related to work or trauma, and if the patient is involved in litigation or a Worker's Compensation claim. It is important to determine if the pain is mechanical, which is associated with activity and relieved by rest, progressive over the course of the day, or nonmechanical, which is independent of activity and often worse at night.

The acute onset of pain in a young athlete is most likely related to a traumatic event and likely to be caused by contusion, muscle strain, or ligamentous sprain. In the older athlete, the acute onset of pain may be related to a much lower energy mechanism of injury. Discogenic pain also becomes much more likely. For chronic pain in the younger athlete, stress fractures and apophysitis must be considered. In individuals under 10 years old or over 60 years old with first-time back pain, the diagnosis of a tumor should also be considered.

The location of the pain—back, lower leg, or both—is important. Pain that radiates into the lower leg or foot is suggestive of nerve root impingement. Nonradiating, localized back pain in the young athlete is rarely discogenic. Back pain can be described by its character, mechanical or nonmechanical, or its location, axial

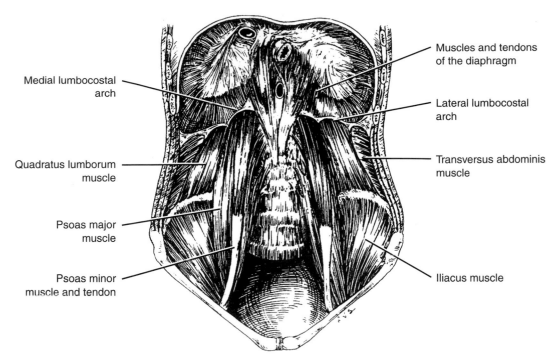

Figure 8–4. The deep muscles of the posterior abdominal wall. *(From Linder HH. Clinical Anatomy 1989. Norwalk, CT: Appleton & Lange; 1989.)*

or radicular. Mechanical pain tends to be associated with activity. It is relieved by rest and is progressive over the course of the day. Nonmechanical pain is independent of activity, is often worse at night, and is not relieved by rest or immobilization; it warrants a more aggressive investigation into other causes such as tumor or infection. Axial pain is most often diffuse and associated with complaints of pain in the paraspinal region. It is not typically associated with paresthesia, numbness, or weakness in a radicular distribution.

Radicular pain is characterized by pain, dysesthesia, paresthesia, or numbness in a dermatomal distribution. A history of axial back pain that precedes leg symptoms is common in radiculopathy due to disk herniation. Clinically evident weakness is often not noticed by pa-

tients at the time of presentation because of its insidious onset and unconscious accommodation to it.[23]

Aggravating and Alleviating Factors

Pain with prolonged sitting may implicate sustained lumber flexion or disk pathology as a cause of the pain. The pain of a herniated disk may find relief by standing. Standing, walking, or running can cause pain in conditions that are worse with hyperextension. Pain during specific activities frequently implies possible overuse injury of muscles, tendons, or bones. Malignancy or infection should be considered in patients with unrelenting pain at rest. Pain from vascular or visceral sources often causes the patient to constantly shift positions in the attempt to alleviate pain, whereas patients with mechanical pain tend to remain in a specific position.

Important information is also gathered in the review of systems that may support the diagnosis of a more serious cause of low back pain. Alteration of bowel or bladder control can be related to cauda equina syndrome or to a tumor. Weight loss and night pain are two other symptoms associated with tumors.

The differential diagnosis should also consider other causes of low back pain (see Table 8-2). Constitutional symptoms should also be determined. Any recent weight loss, history of fevers, chills, or recent infections should be elicited, since tumors or infection are common but often missed as sources of back pain. Relieving and ex-

TABLE 8–1. MUSCLES INVOLVED WITH MOTIONS OF THE LUMBAR SPINE

Forward Flexion	Extension	Lateral Flexion
Psoas major	Latissimus dorsi	Latissimus dorsi
Rectus abdominis	Erector spinae	Erector spinae
External abdominal oblique	Transversospinalis	Transversospinalis
Internal abdominal oblique	Interspinales	Interspinales
Transversus abdominis	Quadratus lumborum	Psoas major External abdominal oblique

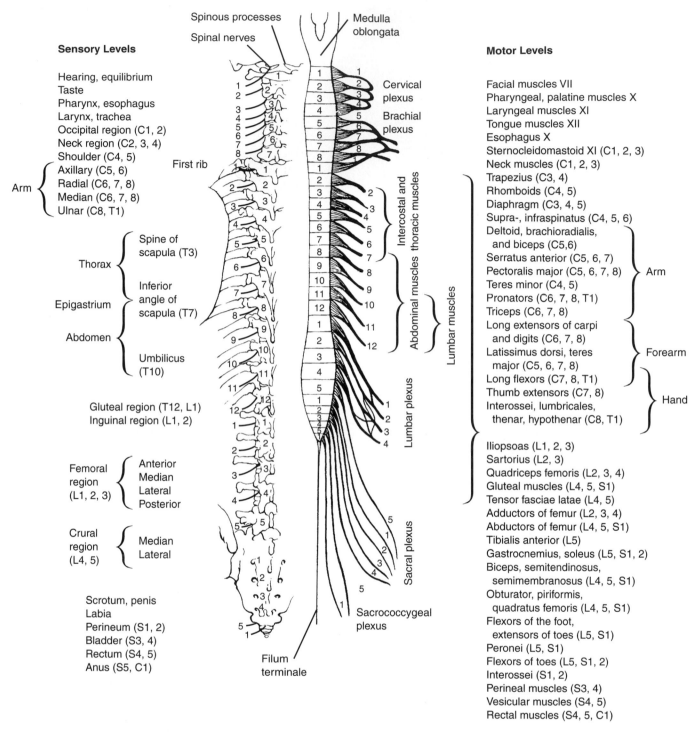

Figure 8–5. Relation of spinal cord to vertebral column. *(From Chusid JG. Correlative Neuroanatomy and Functional Neurology. 19th ed. Norwalk, CT: Appleton & Lange; 1985.)*

acerbating activities and all successful or unsuccessful prior attempts at conservative treatments should also be determined. Other associated events, such as increased pain with menses, needs to be elicited. Hematocolpos secondary to imperforate hymen is an uncommon but reported source of pain in young women.[24]

PHYSICAL EXAM

Observation

The physical examination should begin with observation. Gait abnormalities and posture can be grossly as-

TABLE 8–2. NONMUSCULOSKELETAL CAUSES OF LOW BACK PAIN

Referred Pain from Other Organ Systems:

Aortic dissection	Neoplasm
Abdominal aortic aneurysm	Intraspinal tumors
Gastrointestinal disorders	Metastatic tumors
Pancreatitis	Primary bone tumors
Pancreatic cancer	Neurologic diseases
Ruptured abdominal viscus	Demyelinating diseases
Gynecologic disorders	Neuropathies
Ectopic pregnancy	Transverse myelitis
Pelvic inflammatory disease	Urologic disorders including
Tumors	Prostatitis
Hip pathology	Urinary disorders including
Infections	Nephrolithiasis
Discitis	Pyelonephritis
Epidural abscess	Ureteral colic
Osteomyelitis	Vascular disorders
Metabolic diseases	
Gout	
Hyperparathyroidism	
Osteoporosis	
Paget's disease	

Other Nonmusculoskeletal Causes:

Abusive relationship	Disability seeking
Compensable injury	Drug seeking
Conversion disorder	Psychiatric disorder
Depression	Somatoform disorder

sessed as the patient is brought into the room. Adaptive behaviors in response to weakness and pain may also be evident at this time. Patients must disrobe for a physical examination. Shorts are acceptable for men and a gown open at the back or two-piece bathing suits can be used for women. The overall appearance of the patient can provide valuable information and should not be overlooked. Neck webbing is suggestive of Turner's syndrome. A high arched pallet is associated with a variety of syndromes including Marfan's syndrome. Ear deformities are suggestive of a variety of congenital anomalies.

Posture

Stand behind the patient and observe the curves of the back. Normally there should be gentle concave curves in the cervical and lumbar regions with a gentle convex curve in the thoracic region (see Fig. 8-1). Flattening of the lumbar curve may indicate muscle spasm. Hyperlordosis, the accentuation of the normal concave curve, may have developed to compensate for a protuberant abdomen of pregnancy or obesity, for kyphosis of the thoracic region, or hip flexion contractures. Scoliosis is a lateral curvature of the spine. Structural scoliosis usually involves rotation of the ver-

tebrae and the rotational deformity is accented with forward flexion. A list of the spine is a lateral tilt seen when the spinous process of T1 is shifted off the midline. This condition is a functional scoliosis and disappears with forward flexion.

Leg length discrepancies, chest deformities, either excavatum or carinatum, and high arched feet should also be noted. Attention should then be directed to standing posture in both the frontal and sagittal planes. Pelvis asymmetry is also important to note and document. If the iliac crest cannot be felt, then this should be measured in centimeters from the posterior superior iliac spine or the anterior superior iliac spine. The general nature of the normal and abnormal curves should also be noted.

After observation, the physical examination continues with a gross screening similar to the orthopaedic preparticipation evaluation.[25] This screening will allow a directed evaluation. The patient should perform a toe and heel walk. **Toe walking** (see Fig. 8-6) can be used as a general assessment of S1 motor function; **heel walking** (see Fig. 8-7) is a gross measurement of L4 and L5 motor strength. A **single knee bend** (see Fig. 8-8) is used to assess quadriceps strength, which can be decreased from L3 or L4 nerve root involvement. Referred pain from the hip and knee may present as back pain; therefore, a quick screening should be done by using the **squat test**, sometimes called a bounce test (see Fig. 8-9). A **duck walk test** (see Fig. 8-10) combines movements at the hips, knees, and ankles and can be used to test these joints for gross defects.[26,27] Subtle motor weakness or early fatigu-

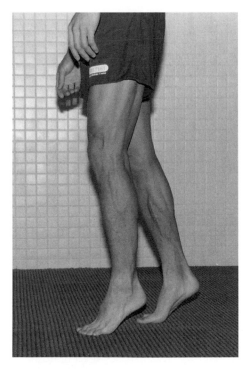

Figure 8–6. Toe walking.

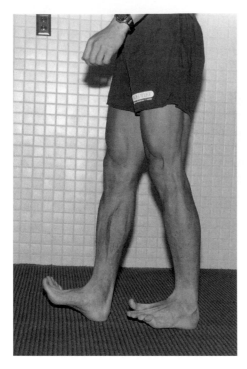

Figure 8–7. Heel walking.

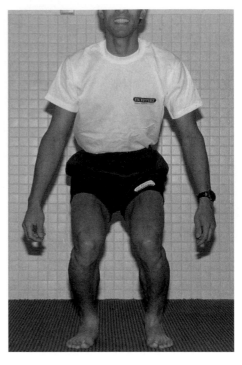

Figure 8–9. Squat test.

ing can often be elicited by repetitive muscle testing and can be a subtle sign of nerve root involvement. A **Trendelenburg sign** may be seen with the patient balancing on one leg. A positive sign is listing of the pelvis away from the weight-bearing leg and may represent glu-

teus medius weakness from coxa vara, fracture of the greater trochanter, or a slipped capital femoral epiphysis. Subtle weakness in the gluteus medius may be elicited by fatiguing the gluteus medius by having the patient do 4 or 5 toe-raises during single stance.[26]

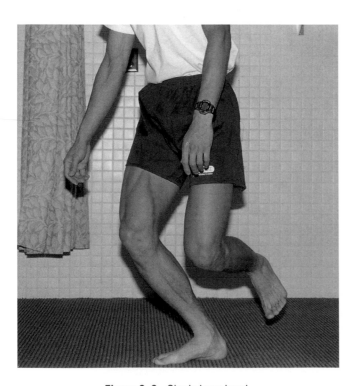

Figure 8–8. Single knee bend.

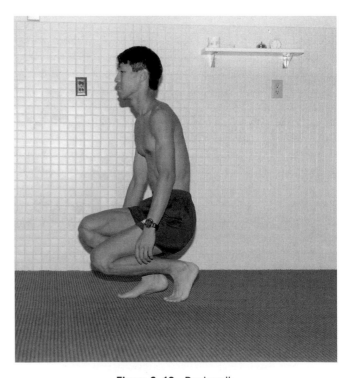

Figure 8–10. Duck walk.

Surface Markings

The skin should be examined for markings and lesions. Lipomas, although usually incidental findings, may be associated with spina bifida, especially if in conjunction with a faun's beard, which is a hairy patch associated with a midline lipoma. Skin tags may indicate neurofibromatosis, especially in conjunction with café-au-lait spots. Port wine stain marks overlying the spine also may indicate spina bifida. Asymmetry or spasm in paraspinal muscles and atrophy of the thighs, legs, and feet should be documented. Surgical scars and skin lesions should also be noted.

Palpation

The midline and paraspinous muscle region should be palpated to elicit tenderness, to note malalignment, and to discover masses. The L4 and L5 interspace lies at the level of the upper border of the iliac crests and serves as a reference point for the palpation exam. The S2 spinous process lies at the level of the posterior superior iliac spines. An area of point tenderness is suspicious for fracture. Step deformity of the spine may be associated with spondylolisthesis or fracture. Pain referred from the back may be reproduced during the palpation of the posterior spine. Coccydynia is a painful coccyx usually caused by a direct blow. To fully palpate the coccyx a rectal examination must be done.

Only the superficial layer of the paraspinal muscles is palpable. The patient lies prone with the head extended, which allows the muscle fascia to relax. Note any tenderness, spasms, or defects. Muscle spasm presents as a rigid, tender prominence. If unilateral, the spasm may cause a scolitic deformity, if bilateral, a loss of the normal sagittal contour of the spine.

The anterior spine may be palpated in a slender patient. The patient should lie supine with the knees bent to relax the abdominal muscles. The aorta lies over the spine until the level of the umbilicus. The scaral promontory (L5 and S1 articulation) is the most easily palpated area of the anterior spine.

Motions

The patient should perform forward flexion and extension and left and right lateral bending, both to permit assessment of the overall range of motion and to determine if pain is provoked by any of these maneuvers. The type of pain should also be noted: low back, referred, or sciatic type. The patient should be instructed to place his or her feet together with knees straight and finger and palms opposed for a forward bending test. The patient then flexes at the waist. The examiner looks from the back for any signs of deformity. Rib prominence is measured from the area of maximum prominence in centimeters. A scoliometer can also be used as an objective measure of the deformity. Forward bending with consistent deviation to one side on repeated testing suggests irritative lesions such as spinal cord tumor, herniated disk, or an osteoid osteoma. Range of motion should also be documented not only for its magnitude, but also for the affect it has on the curve itself and pain elicited. Normal range of motion of the thoracolumbar spine is 85 degrees of flexion, 50 degrees of extension, 40 degrees of lateral bending, and 45 degrees of rotation. Tanner stage should be noted and recorded.[28,29] Pain elicited in extension is suggestive of facet joint arthritis or spinal stenosis. A **Schober test** measures spinal flexibility. With the patient standing, make a mark over the spine at the level of the posterior superior iliac spine (PSIS) (S2 level and mark 10 cm above and 5 cm below the initial mark). When the patient touches the toes, a person with normal flexibility will show an increased distance between the superior and inferior marks of at least 20 cm.[30]

With the patient lying down, hip range of motion should be determined and any hip flexion contractures noted. Leg length should be measured. Abdominal examination should be performed to rule out any intra-abdominal cause of back pain. The flexibility of a kyphotic deformity can be assessed by asking the patient, while lying prone with arms at the sides, to raise the shoulders and head off the table. The examiner can also apply compression to the apex of the scoliotic deformity to get a rough estimation of its flexibility.

The sacroiliac joint mobility should be examined. With the patient standing, the examiner places one thumb over the PSIS on the side to be tested and the other thumb over the sacral spine at the same height. When the patient flexes the hip, the thumb over the PSIS should drop down. Upward motion of the thumb over the PSIS indicates sacroiliac joint fixation.

Neurologic Examination

A complete neurologic examination should also be performed and positive findings explored further (see Table 8-3). Any positive findings on the physical examination should guide subsequent diagnostic studies. Light touch and pinprick deficits should be determined. Note proprioception of both the lower and upper extremities. Proprioception is often lost in both cervical spinal stenosis and neuropathy. A rectal examination should be performed to assess sphincter strength. Abnormal anal wink is suggestive of a sacral root involvement. Reflexes should be tested for evidence of asymmetry and compared to the upper extremities. Hyperreflexia, clonus, and Babinski's sign are important signs of upper motor neuron involvement.

TABLE 8–3. NEUROLOGIC EXAM OF THE LOWER EXTREMITIES

Root	Reflex	Muscles	Sensation
L1, L2	Cremaster	Iliopsoas	Anterior upper thigh
L3	Patellar	Quadriceps	Anterior knee
L4	Patellar	Tibialis anterior	Medial ankle and medial leg
L5	None	Extensor hallicus longus	First dorsal web space and lateral leg
S1	Achilles	Peroneus longus and brevis	Lateral foot
S2 to S4	Anal wink	Toe intrinsics	Perianal and perineal regions

Regional disturbances are considered to be widespread sensory or motor disturbances that do not correspond to specific neuroanatomic lesions. Often both motor and sensory disturbances will involve the same location, such as an entire limb or half of the body. Weakness on formal testing includes giving way or partial cogwheel to resistance. Sensory disturbances are characterized by light touch, pinprick, and other sensory modalities in a nondermatomal pattern that is commonly stocking and glove in nature. There can be overlapping sensory distribution of lumbar nerve roots.

L1 to L3

Iliopsoas weakness is suggestive of L1 and L2 nerve root dysfunction. Absence of the cremasteric reflex, elicited by stroking the inner thigh with the back of a reflex hammer causing the scrotal sac to be pulled upward, is abnormal when other upper motor neuron lesion pathologic reflexes are present. The cremaster muscle is innervated by T12, however; unilateral absence of the reflex is most indicative of lower motor neuron lesions between L1 and L2. Quadriceps strength is decreased with L3 as well as L4 root involvement.

L4

Tibialis anterior strength is associated with L4 motor function. It is tested by resisting ankle dorsiflexion and inversion. L4 root sensation involves the medial ankle and anterior aspect of the shin. Although the patellar reflex is predominately an L4 nerve root function, it also is mediated by L2 and L3 nerves. Thus, the reflex will be present, albeit much diminished, even if the L4 nerve root is severed.

L5

Extensor hallicus longus strength is an indicator of L5 root function. L5 root sensation is distributed over the lateral calf and the first dorsal web space. The posterior

tibial reflex is the most specific for the L5 nerve, but is difficult to elicit and is absent bilaterally in more than 50 percent of patients.

S1 to S4

The peroneus longus and brevis are innervated by the S1 nerve root. These muscles are assessed by resisted plantar flexion and eversion of the foot. The sensory distribution of the S1 nerve root involves the posterior calf, the lateral foot, and the sole. The Achilles tendon reflex is a S1 nerve root. Perianal and perineal sensation should be tested for S2, 3, and 4 nerve root function.

SPECIAL TESTS

A thorough history and back examination will help to limit the differential diagnosis. The remaining possibilities can then be tested by specific provocative tests.[26,31]

Nerve Root Tension Signs

The **straight leg test**, also known as Laségue's test, can be performed with the patient both sitting or lying down with the knees extended and with the pelvis in a stable, fixed position (see Fig. 8–11). The point at which the straight leg raise reproduces radicular symptoms should be noted as well as the symptoms that are produced. The leg is lowered until the symptoms resolve. Radicular pain can often be detected at this lower angle when the foot is then dorsiflexed. The straight leg raise test should only be considered positive when it reproduces pain or numbness in a radicular pattern and should be considered negative if back or thigh pain alone is provoked. The sciatic nerve is completely stretched at 70 degrees and pain after that point is probably due to joint pain from the lumbar or sacroiliac joints.[32] The sensitivity for the single leg straight leg test is 80 percent, but the specificity is only 40 percent.[33] The examiner should then raise both legs in the **bilateral straight leg raise**. If pain is elicited before 70 degrees, the lesion is probably in the sacroiliac joint; if pain is elicited after 70 degrees the lesion is probably in the lumbar spine.

The **crossed straight leg** or well straight leg test is a more sensitive measure of nerve irritability. The asymptomatic leg is elevated and elicits radicular pain in the contralateral symptomatic leg. A positive crossed straight leg test frequently indicates a large disk protrusion, usually medial to nerve root.[32] This test is also called the cross-over sign or the well straight leg test of Fajersztajn. The specificity of a positive test is higher than the ipsilateral straight leg test (75 versus 40 percent), but the sensitivity is much lower (25 versus 80 percent).[33]

The **bowstring test** of the symptomatic leg involves raising the leg until radicular symptoms are elicited. The knee is then flexed until the symptoms are relieved. Compression of the popliteal fossa should reproduce radicular symptoms if the test is positive (see Fig. 8–12).

The **prone straight leg raise test** or femoral stretch test is used to specifically test for nerve root irritation of L3 and L4 (see Fig. 8–13). This should be performed with the knee in extension and should reproduce pain in a radicular pattern. Peripheral pulses should also be noted. Their absence is suggestive of vascular claudication.

Meningeal Signs

Positive **Kernig** and **Brudzinski tests** may indicate meningeal or dural irritation. The tests are performed with the patient supine. A Kernig's sign is pain with neck flexion. Pain with hip flexion is a Brudzinski test.

Upper Motor Neuron Tests

Upper motor neuron tests indicate the loss of normal inhibition of reflexes by the upper motor neurons due to injury. A positive **Babinski's sign** is extension of the great toe and abduction of the other toes with light plantar stimulation. This is also associated with an upper motor neuron lesion, except in infants up to a few weeks old in whom the response is normal. **Oppenheimer's sign** also produces extension of the great toe when a finger is run along the crest of the tibia. This normally causes either no reaction or pain. Clonus can be elicited by a short upper thrust of the ankle and forefoot. This causes repetitive motion of the ankle joint.

Tests for Joint Dysfunction

A positive **one-legged hyperextension test** is suggestive of spondylolysis. The patient stands on one leg and extends the back. The examiner should help the patient maintain balance and be prepared to prevent the patient from falling (see Fig. 8–14). Pain on the support leg is suspicious for an ipsilateral spondylolysis. A positive **pheasant test** is suspicious for spinal segment instability. The examiner places pressure to the posterior lumbar spine on a prone patient while passively flexing the knees until the heels reach the buttocks.

Tests for Malingering

Overreaction during examination can take the form of collapsing, sweating, tremor, disproportionate muscle tension, facial expression, and verbalization. Exaggerated response to venipuncture or myelography can also be significant. Observer bias and cultural variation can affect the interpretation of overreaction, the significance of which must be evenly weighed with the other nonorganic signs found on physical examination.

Nonorganic physical sign testing can be a useful adjunct in the overall assessment of patients with low back pain. The **Waddell signs** provide a simple screening tool to identify individuals who require more formal psychological testing as part of their overall assessment and can be useful in recognizing individuals whose psychological component to their disease may compromise their ultimate surgical outcome.[34] The five types of physical signs are tenderness, simulation, distraction, regional, and overreaction. Three or more positive types of signs are suggestive of malingering, secondary gain, or a significant psychogenic component.

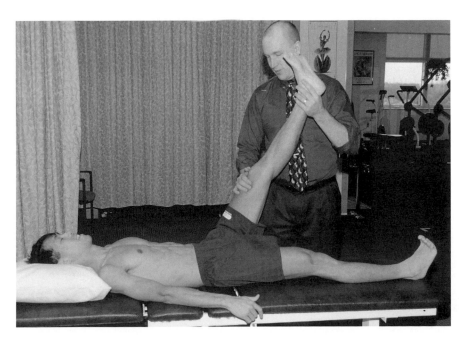

Figure 8–11. Straight leg test.

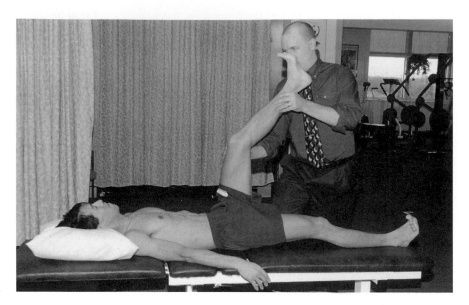

Figure 8–12. Bowstring test.

Nonorganic tenderness is defined as superficial or nonanatomic tenderness. Simulation tests are the axial loading test and the rotation test. The **axial loading test** is positive when vertical loads applied to the top of the head elicits back pain. A positive **rotation test** occurs when rotation of the shoulders and pelvis in the same plane produces back pain. In the presence of root irritation, this maneuver may cause leg pain that does not constitute a positive test for nonorganic pain. Findings that are only present on formal examination, but are absent with casual observation or reexamination using a different provocative maneuver, can suggest a nonorganic

component. The **flip test** is commonly employed to elicit such findings. The straight leg raise test in supine position will be substantially worse than in sitting position. In the **sitting root test**, the patient is asked to flex the neck by placing the chin down against the chest. The knee is extended while the hip is flexed to 90 degrees while the examiner pretends to examine the foot. Patients with true sciatic pain will complain of radicular pain and will sometimes arch backwards to attempt to relieve the pain. In the **Hoover test**, the examiner places a hand under each heel of a supine patient. The patient is asked to do a straight leg lift with one of the legs. If no

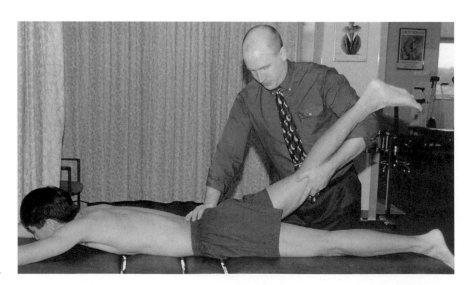

Figure 8–13. Prone straight leg raise test.

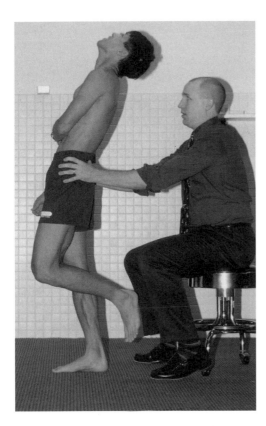

Figure 8–14. One-legged hyperextension test.

pressure is felt or the patient cannot lift the leg, the patient is probably not really trying. If the lifted leg is weaker, the examiner should feel increased pressure under the normal heel because of the increased effort needed to lift the leg.

Other Tests

To test the sacroiliac joint, the hands are placed over the iliac crests with the thumbs on the anterior superior iliac spines (ASIS), then forcibly compressed down and in toward the midline at a 45 degrees angle (see Fig. 8-15). Pain in the sacroiliac joint may be reproduced by this **pelvic squish test**. A **Patrick** or **Faber test** may also reproduce pain in the sacroiliac joint, as well as pain from hip pathology. With the patient supine, the examiner places the foot of the involved side against the medial aspect of the opposite knee. In this position, with the hip flexed, abducted, and externally rotated, inguinal pain indicates hip pathology. At this point, the femur is fixed relative to the pelvis. Pain in the sacroiliac joint is reproduced by stressing the sacroiliac joint by placing one hand over the knee and the other over the oppo-site ASIS and pressing down toward the table (see Fig. 8-16).

HISTORY AND PHYSICAL SUMMARY

A careful, focused history and physical examination is critical to providing good, cost-effective health care. Imaging studies should be ordered only after a differential diagnosis has been generated to minimize unnecessary testing. Individual patient concerns and needs and nonorganic components should be recognized and addressed, since these can have a significant influence on the overall outcome. Attention to detail throughout this process will lead to thorough, efficient diagnosis and management of disorders of the spine.

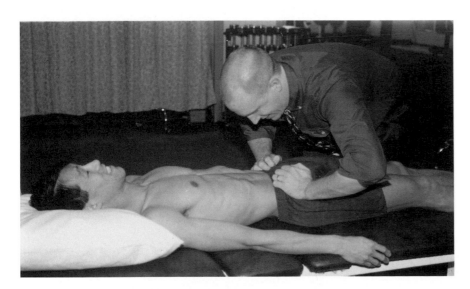

Figure 8–15. Pelvic squish test.

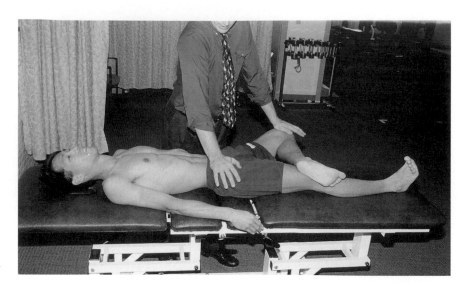

Figure 8–16. Faber test.

DIAGNOSTIC TESTS

X-rays

A complete history and physical usually is sufficient to diagnosis the majority of low back problems. Plain radiographs may be necessary if the examination is suspicious of fracture, infection, or tumor. A standard lumbosacral series usually consists of an anterior posterior (AP), lateral lumbar, and lateral lumbosacral film (see Figs. 8-17 and 8-18). The AP view is used to evaluate the vertebral bodies, facets, pedicles, laminae, and disk spaces. Wedging of the vertebrae is suspicious for fracture. The presence of a bamboo spine is evidence of ankylosing spondylosis. In lumbarization of S1, the S1 vertebral body becomes mobile. Lumbarization is seen in 2 to 8 percent of the population. L5 can also be sacralized, becoming fused to the sacrum or pelvis. The sacralization variant is seen in 3 to 6 percent of the population.

The lateral view is used to evaluate the normal lordotic curves, vertebral bodies, disk spaces, traction spurs, and the slippage of spondylolisthesis. Traction spurs typically occur approximately 1 mm from the disk border, whereas osteophytes occur at the disk-vertebral body border. Traction spurs may indicate an unstable lumbar intervertebral segment.[35] Oblique views are useful primarily to evaluate for possible spondylolysis or spondylolisthesis (see Fig. 8-19).

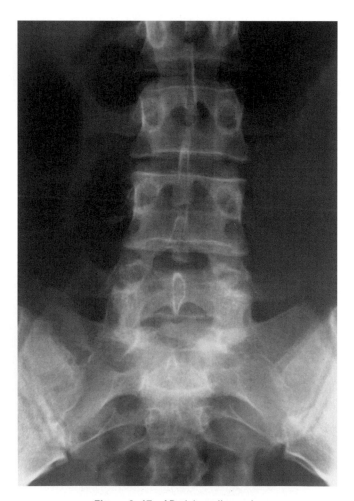

Figure 8–17. AP plain radiograph.

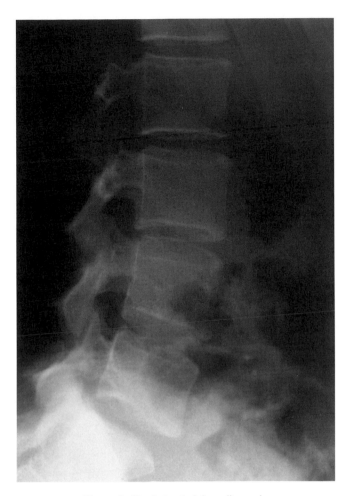

Figure 8–18. Lateral plain radiograph.

Myelogram

A myelogram is useful in the evaluation of a protruding intervertebral disk, a tumor, nerve root entrapment, or spinal stenosis.[36] Water-soluble, nonionic, iodinated contrast solution is instilled into the subarachnoid space (see Fig. 8–20). Side effects of the procedure include headache, stiffness, low back pain, cramps, and lower limb paresthesia. Myelograms are frequently performed in conjunction with CT scans. Myelograms are rarely performed for sport-related back injury and are primarily reserved for patients with neurologic deficits or previous spinal surgery.[2,33,37-39]

Computerized Tomography Scan

Computerized tomography (CT) of the spine provides excellent detail of the bony anatomy (see Figs. 8–21 and 8–22). CT scans will show herniated disks; however, they do not show the internal disk structure or other soft tissue anatomy, such as nerves, as well as MRI.[37] CT scans have the advantage over MRI of being less costly, but have the disadvantage of giving the pa-

tient radiation exposure and are much more costly than plain radiographs or bone scans.[33,40,41] The combination of CT scan and myelography is particularly useful in patients with nerve compression from bony pathology. The diagnostic accuracy of CT scan in the evaluation of disk herniation is approximately 80 percent with plain CT and 90 percent with CT and myelograms.[40] However, studies have also shown that up to one third of asymptomatic patients may also appear to have abnormal disks on CT.[22] Thus, examiners must not order CT scans indiscriminately, but only to confirm a diagnosis made on physical examination and to assist with the treatment plan.

Magnetic Resonance Imaging

MRI has the advantage of being a noninvasive test with no radiation exposure to the patient. Unfortunately, an MRI tends to be the most expensive form of imaging study. MRI is particularly useful in the evaluation of early osteomyelitis, spinal cord tumors, epidural cysts, arteriovenous malformations, and nerve root compression.[33,40] The MRI provides greater detail of soft-tissue

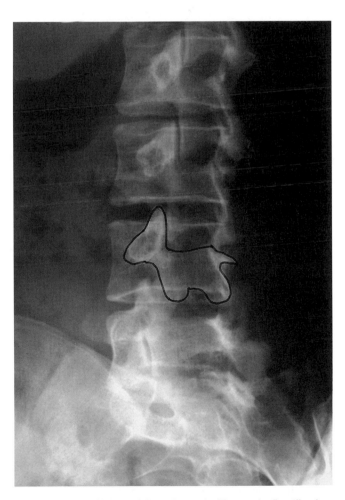

Figure 8–19. Oblique plain radiograph, "Scotty dog" outlined.

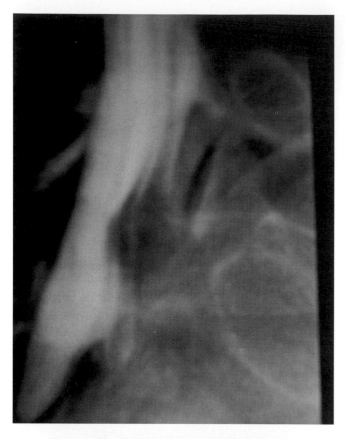

Figure 8–20. Myelogram showing a herniated disk.

structures than CT scans (see Figs. 8–23 and 8–24).[42,43] The MRI is sensitive enough to permit evaluation of the dehydration caused by degenerative disk disease. With the addition of gadolinium contrast, MRI images can lead to differentiation between recurrent disk herniation and epidural scarring.[40] Although there is some evidence that lumbar abnormalities seen on MRI have a higher correlation with frequent low back pain in adolescent patients,[44,45] in adults, a large proportion of asymptomatic individuals may have abnormal findings on MRI.[20,46] Thus, the examiner is cautioned to order an MRI only to confirm a diagnosis made based on the history and physical examination.

Bone Scan

Radionuclide imaging with a technetium (Tc) bone scan provides relatively nonspecific information, but can be useful in directing attention to regions where pathology may exist so that further, more specific testing can proceed. In addition, bone scans are useful in the evaluation of periostitis, reflex sympathetic dystrophy, osteomyelitis, and metastatic disease.[33] The three-phase bone scan consists of the vascular or radionuclide angiogram taken immediately after Tc injection; the blood pool, or soft tissue phase, taken 5 to 10 minutes after injection;

and the delayed, or osseous phase, taken 2 to 5 hours after injection. A positive vascular phase is indicative of soft-tissue inflammation. A positive delayed phase is suspicious for bony pathology. The use of single photon emission computed tomography (SPECT) allows for better anatomic detail.

In the athlete, bone scans are useful in the evaluation of stress fractures, which are often not seen on plain radiographs (see Fig. 8–25). Bone scans are positive 95 percent of the time within 24 hours of the onset of symptoms from stress fractures. In early stress fractures, all three phases are positive. As healing takes place, the vascular, followed by the blood pool images, return to normal. Delayed images can remain positive for 8 to 10 months. Bone scans are especially useful in determining treatment course in spondylolysis.

Electromyogram

An electromyogram (EMG) is not needed for most cases of low back pain. EMG can be useful in distinguishing between peripheral nerve entrapment and nerve root pathology.[7] The sensitivity of EMGs and nerve conduction (NC) studies in diagnosing a herniated disk is 90 percent; however, the specificity is less than 38 percent.[47]

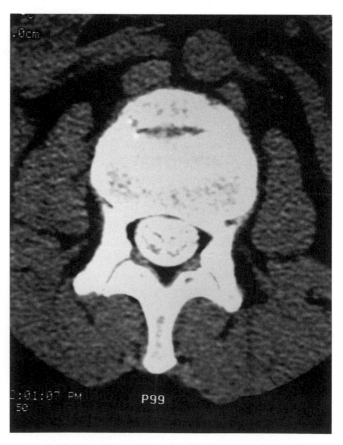

Figure 8–21. CT scan, axial section, showing L2 vertebral compression fracture.

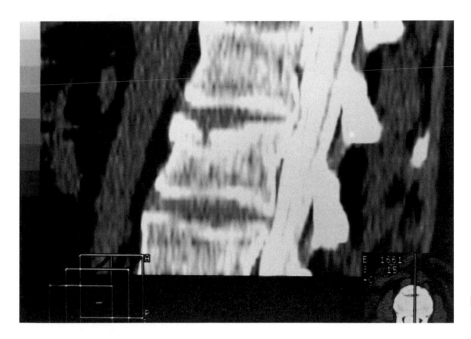

Figure 8–22. CT scan, sagittal view, showing L2 vertebral compression fracture.

EMG may not show positive results until 2 to 3 weeks or more after the initial injury.

SPORTS INJURIES TO THE LUMBAR SPINE—PRESENTATION AND TREATMENT

Spinal injuries have been shown to make up between 2 and 15 percent of all athletic injuries.[48-50] As with nonathletes, the number of individuals who report having back pain is much greater than the number of individuals who actually seek medical help. A survey of football linemen has shown that 75 percent have some type of back pain.[3] The percentage of injury and cause vary from sport to sport, with macrotrauma being most common in high-speed, collision, and acrobatic sports and most frequently affecting the upper spine.[14,50] Microtrauma from repetitive overload tends to be more common in the lower back.[14,50] Although low back pain is common in athletes, most occurrences resolve within 4 to 6 weeks of the onset of symptoms.[4,14,44]

Soft-tissue Injuries

The majority of back pain injuries are minor strains and contusions, most of which are not medically evaluated.[4,14,48,50] Muscle contusion occurs most often in collision and contact sports, but can also be caused by impact with athletic equipment and the playing surface in noncontact sports. Most contusions create minimal disability and resolve quickly with minimal loss of playing time. On examination, an area of ecchymosis and tenderness is usually apparent. Lateral bending to the opposite side usually causes pain. Acute treatment consists of application of ice to the area to minimize bleed-

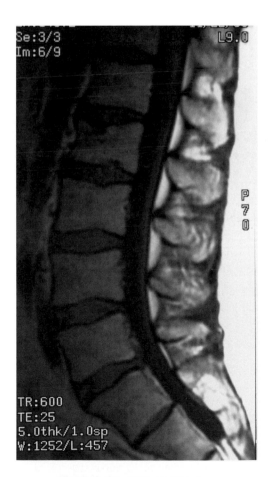

Figure 8–23. MRI, sagittal view.

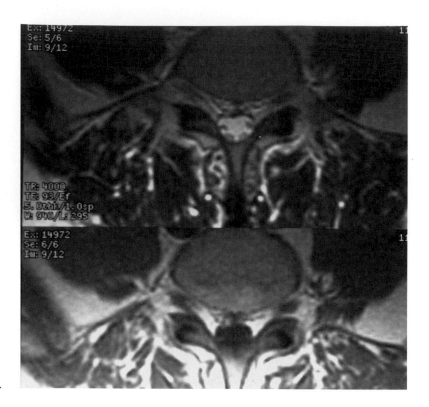

Figure 8–24. MRI, axial sections.

ing. If pain persists after 24 hours, nonsteroidal anti-inflammatory drugs (NSAIDs) are useful. With protection of the contused area, the athlete may return to activity as pain allows after a thorough examination to rule out more serious injuries. A large contusion may mask a fracture or serious internal organ injury, such as a splenic rupture or renal contusion. Injuries sustained after significant impact forces should be carefully followed and not dismissed with a cursory examination. Children in particular are susceptible to renal trauma, with approximately 30 percent of renal trauma being sport related.[51] If renal trauma is suspected, urinalysis should be obtained and the athlete should be told to report any changes in urination. If a fracture is suspected, radiographs should be obtained.

Low Back Strain and Sprain

Muscles strains accounted for up to 27 percent of the low back pain in adults presenting to an outpatient back clinic.[52] Muscle strains are common in sports with extensive twisting motions (e.g., baseball, golf, martial arts), flexion and extension motions (football, gymnastics, rowing), weight-lifting activity (ballet, pairs figure skating), and those that require maintenance of a flexed position for extended periods of time (bicycling). The most common location for the muscle strain is tearing and stretching of the muscle fibers or distal tendons of the paraspinal muscles in the lower lumbosacral or iliac crest areas. Bleeding caused by the tearing of the muscle or ligament fibers often causes a muscle spasm, swelling, and tenderness near the site of the injury.

The patient often gives a history of the immediate onset of pain after a specific incident, although gradual onset from an overuse injury is not uncommon in athletes. The pain is usually aggravated by specific activities. The pain may radiate into the buttock and into the upper posterior thigh. Pain radiating below the knee is rare.

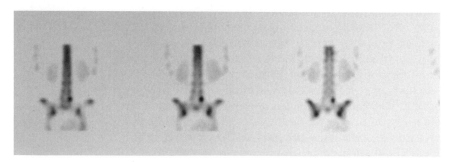

Figure 8–25. Bone scan showing increased uptake of the pars interarticularis region at the L5 level.

Examination of the patient frequently finds muscle spasms, limited range of motion, and occasionally changes in the normal lumbar curve. Most low back strains improve greatly within a few weeks and the majority heal within 2 months.[1,2,30,53] Radiographic studies are rarely needed for acute low back strains. However, if the pain does not respond to treatment, the cause of the pain must be reevaluated and diagnostic studies should be considered, especially in the adolescent athlete, in whom muscle strains accounted for only 6 percent of the low back pain in one series at a pediatric sports clinic.[14,52]

Usually the strains are first or second degree and resolve relatively quickly.[54] First-degree (mild) strains usually have minimal swelling and bruising and minimal loss of motion and function. Second-degree (moderate) strains are characterized by moderate swelling and bruising and are accompanied by significant loss of motion and function. No muscle defect is found on exam in either the first or second-degree strain.[55] The most debilitating pain often is caused by muscle spasm.[48] Acute muscle spasm often responds to ice and stretching. Heat can be useful for the more chronic strain. Usually, mild strains respond to modified activity and rest. In more severe cases, nonsteroidal anti-inflammatory drugs are used. Occasionally, other modalities such as ultrasound and transcutaneous electric nerve stimulation (TENS) can be useful. Muscle relaxants have little direct effect on muscle, but are sometimes useful on a short-term basis in individuals who are having difficulty sleeping because of the back pain, although their side effects often preclude their use.[33] Bedrest should be limited to 2 days.[1,33,56] Long-term bedrest is associated with no greater recovery and, instead, increased muscle atrophy and cardiopulmonary deconditioning.[56,57] Quicker mobilization often results in less total time lost.[56] The use of soft-tissue massage and manipulation is controversial, with some critics warning of possible safety issues in patients with root compression.[7,33,58]

Most athletes may return to sports when pain and range of motion allow. Cardiovascular conditioning and skills drills should be started as soon as tolerated. Specific activities that aggravate back pain should be modified or avoided. The athlete should be started on a strengthening and stretching program to prevent recurrence of the injury.

The best treatment for low back strain is prevention. Prevention includes use of proper lifting and sporting techniques; adequate preseason strengthening and flexibility programs, which include sections for both the abdominal and back muscles; use of proper posture; and adequate preactivity warm-up. Preparticipation exams may note leg length discrepancy, stance, gait, and foot abnormalities, as well as muscle weakness and tightness. Correction of these problems prior to activity may prevent injuries from occurring later in the season. The use of back belts, braces, or corsets is controversial. While some authors recommend them, others have found that they do not have any proven efficacy.[47,48,59-61]

A strain is an injury to the musculotendinous unit, whereas a sprain is an injury to the ligaments. Acute low back sprain presents in a manner very similar to low back strains. On examination, resisted isometric contraction may cause less pain with a sprain then a strain, whereas active motion and passive stretching may cause equal pain. Diagnosis and treatment are similar to that of acute low back strains. The cause of chronic low back sprains, like overuse muscle strains, is often more difficult to isolate. Repetitive activities, as well as poor posture, may be the causes.

Sciatica

Sciatica is severe pain radiating down the leg due to nerve root irritation. The distribution of pain depends on the nerve root or roots involved.[61] L4 root involvement causes pain in the lumbar region and flank with radiation into the medial shin and medial malleolus. L5 root involvement causes radicular pain down the lateral thigh and leg, into the dorsum of the foot, and into the big toe. S1 nerve root involvement causes radicular pain into the buttock, down the posterior thigh, leg, and into the lateral and plantar aspects of the foot. Involvement of each nerve root is also characterized by specific sensory loss, muscle weakness, and deep tendon reflex involvement (see "Neurologic Examination" earlier in the chapter). The L5 and S1 nerve roots are most commonly involved. In athletes over 40 years, sciatica may be from disk herniation, bony hypertrophy, or both. In the athlete over 65 years old, degenerative osteophytic changes are the most likely cause of nerve root irritation.[62] Other causes include spinal stenosis, lumbar facet syndrome, and tumors.[40,63] Sciatica from disk herniation is relatively rare in younger athletes and other etiologies, such as ring apophysitis, should be considered.[14,44,52]

Patients with sciatica often complain of pain aggravated by coughing, laughing, deep breathing, or straining with bowel movements.[1,26] As many as 10 percent of patients with L5 or S1 nerve root irritation experience leg pain with no back pain.[64] The examiner's review of systems should include an evaluation of signs and symptoms of cauda equina syndrome including saddle anesthesia, bilateral leg weakness and pain, loss of bowel or bladder control, and impotence. Saddle anesthesia, reduction of sensation over the buttocks, upper posterior thighs, and perineum, is found in 75 percent of patients with cauda equina syndrome.[7] On examination, these patients frequently have bilateral impairment of motor and sensory functions, as well as loss of anal sphincter tone. Cauda equina syndrome is caused by a large central disk herniation. Back or perianal pain often predominates over radicular symptoms in cauda equina syndrome. Central disk herniation makes up approximately 1 to 2 percent of all disk herniations.[65] In older individuals, this can occur at any level; in younger adults, the herniation is usually at the L4 level.[40] Cauda equina syndrome is a surgical emergency requiring prompt diagnosis and surgical decompression.

In patients with sciatica, but no cauda equina syndrome, spontaneous recovery is usual. Up to half of the patients can be expected to recover in 1 month.[2] Conservative treatment for up to 3 months can be used in individuals with a stable neurologic status without adversely affecting outcome.[66] Thus, diagnostic studies are often not needed in patients with sciatica. For further details on diagnosis and treatment of sciatica, see sections on individual causes.

Herniated Disk

At birth, the water content of the nucleus pulposus is 90 percent, decreasing to 80 percent in young adults, and in some older individuals to less than 70 percent.[62] Thus, the disk is largest and most able to absorb stress in the younger athlete. With age, the annulus fibrosis weakens and is subjected to a larger portion of the stresses.[48,50] The combination of a weakened annulus with a relatively large nucleus pulposus places the middle-aged athlete (aged 30 to 50 years) at relatively high risk for a herniated disk.[54] The combination of the thinning of the annulus fibrosus posteriorly and the weakening of the posterior longitudinal ligament laterally, results in the most common herniated disk in a posterolateral direction. Genetic predisposition, as well as occupational and recreational activities that repetitively load the back, are related to a higher incidence of degenerative disk disease.[67-70]

Herniated disk can be divided into four major subclassifications.[71] A protruded disk refers to the focal asymmetric extension of the nucleus pulposus towards an area of weakness in the annulus, causing a slight deformity of the disk but not rupturing the annulus. A prolapsed disk has protrusion of the nucleus pulposus through all but the outermost fibers of the annulus. In an extruded disk, the nucleus pulposus has traversed the annulus fibrosus and has moved into the canal and may impinge on the adjacent nerve roots. In a sequestrated disk, fragments from the nucleus pulposus have separated from their disk of origin and potentially may migrate (see Fig. 8–26).

A disk herniation most commonly affects a single nerve root. A herniation presents with the involvement of a specific dermatome, reflex, and muscle group. (See

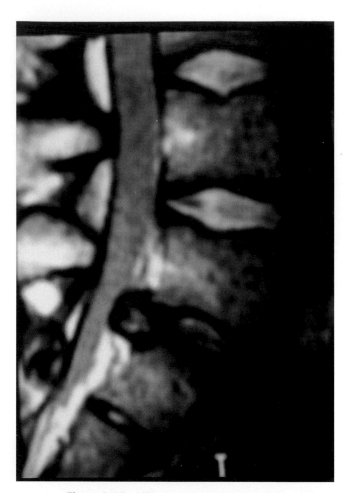

Figure 8–26. MRI scan of sequestrated disk.

the "Sciatica" and "Neurologic Examination" sections earlier in the chapter.) However, a large herniation sometimes will compress two nerve roots.[71]

Although some athletes may remember when they were injured, many athletes with a herniated disk are unable to recall a specific precipitating event. The observant patient will first note low back pain, followed in 24 to 48 hours by radicular pain.[48] Disk herniation occurs at L4 or L5 disks, thus, affecting the L5 and S1 roots, in more than 95 percent of the cases.[47,72] As with sciatic pain, it is important to ask about the signs and symptoms of cauda equina syndrome. In general, the patient will be most comfortable lying down and least comfortable when sitting upright. Patients with a herniated disk may develop a list to alleviate nerve root irritation.[54] In the more common lateral herniation, the patient will lean away from the side with the sciatica. With a medial herniation, the patient lists toward the side with sciatica. The list causes the patient's forward flexion to be off to one side and an asymmetric lateral bend range of motion. Careful muscle strength testing, sensory examination, and reflex testing should be done. An L4 disk herniation usually causes compression of the L5 nerve root with pain caused in the lumbar, groin, and sacroiliac regions, with radiation down the lateral thigh and leg, into the dorsum of the foot; weakness of the extensor hallucis longus and sensory loss on the lateral aspect of the leg and the first dorsal web space is also present (see Table 8-3). An L5 disk herniation usually causes compression of the S1 nerve root, with pain in the lumbar, groin, and sacroiliac regions, with radiation into the buttock, down the posterior thigh and leg, into the lateral foot; weak resisted plantar flexion and foot eversion; sensory loss over the posterior calf, the lateral foot and the sole; and loss of the Achilles tendon reflex. The straight leg test is usually positive; a crossed straight leg test is less often positive but 80 percent specific for a herniated disk.[33] Other useful tests include the bowstring and the prone straight leg tests.

CT and MRI are of little help for the initial evaluation, but may be useful in evaluating patients who do not respond to treatment, patients suspected of having a malignancy or infection, and patients who are surgical candidates.[20,22,46] Usually, treatment of the acute herniated disk includes nonsteroidal anti-inflammatory drugs or analgesics. Muscle relaxants may be useful on a short-term basis in individuals who are having difficulty sleeping because of the back pain.[33] Short periods of bedrest (2 days or less) have been shown to be beneficial to patients with low back pain.[1,33,56] However, prolonged periods of bedrest have adverse affects on an athlete's cardiopulmonary fitness, muscle strength, flexibility, and athletic skills, and therefore, most athletes will refuse complete bedrest. Instead, activities should be modified depending on severity of the symptoms. Continuing cardiopulmonary training may be possible since less than 5 percent of ground reaction stress usually reaches the lumbar spine with running. Alternatively, cross-training in a pool may be possible. Some skill training (shooting free-throws) may be continued. The athlete should have near normal strength and mobility and be able to pass sport-specific functional drills before attempting to return to full sporting activity. The time out before returning to full activity is highly variable depending on severity of the herniation and may range from 6 to 24 or more weeks.

Posture and sporting techniques should be analyzed and corrections made if necessary. A strengthening and stretching program of the abdomen, back, and upper and lower extremities should be initiated under the supervision of an individual trained in rehabilitation techniques. Although of unproven efficacy, some athletes find that limited use of back belts, braces, or corsets during activity is helpful.[47,48,59,60,73] Traction has been shown to transiently reduce the bulging disk.[74,75] Traction may give some athletes prolonged symptomatic relief.[2,54] In general, most patients will have resolution of their symptoms with conservative treatment. However, 5 to 10 percent of patients may eventually require surgery.[66,76] Studies have shown that the long-term results of surgery and conservative treatment are similar.[66,77] However, studies also show that surgery offers a more rapid improvement of symptoms when compared to conservative treatment.[66,78,79] The examiner must take into consideration the fact that many athletes have limited sporting careers and may desire rapid resolution of symptoms, even if it exposes them to more invasive procedures.

Lumbar Scheuermann's Disease and Vertebral Apophysitis

Lumbar Scheuermann's disease, or atypical Scheuermann's disease, is the combination of vertebral end-plate changes and vertebral body wedging that occurs at the thoracolumbar junction or in the upper lumbar segments. Usually only one or two vertebral bodies are involved, most frequently a vertebral body from the T10 to L4 region.[38] Wrestlers and gymnasts seem to be at increased risk.[80] There is a 2 to 1 male to female ratio with peak incidence in the 15 to 17-year-old age group.[81] Signs and symptoms on history, physical, and examination may be subtle in lumbar Scheuermann's disease. Pain may be vague or point-tender over the spine. It is aggravated by activity and relieved by rest. On examination, the patient may have a flat back with hypokyphosis of the thoracic spine and hyperlordosis of the lumbar spine. Radiographs show 3 or more adjacent vertebrae with wedging of 5 degrees or more. Schmorl's nodes, the herniations of the disk into the vertebral end plates and irregularities in the vertebral end plates, may also be found on radiographs. MRI may show the subtle changes in the vertebral end plates.[38,44,45]

Treatment consists of hyperextension bracing (15 to 30 degrees) worn for 18 to 23 hours per day and a stretching and strengthening program with emphasis on hamstring flexibility and back extension exercises. The brace is worn until vertebral body remodeling is visible on plain films, usually a period of 9 to 12 months.[81] In general, the athlete becomes asymptomatic in 4 to 6 weeks and can return to full activity over 3 to 6 months.[14,53]

Vertebral apophysitis, or ring apophysitis, is similar to Scheuermann's disease except the athletes lack the kyphotic deformity. Vertebral apophysitis is a disease that appears almost exclusively in adolescent athletes.[45] Plain radiographic and MRI findings are similar to those found in Scheuermann's disease, without the kyphotic deformity. Treatment and prognosis are also similar.

Facet Syndrome

Facet syndrome is caused by recurrent irritation of the facet joint with attendant synovitis. The underlying disorder is usually bony hypertrophy, osteophyte formation, and disk space narrowing associated with degenerative disk disease. Patients complain of intermittently recurring, episodic, midline low back pain that may be referred to the buttock and the posterior thigh. Acute episodes are treated with nonsteroidal anti-inflammatory drugs and activity modification. Fluoroscopically guided intra-articular or extradural corticosteroid injections have been found to be beneficial in selected patients.[14,54,63] Prevention is aimed at analysis of activity to determine, and then avoid, the aggravating motions and early recognition of recurrences and early treatment.

Spondylolysis and Spondylolisthesis

Most cases of spondylolysis and spondylolisthesis in nonathletes are asymptomatic and are found incidentally in adults.[82] Symptomatic stress fractures are relatively rare in adults, but very common in school-aged athletes, causing 40 to 50 percent of low back pain in children.[52,83,84] Individuals in sports such as gymnastics, ballet, rowing, figure skating, tennis, wrestling, and football, which require repetitive extension and flexion and hyperextension of the back, are at higher risk. Spondylolysis occurs at a markedly increased incidence in young athletes compared to other young patients with low back pain.[85,86]

A spondylolysis is a defect in the pars interarticularis. In athletes, the defect is usually a stress fracture and most frequently occurs at the L4 and L5 levels.[48,87] A spondylolisthesis is the forward displacement of the superior vertebral body in relation to the inferior vertebral body. Spondylolisthesis is graded according to the severity of slippage: grade I represents 0 to 25 percent slippage; grade II, 25 to 50 percent slippage; grade III, 50 to 75 percent slippage; and grade IV, 75 to 100 percent slippage. Spondylolisthesis represents the most severe injury in a spectrum of disease that includes spondylolysis as a moderate injury and pars interarticularis stress reaction as the mildest injury.

The etiology of spondylolysis is multifactorial with genetic predisposition, developmental defects, and repetitive microtrauma all contributing as risk factors.[14,82,87] In athletes, repetitive flexion and extension stresses cause an initial stress reaction in pars interarticularis. Early in the disease, this stress reaction is asymptomatic. However, as the athlete continues the repetitive activity, low back pain gradually occurs and worsens. Eventually, if the athlete continues to play through the pain, a stress fracture occurs. The patient usually has no history of trauma and complains of gradually worsening midline low back pain with activity. Football players may complain of pain with blocking drills and tennis players will complain of pain with serves.[87] Ballet dancers may complain of pain with arabesque. The pain is reproduced by back extension. A positive one-legged hyperextension test (see Fig. 8-14) is especially indicative of ipsilateral spondylolysis. Patients may have pain with forward flexion and rotate away from the side of the lesion and pain with lateral-bend toward the side of the lesion. Many patients also have a hamstring tightness or spasm secondary to a postural reflex to stabilize the segment.[82,87] A step deformity may be palpated over the spine with spondylolisthesis.

Spondylolisthesis is usually visible on a lateral lumbar radiograph (see Fig. 8-27). AP radiograph may show an inverted "Napoleon's hat" sign with spondylolisthesis. Oblique radiographs may reveal a spondylolysis as the classic "Scotty dog" of Lachapele with a collar at the neck and a spondylolisthesis as a decapitated Scotty dog (see Fig. 8-28). However, a spondylolysis may not be visible on plain radiograph for 3 to 6 weeks after the development of the low back pain.[48,53,87] If the clinical index of suspicion is high, the examiner should obtain a three-phase bone scan, which is positive 95 percent of the time within 24 hours of the onset of symptoms from active stress fractures (see Fig. 8-25). CT scanning, MRI, and myelography are not usually necessary.

Treatment of spondylolysis initially consists of modification of activity and control of pain. If the patient has a hot bone scan, the use of a rigid lumbosacral brace in neutral or slight flexion has been advocated as a method to increase speed of recovery.[48,54,87-89] The brace is worn 23 hours a day and is utilized in conjunction with an exercise program. Sporting activity while wearing the brace is allowed when the patient becomes asymptomatic, in most patients 3 weeks after treatment begins.[88-90] Treatment is continued until there is radiologic evidence of healing or the bone scan changes from hot to cold, which takes an average of 6 months.[87] In general, bracing should be continued for at least 3 months.[89] Bracing patients with cold bone scans does not seem to improve treatment outcome.[54,87]

Athletes should not be excluded from sports solely on the basis of spondylolisthesis. Athletes should be warned of the potential risks of future back problems and of increased slippage for individuals with grade II or higher slippage. However, at the present time, there is no evidence that participation in contact sports is related to the progression of slippage in athletes with grade I spondylolisthesis.[48,87] Athletes who continue participation in high-risk activity should be followed with annual radiographs to screen for increased slippage until skeletal maturity is reached, at which point spondylolisthesis usually becomes stable.[87]

Osteoporosis

Osteoporosis, the end stage of low-bone density, results in over a million fractures each year in the United States

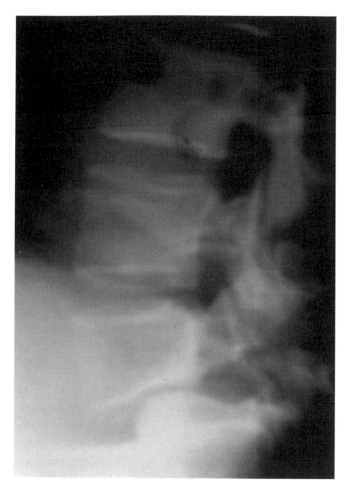

Figure 8–27. Spondylolisthesis of the L5 and S1 level.

with an economic impact of nearly 4 billion dollars.[91] It is critical that women, who suffer most of the morbidity and mortality of osteoporosis, pay particular attention to laying down bone mineral in their early years, as peak mass is attained at approximately age 35, with yearly losses of approximately 1 percent thereafter. Factors that encourage optimal bone mass include dietary calcium intake, weight-bearing exercise, and, in women, estrogen.[92]

Weight-bearing exercise has been traditionally thought to increase bone mineral density and thus, decrease the risk for osteoporosis.[93] Unfortunately, women athletes may find that increased exercise may result in amenorrhea or oligomenorrhea. This side effect may be welcome by athletes, some of whom believe that menstruation diminishes athletic performance.[94] Amenorrhea has been related to decreased bone density in both athletes and nonathletes.[95-97] Amenorrheic female athletes have been shown to have lower bone densities than sedentary women, placing them at risk for stress fractures and eventually for the development of osteoporosis.[96,97] Despite these increased risks, some amenorrheic female athletes, who believe that menstrual periods interfere with their athletic performance, resist reinstatement of menses.[94]

Amenorrhea and oligomenorrhea are found in 10 to 20 percent of female athletes, most frequently in runners, but also in many other sports.[98] The incidence of these menstrual disorders increases in more competitive athletes.[99] Amenorrhea and oligomenorrhea may be caused by a number of common or serious pathologic conditions, which must be ruled out before the diagnosis of exercised-induced menstrual disorder is made.[98,100] These conditions include pregnancy, hyperprolactinemia, hypothyroidism, ovarian failure, and hyperandrogenism.

The cause of exercised-induced amenorrhea and oligomenorrhea is unknown; however, implicated factors include low caloric intake, low percentage of body fat, increased training, and emotional stress.[101-104] Treatment is directed towards correcting these etiologies. However, few athletes are willing to exercise less. Many women athletes also refuse to increase caloric intake, particularly those in sports that place a high value on appearance (gymnastics, figure skating, and dance), in which additional weight is a disadvantage (running and bicycling), or in weight-class sports (martial arts, crew, and weight lifting).

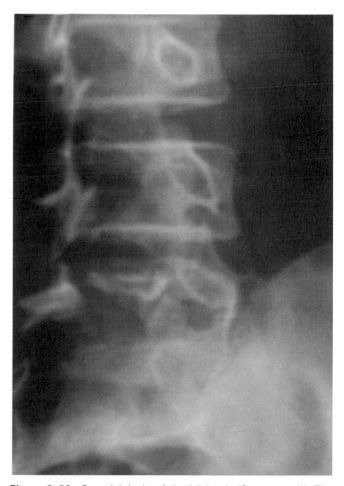

Figure 8–28. Spondylolysis of the L5 level. (Compare with Fig. 8–19.)

Amenorrheic women should take at least 1500 mg of dietary calcium each day. Although some athletes (swimmers and crew) may be participating only minimally in weight-bearing exercise, most female athletes participate in adequate amounts of weight-bearing exercise, which is known to increase bone mineral density in postmenopausal, and to a lesser extent, in menstruating women.[105,106] Thus, for most female athletes, the major concern for bone health may be estrogen production. Estrogen supplementation, either in the form of estrogen replacement therapy or estrogen-containing oral contraceptives, is an alternative for amenorrheic or oligomenorrheic women who will not decrease exercise, increase caloric intake, or both until more normal cycles are achieved.[98] Recent studies linking oligomenorrhea in adolescence and young adulthood with an increased risk of osteoporosis in older women[107-109] suggest that oligomenorrhea should be treated as aggressively as amenorrhea.

Ankylosing Spondylitis

Ankylosing spondylitis is a seronegative spondyloarthropathy with both peripheral and axial skeletal manifestations. It typically presents in young men in their late teens with gradual onset of morning stiffness and vague low back pain. It is aggravated by sudden movements and incompletely relieved by rest. The pain is proportional to activity, and while initially concentrated in the thoracolumbar area, it gradually spreads to affect much of the spine. Pain in the sacroiliac region is not uncommon. On physical exam, the patients have decreased chest expansion and decreased spinal flexibility as measured by a Schober test. Early radiographs are usually negative; later, the first radiologic changes are usually squaring of the vertebral bodies, followed by development of widespread syndesmophytes along the lateral and anterior surfaces of the intervertebral disks, or "bamboo spine." Later, the sacroiliac joints show narrowing and sclerosis and eventually, fusion. Individuals with ankylosing spondylitis usually have the HLA-B27 antigen and a positive bone scan at the sacroiliac joints. Treatment includes modification of painful activities, symptomatic treatment of exacerbation with nonsteroidal anti-inflammatory agents, and postural and breathing exercises.

Referred Pain

Pain can be referred to the lower back by many different diseases and structures (see Table 8-2). These include gastrointestinal disorders, genitourinary disorders, gynecologic disorders, obstetrical disorders, abdominal aortic aneurysm, splenic or hepatic pathology, hip or pelvic pathology, and secondary gain issues.[2]

Piriformis Syndrome

The piriformis syndrome is caused by irritation or impingement of the sciatic nerve by the piriformis muscle. Patients complain of deep pain in the back or posterior hip that often radiates down the leg. Women may complain of dyspareunia.[30] On examination, the patients have sciatic notch tenderness. They have pain to resisted hip external rotation and passive internal hip stretching. Initial treatment is activity modification, nonsteroidal anti-inflammatory agents, and a mobilization program.

Sacroiliac Dysfunction

The sacroiliac joint is among the strongest in the body. Pain from the sacroiliac joint frequently presents as unilateral low back pain and may occasionally cause pain in the thigh. On physical examination, the patient may have tenderness over the sacroiliac joint, posterior superior iliac spine, or buttocks region. The patient may have pain when flexing the hip to bring the knee to the chest. Pain in the sacroiliac joint may be reproduced by a pelvic rock test or Faber test (see Fig. 8-16). The usual treatments include sacroiliac joint mobilization and nonsteroidal anti-inflammatory agents.

Neoplasm

Individuals younger than 50 years make up only 20 percent of patients with neoplasms. The most common spinal tumor is a metastatic carcinoma, usually from cancer of the breast, lung, prostate, gastrointestinal, or genitourinary systems. The most common primary tumor is multiple myeloma. The pain typically has an insidious onset, presenting at waist level or in the midline of the low back, and is aggravated by activity. Night pain, unrelieved by sleep or lying down, is found in almost 90 percent of these patients. Early radiographs may be normal. Bone scans are useful in confirming clinical suspicion of bony tumors or in localizing the area of involvement. CT scan and myelogram are useful in the evaluation of neurogenic tumors.

Infection

Osteomyelitis is usually hematologic in origin. In young patients, a history of a recent respiratory tract infection is common. In older patients, a history of recent urinary tract infection or procedure is common. The combination of pain and fever should raise suspicions about infection, although in many cases, fever is absent or low grade. The pain is usually well localized. It may be aggravated by motion and cause limitation of motion and paraspinal muscle spasm. Early radiographs are often normal. Bone scans are useful in confirming clinical suspicion or in localizing the area of infection. A gallium-labeled or indium-labeled white cell scan is very specific in confirming infection. MRI is also useful in confirming osteomyelitis.

Chronic Low Back Pain

In 2 to 10 percent of individuals, low back pain persists beyond 3 months and can be considered to be chronic low back pain.[1,2,11,40] In these patients, the examiner should carefully repeat the history and physical and reconsider the diagnosis. Secondary gain issues such as disability, pending lawsuits, and drug addiction should be explored. These patients should not be given narcotic medications, which tend to lead to an addicted patient who still has inadequate pain control. Many times, these individuals benefit from a multidisiplanary program of primary care physicians, orthopaedic surgeons, physical therapists, occupational therapists, athletic trainers, nurses, physiatrists, psychologists, psychiatrists, and social workers. A comprehensive program should include pain management, physical and occupational therapy, biofeedback, and counseling. A primary care physician may choose to coordinate independent members of the team or to refer the patient to a chronic pain center which has these elements in place.

BACK INJURIES IN INDIVIDUAL SPORTS

Ballet

Many motions such as arabesque and attitude involve repetitive extension and flexion of the back. Professional and preprofessional ballet dancers spend up to, and sometimes more, than 8 hours a day dancing. These repetitive activities place ballet dancers at high risk for spondylolysis and spondylolisthesis. Male dancers are at risk for low back strain from repetitive lifts of their partners. Placing many dancers at even greater risk for musculoskeletal injury is poor nutrition. Additionally, since most dancers think of themselves as artists first and athletes second, if at all, there is a tendency to forgo any preseason strength training, thus placing themselves at greater risk for injury.

Basketball

Lumbar spine injuries are relatively rare in basketball with the majority of the injuries being contusions, strains, and sprains.[110] Power forwards and centers are at higher risk for back injuries because of their function as rebounders, which exposes them to repetitive twisting and extension and flexion from jumping and increased body contact.

Bicycling

An upright, stationary bicycle places relatively mild stress on the lower back and can be useful as a form of cross-training for injured athletes. Bicycle racing, extended touring, and off-road mountain bicycling can all place the back under considerable stress. These problems tend to be in the upper back, but can occur in the lower back. Proper sizing of rider to bicycle will assist in preventing injury. If the top tube or handlebar stem is too long or the handlebars are too low, the rider is placed in an extended riding position that leads to increased fatigue in the back. This problem is common in individuals with long legs and a shorter torso, and is often seen when females use standard bicycles. Pushing, riding in a high gear at low cadence (less than 60 rpm), increases use of the gluteus maximus and hamstrings, which leads to loss of neutral pelvic tilt and the increased back fatigue. Prolonged seated climbing has a similar effect.[111] Back fatigue can be minimized by alternating handlebar positions while riding, especially when hill climbing, and by maintaining optimal cadence and alternating positions. Slightly lowering tire pressure or use of shock absorbers may decrease the impact from surface obstacles, especially in mountain bicycles.

Football

Low back pain accounts for about 30 percent of the playing time losses in football players.[3,112,113] Low back pain is especially common in interior linemen. A common cause of low back injuries in football is the use of incorrect techniques during strength training sessions.[114,115]

Golf

Spinal injuries are common in golfers, with over 90 percent of tournament-level golfers having a history of spine injury and 10 to 30 percent injured at any one time.[116,117] Many golfers exaggerate the traditional reverse C position in an effort to increase hitting distance. This exaggeration increases the stress on the lower back and predisposes to injury. A more upright finishing position places less stress on the lower back.[115,118] The repetitive twisting motion to one side may place the golfer at risk for lower back overuse injuries.

Gymnastics

Many activities, such as extension walkovers and back flips, require high degrees of hyperextension of the back. Other maneuvers, such as vaulting and dismounts from the balance beam and uneven parallel bars, place tremendous stress on the spine. The rate of spondylolysis in gymnasts is estimated to be between 15 and 30 percent.[119,120] The loading stress of gymnastics place the athlete at risk for lumbar Scheurmann disease.

Racquet Sports

Tennis players have a high incidence of low back pain with almost 40 percent of elite tennis players missing a tennis tournament because of low back pain.[121] The common receiving position with flexed-hip squatting, frequently assumed by tennis players, may lead to iliopsoas tightness, which may cause low back pain. Inadequate flexibility in the shoulder may cause a compensatory overrotation of the lower back during overhead shots and serves. The hyperextension of the back may be minimized during the serve by tossing the ball slightly ahead of the service line.

Swimming

The butterfly stroke's dolphin kick places the low back under stress. Improper mechanics can further aggravate the low back. The use of the above-the-water hand recovery in breaststroke causes hyperextenison of the spine and places these swimmers at increased risk for spondylolysis. The repetitive flexion and extension of flip turns also may place the swimmer at risk for overuse injuries of the lower back.

Track and Field Events

The pole vaulter's back is placed under high stress during jumping.[122] Hammer throwers must be careful to use proper throwing technique, since tremendous forces generated during the prethrow turns place them at risk for low back strains, sprains, and transverse process fractures. The incidence of back injury is relatively low in track events. A survey of runners found the prevalence of low back pain to be between 1.1 and 9 percent.[50]

Volleyball

The flexed-hip posture used during underhand passing stresses the lower back, placing the player at risk for low back strain. The forced hyperextension of the low back during hitting, blocking, and serving stress the posterior elements of the lower spine, placing the player at risk for spondylolysis.

Weight Lifting

One study associates weight lifting with an increased risk of degenerative disk disease,[67] while another found no association.[123] The incidence of low back pain in weight lifters has been estimated to be 40 percent.[124] The weight lifter is especially at risk for low back injury during the shift from spinal flexion to extension when the barbell is lifted overhead, as occurs during both the clean-and-jerk lift and snatch lift.[114] However, some studies have found that with proper technique, the risk of having an injury weight lifting is very low.[125,126]

Wrestling

Most low back injuries in wrestling take place during take-downs and sparring. With the back in hyperextension, sparring wrestlers push and pull each other in a manner similar to the blocking motion used by linesmen in football; this places the wrestler at similar potential risk of low back injury. During take-downs, the wrestler sometimes lifts his opponent off the mat, usually without proper lifting technique.

Other Sports

Baseball and softball players place stress on the lower back region via torsional trunk motions during pitching, throwing, and batting. Pitching places particular stress on the lumbar facets and the sacroiliac joints. Rowers are at risk of back injury since the primary motion of rowing involves the linkage of leg motion through the backs to the arms. Improper rowing technique places the low back at high risk for injury.

Acknowledgments

The authors would like to thank Chris McLaughlin for her assistance with editing this chapter; Sandy Hurth and Chris Gieser for appearing in some of the photographs, as well as Nic Kellner for being the photographer; and Howard S. An, MD, for many of the radiographs.

REFERENCES

1. Gillete RD. A practical approach to the patient with back pain. *Am Fam Physician.* 1996;53:670-676.
2. Wheeler AH. Diagnosis and management of low back pain and sciatica. *Am Fam Physician.* 1995;52:1333-1341.
3. Ferguson RJ, McMaster JH, Stanitski CL. Low back pain in college football lineman. *Am J Sports Med.* 1974;2:63-69.
4. Hainline B. Low back injury. *Clin Sports Med.* 1995; 14:241-265.
5. Pope MH, Novotny JE. Spinal biomechanics. *J Biomech Engineering.* 1993;115:569-574.
6. Papageorgiou AC, Croft PR, Ferry S, et al. Estimating the prevalence of low back pain in the general population: Evidence form the South Manchester back pain survey. *Spine.* 1995;20:1889-1894.
7. Wipf JE, Deyo RA. Low back pain. *Med Clin North Am.* 1995;79:231-246.
8. Loeser JD, Volinn E. Epidemiology of low back pain. *Neurosurg Clin North Am.* 1991;2:713.
9. Kelsey JL, Mundt DJ, Golden AL. Epidemiology of low back pain. In: Jayson M, ed. *The Lumbar Spine and Back Pain.* 4th ed. Edinburgh: Churchill Livingstone; 1992:537-549.
10. Speagler D, Bigos S, Martin N, et al. Back injuries in industry: A retrospective study. 1. Overview and cost analysis. *Spine.* 1986;11:241-245.
11. Klenerman L, Slade PD, Stanley M, et al. The prediction of chronicity in patients with an acute attack of

low back pain in a general practice setting. *Spine*. 1995; 20:478-484.

12. Hart LG, Deyo RA, Cherkin DC. Physician office visits for low back pain: Frequency, clinical evaluation and treatment patterns from a U.S. national survey. *Spine*. 1995;20:11-19.

13. Balagué F, Skovron M, Nordin M, et al. Low back pain in school children: A study of familial and psychological factors. *Spine*. 1995;20:1265-1270.

14. Gerbino PGI, Micheli LJ. Back injuries in the young athlete. *Clin Sports Med*. 1995;14:571-590.

15. Nachemson A. The load in lumbar disc in different positions of the body. *Clin Orthop*. 1966;45:107.

16. Nachemson A, Effström G. Intravital dynamic pressure measurements in lumbar disc. *Scand J Rehabil Med*. 1970.

17. Cavanaugh JM. Neural mechanisms of lumbar pain. *Spine*. 1995;20:1804-1809.

18. Garfin SR, Rydevik B, Lind B, Massie J. Spinal nerve root compression. *Spine*. 1995;20:1810-1820.

19. Jenkins DB. Hollinshead's Functional Anatomy of the Limb and Back. 5th ed. Philadelphia: Saunders; 1981.

20. Boden SD, Davis DO, Dina TS, et al. Abnormal lumbar spine MRI scans in asymptomatic subjects: A perspective investigation. *J Bone Joint Surg*. 1990;72A:403-408.

21. Kliener JB, Donaldson WI, Lurd JG, et al. Extraspinal causes of lumbosacral reaiculopathy. *J Bone Joint Surg*. 1991;73A:817-821.

22. Wiesel SW, Bell GR, Feffer HL, et al. A study of computer-assisted tomography. 1. The incidence of positive CAT scans in an asymptomatic group of patients. *Spine*. 1984;9:549-551.

23. Rothman RH, Rashbaum RF. Pathogenesis of signs and symptoms of cervical disc degeneration. In: *American Academy of Orthopaedic Surgeons, Instructional Course Lectures*. St. Louis: Mosby; 1978:203-215.

24. Letts M, Haasheck I. Hematocolpos as a cause of back pain in premenarchal adolescents. *J Pediatr Orthop*. 1990;10:731-732.

25. Garrick JG. Orthopedic preparticipation screening examination of the young athlete. In: Strauss RH, ed. *Sports Medicine*. 2nd ed. Philadelphia: Saunders; 1991:453-463.

26. Magee DJ. Lumbar spine. In: Magee DJ, ed. *Orthopedic Physical Assessment*. 2nd ed. Philadelphia: Saunders; 1992:247-307.

27. American Academy of Family Physicians, American Academy of Pediatrics, American Medical Society for Sports Medicine, American Orthopaedic Society for Sports Medicine, American Osteopathic Academy of Sports Medicine. Preparticipation physical evaluation (monograph). Kansas City, MO; 1992.

28. Marshall WA, Tanner JM. Variations in pattern of pubertal changes in boys. *Arch Dis Child*. 1970;45:13.

29. Marshall WA, Tanner JM. Variations in pattern of pubertal changes in girls. *Arch Dis Child*. 1969;44:291.

30. Wilhite J, Huurman WW. Thoracic and lumbosacral spine. In: Mellion MB, ed. *The Team Physician's Handbook*. Philadelphia: Hanley & Belfus; 1990:374-400.

31. Hoppenfeld S. Physical examination of the spine and extremities. Norwalk, CT: Appleton-Century-Crofts; 1976.

32. Scham SM, Taylor TKF. Tension signs in lumbar disc prolapse. *Clin Orthop Relat Res*. 1971;75:195.

33. Boyd RJ. Evaluation of back pain. In: Goroll A, May L, Jr AM, eds. *Primary Care Medicine: Office Evaluation and Management of the Adult Patient*. 3rd ed. Philadelphia: Lippincott; 1995:742-751.

34. Waddell G, McCullough JA, Kummel E, Venner RM. Nonorganic physical signs in low-back pain. *Spine*. 1980;5:117-125.

35. Macnab I. The traction spur: An indicator of segmental instability. *J Bone Joint Surg*. 1971;53A:663.

36. Morris EW, DiPaola M, Vallance R, Waddell G. Diagnosis and decision making in lumbar disc prolapse and nerve entrapment. *Spine*. 1986;11:436-439.

37. Albeck MJ, Hilden J, Kjœr L, et al. A controlled comparison of myelography, computed tomography and magnetic resonance imaging in clinically suspected disc herniation. *Spine*. 1995;20:443-448.

38. Greenan TJ. Diagnostic imaging of sports-related spinal disorders. *Clin Sports Med*. 1993;12:487-505.

39. Weisz GM, Lamond TS, Kitchener PN. Spinal imaging: Will MRI replace myelography? *Spine*. 1988;13:65-68.

40. Hackley DR, Wiesel SW. The lumbar spine in the aging athlete. *Clin Sports Med*. 1993;12:465-485.

41. Rosenthal DF, Manken HJ, Bauman RA. Musculoskeletal applications for computed tomography. *Bull Rheum Dis*. 1983;33:1.

42. Haughton V. MR imaging of the spine. *Radiology*. 1988;166:297.

43. Panjabi M, Brand R, White A. Magnetic resonance imaging of the spine: Applications and limitations. *Radiol Clin North Am*. 1985;23:551.

44. Kujala UM, Taimela S, Erkintalo M, et al. Low-back pain in adolescent athletes. *Med Sci Sports Exerc*. 1996; 28:165-170.

45. Erkintalo M, Salminen JJ, Alanen A, et al. Development of degenerative changes in the lumbar intervertebral disc: Results of a prospective MR imaging study in adolescents with and without low-back pain. *Radiology*. 1995;196:529-533.

46. Jensen MC, Brant-Zawadski MN, Obuchowski N, et al. Magnetic resonance imaging of the lumbar spine in people without back pain. *N Engl J Med*. 1994;331:69.

47. Frymoyer JW. Back pain and sciatica. *N Engl J Med*. 1988;318:291-300.

48. Eismont FJ, Kitchel SH. Thoracolumbar spine. In: DeLee JC, Drez D, eds. *Orthopaedic Sports Medicine: Principles and Practice*. Philadelphia: Saunders; 1994:1018-1062.

49. Spenser GW, Jackson DW. Back injuries of the spine. *Clin Sports Med*. 1983;2:191-216.

50. Tall RL, DeVault W. Spinal injury in sport: Epidemiologic considerations. *Clin Sport Med*. 1993;12: 441-448.

51. York J. Sports and the male genitourinary system/kidneys and bladder. *Phys Sportsmed*. 1990;18:116-129.

52. Micheli LJ, Wood R. Back pain in young athletes. *Arch Pediatr Adolesc Med*. 1995;149:15-18.

53. Micheli LJ. Spine and chest wall. In: Johnson RJ, Lombardo J, eds. *Current Review of Sports Medicine*. Philadelphia: Current Medicine; 1994:1-16.

54. Reid DC. Injuries and conditions of the neck and spine. In: Reid DC, ed. *Sports Injury Assessment and Rehabilitation*. New York: Churchill Livingstone; 1992: 784-837.

55. Reid DC. Muscle injury: Classification and healing. In: Reid DC, ed. *Sports Injury Assessment and Rehabilitation*. New York; 1992:85-101.

56. Deyo RA, Diehl AK, Rosenthal M. How many days of bed rest for acute low back pain? *N Engl J Med*. 1986; 315:1064.

57. Gilbert JR, Taylor DW, Hildebrand A, et al. Clinical trial of common treatments for low back pain in family practice. *BMJ*. 1985;66:100.

58. Carey TS, Garrett J, Jackman A, et al. The outcomes and costs of care for acute low back pain among patients seen by primary care practitioners, chiropractors, and orthopedic surgeons. *N Engl J Med*. 1995;333: 913-917.

59. Deyo R. Conservative therapy for low back pain. Distinguishing useful from useless therapy. *JAMA*. 1983;250:1057-1062.

60. The North American Spine Society's Ad Hoc Committee on Diagnositic and Therapeutic Procedures. Common diagnostic and therapeutic procedures of the lumbosacral spine. *Spine*. 1991;16:1161-1167.

61. Smith MJ, Wright V. Sciatica and the intervertebral disc study. *Clin Orthop*. 1977;129:9.

62. Oegema TTJ. Biochemistry of intervertebral disc. *Clin Sports Med*. 1993;12:419-439.

63. Helbig T, Lee CK. The lumbar facet syndrome. *Spine*. 1988;13;61-64.

64. Friis M, Gulliksen GC, Rasmussen P, et al. Pain and spinal root compression. *Acta Neurochir*. 1977;39:241-249.

65. Raaf J. Some observations regarding 905 patients operated upon for protruded lumbar intervertebral discs. *Am J Surg*. 1959;97:388-399.

66. Weber H. Lumbar disc herniation. A controlled, prospective study with ten years observation. *Spine*. 1983;8: 131-140.

67. Videman T, Sams S, Battié MC, et al. The long-term effects of physical loading and exercise lifestyles on back-related symptoms, disability, and spinal pathology among men. *Spine*. 1995;20:699-709.

68. Battié MC, Vidman T, Gibbons LE, et al. Determinants of lumbar disc degeneration: A study relating lifetime exposures and magnetic resonance imaging findings in identical twins. *Spine*. 1995;20:2601-2612.

69. Haher TR, O'Brien M, Kauffman C, Liao KC. Biomechanics of the spine in sports. *Clin Sports Med*. 1993; 12:449-464.

70. Frymoyer JW, Pope MH, Clements JH, et al. Risk factors in low-back pain. *J Bone Joint Surg*. 1983;65A:213-218.

71. MacNab I. *Backache*. Baltimore: Williams & Wilkins; 1977.

72. Deyo RA, Loeser J, Bigos SJ. Herniated lumbar intervertebral disc. *Ann Intern Med*. 1990;112:1990.

73. Cirello VM, Snook SH. The effect of back belts on lumbar muscle fatigue. *Spine*. 1995;20:1271-1278.

74. Mathews J. Dynamic discography: A study of lumbar traction. *Ann Phys Med*. 1968;9:275.

75. Kane MD, Karl RD, Swain JH. Effects of gravity facilitated traction on intervertebral dimensions of the lumbar spine. *J Orthop Sports Phys Ther*. 1985;6:281.

76. Bush K, Cowan N, Katz DE, Gisher P. The natural history of sciatica associated with disc pathology. *Spine*. 1992; 17:1205-1212.

77. Saal JA, Saal JS. Nonoperative treatment of herniated lumbar intervertebral disc with radiculopathy. An outcome study. *Spine*. 1989;14:431-437.

78. Hoffman RM, Wheeler KJ, Deyo RA. Surgery for herniated lumbar discs: A literature synthesis. *J Gen Intern Med*. 1993;8:487.

79. Hall S, Bartleson JD, Onofrio BM, et al. Lumbar spinal stenosis: Clinical features, diagnostic procedure, and results of surgical treatment in 68 patients. *Ann Intern Med*. 1985;103:271.

80. Swärd L, Hellström M, Jacobsson B, Karlsson L. Vertebral ring apophysis injury in athletes: Is the etiology different in the thoracic and lumbar spine? *Am J Sports Med*. 1993;21:841-845.

81. Yancey RA, Micheli LJ. Thoracolumbar spine injuries in pediatric sports. In: Staniski CL, DeLee JC, Drez D, eds. *Pediatric and Adolescent Sports Medicine*. Philadelphia: Saunders; 1994:162-174.

82. Stinson JT. Spondylolysis and spondylolisthesis in the athlete. *Clin Sports Med*. 1993;12:517-528.

83. Hardcastle RH. Repair of spondyloysis in young fast bowlers. *J Bone Joint Surg (Br)*. 1993;75:398-402.

84. Jackson DW. Low back pain in young athletes: Evaluation of stress reaction and discogenic problems. *Am J Sports Med*. 1979;7:364.

85. Cirillo J, Jackson DW. Pars interarticularis stress reaction, spondylolysis, and spondylolisthesis in gymnasts. *Clin Sports Med*. 1985;4:95.

86. Hellstrom M, Jacobsson B, Sward L, et al. Radiologic abnormalities of the thoracolumbar spine in athletes. *Acta Radiol*. 1990;31:127.

87. Madelbaum BR, Gross ML. Spondylolysis and spondylolisthesis. In: Reider B, ed. *Sports Medicine in the School-age Athlete*. 2nd ed. Philadelphia: Saunders; 1996:44-156.

88. Steiner ME, Micheli LJ. Treatment of symptomatic spondylolysis and spondylolisthesis with the modified Boston brace. *Spine*. 1985;10:937-943.

89. Micheli LJ, Hall JE, Miller ME. Use of a modified Boston brace for back injuries in athletes. *Am J Sports Med*. 1980;8:351-356.

90. Micheli LJ. Back injuries in gymnastics. *Clin Sports Med*. 1985;4:85.

91. National Institutes of Health. Consensus Development Conference on Osteoporosis. Washington, DC: U.S. Government Printing Office; 1984. Pub no. 421-132: 46 ed.

92. Snow-Harter CM. Bone health and prevention of osteoporosis in active and athletic women. *Clin Sports Med*. 1994;13:389-404.

93. Nilson ME, Fisher EC, Catsos PD, et al. Bone density in athletes. *Clin Orthop Relat Res*. 1971;77:179-182.

94. Shangold MM. Gynecologic concerns in exercise and training. In: Shangold MM, Mirkin G, eds. *Women and Exercise.* 2nd ed. Philadelphia: Davis; 1994:223-233.

95. Myburgh KH, Bachrach LK, Lewis B, et al. Low bone mineral density at axial and appendicular sites in amenorrheic athletes. *Med Sci Sports Exerc.* 1993;25:1197-1202.

96. Cann CE, Martin MC, Genant HK, Jaffe RB. Decreased spine mineral content in amenorrheic women. *JAMA.* 1984;251:656-659.

97. Drinkwater BL, Nilson K, Chestnut CHI, et al. Bone mineral content of amenorrheic and eumenorrheic athletes. *N Engl J Med.* 1984;311:277-281.

98. Shangold M. Menstruation and menstrual disorders. In: Shangold M, Mirkin G, eds. *Women and Exercise: Physiology and Sports Medicine.* 2nd ed. Philadelphia: Davis; 1994:152-171.

99. Sanborn C, Martin B, Wagner W. Is athletic amenorrhea specific to runners? *Am J Obstet Gynecol.* 1982;143:859-861.

100. Marshall L. Clinical evaluation of amenorrhea. In: Agostini R, ed. *Medical and Orthopedic Issues of Active and Athletic Women.* Philadelphia: Hanley & Belfus; 1994:152-163.

101. Shangold M. Menstrual irregularity in athletes: Basic principles, evaluation and treatment. *Can J Appl Sport Sci.* 1982;7:68-73.

102. Schwartz B, Cumming D, Riordan E, et al. Exercise-associated amenorrhea: A distinct entity? *Am J Obstet Gynecol.* 1981;141:662-670.

103. Sanborn C, Albracht B, Wagner WW Jr. Athletic amenorrhea: Lack of association with body fat. *Med Sci Sports Exerc.* 1987;19:207-212.

104. Loucks A. Effects of exercise training on the menstrual cycle: Existence and mechanisms. *Med Sci Sports Exerc.* 1990;22:275-280.

105. Adami S. Optimizing peak bone mass: What are the therapeutic possibilities? *Osteroporosis Int.* 1994;4:27-30.

106. Chestnut CH. Bone mass and exercise. *Am J Med.* 1993;95:34S-36S.

107. Snow-Harter C. Athletic amenorrhea and bone health. In: Agostini R, ed. *Medical and Orthopedic Issues of Active and Athletic Women.* Philadelphia: Hanley & Belfus; 1994:164-168.

108. Micklesfield L, Lambert E, Fataar A, et al. Bone mineral density in mature, premenopausal ultramarthon runners. *Med Sci Sports Exerc.* 1995;27:688-696.

109. Alekal L, Clasey J, Fehling P, et al. Contributions of exercise, body composition and age to bone mineral density in premenopausal women. *Med Sci Sports Exerc.* 1995;27:1477-1485.

110. Herskowitz A, Selesnick H. Back injuries in basketball players. *Clin Sports Med.* 1993;12:293-306.

111. Mellion MB. Neck and back pain in bicycling. *Clin Sports Med.* 1994;13:137-164.

112. Saal JA. Rehabilitation of football players with lumbar spine injury. *Physician Sport Med.* 1988;16:61.

113. Semon RL, Spengler D. Significance of lumbar spondylosis in college football players. *Spine.* 1981;6:172.

114. Watkins RG, Dillion WM. Lumbar spine injuries. In: Fu FH, Stone DA, eds. *Sport Injuries, Mechanisms, Prevention, and Treatment.* Baltimore: Williams & Wilkins; 1994.

115. MaCarroll JR. Golf. In: Fu FH, Stone DA, eds. *Sports Injuries: Mechanisms, Prevention, and Treatment.* Baltimore: Williams & Wilkins; 1994:375-381.

116. McCarroll JR, Gioe TJ. Professional golfers and the price they pay. *Physician Sports Med.* 1982;10:64-70.

117. Spencer CW, Jackson DW. Back injuries in athletes. *Sports Neurology.* Rockfield, MD: Aspen; 1989:159-177.

118. Hosea TM, Gatt CJ. Back pain in golf. *Clin Sports Med.* 1996;15:37-53.

119. Rossi F, Dragoni S. Lumbar spondylolysis: Occurrence in competitive athletes. *J Sports Med Phys Fitness.* 1990;30:450-452.

120. Rossi F. Spondylolysis, spondylolisthesis and sports. *J Sports Med Phys Fitness.* 1978;18:317-340.

121. Marks MR, Haas SS, Wieses SW. Low back pain in the competative tennis player. *Clin Sports Med.* 1988;7:277.

122. Gainor BJ, Hagen RJ, Allen WC. Biomechanics of the spine in the polevaulter as related to spondylolisthesis. *Am J Sports Med.* 1983;11:53-57.

123. Mundt DJ, Kelsey JL, Golden AL, et al. An epidemiologic study of sports and weight lifting as possible risk factors for herniated lumbar and cervical discs. The Northeast Collaborative Group on Low Back Pain. *Am J Sports Med.* 1993;21:854-860.

124. Aggrawal ND, Kaur R, Kumar S, et al. A study of changes in weight lifters and other athletes. *Br J Sports Med.* 1979;13:58-61.

125. Risser WL, Risser JM, Preston D. Weight-training injuries in adolescents. *Am J Dis Child.* 1990;144:1015-1017.

126. Risser WL. Weight-training injuries in children and adolescents. *Am Fam Physician.* 1991;44:2104-2108.

Management and Rehabilitation of Athletic Lumbar Spine Injuries

John G. Lachacz

Treatment of the lumbar spine is based on understanding many components: functional anatomy, spinal biomechanics, soft-tissue healing, adaptive changes of the musculoskeletal and cardiovascular tissues, and the influence of the nervous system on motor behavior. Thorough discussion of each of these components would take a book in itself, so instead, key parts of each component are used in this section to develop a comprehensive treatment plan. The best treatment plan emphasizes patient self-management with active techniques (patient performed). Passive techniques, performed by the rehabilitation specialist, are used only as adjuncts to self-administered active techniques. Athletes are self-motivated to adhere to treatment plans, and the rehabilitation specialist is challenged to return athletes back to their sport as quickly as possible to fulfill individual and team expectations. The timing of return must combine maximum functional restoration with minimal potential for reinjury.

Treatment of the athlete's lumbar spine can be very complex due to detailed neuroanatomy and osteokinematics, yet mechanical low back pain can be treated just as can treatment of mechanical pathology of the extremities. Many years ago, an ankle sprain would be treated by casting for weeks. Now, because the ill effects of immobilization are understood, protected range-of-motion exercise is begun immediately, and stresses are progressively increased throughout the entire rehabilitation program. The ill effects of immobilization are cartilage degeneration and a proliferation of fibrofatty connective tissue within the joint that becomes adherent to exposed synovial and cartilage surfaces.[1] Treatment of an ankle does not cease once it is pain free, but continues until maximum function is regained. This is the same for the lumbar region. This chapter gives some general guidelines on treating athletes with low back injuries. However, each program needs to be individualized to maximize the athlete's return to activity.

RESEARCH FINDINGS

Despite the tremendous advances that have been made in imaging techniques, surgical procedures, and rehabilitation techniques, the number of people disabled by back pain increased by 168 percent from 1971 to 1981. This form of disability increased 14 times faster than the population increased.[2] Although physical therapy procedures have been described for the treatment of low back pain, their efficacy remains unclear. Unfortunately, there are many barriers to research in low back pain, such as lack of instruments to measure spinal motion, spinal muscle performance, pain, and functional capacity. It is difficult to manage research when 60 percent of patients return to work in 1 week and 80 percent return in less than 6 weeks.[3] As many as 90 percent of low back patients recover within 3 months, regardless of treatment.[4] Finally, other variables are difficult to control in matching subjects with a precise pathoanatomic diagnosis. Physiologic effects, placebo effects, and the potential for secondary gain will also impact the ability to research efficacy of treatment.

CURRENT TRENDS

The current rehabilitation emphasis for patients with low back pain is health, wellness, and active participation in rehabilitation using self-management techniques. Functional restoration is emphasized over pain reduction. Where bedrest for acute low back pain once was 7 days, the maximum is now 2 days, if any.[5] Surgical intervention plays a far smaller role today than it did in the 1970s, when there was 400 percent more spinal surgery in the United States than anywhere else in the world.[3]

Treating mechanical low back pain with activity decreases the disability, whereas treating the patient with prolonged rest, analgesics, and minimal activity increases the disability. Linton and associates demonstrated that early active physical intervention for patients suffering their first episode of acute musculoskeletal pain significantly decreased the incidence of chronic pain.[6] Active treatment helps minimize the potential for the development of chronic pain syndrome.[7] Sixty to seventy percent of patients with low back pain have recurrent episodes, in which the episodes become more frequent and more painful. So the challenge is to prevent the future episodes.[4]

The fundamental theme of treatment for the athlete with low back pain is the process of restoring the function. This involves not only regaining full, pain-free range of motion, but also effecting a behavioral change in the athlete. Patient education is the keystone with the athlete sharing responsibility for his or her care and avoiding dependency on the rehabilitation specialist.

Research, such as the work by Deyo and associates on days of bedrest and MeKenzie's techniques, has changed our approach to treating low back pain, but the Federal Agency for Health Care Policy and Research (AHCPR) clinical practice guideline number 14 on acute low back problems in adults may be the most influential on practice. This may dictate treatment, as some insurance companies use reimbursement guidelines selectively.[5,8,9] Due to a diversity of opinions on this document, the final effect on rehabilitation specialists is unclear. The rehabilitation specialist must retain professional judgment in selecting the best treatment for the athlete. The specialist must continue to read new outcome studies and increase his or her knowledge base. Finally, managed care and shrinking health care dollars have minimized the number of visits with patients and they have become more responsible, active participants in their own care. Rehabilitation specialists must continue to push the preservation of the athletes' rights to access of all clinical tools necessary to rehabilitate.

EXAMINATION

The subjective examination can be the single most important event in the examination process. Despite time demands in the clinic or training room, it is critical to make time to listen to the athlete. The athlete's history can dramatically assist in determining his or her condition and thus, hasten a return to sports. Frequently, the history may tell the examiner the exact pathology and the athlete may tell the examiner the solution, if permitted.

The objective examination has been presented earlier in this chapter, but some additional tests more related to rehabilitation issues are suggested. The examiner must emphasize function in the evaluation, look not only at straight plane range of motion, but also the diagonal range of motion. The examiner should use repeated range-of-motion testing to see the change in quantity and quality of motion. Everyday life requires many repetitions of flexion, which the examiner must attempt to reproduce. Evaluating neck pain in a painter who has pain while

painting ceilings demands seeing repeated or sustained cervical extension. The "think function" principle can be applied to strength testing as well. Examiners also need to look at endurance, habitual postures, and body mechanics. They must identify the athlete's ability to maintain a balanced alignment with static positioning and with dynamic activities.

One useful tool to add to the examination for the athlete is the lumbar protective mechanism test.[10,11] The goal is to educate and train the athlete's muscles to stabilize the lumbar spine in a pain-free neutral position using neuromuscular control. It is based on the premise that the spine will be less traumatized if an efficient alignment is used. This gives the athlete's lumbar spine an effective base of support and exhibits an inherent ability to brace or stabilize the spine during activities. The ability to brace or stabilize the lumbar spine, either consciously or by reflex, is the definition of the lumbar protective mechanism. The first test of the lumbar protective mechanism is the vertical compression test (see Fig. 8–29). The athlete stands in a comfortable, natural

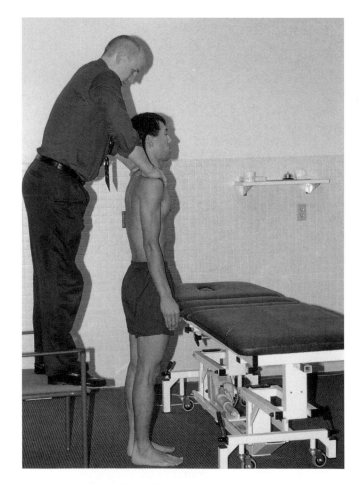

Figure 8–29. Vertical compression test.

stance while the examiner applies vertical pressure down through the shoulders, feeling for any give or buckling in the spine. This test allows the examiner to see how the loaded spine reacts: noting the vertical alignment and positional relationship of pelvis, lumbar, and thoracic spine. Is there a postural deviation or weakness? Does the athlete have pain during or after the test? Typical deviations are an increased lumbar lordosis and anterior shear of the pelvis. These deviations inhibit the trunk muscles from bracing or stabilizing in midrange. Other tests of the lumbar protective mechanism involve principles of proprioceptive neuromuscular facilitation (PNF), such as diagonal patterns and manual contact.[12,13] These tests are performed like the vertical compression test, applying pressure to evaluate the standing athletes spine (see Figs. 8-30 and 8-31). Resistance can be applied in a variety of directions: anterior, posterior, and diagonally. The test can also be performed with the athlete braced against the table at proximal femur level. The athlete can stand in a natural stance or a straddled stance. No instructions are given to the athlete initially, allowing the examiner to see their natural response, evaluating the quality, initiation, strength, and endurance of the contraction. Good spinal stability is indicated by isometric, not concentric contraction. As the athlete's timing to the response normalizes, the examiner's resistance can increase to work on overall strength and endurance. Further testing can be done in functional positions such as pushing (see Fig. 8-32) or a basketball player's defensive stance.

Observation and palpatory examination also must be performed thoroughly, taking the time needed to observe the athlete in multiple positions, as well as through the range of motion. Look for functional asymmetry such as leg length discrepancy, pelvic obliquity, muscle imbalance, and postural disorders. Many athletes, owing to the specific functions of their sport, will have lumbar paraspinal imbalance. Hypertrophic paraspinals will be hypomobile and hypomobile soft tissues can result in hypomobile lumbar spines. Observing this muscle imbalance will direct the palpatory exam to these hypertrophied tissues and to examining the junctional zone of T12 and L1, and L5 and S1, where the line of forces falls through and the greatest amount of forces is found. While this is not the only area for examination, it gives some initial clues to begin treatment.

ACUTE TREATMENT

Following a thorough examination, a game plan must be established with specific objectives. The final goal

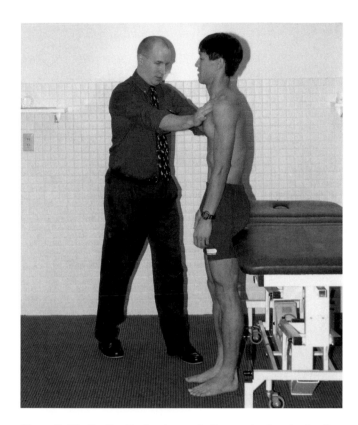

Figure 8–30. Testing the lumbar protective mechanism in standing with diagonal anterior-posterior resistance.

is to restore maximum function to the athlete, with a number of other objectives to be reached along the way. The initial objective is to control and resolve pain and swelling using modalities such as hot pack, electrical stimulation, and ultrasound. These have value in the acute or reinjury state, but they should be used sparingly to prevent dependence by the athlete and to encourage active participation in the management of the back injury. Ice is strongly encouraged the first 48 to 72 hours following a mechanical low back injury and should be used longer if achy, resting pain continues.[14] The duration of ice application time is 20 to 30 minutes every 2 hours, varying for depth and type of tissue.[15]

After the initial 48 to 72 hours, cryokinetics can be used.[16] Cryokinetics is the use of ice and exercise through the range of motion. The ice will minimize the effects of new microtrauma secondary to the treatment. In the acute state, cryokinetics should be used with passive and progress to active assisted range-of-motion activity. This will initiate the process of restoring normal lumbar osteokinematics, as well as arthrokinematics. For this treatment, the athlete is prone with the ice applied. They are progressively moved through the available flex-

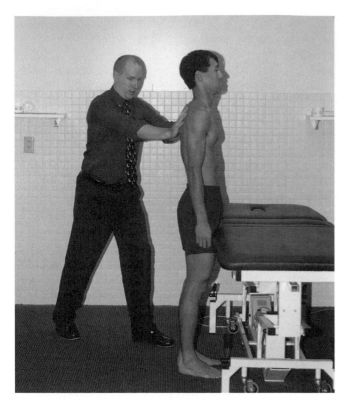

Figure 8–31. Testing the lumbar protective mechanism in standing with diagonal posterior-anterior resistance.

ion and extension ranges on an adjustable bivalve table. Care should be taken not to exceed the points of discomfort.

While ice is applied, electrical stimulation can also be administered to decrease pain, swelling, and muscle spasm. The electrical stimulation will help with the first objective of reducing pain and swelling, while promoting an optimal healing environment and tissue remodeling. Electrical stimulators include high-voltage pulsed stimulation (HVPS), transcutaneous electrical nerve stimulation (TENS), interferential current (IFC), and microamperage nerve stimulation (MENS). Efficacy of and preference for stimulators varies; until long-term outcome studies are completed, examiners should use what works best in their hands. Ultrasound used in a pulsed, nonthermal mode can also assist the healing process during the acute state.[14,17,18]

Progression to the next stage calls for educating the athlete on the anatomy and biomechanics of the lumbar spine. Understanding the normal range of motion and lumbar mechanics permits him or her to take an active approach in the treatment and, knowing his or her limits, to minimize destructive behavior throughout the treatment. In other words, teach the athlete what positions

and movements are best and those that can hamper the healing process.

MANUAL TREATMENT TECHNIQUES

Treatment approaches use manual and active techniques that create forces in and around the lumbar region to promote healing without being destructive. Manual techniques include massage, soft-tissue mobilization, myofascial techniques, joint mobilization, rolfing, and acupressure. Active techniques include contract and relax, flexion and extension protocols, muscle energy, strain and counterstrain, and stabilization protocols.

Soft-tissue mobilization is an excellent technique for beginning rehabilitation. This hands-on technique allows the athlete to quickly gain confidence in the examiner, establishing the basis for good two-way communication. Other manual and active techniques discussed lead to physiologic responses including influence on the fluid dynamics of the injured area, generation of afferent input into the central nervous system, and modification of the connective tissues.[19] Many other good techniques not discussed here also can be useful tools such as Feldenkrais

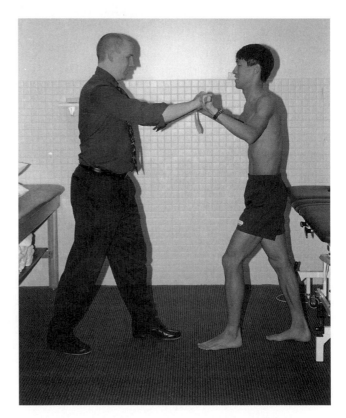

Figure 8–32. Testing the lumbar protective mechanism during a resisted activity.

techniques, Travell trigger points, Aston patterning, Trager approach, and many others.[20,21] The key to effective treatment is not to be limited to one technique but, understanding the similarities of many techniques, to select a particular technique that facilitates the quickest return for the athlete.

Soft-tissue Mobilization

Following a thorough examination, soft-tissue mobilization can play a valuable role in treating any identified soft-tissue dysfunctions. Frequently, the soft tissues of the body are found to be in an inefficient state of mobility and tone, which causes, precipitates, and perpetuates many symptoms of the lumbar spine.[22] A common reason for the development of inefficient soft tissues is poor posture. This results in a change of the plumb line through the vertebra creating more force and weight anterior or posterior to the joint. The body weight is counterbalanced by passive tension in the soft tissue. A joint can be stable only if there is equilibrium between the forces acting on it.[22] Without equilibrium, there is poor attenuation of forces and abnormal firing patterns of muscles. This leads some muscles to become facilitated with trigger points and ligamentous creep, possibly resulting in osteophytes and instability.[22,23] Poor posture can also delay healing of lesions. Soft-tissue mobilization is one component of rehabilitation needed to equalize the forces.

Muscular and postural imbalances result from muscle weakness due to shortening, joint restrictions due to soft-tissue restrictions, fascial restrictions, problems with self-image, and body language. This can result in injury, degeneration of joints, local vascular disturbances, visceral-somatic responses, and somatic-visceral responses.[24] The postural imbalance will create immobilization in some joints due to certain tissues restricting range of motion.[25] This holding pattern places the facet joints in a different resting position, and will cause the muscles around them to become imbalanced. If the joints and soft tissues are maintained in an immobile, shortened range, chronic abnormal neural feedback and compensatory structural changes in those tissues may result.

One last component of back injury that can be addressed with the use of soft-tissue mobilization is scar tissue adhesions. This scar tissue can develop from callous formation following a fracture, or from soft-tissue trauma. The trauma could be from a specific injury, a laceration, or surgical incision. Fractures will result in callous formation affecting the connective tissues matrix from bone level to fascial level. This scar tissue is an irregular mass of connective tissue with poor extensibility. According to Wolf's law, bone adapts to the stresses applied; so does other connective tissue such as fascial, ligament, tendon, and capsule. Examiners must apply a gentle external manual force to the myofascial unit to assist the tissues into a lengthened more functional direction.[22,26]

If the appropriate remodeling stimuli are not applied during the healing stage, the scar will be inextensible and nondynamic.[22,26] This scar tissue can produce localized adhesions, resulting in a loss of normal mobility of structures and articulations in the surrounding region.[27] In normal, healthy connective tissue, the three-dimensional mobility is called normal play.[11] When this normal play does not exist, normal extensibility, accessory mobility, and biomechanical function of the tissue is limited. This state of dysfunction is called restricted or decreased play.[11] To identify the dysfunctions, a skilled evaluation must be completed. One component is skilled palpation. To proceed with good soft-tissue mobilization, fine tuning of palpation skills is needed, as discussed in the following section.

Palpatory Evaluation
The techniques described here with his permission, were developed by Greg Johnson of the Institute of Physical Art, Milwaukee.

Superficial Assessment. Evaluation guides examiners to the general area of dysfunction. The soft-tissue assessment of that area begins superficially. These dysfunctions can exist in single or multiple connective tissue layers. It is best to clear the dysfunction in the top layer before diving into the deep layers. Too many examiners are divers, palpating the deep layers immediately using excessively heavy pressure. A key to remember is, if you can't feel the dysfunction initially, lighten your pressure, which yields better sensitivity, rather than increasing your pressure. Any tenderness elicited by appropriate palpation is often indicative of tissue dysfunction.[22]

Motion Palpation. Palpation evaluation is comprised of motion palpation and passive palpation. Motion palpation is observing and feeling for compliance of the tissues as they are shortened and lengthened. For example, as the athlete is standing completing right lumbar sidebending, the right lumbar paraspinals and associated soft tissues must fold like an accordion to allow full range of motion. Subsequently, the left-sided soft tissues must lengthen. The evaluation can be done actively or passively, with the patient in a variety of positions.

Passive Palpation. Passive palpation is done to evaluate tissue end feel, excursion, and recoil. Tissue end feel, as described by Cyriax, is the quality of tension felt when the tissue is manually deformed, through direct pressure, to its physiologic or accessory end-range.[28] In normal tissues, the end feel is springy like a new rubber band. The amount of play in soft tissues can vary throughout the body, but the end feel is consistently springy.[22] Dysfunctional tissues have a hard end feel. Locating the degree of dysfunction, the direction in which it is most limited, and its epicenter of exact depth, will allow an examiner to be more specific and less invasive with treatment.[11]

Excursion. Excursion is evaluated by either direct pressure to the tissues or through elongation of the tissues by joint motion. The soft-tissue restriction may be felt through the full range of motion or only in isolated portions. Again, locating the epicenter at the specific part of the range will improve treatment. Elasticity of the tissues is evaluated through the range of motion and recoil is evaluated upon return to the resting position.[22]

Treatment Strategy

The soft-tissue treatment progression is based on a layer progression beginning with the skin and superficial fascia. The skin should first be evaluated for temperature, moisture, and texture to determine the condition of the underlying tissues. In the acute situation, the tissues will be warm and a slight rise in moisture maybe noted. In a chronic situation, the tissues will be dry, smooth, and shiny.

To evaluate and treat the tissues for mobility, extensibility, end feel, and elasticity requires the use of the following skills. First, there is skin sliding or palm sliding to help identify the location of the restriction and identify its direction of restriction (see Fig. 8-33). The general technique is to use the entire palm surface in addressing the skin's ability to slide on the underlying tissue. To be more specific, use the fingertips, which being more sensitive, may help in locating distant restrictions. These techniques must be performed in all directions, not just the direction of the overlying muscle.

The next skin technique is finger gliding using the middle finger or thumb to address the ability to glide through the skin. In normal tissue, the finger slides with ease like skiing downhill on fresh snow. Restrictions will feel like hitting wet snow. Normally, as the finger slides it creates a wave of skin in front of the finger (see Fig. 8-34.)

The last skin assessment and treatment technique is skin rolling. The skin and subcutaneous fascia is lifted between the index finger, middle finger, and the thumb (see Fig. 8-35). This test is done bilaterally, looking for differences in skin pliability and thickness. This is especially helpful over bony prominences to see the skin's ability to lift from the underlying tissues.

The next step is evaluating and treating around the bony contours. Due to multiple soft tissue attachments to the bone, this is a frequent site of dysfunctions, as well as a major site of pain due to the highly innervated periosteum. Frequent structures of pathology are around the iliac crest, sacral sulcus, the lower border of the rib cage, and the groove between the

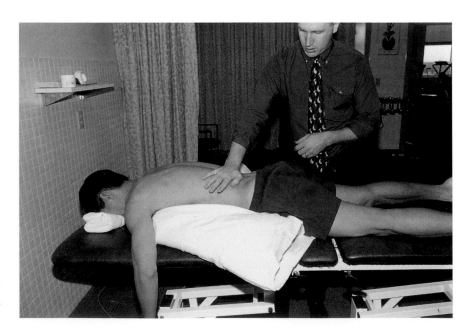

Figure 8–33. Skin sliding/palm sliding a general technique for skin and superficial fascia assessment.

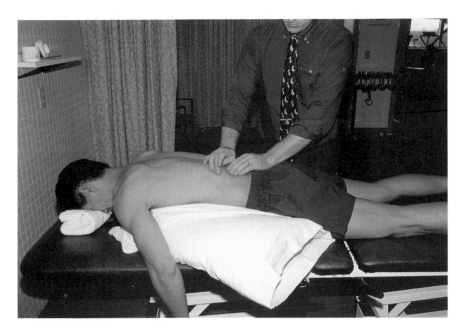

Figure 8–34. Finger gliding for skin and superficial fascia assessment.

spinous and transverse processes. Slide your fingers parallel along the edges of the bone feeling for restricted mobility at the various tissue depths (see Figs. 8-36 and 8-37).

The myofascial tissue is next to evaluate and treat. Look at muscle tone, play, and functional excursion. Frequently, an examiner will see increased muscle tone with dysfunctions indicating the muscle's inability to fully relax. The tissue will feel denser and is frequently tender to palpation. The increased tone can affect the entire muscle versus specific points only. Be specific

with palpation to locate the exact depth and direction of the increased tone. Muscle play is the accessory mobility of muscle in relation to other muscles or adjacent structures. To evaluate and treat, use perpendicular (transverse) mobilization and parallel (longitudinal) mobilization, which is discussed in the next section. Again, identify the specific depth and direction of the restriction. Muscle functional excursion looks at the length of the muscle between its origin and insertion. Contract and hold relaxation techniques work well to regain normal length.[13] Also, look at the arc of motion

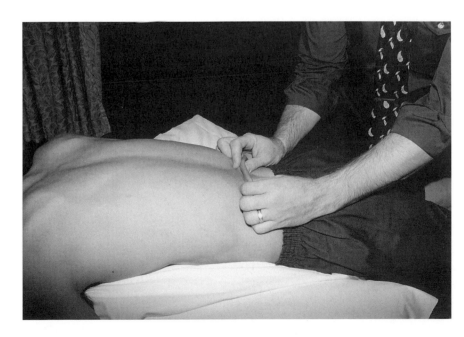

Figure 8–35. Skin rolling.

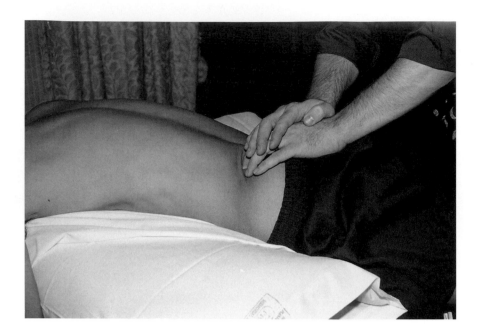

Figure 8–36. Assessment of bony contours.

with varying rotation. With the use of proprioceptive neuromuscular facilitation, an examiner can observe the recruitment and sequencing patterns of these soft tissues.[12,13] Improvement in neuromuscular control helps with long-term maintenance of the soft tissues.[12] After the soft tissues are normalized, joint mobilization is used to return normal joint mechanics. With the neuromuscular control regained, treatment can then be completed by normalizing body mechanics and working on conditioning exercises.[11,26] These final steps will be discussed in a later chapter.

Treatment Techniques

The functional orthopedic treatment techniques that are most effective are direct sustained pressure, unlocking spiral, and direct oscillations.[11,26] These techniques can be used with an assisting hand to shorten or lengthen the surrounding tissues, as well as performing associated oscillations. The assisting hand facilitates relaxation to help normalize the soft tissues. Most often, the treatment begins with the patient in a relaxed position, well supported, while maintaining a good breathing pattern. The final progression is functional mobilization using the

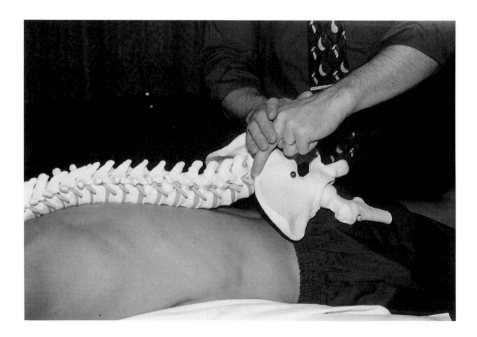

Figure 8–37. Assessment of bony contours.

treatment techniques during passive, active, or resistive motions.

The first technique is sustained pressure. This can be applied in a diffuse manner by using the forearm, heel of the hand, or elbow. Focal pressure may be applied using fingers or thumb. This sustained pressure is applied in the direction of the restriction with a push or a pull. Hold the pressure on the same level until you feel the restriction release, then reevaluate. If the restriction does not release, use the other hand to shorten or lengthen the surrounding tissues. When the restriction softens the slack must be taken up, first by the treating hand and then by the assisting hand, if an assisting technique is being used. Also, the assisting hand can oscillate the legs for optimal relaxation (see Fig. 8-38).

If the restriction does not respond to a gentle push or pull, then attempt an unlocking spiral. Maintaining finger tip pressure against the restriction, apply a clockwise or counterclockwise motion to identify the direction that the tissue rotates with the greatest ease. While holding in the more easily rotated position, take up the slack to complete the technique. Reevaluate and check to see if the restriction has also resolved towards the most restricted direction and treat appropriately (see Fig. 8-39).

Other techniques are parallel and perpendicular mobilization. Parallel mobilization is longitudinal pressure along the side of the muscle belly, such as along bony contours or between two muscles (see Fig. 8-40). Perpendicular mobilization is transverse pressure to the muscle belly to improve its play (see Fig. 8-41).

Strumming like a guitar string is another technique of transverse pressure, but done in a repeated, rhythmic deformation of the muscle belly to reduce its tone (see Fig. 8-42).

Throughout these techniques, the assisting hand can implement oscillations to help the tissues release. In the lumbar region, for example, while the treating hand sustains pressure along the muscle belly and at the appropriate layer, the assisting hand can create a repeated rhythmic motion by gently rocking the pelvis or leg resulting in an indirect oscillation. The treating hand can also implement direct oscillations with most techniques. The speed of oscillation will vary with the depth of the restriction and size of the patient. Finally, the patient can actively create small-amplitude pelvic motions to facilitate relaxation.

The contraindications for soft-tissue mobilization include, but are not limited to, malignancy, fracture, osteoporosis, osteomyelitis, hemorrhage sites, aneurysm, acute rheumatoid arthritis, advanced diabetes, inflammatory skin condition, inflammatory state of fibromyalgia, and any increased symptoms.

The purpose of soft-tissue mobilization is to release increased muscle tone, rid fascial tissue of restrictions, decongest tissues, increase blood flow, decrease pain, and alter the facilitated segment. In addition to the mechanical effect of soft tissue mobilization, there is also a psychological benefit from the laying on of hands. There are neurophysiologic effects from the motions produced that, by excitation of sensory receptors, may provide pain relief and reduce muscle holding. Soft-tissue mobilization will achieve optimal results if com-

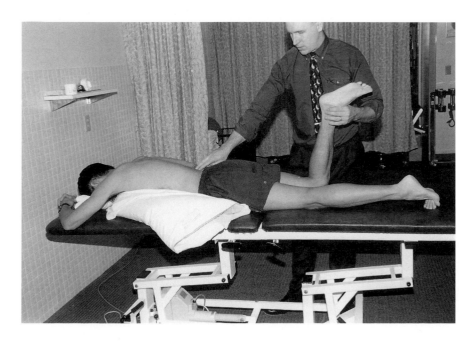

Figure 8–38. Sustained pressure.

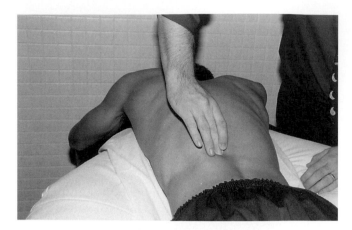

Figure 8–39. Unlocking spiral.

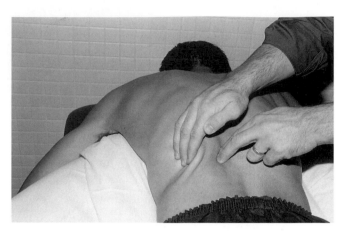

Figure 8–41. Perpendicular mobilization

bined with other manual therapy techniques, good patient education, and a high-quality exercise program that optimizes stabilization and conditioning. A primary factor in the long-term effectiveness of treatments will be educating the patient to minimize stressful positions.[22]

Joint Mobilization

Joint mobilization may be indicated if the soft tissues have been returned to normal play, tone, and extensibility but a functional deficit remains. Joint mobilization, as described by Paris, is the skilled passive movement of a joint.[30] An evaluation of the suspected target area will guide the examiner's hands to the joint needing treatment. For example, if during the evaluation of the lumbar spine, the lumbar lordosis will not reverse during forward bending, while side-bending is unaffected, soft-

tissue restrictions should be suspected. If side-bending is also limited, there may be facet joint dysfunction causing the motion restriction. During side-bending, the lumbar spine should show a smooth curve representing good segmental mobility. Restricted segments will be represented by deviations from this smooth curve. Do not forget to look for adequate soft-tissue folding on the approximated side, while soft-tissue lengthening occurs on the opposite side. Another tool to use in evaluation is overpressure. Pressure is applied at the end of an active range to address the end feel. The restriction may be caused by the elastic resistance of muscle, the firmness of capsule, or the relative hardness of adhesions.[30] In an evaluation look at a variety of motions. Beside the standard flexion, extension, side-bending, and rotation also look at pelvic shear and diagonal motions. For details beyond the scope of this section refer to the writings of Cyriax, Grieve, Kaltenborn, Maitland, and Paris.[28,31-34]

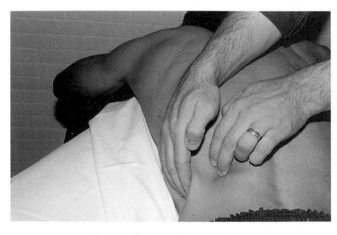

Figure 8–40. Parallel mobilization.

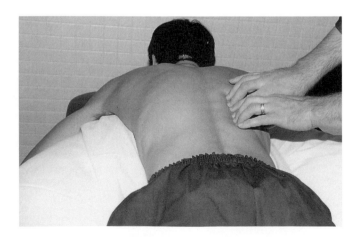

Figure 8–42. Strumming.

The goal of this section is to provide an overview of additional evaluation and treatment techniques to improve joint mobility. Joint mobilization is used to increase the quality and quantity of pain-free, functional range of motion. For best results with joint mobilization, the specific restriction must be identified. Passive intervertebral motion (PIVM) testing is a tool to find the specific joint restriction. PIVM testing can be completed on each individual lumbar segment through all available planes to evaluate their range of motion and can be given a respective grade. In recording mobility, Paris uses a 0 to 6 scale.[35]

Grade	Description	Criteria
0	Anklyosis	No detectable movement within segment
1	Considerable restriction	Significant decrease in expected range and resistance
2	Slight restriction	Limitation expected in range and minimal resistance
3	Normal	Expected range of motion for body type and uniform
4	Slight increase	Mild increase in range
5	Considerable increase	Excessive range, but restricted eventually by capsule
6	Unstable	Excessive range and no capsule restraint

Testing PIVMs by palpation enhances the evaluation of joint motion of the target area. Findings lead to initiation of treatment. Look at all aspects of motion, quality, quantity, and overpressure. Assess the capability of the tissues to tolerate stresses of overpressure at end range. Speeds of techniques vary, with slower speeds being most effective for the evaluation. If after the first gentle movement, there is no pain or restriction, the next movement can be applied with greater depth. After 2 or 3 oscillations to one vertebra proceed to the next anatomic level for comparison. This test will detect abnormalities or pain versus normal mobility. Due to the wide variety of PIVM testing and mobilization techniques, this section will present those thought to be most appropriate. The PIVM positions are described. The mobilization techniques that use the same positions are described after PIVM testing with specific illustrations.

Passive intervertebral motion testing for flexion and extension of T11 and S1 is completed in the sidelying position. Facing the athlete, grasp under his or her top leg to flex and extend the hip, moving the lumbar spine respectively. While creating the lumbar movement, the examiner's other hand is palpating the underside of the targeted interspinous space. The tip of the underside index or middle finger faces upward evaluating that segment's mobility. Evaluation of each interspinal segment is essential.

Side-bending or lateral flexion is also tested in the sidelying position. Allow the tibias to drop over the side of the table with hips and knees at 90 degrees of flexion to create side-bending of the lumbar spine. With the other hand, palpate on the interspinous space with the pad of the middle finger. An alternate position for side-bending testing in sidelying is to rock the pelvis upwards to create side-bending.

Rotation can be accomplished in multiple positions. For a beginner, a prone lying position can be used. Grasp the ASIS and lift upwards to create lumbar rotation.

Maitland describes two types of joint mobilization to achieve normal range. The first is passive oscillatory movements performed either smoothly and slowly (1 every 2 seconds) or quickly (3 per second) with small or large amplitude applied in any part of the total range of movement. This oscillatory movement can be performed while the joint is compressed or distracted. Remember that examining movements are usually performed at a slower speed than they are when used as treatment technique. The second passive movement is sustained stretching. This may be performed with or without tiny amplitude oscillations at the limit of the range. Within these two oscillation techniques, Maitland developed four grades of oscillations.[31]

- Grade I: Small-amplitude movement near the starting position of the range.
- Grade II: Large-amplitude movement performed within the range that is free of any stiffness or muscle spasm.
- Grade III: Large-amplitude movement performed up to the limit of range.
- Grade IV: Small-amplitude movement stretching into stiffness or muscle spasm at the limit of range.

For athletes who have pain with lumbar extension, a treatment that may be used is posterior–anterior central vertebral pressure on the spinous process. The athlete is positioned prone with arms relaxed. The examiner uses the ulnar border of the hand between the pisiform and the hook of the hamate to contact the spinous process of the vertebra to be mobilized. The examiner needs to monitor his or her body mechanics over the athlete. Positioning of the shoulders over the vertebra, elbows slightly flexed, and the wrist fully extended is the correct or desired alignment of the treating clinician. If treating the right side of the athlete use the right

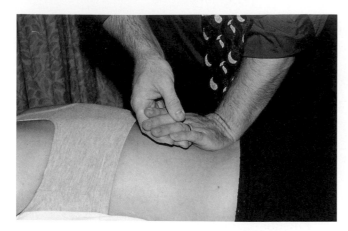

Figure 8–43. Posterior-anterior central vertebral pressure.

hand. Use the left hand to cup over the right hand for re-inforcement. To create the movement at each vertebra the examiner moves his or her body weight forward over the target vertebra creating a rocking movement of the trunk (see Fig. 8-43). Under normal conditions, there is no tenderness with posterior–anterior maneuvers and movement is equal segmentally in the lumbar spine, with the exception of L5 which has less mobility. If pain or protective muscle spasm is felt, then posterior–anterior mobilization can be used as a treatment. All treatment should not provoke an increase of the patient's symptoms. In addition, this technique is useful when the athlete has lumbar pain evenly distributed on both sides.[31,36]

Another technique using the spinous process to evaluate and treat side-bending mobility is transverse verte-bral pressure. This technique is also used to treat the athlete who has unilateral pain, especially for the upper lumbar spine. The athlete lies prone with arms relaxed. The thumbs are placed against the side of the spinous process. The pad of the top thumb should be over the nail of the bottom thumb. The fingers are placed over the athlete's back to stabilize the thumb position. Pressure is applied to the thumbs through the arms held horizontally (see Fig. 8-44). To make this a stronger technique to stretch the joint, oscillate the ipsilateral leg as you apply pressure. Take up the slack as the leg is initially abducted, and then complete the mobilizing oscillations (see Fig. 8-45).[31,36] For evaluation, both sides are tested. For treatment of unilateral pain, stand on the nonpainful side to open the painful side.

The technique for rotation uses the transverse process and is called posterio–anterior unilateral verte-bral pressure. This technique is good for treating muscle spasm of the deep intrasegmental muscles. The athlete is prone with the arms relaxed. The examiner will evaluate both sides, but for treatment address the side of the unilateral muscle spasms or pain. The thumbs are placed next to the spinous process and pointing to each other. The fingers are placed on the back to stabilize the thumbs. Again the examiner's shoulders are over the vertebrae and their trunk is rocked to create the force. Apply the pressure slowly to sink through the muscle bulk, using the thumb pads to feel the transverse process (see Fig. 8-46).[31] An alternate technique to increase rotation is to use the pelvis. The palpating finger is placed between the spinous process to feel the rotation. Grasp the ASIS on the opposite side and pull up, feeling the rotation on the lower spinous process that will be moving

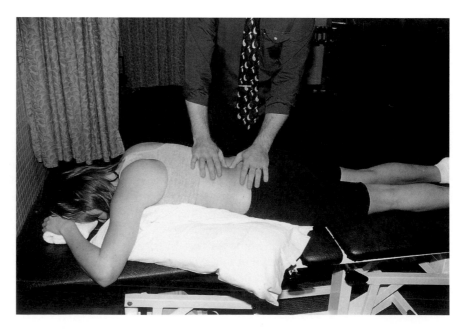

Figure 8–44. Transverse vertebral pressure.

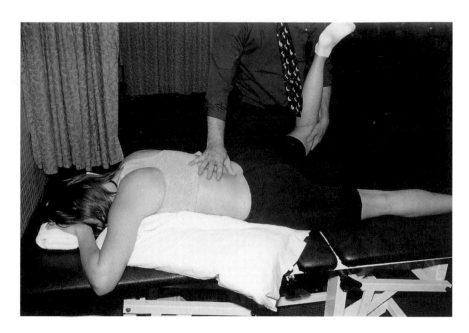

Figure 8–45. Transverse vertebral pressure, using the right leg to apply stronger pressure.

towards the middle finger (see Fig. 8-47).[32] Rotation can also be accomplished using the legs with the knees at 90 degrees (see Fig. 8-48).[32]

The prone techniques using the spinous process address extension and side-bending or lateral flexion, while the transverse process techniques address rotation. Next are sidelying techniques for flexion, side-bending, and rotation mobility. For side-bending, the athlete is lying on the left side with the hips and knees flexed, placing the lumbar spine in a neutral (midway between flexion and extension) position. The examiner

stands facing the athelte's feet with the athlete on his or her left side, grasps the feet with the left hand, and braces the athlete's knees on the examiner's hip. With the middle finger of the right hand the examiner palpates the space on the top side between the spinous process. Keeping the athlete's hips and knees at right angles, the examiner slowly lowers the feet off the table to create left side-bending (see Fig. 8-49), and then raises the feet to create right side-bending (see Fig. 8-50).[32,36] Maitland's treatment approach is to use force on the athlete's pelvis and upper thigh to laterally flex

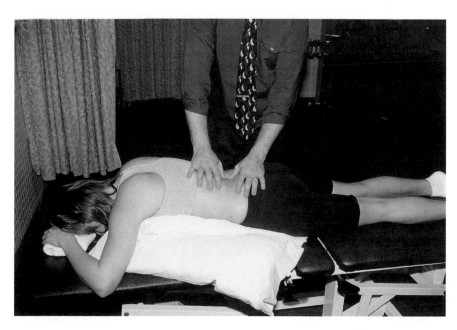

Figure 8–46. Posterior-anterior unilateral vertebral pressure.

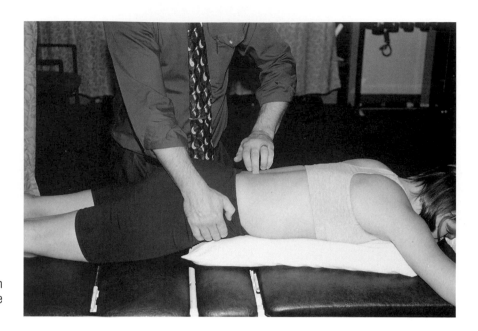

Figure 8–47. Lumbar rotation mobilization with the use of the anterior-superior iliac spine (ASIS).

the lumbar spine from below while palpating the underside of the interspinous space of the segment being evaluated (see Fig. 8-51).[31] Once the restriction is localized to a segment, mobilization can be done by oscillating with the legs or the treating hand.

The sidelying position can also be used to evaluate and treat the motions of flexion and extension. The athlete is positioned on his or her right side facing the examiner with hips and knees flexed to 90 degrees. The examiner grasps the athlete's flexed legs. The knees rest on the ex-

aminer's hip. The left hand palpates the interspinous space with the pad of the middle finger. The same arm can prevent any rotation of the thorax. Passive flexion of the lumbar spine is produced by rocking the athlete's knees toward his or her chest (see Fig. 8-52). Move the hips toward the direction of extension to create lumbar extension (see Fig. 8-53). Many examiners find both knees difficult to control and will therefore use the top leg only.[31,32]

Rotational forces are easily applied in the described position and extreme care must be taken. The examiner

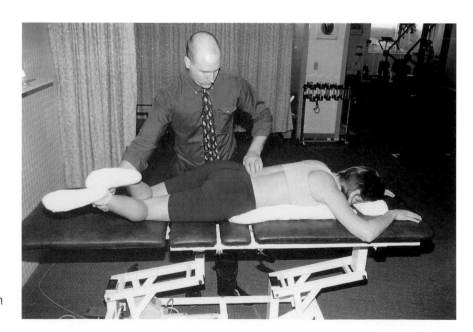

Figure 8–48. Lumbar rotation mobilization with the use of the legs in the prone position.

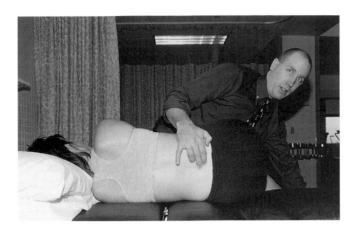

Figure 8–49. Left side-bending mobilization using the legs.

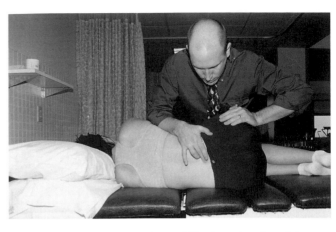

Figure 8–51. Side-bending mobilization using the pelvis.

must understand what he or she is doing to the athlete and be in control. The athlete lies on their right side. The athlete's left arm can rest on his or her abdomen. For better visual demonstration, Figure 8-53 shows the left hand behind the athlete. The examiner can flex both legs, or just the top leg. The leg is flexed until movement is palpated at the interspinous space of the segment being evaluated. Lift the athlete's right arm towards the ceiling to gain additional rotation. The examiner's left arm maintains the rotation just gained. Oscillations then can be completed with the treating hand (see Fig. 8-54).[31,32,36] Other advanced mobilization techniques can be performed in the sidelying position, but are beyond the scope of this chapter.

Contraindications for joint mobilization are pregnancy, malignancy, tuberculosis, osteomyelitis, active osteoporosis, fracture, acute arthritis, and disk prolapse with serious neurologic changes. For a practitioner with minimal mobilization skill, the list may also in-clude disk prolapse and herniation, spondylolysis, spondylolisthesis, scoliosis, and hypermobility.[30] As this list is not all inclusive, good judgment must be used.

Mobilization of the Nervous System

An examiner should be able to form a good impression of what to expect on the physical examination after completing the subjective questioning. Maitland expressed it as making the features fit. In the acute and subacute phases, the pain will fit the physical findings. In the chronic state, pain can take on a life of its own and all subjective complaints may not fit the objective findings. Clinicians need to assist the athlete in correcting the physical findings and preventing recurrences. Understading the symptoms and their physical mechanisms will help clinical reason-

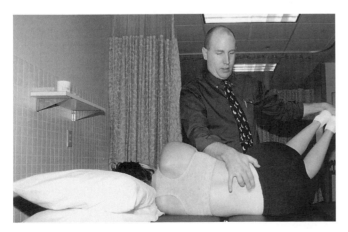

Figure 8–50. Right side-bending mobilization using the legs.

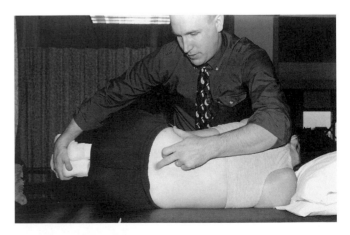

Figure 8–52. Flexion mobilization of the lumbar spine.

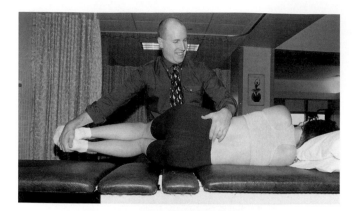

Figure 8–53. Extension mobilization of the lumbar spine.

ing as the examination progresses to neurodynamic evaluation.

Butler states that the cause of symptoms can be categorized into five mechanisms.[37] The first is peripheral nociceptive or nerve end pain. The nociceptors are activated by musculoskeletal and visceral structures. The main source is inflammation in target tissues such as spinal joints, dura, and nerve root sheaths. Responses to painful stimulation will usually be repeatable, and will settle after the stimulus.

The second mechanism is peripheral neurogenic, which may be seen with mechanical back pain. The radicular (nerve root) symptoms originate in neural tissue outside the central nervous system. Examples are dorsal root ganglion, peripheral and cranial nerves, plus their connective tissues. The pain is mechanically patterned. Mobilizing these lesions can result in swelling.

The third mechanism is central, located in the central nervous system. The symptoms are due to abnormal sensitivity of the central nervous system. Pain may be termed pathological because the pain does not behave with stimulus predictability. One example is that move-

ment may not cause pain consistently. Another example is sudden stabs of unprovoked pain.

The fourth mechanism is autonomic and motor pathways. Autonomic pathways can produce the symptoms of sweating, swelling, skin redness, and sustained pain whereas, motor pathways can produce muscle spasms. Due to the autonomic nervous system involvement and its sympathetic trunk location just anterior to the ever moving costotransverse joints, it may be necessary to mobilize the thoracic spine. There may be a protective muscle spasm.

The last component is affective, in which there are psychological components of pain. A clinical impression of the dominant mechanisms must be reached to develop the most effective treatment. Great variations in pain can be expected.

Important features of the nervous system biomechanics are its mobility and the continuous tract nature of the central and peripheral nervous system. Performing a straight leg raise shows how the nervous system's mobility can act independently or dependently of the structures it spans. A normal straight leg raise produces tension in the calf and foot, but no activity in the foot's nonneural structures. A straight leg raise with ankle dorsiflexion will place the neural structure in the calf and foot dependent on the hip joint position. Other features of the nervous system must be understood prior to attempting the neurodynamic testing. Further reading of Maitland,[31] Butler,[37] and others will greatly enhance examiner knowledge.

Neurodynamic testing, previously called tension tests, looks at the mechanics and physiology of the nervous system as they relate to one another.[38] The base testing for the trunk includes passive neck flexion (PNF), straight leg raise (SLR), slump test, and prone knee bend (PKB). Look for the reproduction of symptoms and the resistance encountered. Watch for antalgic posture, such as hip-hiking during straight leg raise. Many variations of the base tests have been developed, although base tests should be mastered before progressing to other tests. All tests should be done bilaterally for comparison.

The first test is passive neck flexion. This is done in the supine position without a pillow and the athlete's arms at his or her side. After asking the athlete to lift the head off the table a few inches, the examiner grasps the head to passively flex the neck with the chin headed for the chest (see Fig. 8–55). The test should be painless outside of a mild pulling sensation at the cervicothoracic junction. This is indicated for all possible spinal disorders. It is often positive for low back pain. The neural structures tested are the pons, spinal cord, and meninges. If this test produces lumbar pain, then the source of pain lies within the nervous system.[39]

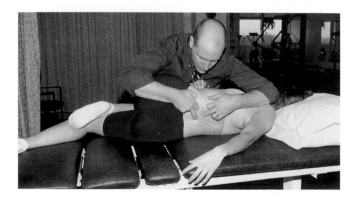

Figure 8–54. Lumbar rotation mobilization in the sidelying position.

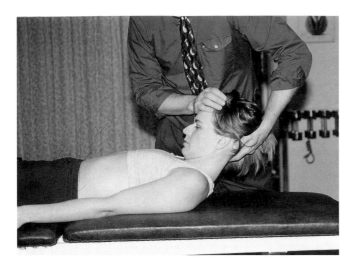

Figure 8–55. Passive neck flexion.

The next neurodynamic test is prone knee bend, a good test for upper lumbar symptoms, as well as for the knee, anterior thigh, and hip. As upper lumbar radiculopathy is less common than lower lumbar radiculopathy, this test is not done as frequently as it should be. The athlete lies prone in a consistent position. The examiner grasps the anterior distal tibia and flexes the knee (see Fig. 8-58). The normal range of motion is heel near the buttocks and symptom response in the quadriceps. Watch for postural deviations such as rotation or the buttocks lifting up. Determine where the pain is from: muscle, fascia, or nervous system.

The last base test is the slump test, a test Maitland has studied normatively and has popularized in manual therapy. This test is a logical progression after the PNF and the SLR. The following is a description of the slump test for an athlete with a nonirritable disorder. Symptoms need to be monitored throughout the test, and the range of movement is estimated after each segment.

The athlete sits at the very edge of the table with the knees together to allow an easily repeatable position. The athlete's hands are behind the back and linked together. The examiner stands at the side of the athlete (see Fig. 8-59). The athlete is then asked to slump (slouch), while the examiner maintains the cervical spine in neutral position. Overpressure may be applied to encourage maximum thoracic and lumbar flexion, but not to increase hip flexion (see Fig. 8-60). Maintaining the first two positions, the athlete actively places the chin on the chest and the examiner can apply overpressure (see Fig. 8-61). In uninjured athletes, pain will be felt 50 percent of the time in the area of T8 and T9. The athlete then actively extends each knee starting with the uninvolved side (see Fig. 8-62). Pain in the ham-

The second test is the straight leg raise. The test is performed in the supine position with the athlete's trunk and hips in neutral position. The examiner grasps under the distal achilles tendon placing the other hand on the anterior aspect of the distal femur. The leg is lifted into true hip flexion of the saggital plane and the knee maintained in extension (see Fig. 8-56). Be consistent in your testing. Use the same position, force, and no pillow under the neck for all the athletes tested. As with all neurodynamic tests, feel the quality of range, symptom response, and resistance encountered. There is a wide range of normal response through the range of motion. Typical symptoms are tension in the posterior hamstring, posterior knee, and calf. Dorsiflexion of the ankle can also be added (see Fig. 8-57).

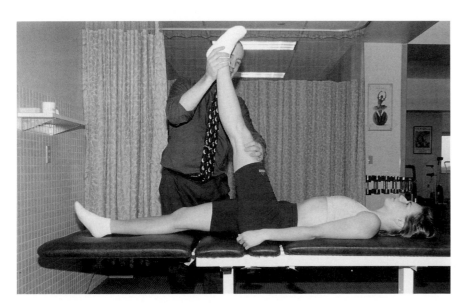

Figure 8–56. Straight leg raise.

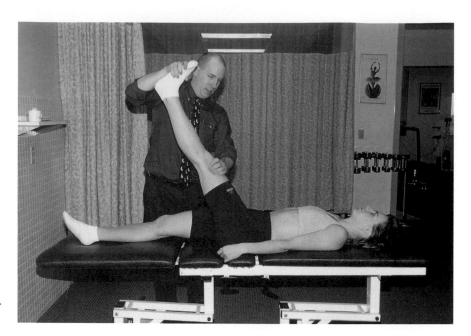

Figure 8–57. Straight leg raise with ankle dorsiflexion superimposed.

string and popliteal area is common, and a limitation of knee extension is seen frequently. The athlete then actively dorsiflexes the ankle (see Fig. 8-63). The next step is to release cervical flexion and carefully assess the response (see Fig. 8-64). With the release of cervical flexion, there is a decrease of symptoms and an increase in knee extension.

The nerve tension tests need to be completed slowly to maintain optimal positioning and to prevent further injury to the neurologic system. As the name implies, tension test is exactly how the test is completed and how treatment is initiated. Through the years, the name has changed to dynamic test to imply that tension is not the only way to treat this area. Neurogenic pain is normally treated aggressively, while central pain needs to be teased along. For instance, instead of both ends of the chain placed on maximum tension, place one end on tension while the other end is off tension. Then si-

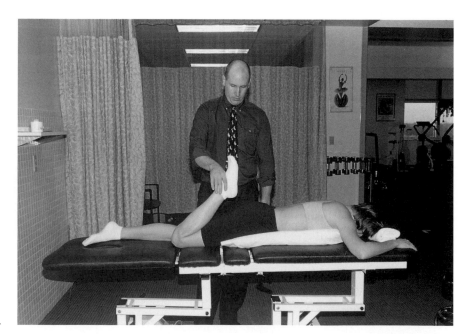

Figure 8–58. Prone knee bend.

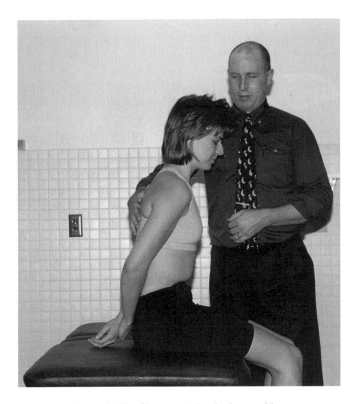

Figure 8–59. Slump test, beginning position.

minimal muscle twitch to a maximum muscle contraction. The duration of the effort by the athlete may vary from a fraction of a second to a sustained effort lasting several seconds. Any of three types of muscle contraction may be used, but always begin with isometric. Isometric contraction results in tension of the muscle without shortening or lengthening. The second contraction is concentric, resulting in shortening of the muscle. The third contraction is eccentric, during which the muscle lengthens. Isometric muscle energy techniques primarily reduce the tone in a hypertonic muscle and normalize its resting length. Hypertonic muscle and shortened muscles are frequently identified as the major component of restricted motion of an articulation. As a result of the muscle contraction needed to do muscle energy techniques, the athlete may have some muscle soreness 12 to 36 hours after the first treatment. The muscle spindle and the reciprocal inhibition reflexes are two specific reflex mechanisms that allow muscle energy techniques to be worked by altering the muscle physiology.

Key factors essential for any successful muscle energy procedure include the following.

1. Accurate diagnosis of the restriction.
2. Accurate patient positioning to control joint positioning by engaging the restrictive barrier in

multaneously reverse the two ends to assist the neurologic system in sliding. Lastly, another treatment technique is to place one end on tension, while the other end is actively placed on and off tension, while the therapist traces along the nerve tract to detect adherences and subsequently treat with soft-tissue techniques. Be gentle and constantly talk to the athlete to monitor.

ACTIVE TREATMENT TECHNIQUES

Muscle Energy

Osteopathic muscle energy technique is a manual therapy treatment procedure that involves the voluntary use of the athlete's muscles from a precisely controlled position in a specific direction against a distinctly executed counterforce.[40-42] This is an active technique that can be used to lengthen a shortened or contracted muscle, to strengthen a physiologically weakened muscle, to reduce localized edema, or to mobilize restricted joint motion.

Muscle energy procedures can influence any articulation in the body that can be moved by voluntary muscle action either directly or indirectly. The amount of force or effort applied by the athlete may vary from a

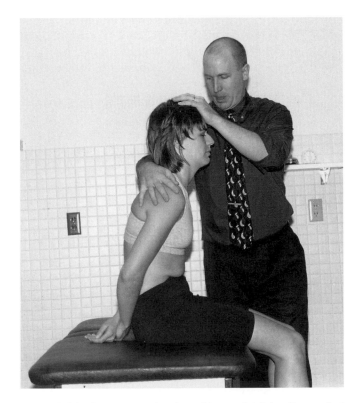

Figure 8–60. Slump test, slouch position, maintaining the cervical spine in neutral.

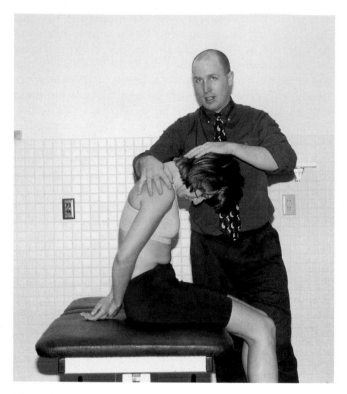

Figure 8–61. Slump test, full cervical flexion is added, plus overpressure is applied.

tant that the athlete and the examiner be balanced, with the examiner in control to optimize the localization of the technique.

The advantage of muscle energy technique over a thrust manipulation is that it is easier to get the patient to cooperate and relax. Furthermore, muscle energy seems clinically more effective, applicable, and safer in acute situations. Muscle energy does, however, require very sensitive palpatory skill to constantly monitor the involved joint.

There are other approaches to muscle energy than the osteopath's techniques. One example is what Johnson teaches in his functional mobilization course for the lower quadrant.[44] Differences in his techniques are that the athlete is in a weight-bearing position (a functional position), during the evaluation and treatment rather than a recumbent position. Second, the end feel of the transverse process is evaluated, not just the depth of the transverse process. For example, to test lumbar forward bending the athlete is in the functional weight-bearing position of sitting. The examiner is positioned behind the athlete palpating the transverse processes with the thumbs to assess the segment's mobility and end feel during physiologic motions. The athlete is instructed to roll forward. In the normal state, both transverse processes move posteriorly and at end

all three planes (flexion and extension, side-bending left and right, rotation left and right).
3. Appropriately applied counterforce (direction and duration).
4. Appropriate patient effort in the correct direction.
5. Complete relaxation after the muscle effort.
6. Repositioning to the new restrictive barrier in all three planes.
7. Repetition of steps 1 through 6.
8. Retest.[40,43]

The examiner places the athlete in the correct position, and directs the athlete to contract the muscle. The amount of force utilized is graded from a few ounces to several pounds. For instance, with an isometric contraction the force is light to moderate, nearing 1 pound of force. For an isotonic contraction the force is hard to maximal at approximately 3 pounds of force. To gain maximum benefit, it is very important to pause after the contraction before additional stretch is attempted, then reposition to repeat the technique. The duration of the contraction is sustained for 3 to 6 seconds with 3 to 6 repetitions. When using an isotonic contraction, the muscle should contract over its total range. It is impor-

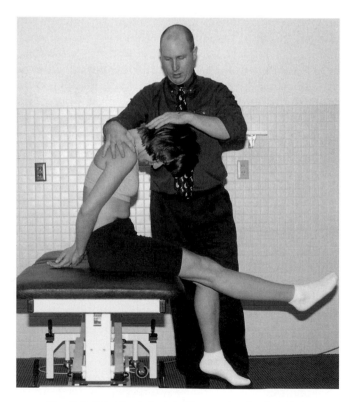

Figure 8–62. Slump test, full knee extension is added.

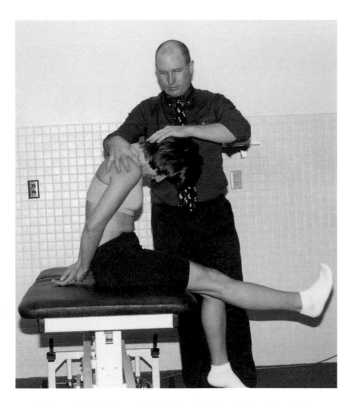

Figure 8–63. Slump test, full ankle dorsiflexion is added.

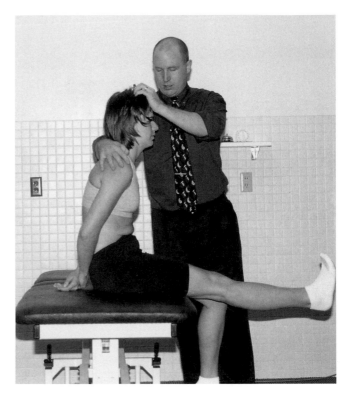

Figure 8–64. Slump test, release cervical flexion.

range have a springy end feel (see Fig. 8-65). In a dysfunctional state, one or both transverse processes will remain forward and easily palpated. End feel testing is very important to detect greatest dysfunction. While continuing to monitor at the transverse process for end feel, assist the athlete in a left forward bending diagonal (see Fig. 8-66). Then assist the athlete in a right forward bending diagonal. Once the side and diagonal of hardest end feel is identified, functional mobilization is applied. Place the athlete in the position where the transverse process has the hardest end feel and resist trunk flexion in that diagonal using a combination of isotonics (see Fig. 8-67). A combination of isotonics is using whatever type of contraction (isometric, isotonic, or eccentric) is needed to get optimal results. Retest end feel and treat to equalize the transverse processes. To test and treat for lumbar extension have the athlete sit. Instruct to backward bend by rolling forward on the pelvis and letting the belly move and relax forward, then backward bend from the upper back. In the efficient state, both transverse processes move forward and have a springy end feel. If dysfunctional, one or both transverse processes will remain more posterior. Be sure the psoas muscle is not the reason for this dysfunction before proceeding. Initially, test the transverse processes in backward bending (see Fig. 8-68). Assist the athlete in a right

extension diagonal and monitor at the transverse process (see Fig. 8-69). Left diagonal is then tested. If the right diagonal produces the hardest end feel, place the athlete in the dysfunctional position to the right. The athlete should push down into the left foot to stabilize the body on the chair and resist right extension placing the examiner's hand on the scapula. Monitor with

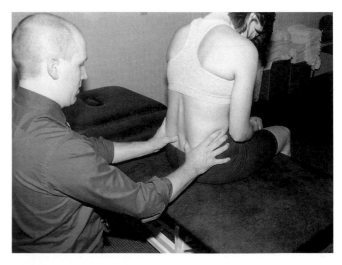

Figure 8–65. Lumbar flexion in sitting, assessing the transverse processes.

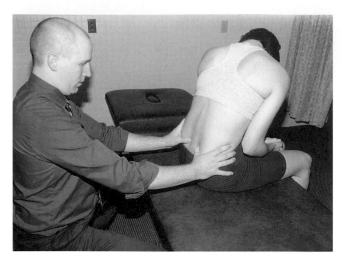

Figure 8–66. Lumbar flexion with left diagonal in sitting, assessing the transverse processes.

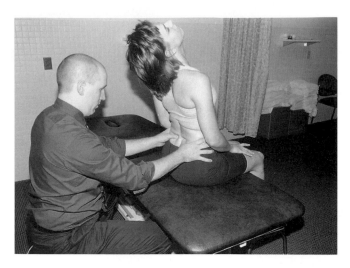

Figure 8–68. Lumbar extension in sitting assessing the transverse processes.

the other hand at the transverse process (see Fig. 8–70). The restriction may not resolve with resistance on the right. The examiner can try resistance on the left.

The specific techniques and classification system that osteopaths have taught other health care professionals is very complex and detailed, yet very successful. To learn their techniques, further reading such as Greenman's *Principles of Manual Medicine* is recommended.[40]

McKenzie Exercises

Prior to McKenzie's contribution to the treatment of low back pain, flexion or William's exercises were a

commonly used tool. Some diagnoses such as spondyloysis, spondylolisthesis, spinal stenosis, and severe lumbar degenerative joint disease, respond well with flexion exercises as rehabilitation begins, but many other diagnoses have an increase of symptoms with flexion exercises. Through trial and error, McKenzie developed the use of extension to centralize the patient's pain. Not all patients improve with extension, and therefore, other positions and movements were identified to centralize pain. McKenzie describes the centralization phenomenon as a result of the performance of certain repeated movements or changes of position to move the radiating pain from the periphery

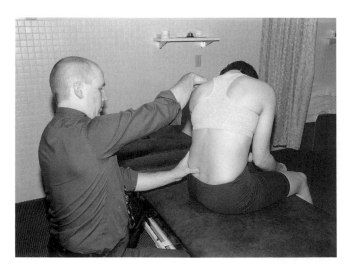

Figure 8–67. Lumbar flexion with left diagonal and resisting trunk flexion.

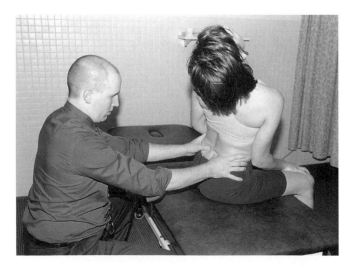

Figure 8–69. Lumbar extension with right diagonal in sitting, assessing the transverse processes.

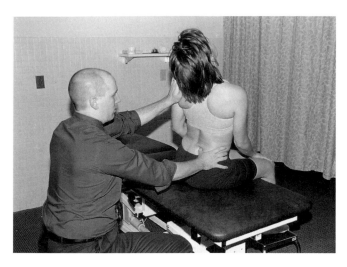

Figure 8–70. Lumbar extension with right diagonal and resisting trunk extension.

towards the center of the spine.[8] The repeated movement uses a similar basis as Codman's exercises for the shoulder. McKenzie principles are used not only for disk pathology and patients with radiating leg pain, but also for mild lumbar strains. The key is the analysis and subsequent effect of this mechanical stress on the pain pattern.[19] These techniques work well with a young posture pathology, but are less effective with an old, stiff spine.

Making a specific diagnosis regarding low back pain is difficult. McKenzie uses an alternate classification system rather than aiming for a specific diagnosis based on a particular pathology. He bases the system on the premise that low back pain is caused by mechanical deformation of soft tissues containing nociceptive recep-

tors. He divides back pain into three syndromes: postural, dysfunction, and derangement.

Postural Syndrome

This is caused by mechanical deformation of soft tissues as a result of postural stresses. It is characterized by intermittent pain brought on by particular postures or positions maintained for a period of time. The pain ceases with a change of position. There is no deformity. Treatment involves postural correction and education.

Dysfunction Syndrome

This is caused by mechanical deformation of soft tissues by adaptive shortening. It is characterized by intermittent pain and partial loss of movement. Pain occurs at or before end range stretch and ceases when the stress is released. There is no deformity. Treatment involves postural correction and stretching of shortened structures. Frequently, there is loss of extension in standing. The press-up is a passive exercise used as a mobilization tool (see Fig. 8–71).

Derangement Syndrome

This is caused by mechanical deformation of soft tissues as a result of internal derangement, for example, alteration of the position of the nucleus within the disk. Various degrees are possible. It is usually characterized by constant pain, partial loss of motion, and deformities such as kyphosis or scoliosis.

McKenzie identifies seven derangement syndromes. Treatment is based on the centralization principle, where the performance of certain repeated movements or the adoption of certain positions moves a radiating pain away from the periphery and towards the midline of the spine. Treatment begins with postural

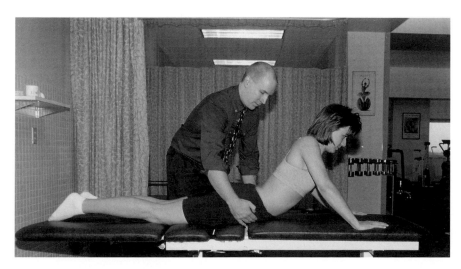

Figure 8–71. Press-up.

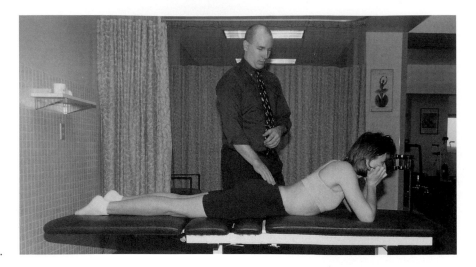

Figure 8–72. Prone on elbows.

correction and education. If a lateral shift is present, it must be taken care of first. Next, progress from prone on elbows to a press-up to centralize the pain (see Fig. 8-72). If prone on elbows is too painful, begin with extension in the standing position. A lateral shift or a functional rotoscoliosis is when the athlete is seen to list or tilt to one side, this usually occurs at about the level of L4 and L5. Frequently, a compensatory curve is seen at a much higher level. Approximately 9 out of 10 subjects exhibiting a shift do so away from the painful side. The incidence of neurologic deficit is higher for those who shift toward the painful side. To correct a lateral shift, the examiner stands on the side of the shift. On that side, the athlete bends his or her elbow to 90 degrees. The examiner encircles the patient's trunk, clasping his or her hands about the pelvis. Next, the examiner presses his or her shoulder against the athlete's elbow, pushing away the athlete's rib cage, while at the same time drawing his or her pelvis towards the examiner (see Fig. 8-73). This will reduce the lateral shift. The athlete must be questioned continually regarding pain, with the focus being centralization of pain.[8] Once the shift has been corrected, then extension must be restored. Extension can be restored with the use of a prone press-up. Whether this is an exercise or active mobilization technique can be debated, but the key is to alter the patient's pain and restore function. Do not attempt to exercise with a lateral shift; it must be reduced first. A lumbar roll will help maintain extension. For further details read McKenzie: *The Lumbar Spine: Mechanical Diagnosis and Therapy*.[8]

Flexibility

The goal is not only to return the athlete to competition as quickly and as safely as possible, but to prevent re-injury. If flexibility is not addressed, there will be a greater likelihood of further injury down the road. Because the lumbar spine exists in a kinematic chain relationship with the lower extremities, normal intervertebral mobility is dependent on normal connective and contractile tissue extensibility. To maintain normal range of motion and to minimize stress to the joints and surrounding tissue, normal flexibility must be maintained. Muscles that need to be addressed will be evident after the functional examination.

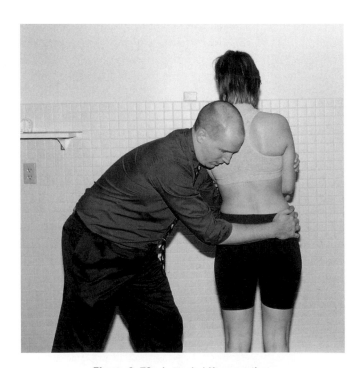

Figure 8–73. Lateral shift correction.

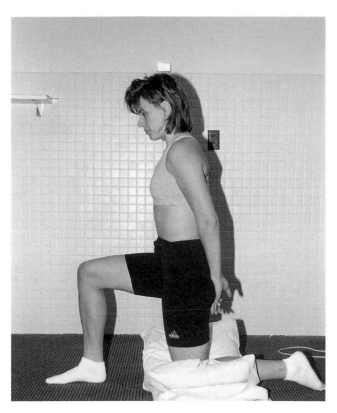

Figure 8–74. Iliopsoas stretch.

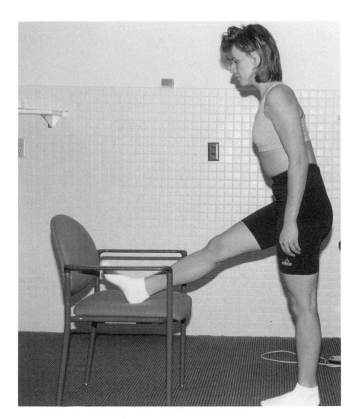

Figure 8–75. Hamstring stretch.

According to Janda, muscles do not respond to dysfunction in a random occurrence, but respond in a characteristic manner.[45] Postural or tonic muscles respond to dysfunction by facilitation, hypertonicity, and shortening. For example, the postural muscles around the hip and back that shorten are the iliopsoas, piriformis, hamstrings, quadratus lumborum, lumbar erector spinae, hip adductors, and the tensor fascia latae. The dynamic or phasic muscles respond by inhibition, and therefore become hypotonic and weak. For example, around the hip and back, the dynamic muscles that weaken are the gluteus medius and maximus, rectus abdominals, and obliques. The abdominals become weak while the lumbar erector spinae shorten limiting lumbar flexion. According to Janda, first the lumbar flexion mobility must be regained, after which treatment proceeds to strengthen the abdominals. By stretching a previously inhibited muscle to regain normal length, a spontaneous muscle disinhibition will occur.[45] Sahrman teaches that the most effective way of lengthening a short muscle is by working its antagonist that is too long.[46] In this example, then, don't stretch first, but strengthen the lengthened lower abdominals. This strengthening will lengthen the short lumbar paraspinals.

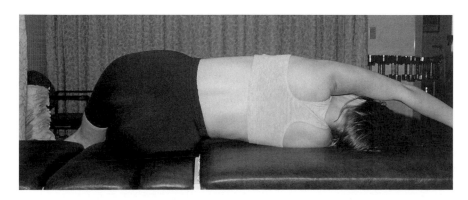

Figure 8–76. Quadratus lumborum stretch.

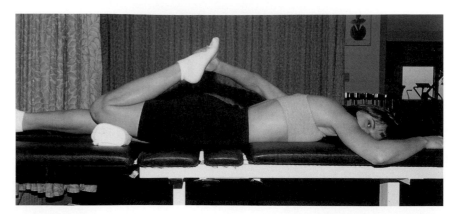

Figure 8–77. Quadriceps stretch.

Stretching needs to be held for 30 seconds and completed frequently throughout the day, such as 4 times per day.[47] In addition, many athletes' collagen properties will not allow a significant change in length to occur from stretching. Therefore, it is recommended that soft-tissue techniques be added while the athlete stretches. The illustrated stretches are for the iliopsoas (see Fig. 8-74), hamstrings (see Fig. 8-75), quadratus lumborum (see Fig. 8-76), quadriceps (see Fig. 8-77), piriformis (see Fig. 8-78), and iliotibial band (see Fig. 8-79).

Stabilization Exercises

The major task in rehabilitation is to educate the athlete on how to move without creating destructive forces to the spine. To accomplish this, the athlete must be taught a precise exercise program to fit his or her specific deficits. The athlete must be taught to correct faulty postural habits and movement patterns. Athletes generally feel better when exercising and learn best by doing.[48] This learning process requires repetition and positive feedback.[13] The exercise program must be individualized. The athlete cannot simply be given a flexion or extension exercise sheet and be sent away. Friedrich and colleagues compared the success of home exercise programs based on instruction. The first group was given a brochure of exercises, while the second group received supervised instruction from a professional. The results on a rating scale evaluating the correctness of exercise performance at follow-up showed that the supervised group performed better than the brochure group. In addition, there was a stronger correlation between the quality of exercise performance and decrease in pain in the supervised group. The brochure group completed the exercises correctly only 50 percent of the time.[49] The final objective is to teach the athlete how to stabilize the trunk, rather than using the trunk muscles as prime movers.[7] A variety of authors have defined stabilization as maintaining the spine in a pain-free, balanced, neutral posi-

tion through continuous fine adjustments in muscle tension in response to fluctuating load.[10,11,48,50] Saal and Saal describe stabilization with terms such as muscle fusion and corseting, in which the soft tissues maintain a corseting effect to brace the lumbar spine and protect the individual segments from repetitive microtrauma.[51] The goal of this concept is to teach the athlete how to self-brace, or stabilize. Static stabilization was initially developed to protect an unstable segment from stress.[52] Static stabilization is completed in the early stages of rehabilitation and must be likened to placing a shoulder in a sling. The next stage is dynamic or functional stabilization, which is the ability to move and function normally through postures and activities without creating undue segmental stress.[52] This teaches the

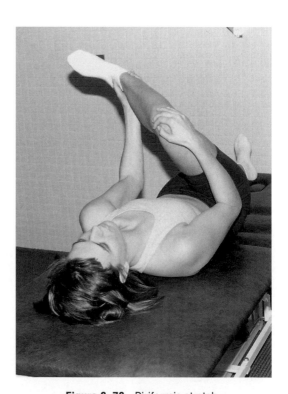

Figure 8–78. Piriformis stretch.

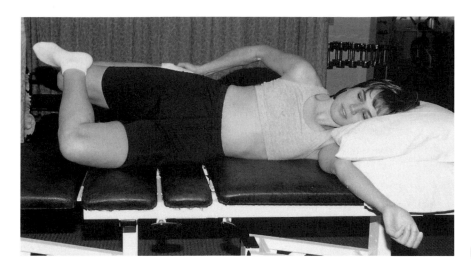

Figure 8–79. Iliotibial band stretch.

athlete to move their spine segmentally, while staying away from end ranges. The desired goal of any stabilization program must be to produce stability during functional activities while allowing for normal motion of the previously unstable segment. Prior to stabilization, many athletes will need to work on different exercises to decrease their pain and decrease their mechanical faults. This section provides some exercise ideas for initial treatment prior to stabilization.

For the athlete who has pain with flexion clinically and functionally, extension principles previously discussed by McKenzie can be used. In addition, prone arm lifts in a pain-free position to recruit the lumbar paraspinals may be used. The athlete needs to learn how to flex at the hip, stretching the gluteus maximus. This will minimize the stress on the lumbar spine. The athlete can stretch the gluteus maximus with a knee-to-chest exercise in the supine position with a towel roll under the lumbar spine to prevent flexing at the lumbar

spine (see Fig. 8–80). Partial rocking back on hands and knees is a good exercise the athlete can control.

An exercise for the athlete who has pain with lumbar extension is a posterior pelvic tilt using the lower abdominals. Encourage posterior pelvic tilt in a variety of positions, especially functional positions. Start in the supine hook lying position while performing a posterior pelvic tilt. Have the athlete slowly slide one heel down the table maintaining the pelvic tilt. Knee-to-chest exercise can also be done in this scenario.

For the athlete who has pain with lumbar rotation, which is seen frequently due to the amount of lumbar rotation needed in sports, it is encouraged to clear any straight-plane dysfunction first. For rotational pain, an exercise idea is a posterior pelvic tilt in the supine position with knees bent. Next, have the athlete slowly allow the bent knee to fall out (hip external rotation) without losing the posterior pelvic tilt. Pelvic clock exercises can be used in the supine position. Encourage athletes to ad-

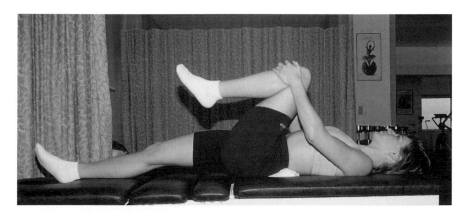

Figure 8–80. Gluteus maximus stretch.

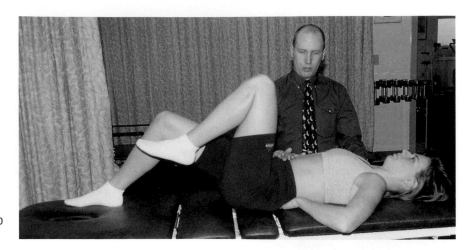

Figure 8–81. Marching using the hands to monitor the lumbar spine in neutral position.

dress the weakness of the hip rotators as well as the hip adductors and abductors.

The next stage is to begin the stabilization program. Bracing is the athlete's ability to selectively recruit the lower trunk muscles to stabilize the lumbar spine. The initial assessment can be done with the athlete supine and hook lying. The examiner can apply pressure to the walls of the trunk and ask the athlete to contract these muscles. If the response is inefficient, the athlete is placed on a stabilization program.[11] Hook lying is a good position to begin the stabilization program. One way to help facilitate contraction of the lower trunk muscles is to isometrically resist hip flexion at 90 degrees of flexion. At the same time the athlete attempts to brace, the examiner's fingers can be placed deep into the soft tissues of the trunk for the athlete to push out against. Bracing should be completed in the most pain-free position, the neutral position. Neutral is defined as half way between flexion and extension of the lumbar spine. The definition is broad to fit the patient's symptoms, pathology, and current musculoskeletal restrictions.[53] The neu-

tral position should not be at end ranges of a segment. Bracing can be completed in supine, standing, standing with each leg at different heights of a step, sitting, getting up from a chair, and the four-point position. Once bracing is mastered in these positions, arm and leg movements can be superimposed. Next, the athlete can proceed to functional positions. Meticulous technique is important for the performance of this exercise. An important factor initially is to obtain good stabilization at the specific individual segment of the lumbar spine where the pathology exists. Accomplishing individual segment stability can be nicely done in the four-point position. Stabilization programs have produced good outcomes in the mid to high 80 percentile for patients with radiculopathy.[50]

The athlete needs to learn stabilization so that it becomes a natural response or natural position. Once the response can be elicited on command and endurance has been developed, the program can progress to extremity movement. In the supine position with the knees bent and the athlete bracing, have the athlete

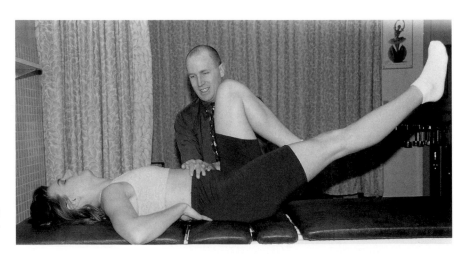

Figure 8–82. Marching with the lumbar spine in neutral and superimposed with single leg extension.

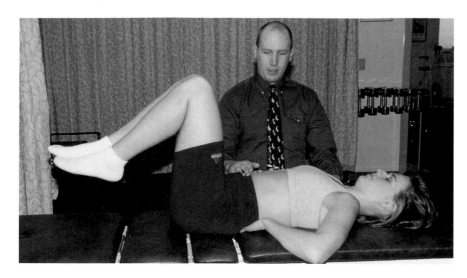

Figure 8–83. Double leg lowering with the lumbar spine in neutral.

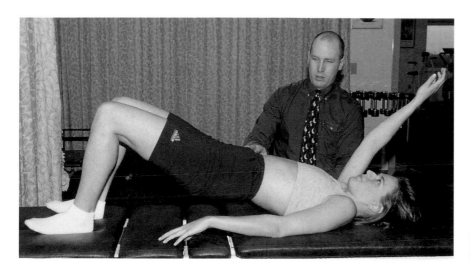

Figure 8–84. Bridging with the lumbar spine in neutral and superimposed with single arm raise.

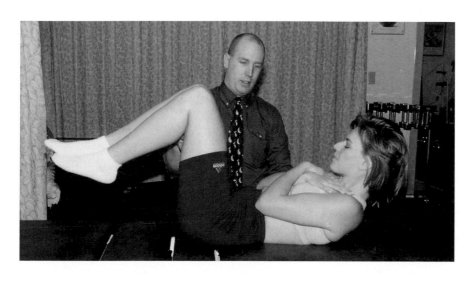

Figure 8–85. Sit-up.

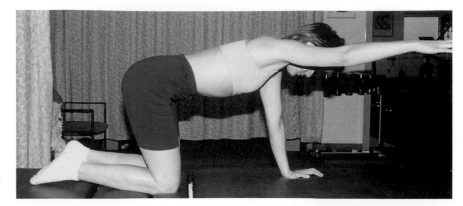

Figure 8–86. Four-point position, with single arm raise.

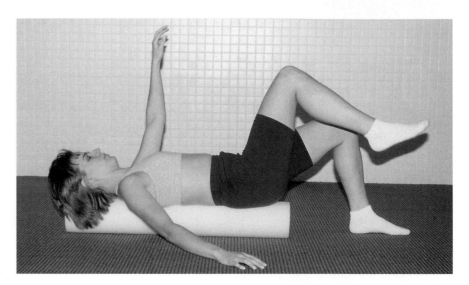

Figure 8–87. Foam roll, arm and leg raise.

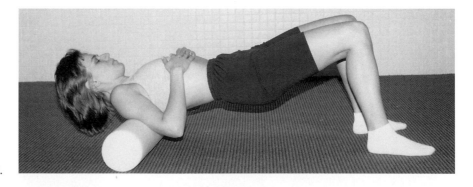

Figure 8–88. Foam roll, bridging.

march in place taking tiny steps (see Fig. 8-81). While marching in place, the athlete can superimpose arm movement. The progression is designed to improve the strength and endurance of the lower trunk and abdominal muscles in both the open and closed kinetic chain.[10] From marching, the athlete can progress to single leg raises beginning with the knees bent at 90 degrees. He or she can progress to full knee extension and raise the leg up and then down before returning to the initial position. This is repeated with the opposite leg (see Fig.

8-82). This step is to progress to bilateral leg lowering (see Fig. 8-83). To progress into closed kinetic exercise, bridging can be done in the supine position. When bridging is mastered, the workload can be increased by raising one arm at a time, and then one arm and one leg at a time (see Fig. 8-84). The final supine position exercises are sit-ups, which can be done in multiple positions and must be individualized (see Fig. 8-85). The last of the basic postural control portion of the stabilization exercises are completed in the prone position. The next progression is in four-point beginning with individual arm and leg raises and progressing to alternating the opposite arms and legs (see Fig. 8-86).

The program can be advanced with weights or rubber tubing. For the injured athlete, encourage rotational exercises with cable resistance or rubber tubing devices. Encourage PNF techniques for enhancing neuromuscular facilitation and reeducation.[30] The program can be progressed to work on bracing and balance on foam rolls and swiss balls (see Figs. 8-87 through 8-95).[55,56]

In addition to the stabilization program, the athlete is placed on a general conditioning and strengthening program to address any other weakness identified. Normal athletic performances typically require a high level of aerobic capacity that is frequently compromised secondary to inactivity following a spinal injury.[57] If aerobic conditioning is not addressed, the athlete may fatigue early resulting in altered mechanics and possible subsequent reinjury. Aerobic conditioning is very important early in the rehabilitation especially with activities that do not load the spine heavily, such as pool therapy.[58,59]

A brief summary of the exercise progression follows.[52,60]

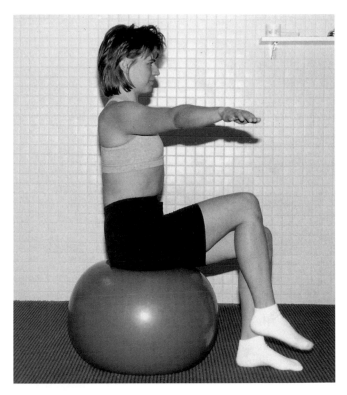

Figure 8–89. Swiss ball, sitting with arm and leg raise.

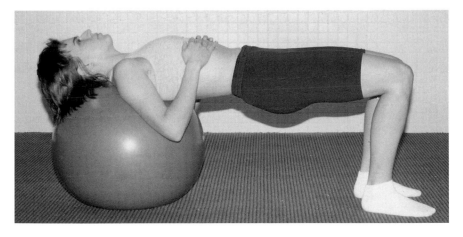

Figure 8–90. Swiss ball, bridging.

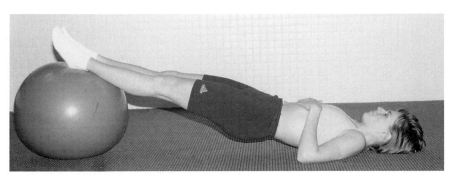

Figure 8–91. Swiss ball, supine on floor with feet on the ball and bridge.

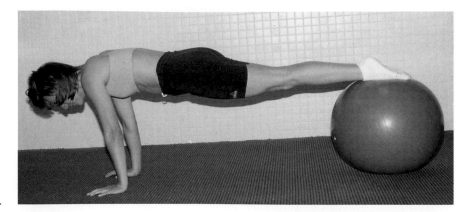

Figure 8–92. Swiss ball, four-point position.

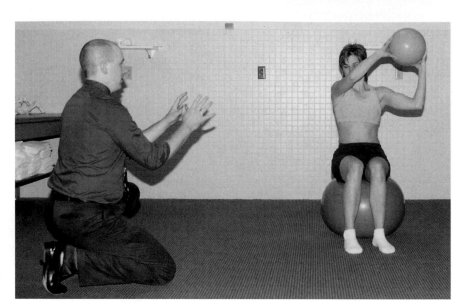

Figure 8–93. Swiss ball, sitting with ball throw in a diagonal pattern.

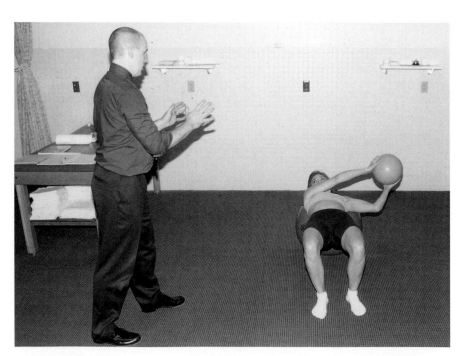

Figure 8–94. Swiss ball, bridge with ball throw in a diagonal pattern.

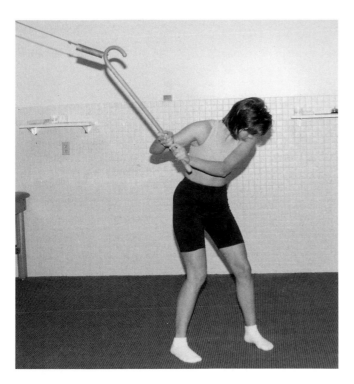

Figure 8–95. Tubing exercise in a functional position: "Batter up."

- Level 1: Education—back school.
- Level 2: Static-stabilization—muscular fusion. Abdominal bracing: supine, standing, stairs, sitting, four-point, kneeling, squats. Partial sit-ups.
- Level 3: Advanced pelvic stabilization: marching, single-leg raise, bridge, bridge with extremity movement, bilateral leg lowering, four-point with extremity movement, and diagonal sit-ups.
- Level 4: Foam roll and swiss ball exercises in multiple positions and degrees of difficulty.
- Level 5: Dynamic stabilization: functional positions with multiple degrees of resistance.

CONCLUSION

This chapter provides the methods necessary to effectively treat the injured athlete's back. Initially stressed is the importance of listening to the athlete to obtain the specific mechanism of injury and what symptoms are currently present. This is a great time to pick up on the learning style of the athlete, which will assist in the treatment approach. Specific treatment techniques follow with an emphasis on manual therapy. The power of touching the athlete yields so much information. Work with the athletes, do not just give out exercise sheets. Finally, the section is completed with a flexibility and stabilization program with a variety of options for each individual objective finding. Teach the athlete what needs to be accomplished, so the athlete can self-manage the condition. Use the body's ability to heal itself.

REFERENCES

1. Akeson W, Woo S, Amiel D, et al. The connective tissue response to immobility: Biomechanical changes in periarticular connective tissue of the immobilized rabbit knee. *Clin Orthop.* 1973;93:1
2. Hazard R, Fenwick J, Kalisch S. Functional restoration with behavioral support: A one year prospective study of patients with chronic low back pain. *Spine.* 1989;14:157.
3. Beattie P. Low back, SI joint, and hip course notes. St. Louis; 1993.
4. Donelson RG. The McKenzie method. In: White AH, Anderson R, eds. *Conservative Care of Low Back Pain.* Baltimore: Williams & Wilkins; 1991.
5. Deyo RA, Diehl AK, Rosenthal M. How many days of bed rest for acute low back pain? *N Engl J Med.* 1986; 315:1064–1070.
6. Linton SJ, Helsing A, Anderson D. A controlled study of effects of an early intervention on acute musculoskeletal pain problems. *Pain.* 1993;54:353–359.
7. Porterfield JA, DeRosa C. Treatment of lumbopelvic disorders. In: Porterfield JA, DeRosa C, eds. *Mehanical Low Back Pain.* Philadelphia: Sanders; 1991.
8. McKenzie RA. *The Lumbar Spine: Mechanical Diagnosis and Therapy.* Waikanae, NZ: Spinal Publications; 1981.
9. Bigos S, Bowyer O, Braen G, et al. *Acute Low Back Problems in Adults.* Clinical Practice Guideline no. 14. Rockville, MD: Agency for Health Care Policy and Research, Public Health Services, U.S. Dept. of Health and Human Services; 1994. ANCPR 95-0642.
10. Saliba VL, Johnson GS. Lumbar Protective Mechanism. In: White AH, Anderson R, eds. *Conservative Care of Low Back Pain.* Baltimore: Williams & Wilkins; 1991.
11. Johnson GS. Functional orthopedics I, course outline. Milwaukee: Institute of Physical Art; 1990.
12. Saliba VL. PNF 1 course notes. Chicago: Institute of Physical Art; 1992.
13. Knott M, Voss DE. *Proprioceptive Neuromuscular Facilitation.* 2nd ed. London: Balliese, Daintily & Cogs; 1968.
14. Michlovitz SL. *Thermal Agents in Rehabilitation.* 2nd ed. Philadelphia: Davis; 1990.
15. Ho SW, Illgen RL, Meyer RW, et al. Comparison of various icing times in decreasing bone metabolism and blood flow in the knee. *Am J Sports Med.* 1995;23:74–76.
16. Timm KE. Management and rehabilitation of athletic lumbar spine injuries. In: Timm KE, Malone TR, eds. *Back Injuries and Rehabilitation.* Baltimore: Williams & Wilkins; 1989.
17. Nelson RM, Currier DP, eds. *Clinical Electrotherapy.* Norwalk, CT: Appleton & Lange; 1987.
18. Prentice WE. *Therapeutic Modalities in Sports Medicine.* St. Louis: Times Mirror/Mosby College Publishing; 1990.
19. De Rosa CP, Porterfield JA. A physical therapy model for the treatment of low back pain. *Phys Ther.* 1992;72:261–272.

20. Miller B. Alternative somatic therapies. In: White AH, Anderson R, eds. *Conservative Care Of Low Back Pain.* Baltimore: Williams & Wilkins; 1991.

21. Travell JG, Simons DG. Myofascial pain and dysfunction. *The Trigger Point Manual.* Baltimore: Williams & Wilkins; 1983.

22. Johnson GS. Soft tissue mobilization. In: White AH, Anderson R, eds. *Conservative Care Of Low Back Pain.* Baltimore: Williams & Wilkins; 1991.

23. Janda V. Muscles, central nervous motor regulation and back problems. In: Korr IM, ed. *The Neurologic Mechanisms in Manipulative Therapy.* New York: Plenum; 1977.

24. Grodin A. Soft tissue mobilization, course outline. Eau Claire, WI; 1983.

25. Grodin A. Soft tissue techniques. In: Grodin A, Myerson G, Malone TR, eds. *Soft Tissue Mobilization.* Baltimore: Williams & Wilkins; 1989.

26. Nikolaou PK, MacDonald BL, Glisson RR. Biomechanical and histological evaluation of muscle after controlled strain injuries. *Am J Sports Med.* 1987;15:9-14.

27. Malone TR. *Muscle Injury and Rehabilitation.* Baltimore: Williams & Wilkins; 1988.

28. Cyriax J. Diagnosis of soft tissue lesions. In: Cyriax J, ed. *Textbook of Orthopedic Medicine.* 8th ed. Baltimore: Williams & Wilkins; 1984.

29. Johnson GS. Functional orthopedic II, course outline. Milwaukee: Institute of Physical Art; 1991.

30. Paris SV. Mobilization of the spine. *Phys Ther.* 1979;59:8.

31. Maitland GD. *Vertebral Manipulation.* 5th ed. London: Butterworths; 1986.

32. Paris S. S-1 course notes. Milwaukee: Institute for Graduate Health Sciences; 1984.

33. Kaltenborn FM. *Mobilization of the Extremity Joints.* 3rd ed. Oslo: Olaf Norlis; 1980.

34. Grieve GP. *Common Vertebral Joint Problems.* Edinburgh: Churchill Livingstone; 1981.

35. Gonnella C, Paris SV, Kutner M. Reliability in evaluating passive intervertebral motion. *Phys Ther.* 1982;62:436-444.

36. Synenham RW. Manual therapy techniques for the thoracolumbar spine. In: Donatelli RA, Wooden MI, eds. *Orthopedic Physical Therapy.* New York: Churchill Livingstone, 1994.

37. Butler DS, Jones MA. *Mobilization of the Nervous System.* Melbourne: Churchill Livingstone; 1991.

38. Butler DS. Mobilization of the nervous system. Course notes, level II. Dubuque: 1995.

39. Shacklock M. Mobilization of the nervous system. Course notes, level I. Madison: 1994.

40. Greenman PE. *Principles of Manual Medicine.* Baltimore: Williams & Wilkins; 1989.

41. Hartenburg J. Muscle energy for cervical and lumbar. Course notes. Green Bay, WI: 1992.

42. Bourdillon JF, Day EA, Bookhout MR. *Spinal Manipulation.* 5th ed. London: Butterworth Heinemann; 1994.

43. Graham KE. *Outline of Muscle Energy Techniques.* Oklahoma College of Osteopathic Medicine and Surgery; 1985.

44. Johnson G. Functional mobilization of the lower quadrant. Course notes. Milwaukee: 1996.

45. Bookhout MR. Exercises as an adjunct to manual medicine. Sept. 17-18, 1994, Eau Claire, WI.

46. Caldwell C. Diagnosis and treatment of muscle imbalances and musculoskeletal pain syndromes, level II. Course notes. Milwaukee: 1995.

47. Bandy WD, Irion JM. The effect of time on static stretch on the flexibility of the hamstring muscles. *Phys Ther.* 1994;74:845-852.

48. White AH. Stabilization of the lumbar spine. In: White AH, Anderson R, eds. *Conservative Care of Low Back Pain.* Baltimore: Williams & Wilkins; 1991.

49. Friedrich M, Cermak T, Maderbacher P. The effect of brochure use versus therapist teaching on patients performing therapeutic exercise and on changes in impairment status. *Phys Ther.* 1996;76:1082-1088.

50. Saal JA, Saal JS. Nonoperative treatment of herniated lumbar intervertebral disc with radiculopathy. *Spine.* 1989;14:4.

51. Saal JA, Saal JS. Rehabilitation of the patient. In: White AH, Anderson R, eds. *Conservative Care of Low Back Pain.* Baltimore: Williams & Wilkins; 1991.

52. Paris SV. Stabilization: Whole spine stabilization. Course notes. Institute of Physical Therapy; 1994.

53. Robison R. Low back school and stabilization: Aggressive conservative care. In: White AH, Schofferman JA, eds. *Spine Care.* St. Louis: Mosby; 1995.

54. Dynamic lumbar stabilization program. San Francisco Spine Institute. Videotape.

55. Irion JM. Use of the gym ball in rehabilitation of spinal dysfunction. *Orthop Phys Ther Clin.* 1992;1,2:10-22.

56. Hauswirth BE. Integrating function: The foam roll approach. Fall conference, Wisconsin Physical Therapy Association, Madison, October 1996.

57. Saal JA. Rehabilitation of football players with lumbar spine injury. *Phys Sports Med.* 1988;16:9.

58. Jackson C, Brown M. Analysis of current approaches and a practical guide to exercise prescription. *Clin Orthop.* 1983;179:46.

59. Jackson C, Brown M. Is there a role for exercise in the treatment of patients with low back pain? *Clin Orthop.* 1983;179:38.

60. Robison R. The new back school prescription: Stabilization training, part I. *Sine State Art Rev.* 1991;5:349.

Chapter 9

The Shoulder

Common Pathologies

Andrew J. Cosgarea and Wayne J. Sebastianelli

As humans assumed an upright posture during evolutionary development, a tremendous change took place in the functional requirements of the shoulder joint. It was no longer needed to provide propulsion and bear weight, but rather, to position the hand in space so that humans could use tools. To meet these prehensile needs, the shoulder adapted by developing the greatest range of motion of any joint in the body. This motion allowed humans to manipulate the environment, but was achieved with a concurrent loss of inherent stability.[1] Galen, a Greco-Roman physician and the acknowledged father of sports medicine, described this relationship as "antagonism between diversity of movement and safety of construction."[2]

Functional requirements of the shoulder vary with specific sports and occupations. For manual laborers and sport weight-lifters, the shoulder partially resumed a weight-bearing function. The large forces generated with lifting weights can lead to compressive failure at the acromioclavicular joint, pathologic glenohumeral joint translation, and attritional changes in the rotator cuff. Throwing sports, like baseball and football, require rapid acceleration and deceleration forces. This places supraphysiologic stresses on the soft-tissue stabilizing structures of shoulder. Although adaptive changes usually take place, failure may be manifested as instability, impingement, and rotator cuff tears. Appreciation of the shoulder's ability to respond to a great variability in functional needs requires an understanding of the anatomy, biomechanics, and common pathologic processes of the shoulder.

ANATOMY

Discussion of shoulder anatomy generally includes consideration of the glenohumeral (GH), scapulothoracic (ST), acromioclavicular (AC), and sternoclavicular (SC) joints. Twenty muscles act on the shoulder girdle.[3] Together they function through the glenohumeral joint to position the upper arm in space. There is very little intrinsic glenohumeral stability because the diameter of the humeral head is nearly twice that of the glenoid. Only a small portion of the humeral head is in contact with the glenoid fossa at any point (see Fig. 9-1). The glenoid labrum is a fibrous structure attached to the periphery of the glenoid rim that acts as a "chock block" by doubling the depth of the glenoid fossa[4] and forming a peripheral buttress. The shoulder capsule attaches to the labrum at the glenoid rim to capture the humeral head. Glenohumeral ligaments are distinct condensations of the capsule demonstrable both clinically and histologically. The superior, middle, and inferior glenohumeral ligaments are located anteriorly and inferiorly in the capsule and function to stabilize the glenohumeral joint. The inferior glenohumeral ligament (IGHL) has anterior (AIGHL) and posterior (PIGHL) components that have been likened to a hammock supporting the humeral head (see Fig. 9-2). The AIGHL is positioned anatomically to tighten as the humerus is abducted and externally rotated, making it the primary restraint to anteroinferior translation in that position.

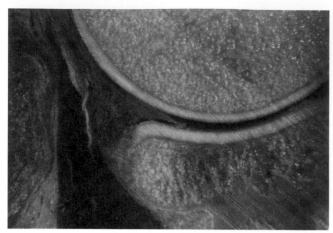

Figure 9–1. Photograph of glenohumeral anatomy. *(From Rockwood CA, Matsen FA III. The Shoulder. Philadelphia: Saunders; 1990:14. With permission.)*

The distal clavicle articulates with the acromion process of the scapula at the diarthrodial acromioclavicular joint. The AC joint is reinforced by the two coracoclavicular (CC) ligaments (see Fig. 9–3). The trapezoid and the conoid ligaments stabilize the distal clavicle to the coracoid process of the scapula. The clavicle protects the underlying neurovascular structures, serves as the attachment point for many muscles, and acts as a fulcrum separating the shoulder from the chest. The sternoclavicular (SC) joint anchors the medial clavicle to the chest wall. It consists of an incongruous articulation enveloped by a fibrous capsule with various fascial condensations. In addition to the anterior and posterior sternoclavicular and the interclavicular ligaments, the SC joint is reinforced by costoclavicular ligaments (see Fig. 9–4).

The scapula attaches to the humerus through the glenoid at the GH joint, to the clavicle at the coracoid process through the AC and CC ligaments, and to the posterior chest wall through muscular attachments. It is positioned in a plane 45 degrees to the plane of the torso and is tethered by the scapular muscles, which control its stability and motion. The four muscles of the rotator cuff arise from the scapula and attach to the tuberosities of the humerus.

BIOMECHANICS

Normal shoulder function requires a complex series of events occurring simultaneously and synchronously to exert a force over a long lever arm through a great degree of motion. At the same time, the slippery humeral head must be balanced on the relatively flat glenoid fossa. Pathologic glenohumeral motion is limited by static (bone, labrum, capsule) and dynamic (muscle)

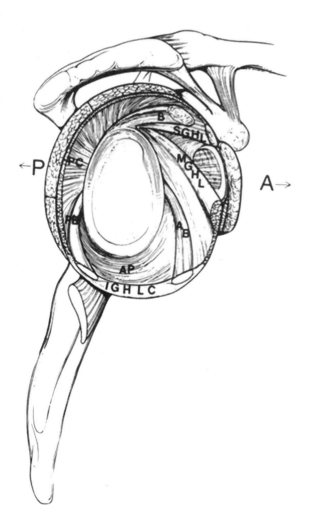

Figure 9–2. The inferior glenohumeral ligament (IGHL) hammock. *(From O'Brien SJ, Neves MC, Arnoceky SP. The anatomy and histology of the inferior glenohumeral ligament complex of the shoulder. Am J Sports Med. 1990;18:449–456. With permission.)*

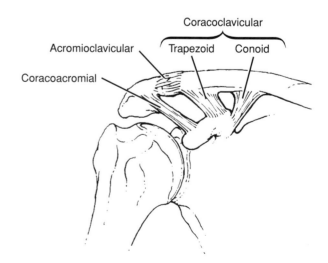

Figure 9–3. The acromioclavicular joint. *(From Jobe FW. Operative Techniques in Upper Extremity Sports Injuries. St. Louis: Mosby-Year Book; 1996:342. With permission.)*

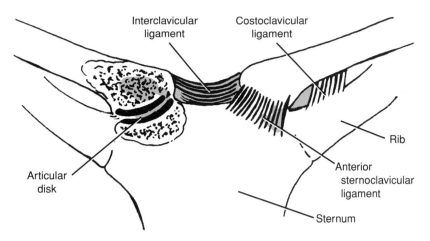

Interclavicular ligament

Costoclavicular ligament

Articular disk

Anterior sternoclavicular ligament

Rib

Sternum

Figure 9–4. The sternoclavicular joint. *(From Hollinshead WH. Functional Anatomy of the Limbs and Back. Philadelphia: Saunders; 1951:89. With permission.)*

constraints. The shoulder exhibits a great degree of flexibility coupled with very little inherent stability. The labrum deepens the glenoid somewhat, but the capsule is the primary contributor to the stability of the glenohumeral joint. The inferior glenohumeral ligament is the most important component of the capsulolabral complex. But glenohumeral ligaments can only restrict translation in the limited range where they are placed under tension. Normal passive glenohumeral translation typically approaches 1 cm in the anterior and posterior directions, and exceeds 1 cm inferiorly.[3]

Dynamic constraints help prevent pathologic glenohumeral translation despite limitations of the static constraints. These include the rotator cuff muscles, deltoid, and scapular muscles. Normal glenohumeral motion requires the synchronous activation of the deltoid and rotator cuff muscles. With shoulder abduction, the supraspinatus muscle initiates elevation, augmented by deltoid muscle function as the abduction angle increases. Infraspinatus, teres minor, and subscapularis activation functions to depress the humeral head, preventing superior migration and keeping the humeral head centered on the glenoid. The glenoid follows the humerus through scapular muscle function to minimize shear at the glenoid. Muscular control of the scapula assures that joint forces are generated so as to minimize humeral head translation and resultant glenohumeral subluxation. Spatial poisoning of the scapula and glenohumeral joints is task dependent. Shoulder abduction involves a combination of glenohumeral and scapulothoracic motion. On average, there are 2 degrees of glenohumeral elevation for every degree of scapulothoracic elevation, although the actual ratio varies during any portion of the arc.[5] The optimum position when restraining ligaments are taut and the glenohumeral joint is stable depends on the direction and magnitude of the forces generated during a given task.

Acromioclavicular stability is imparted through a thick joint capsule described collectively as the AC ligament. The medial acromial and lateral clavicular joint sur-

faces are not covered by true articular cartilage, but rather separated by meniscoid tissue. The biomechanical role of the meniscus is not well understood.[5] Relatively little motion normally occurs through the AC joint. Sequential ligament sectioning studies[6] have shown that the AC ligaments act to restrain posterior translation at both low and high degrees of displacement. Superior translation is restrained by the AC ligament at low degrees of displacement, but at larger degrees, the primary restraints to superior translation are the CC ligaments, particularly the coronoid ligament (see Fig. 9–5). The trapezoid ligament is uniquely positioned to resist axial compression of the clavicle at the AC joint. The forces can be very high, leaving the distal clavicular articular surface prone to compressive failure as seen in osteolysis.

The clavicle acts as a lateral fulcrum separating chest wall muscles from the midline. It rotates and elevates synchronously with the scapula so that with scapulothoracic translation, motion occurs through the sternoclavicular joint.[5] Ligamentous contributions to sternoclavicular stability are complex and vary depending on position and loading configuration.[7]

Smooth scapulothoracic motion requires synchronous function of the scapular muscles. The serratus anterior holds the medial scapular edge against the chest wall, while the trapezius rotates and elevates the scapula. Loss of serratus function allows the medial scapula to separate from the chest wall and leads to scapular winging. Loss of trapezius function results in painful drooping of the shoulder. In both cases, loss of muscle function interrupts the intricate balance necessary for smooth scapulohumeral rhythm.

ACROMIOCLAVICULAR INJURIES

Degenerative arthritis of the AC joint has been postulated to be age related,[8] or it may be secondary to trauma as in AC separation and intra-articular fractures. Patients with these injuries report localized or diffuse shoulder

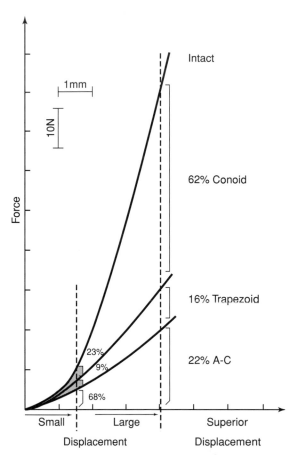

Figure 9–5. Graph of the acromioclavicular and sternoclavicular ligament contributions from Fakuda. *(From Fakuda K, Craig E, An K, et al. Biomechanical study of the ligamentous system of the acrioclavicular joint.* J Bone Joint Surg. *1986;68A:434–440. With permission.)*

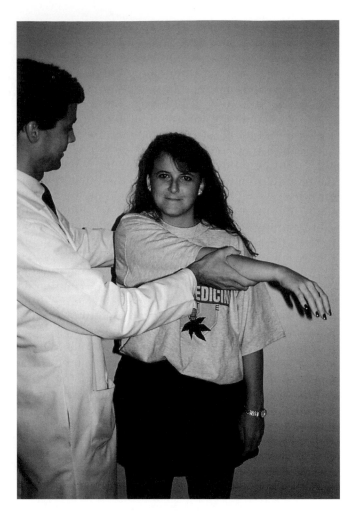

Figure 9–6. Photograph demonstrating the adduction sign.

pain. Trapezial pain secondary to muscle spasm is a common complaint. Subacromial impingement symptoms may coexist independently or secondary to AC joint osteophytes that reduce the size of the supraspinatus outlet. Patients report pain particularly with push-ups, dips, and bench presses. They are often unable to sleep on the affected side. Patients are typically point tender at the AC joint, and shoulder cross-body adduction maneuvers predictably exacerbate symptoms (see Fig. 9-6). Radiographs show joint space narrowing, sclerosis, and osteophytes on both sides of the joint (see Fig. 9-7). Because radiographically apparent AC joint arthritis may be asymptomatic, a diagnostic injection can be useful when other shoulder pathology coexists. Initial treatment consists of activity modification, nonsteroidals, and occassional corticosteroid injections. If symptoms fail to improve after prolonged conservative treatment, surgery may be indicated. Open excision of the distal clavicle (Mumford procedure) is the "gold standard."[9] Good results have also been described with arthroscopic resection.[10]

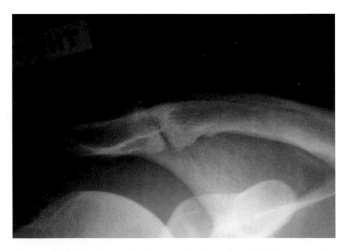

Figure 9–7. Radiograph of acromioclavicular joint degenerative changes.

In contrast to AC joint arthritis, osteolysis primarily involves the distal clavicle. It is seen most commonly in weightlifters and those with heavy lifting occupations. Distal clavicular osteolysis may follow a traumatic event, but is usually secondary to repetitive microtrauma. Pain is exacerbated by overhead lifting and adduction maneuvers. Tenderness is localized to the distal clavicle and AC joint. X-rays show osteopenia and loss of bone detail (see Fig. 9–8). The diagnosis is usually clinically apparent, but may be confirmed by diagnostic injection or bone scan.[11-13] The mainstay of conservative treatment is activity modification. Oral nonsteroidals and corticosteroid injections can be helpful. In patients who fail to respond to conservative treatment or choose not to follow activity modification recommendations, surgical excision of the distal clavicle is indicated. In contrast to the arthritic AC joint, the osteolytic distal clavicle is well suited to arthroscopic resection. The bone is soft and the joint space is not restricted by osteophytes. Arthroscopy minimizes injury to the deltoid muscle and AC ligaments,[14] decreasing recovery time. Arthroscopic resection can be performed through the subacromial space in conjunction with glenohumeral arthroscopy or as an isolated procedure, using small portals just inferior and superior to the AC joint. Isolated AC joint arthroscopic resection further minimizes surgical trauma.[10] Good results have also been reported with open techniques.[11,13]

In contrast to AC joint arthritis and distal clavicular osteolysis, AC separation occurs as a result of an acute traumatic episode. The injury is usually caused by a direct blow to the anterolateral shoulder. In the majority of significant AC separations, the distal clavicle displaces superior and posterior. Pain and deformity are immediate and depend on the degree of the ligamentous injury. AC separations are commonly classified into six types (see Fig. 9–9). Clinical evaluation involves determination of the stability of the AC joint using stress x-rays, if the extent of injury is not otherwise apparent. Grades 1 and 2 separations are treated nonoperatively, grades 4, 5, and 6 usually require surgery. Treatment of grade 3 sprains remains controversial. Good results have been reported after both surgical[15,16] and nonsurgical treatment.[17] Early repair is recommended if surgical treatment is selected.[16] If AC arthritis develops, or when the prominent distal clavicle is symptomatic, distal clavicle resection can be performed later.

ROTATOR CUFF PATHOLOGY

Rotator cuff disease involves a spectrum of pathology including tendonitis, subacromial bursitis, impingement syndrome, and partial and full-thickness tears. Overuse is an important factor in most cases. A single isolated traumatic event without preexisting pathology is unusual. Symptoms vary from minor discomfort to profound shoulder weakness and severe disabling pain.

Impingement Syndrome

The degree of cuff pathology has been shown to follow a continuum. Neer described the impingement syndrome as occurring in three stages. Stage one is characterized by subacromial edema and hemorrhage, stage two by fibrosis and tendonitis, and stage three by rotator cuff tears and bony changes.[18] The term "impingement" suggests that the rotator cuff tendons and subacromial bursal tissue are entrapped in the subacromial space between the bony acromial roof and humeral head. The coracoacromial ligament contributes to the acromial roof as it runs from the tip of the coracoid to the anterior acromion. Impingement occurs when the space available for the soft tissue decreases or the need for soft-tissue space increases.

Mechanical factors felt to predispose a person to impingement include the presence of a bony spur at the anterior edge of the acromion, AC joint osteophytes, and an elevated acromial tilt angle (see Fig. 9–10).[19] Trauma to the rotator cuff tendons (tendonitis, partial or full thickness tear) or subacromial bursa (hemorrhagic bursitis) can cause inflammation and secondary swelling of the soft tissue leading to decreased subacromial soft-tissue space. Impingement syndrome is typically seen in middle-aged patients with chronic shoulder symptoms. It may also occur secondary to glenohumeral subluxation, especially in the younger, more active population. Rotator cuff tendonitis and subacromial bursitis is common in athletes involved in repetitive shoulder sports like swimming and baseball pitching, especially in youngsters who have increased physiologic laxity.

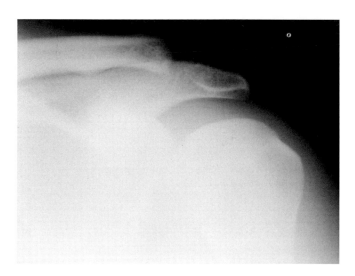

Figure 9–8. Radiograph of osteolysis of distal clavicle.

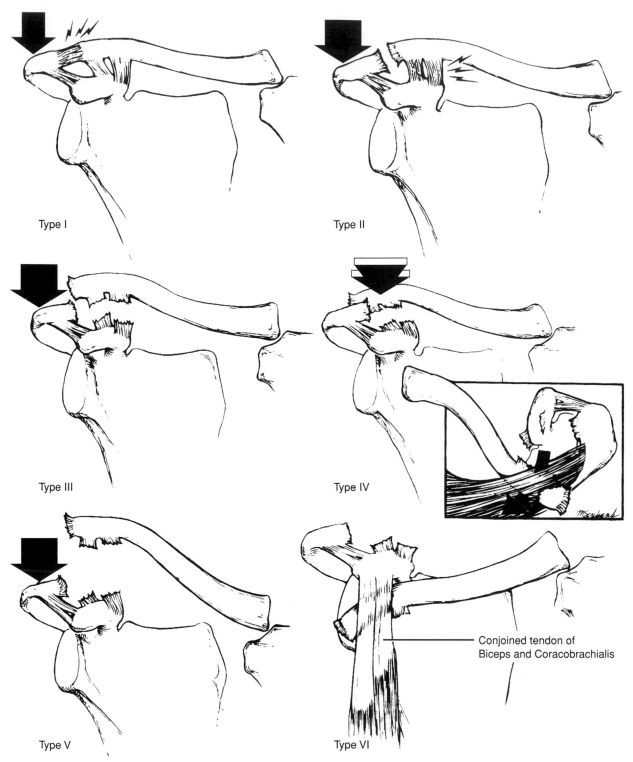

Type I

Type II

Type III

Type IV

Type V

Type VI

Conjoined tendon of
Biceps and Coracobrachialis

Figure 9–9. Diagram of acromioclavicular joint separation classifications. *(From Rockwood CA, Green DP. Fractures in Adults. 3rd ed. Philadelphia: Lippincott; 1991:1193. With permission.)*

The diagnosis of impingement syndrome can usually be determined based on history. Patients report pain with activities requiring forward elevation and internal rotation. They describe pain over the acromion or down the anterior and lateral arm to the deltoid insertion. On ex-amination, patients are found to have pain and crepitation with forward elevation and internal rotation maneuvers. Subacromial lidocaine injection (the impingement test) confirms the presence of pathology in the subacromial space. Radiographic evaluation, including the supra-

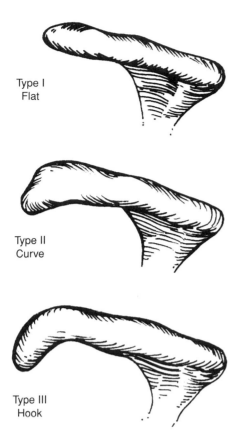

Type I
Flat

Type II
Curve

Type III
Hook

Figure 9–10. Diagram of acromial morphology classifications. *(From Rockwood CA, Lyons FR. Shoulder impingement syndrome: Diagnosis, radiographic evaluation, and treatment with a modified Neer acromioplasty. J Bone Joint Surg. 1993;75A:409–424. With permission.)*

spinatus outlet view, can be helpful in determining bony predisposition to impingement, although the diagnosis should be made on a clinical basis. Initial treatment consists of modalities to decrease inflammation, in addition to rotator cuff strengthening exercises to improve stability. Activity modification, ice, nonsteroidal anti-inflammatories, and corticosteroid injections are the mainstay of conservative treatment.

Surgical intervention is indicated only when prolonged nonoperative measures fail. The gold standard for partial acromioplasty is open resection of the anterior third of the acromion,[20] but the procedure should also address other causes of impingement including the coracoacromial ligament and any AC joint osteophytes that may be present. Similar good results have been obtained with arthroscopic techniques with the added benefit of limited surgical trauma.[21]

Rotator Cuff Tears

The reported incidence of rotator cuff tears found in cadaver dissection studies varies from about 5 to 25 per-

cent and increases with age. Partial-thickness tears are twice as common as full-thickness tears.[22] The etiology of rotator cuff tears has been debated extensively. Neer described a progression of rotator cuff disease occurring through repetitive damage to the supraspinatus as it is compressed between the acromion and humeral head.[18] Other factors felt to predispose a person to rotator cuff failure include a localized area of hypovascularity near the supraspinatus insertion and the detrimental effect of aging on biomechanical tendon properties.

Patients with cuff tears frequently report previous episodes of tendonitis or bursitis. Minor tendon fiber damage may progress with each episode. Patients may report general shoulder discomfort, as well as night pain and inability to sleep on the affected shoulder. Eventually, only a relatively minor acute injury may be necessary to cause complete failure. Although trauma is often associated with a sudden increase in symptoms, significant pre-existing pathology probably predates the acute episode, especially in the older population. Full-thickness tears in younger patients generally require significant trauma and more frequently represent isolated pathology (see Fig. 9-11). Patients with full-thickness tears typically have weakness and pain with resisted motion. Weakness may be due to tendon fiber failure or disuse atrophy.[22] When the rotator cuff fails, upward displacement of the humeral head leads to roof impingement. The long head of the biceps tendon is in the impingement region and is at risk for rupture. Chronic cuff deficiency may also lead to cuff-tear arthropathy. This arthritic condition is thought to be caused by rubbing of the superiorly displaced humeral head on the undersurface of the acromion, as well as loss of normal joint nutrition (see Fig. 9-12).

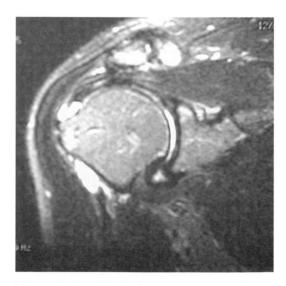

Figure 9–11. MRI of full-thickness rotator cuff tear.

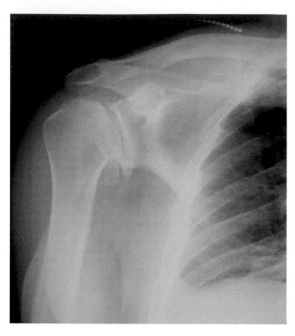

Figure 9–12. Radiograph of glenohumeral degenerative changes.

Not all patients with rotator cuff tears have profound weakness. Many patients with partial or even full-thickness tears may be minimally symptomatic. On the other hand, even partial-thickness rotator cuff tears can be symptomatic when they are associated with impingement. Because of this variable clinical picture, it is often necessary to determine the extent of cuff pathology with an arthrogram or magnetic resonance imaging (MRI). Initial treatment consists of conservative measures to modulate inflammation and decrease impingement. If conservative measures fail, arthroscopic subacromial decompression and minor debridement of a partial-thickness tear is indicated. Patients should be instructed in activity modification and cuff-strengthening exercises to protect what remains. Most patients with symptomatic full-thickness rotator cuff tears require formal surgical repair. Open repairs are generally performed in conjunction with open partial acromioplasty. Arthroscopic repair techniques have shown some promise with small tears, but long-term results are limited.

LABRAL TEARS

The importance of the anterior labrum in glenohumeral stability has long been recognized. The presence of the peripheral labrum increases the surface area of the glenoid, improves glenohumeral congruity, and serves as a capsular attachment point. The capsuloligamentous structures attach at the labrum, and local separation (Bankart lesion) is frequently seen after anterior dislocation. Labral

separation decreases the concavity of the glenoid[4] and compromises the stability of the glenohumeral joint.

The superior labrum is functionally important in serving as the anchor for the long head of the biceps on the glenoid rim.[23] Superior labrum anterior and posterior lesions (SLAP) are areas of variable superior labrum pathology (see Fig. 9–13). Damage may involve only minor fraying, or extensive detachment of the entire superior labrum and biceps insertion. Patients complain of pain, popping, and catching. On examination weakness, crepitation, and increased glenohumeral translation are frequently demonstrable.[24] The diagnosis can sometimes be confirmed with MRI, although physical examination is more accurate.[25]

Surgical treatment is reserved for patients with symptomatic labral tears who fail to respond to adequate conservative treatment. The operative procedure depends on the exact type of SLAP lesion. Debridement is generally successful with minor tears. But since occult glenohumeral instability is frequently present in patients with labral tears, formal repair with anchor fixation is often necessary.[26-28]

GLENOHUMERAL INSTABILITY

The first known depiction of a shoulder dislocation dates back to 1200 BC. Hippocrates later described different types of dislocations, reduction maneuvers, and treatment.[29] He proposed scarification of the anterior shoulder soft-tissue structures using a red hot poker in the axilla, a concept not entirely different from many modern reconstructive techniques. Shoulder instability poses a significant problem to the athlete not only due to the initial event, but particularly with chronic recurrent instability episodes.

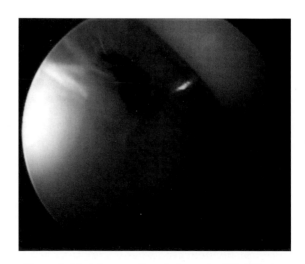

Figure 9–13. Intraoperative photograph of SLAP lesion.

ANTERIOR INSTABILITY

The shoulder is the most commonly dislocated joint in the body. The incidence of anterior dislocation was estimated at approximately 1.7 percent in a random study of the Swedish population.[30] With every dislocation episode, patients are more likely to redislocate. The youngest patients are most likely to develop chronic recurrent dislocations. The vast majority of dislocations occur as an acute traumatic injury. The classic mechanism of injury is forced shoulder abduction and external rotation. In contrast to acute traumatic dislocations, atraumatic dislocations are relatively rare. They can occur as a consequence of a minor incident such as rolling over during sleep. These patients frequently have hypermobile joints. Voluntary dislocators may or may not have associated psychological problems. Recommended treatment and overall prognosis are related to etiology. The best outcomes are seen in patients with traumatic etiologies. Surgical results are poor in voluntary dislocators, especially when a psychological component is involved.

The patient with an acute anterior dislocation presents with classic physical findings. Typically, they have moderate to severe pain and the affected arm is held at the side slightly abducted. There is a fullness appreciated in the anterior shoulder and the acromion process is prominent. Axillary nerve injuries are relatively common and usually represent neuropraxias, which resolve hours or days after shoulder reduction. Vascular injuries are less common, but may occur with major trauma or in older patients with less compliant vessels. After documenting neurovascular status and obtaining x-rays when possible, any of several different reduction techniques can be performed. Patients with recurrent instability typically have positive apprehension and relocation tests. Treatment following dislocation generally involves a short period of immobilization followed by a progressive strengthening program. High-quality therapy following injury and surgery is paramount.

Surgical reconstruction is generally reserved for individuals with recurrent dislocations who have failed conservative treatment or those in sports or occupations at high risk for recurrent dislocation. Surgical procedures are directed at correction of the actual anatomic defect. Numerous investigators have tried to identify a single lesion associated with anterior dislocations. Bankart felt that the essential lesion was the detached anterior glenoid labrum.[31] Other authors have cited capsular redundancy or rupture, rotator cuff injury, glenoid fractures, and many other causes. Most recent authors cite some combination of capsular laxity, labral pathology, and glenohumeral ligament damage.

More than 100 operations have been described to treat anterior shoulder dislocations.[29] With so much uncertainty over the exact cause of instability, it is easy to understand why there have been so many different operations advocated. Currently, open capsular shift and Bankart reconstructions are the most popular procedures performed in the United States. Redislocation rates following surgery are generally 5 percent or less. Some authors have shown good results with arthroscopic techniques, although they are technically difficult and long-term results are limited. Even with surgical reconstruction, postoperative rehabilitation is important to assure successful outcome.

Shoulder instability is defined as pathologic glenohumeral translation. "Normal" translation varies from individual to individual based on both intrinsic and environmental factors. Athletes in some sports are noted to have relatively loose shoulders. Subluxation is pathologic translation without frank dislocation. Recurrent subluxation can lead to secondary impingement, and is especially common in throwing sports. Some authors have advocated capsuloligamentous reconstruction in baseball pitchers when nonoperative treatment fails.[32,33]

POSTERIOR INSTABILITY

Dislocations are estimated to occur posteriorly approximately 2 percent of the time. They may occur from an anterior blow, a fall on a flexed and adducted arm, or from shock therapy or seizures. The clinical presentation is usually less impressive than anterior dislocations. Patients have an anterior shoulder flattening, prominence of the coracoid, and fullness posteriorly. They have limited forward elevation and external rotation. Detachment of the posterior labrum, capsular laxity, glenoid insufficiency, and increased retroversion have all been implicated as causes. The treatment of choice is physical therapy.

Most orthopedists have limited experience with surgical reconstruction for posterior instability. Posterior reconstruction is more difficult because of flimsier quality of the capsule and less familiarity with the posterior approach. A number of operations have been proposed most of which utilize the same principles as the anterior reconstructions. There is a fairly high recurrence and complication rate associated with posterior reconstruction. A voluntary component is relatively common in patients with recurrent posterior instability. Reasonable results have been reported with an open posterior capsular shift procedure when posterior capsular redundancy is corrected. Posterior subluxation is increasingly becoming recognized as a source of pain particularly in throwers and football lineman. Clinical findings are subtle and the diagnosis may be difficult. Provocative maneuvers may elicit pain and reproduce the patient's symptoms. Extensive, high-quality physical therapy is indicated before surgical reconstruction is entertained.

MULTIDIRECTIONAL INSTABILITY

Patients with multidirectional instability (MDI) experience subluxation or dislocation in more than one direction. Most have an atraumatic etiology,[34] and many have a voluntary component. Systemic ligamentous laxity is felt to play a big role and is manifested by hyperextension of the knee and elbow as well as hypermobility of the thumb and shoulder. Most patients with MDI have a primary direction in which instability episodes occur.[35] The primary complaint is often pain and not necessarily instability episodes. Patients may present with neurologic symptoms or have episodes of "dead arm syndrome." The classic clinical finding is the sulcus sign. Surgery is indicated only after failure of extensive physical therapy. The open inferior capsular shift is the most popular procedure currently.

REFERENCES

1. O'Brien SJ, Arnoczky SP, Warren RF, Rozbruck SR. Developmental anatomy of the shoulder and anatomy of the glenohumeral joint. In: Rockwood CA, Matsen FA, eds. *The Shoulder*. Philadelphia: Saunders; 1990:1–33.
2. Jobe CM. Gross anatomy of the shoulder. In: Rockwood CA, Matsen FA, eds. *The Shoulder*. Philadelphia: Saunders; 1990:1–33.
3. Simon SR, Alaranta H, An K, et al. Kinesiology. In: Simon Sr, ed. *Orthopaedic Basic Science*. Rosemont, IL: American Academy of Orthopedic Surgeons; 1994:523–535.
4. Pagnani MJ, Warren RF. Stabilizers of the glenohumeral joint. *J Shoulder Elbow Surg*. 1994;3:173–190.
5. Flatow EL. The biomechanics of the acromioclavicular, sternoclavicular, and scapulothoracic joints. *Instr Course Lect*. 1993;42:237–245.
6. Fukuda K, Craig E, An K, et al. Biomechanical study of the ligamentous system of the acromioclavicular joint. *J Bone Joint Surg*. 1986;68A:434–440.
7. Dempster WT. Mechanisms of shoulder movement. *Arch Phys Med Rehab*. 1965;46A:49–70.
8. DePalma AF. *Degenerative Changes of the Sternoclavicular and Acromioclavicular Joints in Various Decades*. Springfield, IL: Thomas; 1957.
9. Mumford EB. Acromioclavicular dislocation: A new operation. *J Bone Joint Surg*. 1941;23:799–801.
10. Flatow EL, Duralde XA, Nicholson GP, et al. Arthroscopic resection of the distal clavical with a superior approach. *J Shoulder Elbow Surg*. 1995;4:41–50.
11. Cahill BR. Osteolysis of the distal part of the clavicle in male athletes. *J Bone Joint Surg*. 1982;64A:1053–1058.
12. Scavenius M, Iversen BF. Nontraumatic clavicular osteolysis in weight lifters. *Am J Sports Med*. 1992;20:463–467.
13. Slawski DP, Cahill BR. Atraumatic osteolysis of the distal clavicle: Results of open surgical excision. *Am J Sports Med*. 1994;22:267–271.
14. Gartsman GM, Combs AH, Davis PF, Tullos HS. Arthroscopic acromioclavicular joint resection. *Am J Sports Med*. 1991;19:2–5.
15. Weaver JK, Dunn HK. Treatment of acromioclavicular injuries, especially complete acromioclavicular dislocation. *J Bone Joint Surg*. 1972;54A:1187–1194.
16. Weinstein DM, McCann PD, McIlveen SJ, et al. Surgical treatment of complete acromioclavicular dislocations. *Am J Sports Med*. 1995;23:324–331.
17. Wojtys EM, Nelson, G. Conservative treatment of grade III acromioclavicular dislocations. *Clin Orthop*. 1991;268:112–119.
18. Neer CS. Impingement lesions. *Clin Orthop*. 1983;173:70–77.
19. Rockwood CA, Lyons FR. Shoulder impingement syndrome: Diagnosis, radiographic evaluation, and treatment with a modified Neer acromioplasty. *J Bone Joint Surg*. 1993;75A:409–424.
20. Neer CS. Anterior acromioplasty for the chronic impingement syndrome in the shoulder. A preliminary report. *J Bone Joint Surg*. 1972;54A:41–50.
21. Altchek DW, Warren RF, Wickiewicz TL, et al. Arthroscopic acromioplasty: Technique and results. *J Bone Joint Surg*. 1990;72A:1198–1207.
22. Matsen FA, Arntz CT. Rotator cuff tendon failure. In: Rockwood CA, Matsen FA, eds. *The Shoulder*. Philadelphia: Saunders; 1990:647–677.
23. Snyder SJ, Banas MP, Karzel RP. An analysis of 140 injuries to the superior glenoid labrum. *J Shoulder Elbow Surg*. 1995;4:243–248.
24. Terry GC, Friedman SJ, Uhl TL. Arthroscopically treated tears of the glenoid labrum: Factors influencing outcome. *Am J Sports Med*. 1994;22:504–512.
25. Lui SH, Henry MH, Nuccion S, et al. Diagnosis of glenoid labral tears: A comparison between magnetic resonance imaging and clinical examination. *Am J Sports Med*. 1996;24:149–154.
26. Banas MP, Miller RJ, Totterman S. Relationship between the lateral acromion angle and rotator cuff disease. *J Shoulder Elbow Surg*. 1995;4:454–461.
27. Bigliani LU, Ticker JB, Flatow EL, et al. The relationship of acromial architecture to rotator cuff disease. *Clin Sports Med*. 1991;10:823–838.
28. Gartsman GM. Arthroscopic acromioplasty for lesions of the rotator cuff. *J Bone Joint Surg*. 1990;72A:169–180.
29. Matsen FA, Thomas SC, Rockwood CA. Glenohumeral instability. In: Rockwood CA, Matsen FA, eds. *The Shoulder*. Philadelphia: Saunders; 1990:526–622.
30. Hovelius L. Incidence of shoulder dislocation in Sweden. *Clin Orthop*. 1982;166:127–131.
31. Bankart AS. The pathology and treatment of recurrent dislocation of the shoulder joint. *Br J Surg*. 1939;26:23–29.
32. Jobe FW, Giangarra CE, Kvitne RS, Glousman RE. Anterior capsulolabral reconstruction of the shoulder in athletes in overhand sports. *Am J Sports Med*. 1991;19:428–434.
33. Rubenstein DL, Jobe FW, Glousman RE, et al. Anterior capsulolabral reconstruction of the shoulder in athletes. *J Shoulder Elbow Surg*. 1992;1:229–237.
34. Altcheck DW, Warren RF, Skyhar MJ, Ortiz G. T-plasty modification of the bankart procedure for multidirectional instability of the anterior and inferior types. *J Bone Joint Surg*. 1991;73A:105–112.
35. Mallon WJ, Speer KP. Multidirectional instability: Current concepts. *J Shoulder Elbow Surg*. 1995;4:54–64.

Treatment and Rehabilitation for Rotator Cuff Tendinitis, Bicipital Tendinitis, and Acromioclavicular Sprains

Paul K. Canavan

ROTATOR CUFF TENDINITIS

There is little written about treatment and rehabilitation of tendinitis in general. Choice and progression of treatment is dependent on many factors, primarily whether it is an acute tendinitis or a chronic tendinitis. Chronic tendinitis may be related to instability (see Fig. 9-14). The next section of this chapter discusses shoulder instability. Other factors that should be taken into account while developing an individualized plan of rehabilitation are patient goals, prior activity level, age, past and present medical conditions, present cardiovascular fitness level, prior experience with conditioning, present strength level, range of motion, and access to equipment.

Before treating and development of a plan, one should know what is "normal" for muscle activity with functional-type activities.[1] Also, knowledge of what happens to muscle activity for the people who have rotator cuff tendinitis is important. In the presence of supraspinatus tendinitis, it has been shown that there is decreased activity of the middle deltoid at the angle of 45 degrees of abduction. This may happen to avoid impinging the supraspinatus tendon.[2] Swimmers with painful shoulders have been shown to have no difference in activity level of the supraspinatus compared to their nonpainful shoulder. There was decreased activity of the anterior and middle deltoid at the point of hand entry into the water.[3] Scapular stabilizing muscles, the serratus anterior and rhomboids, play an important role in the proper force couple and correct arthrokinematics with upper extremity movements.

When an athlete first develops tendinitis in the shoulder, resting the involved upper extremity for 3 days is essential to prevent a chronic condition. Primary treatment includes rest, anti-inflammatory medication, ice, and avoidance of above-the-head activities and heavy lifting for 5 to 7 days. After approximately 5 days, based upon each individual's unique situation, light isometrics and rhythmic stabilization exercises should be performed. The next section of this chapter has a thorough criteria-based progression for rehabilitation. Knowledge of how muscles work during rehabilitation is also necessary.[4] Modalities and manual techniques are also used in the treatment of rotator cuff tendinitis.[5,6]

Development of a Plan and Prevention

One or many factors can be involved in rotator cuff tendinitis, including poor technique; muscular fatigue; muscular imbalance; shoulder range-of-motion limitations; lack of flexibility in the hip flexors, gastrocnemius, soleus, or low back; improper practice regimens; cervical and scapular tightness; decreased proprioceptive ability; glenohumeral instability; general fatigue; and (possibly) vibration. Significant exposure to vibration combined with a traction-type movement may play a role in development of some shoulder problems. This may be found in athletes who play tennis who have the tension of the string changed and perform repeated strokes or a baseball player who hits batting practice everyday with an aluminum bat. Vibration has previously been shown to be associated with shoulder pain.[7] A change in the grip size and type may also play a role.

Decreased proprioception may also play a role in instability and shoulder pain.[8] When proprioceptive ability is lacking then vision of the limb partially substitutes for the deficiency.[9] Therefore, in rehabilitation some exercises should be done with the eyes closed. Muscular fatigue also has been shown to diminish proprioceptive ability.[10] Directional errors may be a result of errors in the planning process.[11] This internal (planned) model may be updated using proprioceptive information.[9]

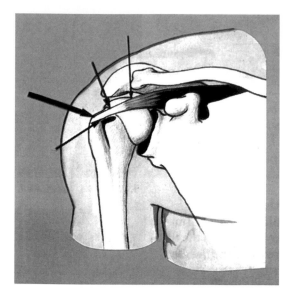

Figure 9–14. Rotator cuff tendinitis. *(From Cyriax JH, Cyriax PJ. Illustrated Manual of Orthopaedic Medicine. London: OM Publications; 1983. With permission.)*

Proprioception and kinesthetic awareness is a complex subject and is continuing to be researched. Use of electromyography (EMG), biofeedback, visual feedback (mirror), and use of patterned electrical muscular stimulation[12] may help reestablish normal arthrokinematics with individuals who have abnormal kinematics.

After identifying the possible causes, one needs to address each weakness and create an individualized rehabilitation program to fit the injured athlete. This will allow that particular athlete to progress in the most efficient manner to return him or her back to competition. The importance of prevention cannot be overemphasized.

BICIPITAL TENDINITIS

Bicipital tendinitis may be related to shoulder laxity and instability (see Fig. 9-15). Tendinitis at the proximal end of the biceps may be related to traction overload tendinitis.[13] The biceps' long head acts as a humeral stabilizer as well as a decelerator of elbow extension. When there is increased translation of the humeral head with activities, more stress is placed on the biceps and ligamentous structures.

Activities that include repeated shoulder abduction with external rotation, such as throwing, may result in impingement of the biceps tendon in the bicipital groove beneath the acromion.[14] Some possible causes of discomfort that have been observed with ultrasound include synovitis or effusion of the bicipital groove, mineralization of the transverse ligament, subluxating biceps tendon, and cysts of the tendon.[15]

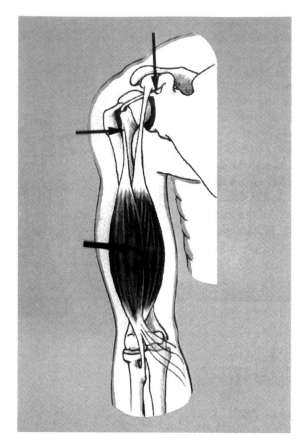

Figure 9–15. Bicipital tendinitis. *(From Cyriax JH, Cyriax PJ. Illustrated Manual of Orthopaedic Medicine. London: OM Publications; 1983. With permission.)*

Primary treatment should include ice, rest, and anti-inflammatory medication. Rest of approximately 7 days may be needed followed by gradual progression back to activity. Exercise including shoulder elevation with the forearm in supination and elbow curls with the shoulder elevated with emphasis on the eccentric phase of the exercise should be utilized. In chronic cases, steroid injections and therapeutic modalities have also been used. Surgical intervention may be needed as biceps tendinitis may be the secondary problem.

ACROMIOCLAVICULAR SPRAINS

Injuries to the acromioclavicular (AC) joint are common in sports, especially when there are increased possibilities of falling onto the ground (football) or slamming into the boards (ice hockey). Literature strongly favors the conservative approach in treating AC joint injuries. The treatment protocols in Table 9-1 have time frames attached to them; however, each individual's progression should be based on pain, successful completion of exercises, and tissue healing time. It is best to be conservative in treating individuals with AC joint injuries, as progress-

TABLE 9–1. ACROMIOCLAVICULAR JOINT REHABILITATION PROTOCOL

Type I

Days 1 to 4	Sling use, as needed per patient's complaints of pain and discomfort. Ice, anti-inflammatory medication, light pendulum exercises as tolerated. Use of home electrical stimulation unit. Passive range-of-motion exercise (PROM).
Days 3 to 7	Initiation of active range-of-motion exercises (AROM), as tolerated. Aerobic conditioning as tolerated, avoiding irritation to the shoulder joint. Initiation of light isometric exercises.
Days 6 to 12	Addition of concentric strengthening exercises with no greater than 5 pounds. Avoid shoulder horizontal adduction and full-range shoulder elevation exercises.
Days 10 to 14	Greater addition of light progressive resistive exercises (PREs). Return to activities such as jogging and sport-type activities, avoiding contact with other players or the ground. Full AROM and light PREs as tolerated.
After day 14	Gradual return to full functional activities as tolerated, avoiding direct contact and tumbling for 1 more week.

Type II

Weeks 2 to 5	Use of sling and/or immobolizer as tolerated. Avoiding sleeping on the involved side.
Days 5 to 8	Initiation of PROM exercise in supine as tolerated. Light standing pendulum exercise. Continue use of ice, medication, home electrical stimulation unit.
Days 7 to 14	Initiation of light isometrics in all directions. Initiation of active assistive range-of-motion exercises (AAROM) with bilateral arms and use of therapeutic cane in supine. Pulley exercise as tolerated.
Weeks 2 to 3	Progression from AAROM to AROM with bilateral to single upper extremity in supine to initiation of AAROM in sitting with bilateral upper extremities with use of cane.
Weeks 3 to 5	Gradual transition to AROM in sitting. Addition of light concentric exercises avoiding horizontal adduction and full active elevation. Addition of light manual resistance, as tolerated.
Weeks 5 to 8	Gradual progression with resistance exercises. Use of upper extremity ergometer. Initiation of jogging, running, and gradual progression to sport-type activities. Avoiding quick forceful shoulder movements and contact activities.
Weeks 7 to 9	Gradual progression to activities, as tolerated.

Type III
Use Type II protocol, delaying by 2 weeks or greater after the weeks 2 to 3 phase.

---

ing an athlete back to competition too soon could lead to chronic shoulder pain in the future. AC sprains were discussed in the previous section. Table 9–1 gives a baseline on how to progress; many other treatments and exercises can be performed.

REFERENCES

1. Moynes DR, Perry J, Antonelli DJ, Jobe FW. Electromyography and motion analysis of the upper extremity in sports. *Phys Ther.* 1986;66:1905-1911.

2. Michaud M, Arsenault AB, Gravel D, Tremblay G, Simard TG. Muscular compensatory mechanism in presence of a tendinitis of the supraspinatus. *Am J Phys Med.* 1987;66:109-121.

3. Scovazzo ML, Browne A, Pink M, Jobe FW, Kerrigan J. The painful shoulder during freestyle swimming. *Am J Sports Med.* 1991;19:577-582.

4. Townsend H, Jobe FW, Pink M, Perry J. Electromyographic analysis of the glenohumeral muscles during a baseball rehabilitation program. *Am J Sports Med.* 1991;19:264-272.

5. Gieck JH, Saliba E. Therapeutic ultrasound: Influence on inflammation and healing. In: Leadbetter WB, Buckwalter JA, Gordon SL, eds. *Sports-induced Inflammation.* Park Ridge, IL: American Academy of Orthopedic Surgeons; 1990:479-492.

6. Knight KL. Cold as a modifier of sports-induced inflammation. In: Leadbetter WB, Buckwalter JA, Gordon SL, eds. *Sports-induced Inflammation.* Park Ridge, IL: American Academy of Orthopedic Surgeons; 1990:463-475.

7. Stenlund B, Goldic I, Hagberg M, Hagstedt C. Shoulder tendinitis and its relation to heavy manual work and exposure to vibration. *Scand J Work Envin Health.* 1993;19:43-49.

8. Warner JJ, Lephart S, Fu FH. Role of proprioception in pathoetiology of shoulder instability. *Clin Orthop.* 1996; 330:35-39.

9. Ghez C, Sainburg R. Proprioceptive control of interjoint coordination. *Can J Phys Pharm.* 1995;73:273-284.

10. Voight ML, Hardin JA, Blackburn TA, Tippett S, Canner CG. The effects of muscle fatigue on and the relationship of arm dominance to shoulder proprioception. *J Orthop Sports Phys Ther.* 1996;23:348-352.

11. Gordon J, Ghilardi MF, Ghez C. Accuracy of planar reaching movements, Independence of direction and extent variability. *Exp Brain Res.* 1994;99:97-111.

12. Palermo FX. Patterned electric stimulation vs. shoulder pain in chronic and acute hemiplegia. *Abs Neurol.* April 1987.

13. Wolf WB. Shoulder tendinoses. *Clin Sports Med.* 1992; 11:871-890.

14. Hunter SC, Poole RM. The chronically inflamed tendon. *Clin Sports Med.* 1987;6:371-388.

15. Wurnig C. Sonography of the biceps tendon (German). *Z Orthop Ihre Grenzgeb.* 1996;134:161-165.

SELECTED READING

Becker DA, Cofield RH. Tenodesis of the long head of the biceps brachii for chronic bicipital tendinitis. Long term results. *J Bone Joint Surg.* 1989;71:376–381.

Clancy WG. Tendon trauma and overuse injuries. In: Leadbetter WB, Buckwalter JA, Gordon SL, eds. *Sports-induced Inflammation.* Park Ridge, IL: American Academy of Orthopedic Surgeons; 1990:609–618.

Clancy WG, Hagan SV. Tendinitis in golf. *Clin Sports Med.* 1996;15:27–34.

Dias JJ, Gregg PJ. Acromioclavicular joint injuries in sport. Recommendations for treatment. *Sports Med.* 1991; 11:125–132.

Erickson SJ, Fitzgerald SW, Quinn SF, et al. Long bicipital tendon of the shoulder: Normal anatomy and pathological findings on MR imaging. *Am J Roentg.* 1992;158: 1091–1096.

Fisk J, Lackner JR, DiZio P. Gravitoinertial force level influences arm movement control. *J Neurophys.* 1993;69:504–511.

Fye I, Stanish WD. The use of eccentric training and stretching in the treatment and prevention of tendon injuries. *Clin Sports Med.* 1992;11:601–623.

Gartner J. Tendinosis calcarea: Results with needling (German). *Z Orthop Ihre Grenzgeb.* 1993;131:470–473.

Griffin JE, Echrenach JL, Price RE, Touchstone JC. Patients treated with ultrasonic driven hydrocortisone and with ultrasound alone. *Phys Ther.* 1967;47:594–601.

Kibler WB, Chandler TJ, Pace BK. Principles of rehabilitation after chronic tendon injuries. *Clin Sports Med.* 1992; 11:661–671.

Loew M, Jurgowski W. Initial experiences with extracorporeal shockwave lithotripsy (ESWL) in treatment of tendinosis calcarea of the shoulder (German). *Z Orthop Ihre Grenzgeb.* 1993;131:470–473.

Sainburg RL, Poizner H, Ghez C. Loss of proprioception produces deficits in interjoint coordination. *J Neurophys.* 1993;70:2136–2147.

Wojtys EM, Neslson G. Conservative treatment of grade III acromioclavicular dislocations. *Clin Orthop.* 1991;268: 112–119.

Rehabilitation of Rotator Cuff Dysfunction and Glenohumeral Instability

Turner A. "Tab" Blackburn, Jr. and J. Allen Hardin

SHOULDER IMPINGEMENT SYNDROME

Shoulder impingement syndrome, first described by Charles Neer in 1972, is characterized as a continuum beginning with an inflammatory process, progressing to fibrosis, and ending in rotator cuff rupture. Impingement was defined by Matsen and Arntz as the encroachment of the acromion, coracoacromial ligament, coracoid process, or the acromioclavicular joint on the underlying rotator cuff mechanism as the glenohumeral joint is moved. The structures that become compromised during mechanical impingement include the supraspinatus tendon, the long head of the biceps tendon, the subacromial bursa, and less frequently, the infraspinatus tendon. Neer categorized impingement lesions into three progressive stages. In stage 1, reversible edema and hemorrhage are present in patients typically under 25 years of age. Stage 2 consists of fibrosis and tendinitis affecting the rotator cuff of patients ages 25 to 40. Stage 3 includes resultant bone spurs and tendon ruptures in individuals typically over the age of 40.

Etiologic Classification

Etiologic factors have been similarly categorized, described as either extrinsic or intrinsic, primary or secondary, or perhaps most appropriately, as either structural or functional. Extrinsic causes occur from an outside structure causing repetitive mechanical impingement on the rotator cuff tendons. These may be primary, such as those associated with alterations on the undersurface of the acromion and variations in the shape of the acromion, or secondary, such as those resulting from glenohumeral instability and scapulothoracic instability. Primary impingement is the mechanical obstruction of the rotator cuff tendons under the coracoacromial arch. Secondary impingement is the relative decrease in subacromial space due to another pathology or condition. Intrinsic causes are commonly degenerative in nature, often associated with inflammatory changes within the rotator cuff from overstress impingement of the tendons and diminished blood supply. Yet another classification of mechanisms of shoulder impingement syndrome differentiates between structural and functional etiologic factors. Structural factors such as congenital abnormalities or degenerative changes in the subacronial arch can occur. Functional causes include abnormal scapular position or motion, glenohumeral capsular hyper- or hypomobility, cervical spine dysfunction, or postural deviations. Structural and functional etiologic factors are outlined in Table 9-2.

Some of the effects of impingement may further intensify the impingement syndrome, creating a self-perpetuating process. Hence, Keirns stated that shoulder impingement syndrome "is a continuum that can begin anywhere in the sequence and can formulate a vicious succession." Figure 9-16 details the impingement cycle facilitated by this process, as described by Keirns.

Understanding the etiology of the impingement is requisite to its successful treatment. As with any pathologic condition, determining and treating the cause, not just the symptoms, is fundamental for appropriate rehabilitation. Distinguishing whether the mechanical impingement is of structural or functional origin is essential. The diagnosis of impingement without investigation of the causal relationship is incomplete, for without this, an appropriate rehabilitation plan cannot be established. For example, if a diagnosis of impingement syndrome secondary to hypermobility is made, treatment should focus on the primary diagnosis of glenohumeral instability.

Mechanism of Injury

Impingement syndrome of the shoulder is most often the result of the cumulative effect of multiple passages of the rotator cuff tendons beneath the coracoacromial arch. The relative size of the subacromial space is frequently a precursor to the process. Reduction in available space

TABLE 9–2. FACTORS POTENTIALLY INCREASING ROTATOR CUFF IMPINGEMENT

Structural

Acromioclavicular Joint
  Congenital abnormality
  Degenerative spurs

Acromion
  Unfused (bipartite acromion)
  Abnormal shape (flat or overhanging)
  Degenerative spur
  Nonunion of fracture
  Malunion of fracture

Coracoid
  Congenital abnormality
  Posttraumatic or postsurgical change in shape or location

Bursa
  Primary inflammatory bursitis (e.g., rheumatoid arthritis)
  Chronic thickening from previous injury/inflammation/injection
  Pins, wires, sutures, and other foreign materials projecting into the bursal space

Rotator Cuff
  Thickening related to chronic calcium deposits
  Thickening from retraction of partial-thickness tears
  Flaps and other irregularities of upper surface due to partial or complete tearing
  Postoperative or posttraumatic scarring

Humerus
  Congenital abnormalities or fracture malunions producing relative or absolute prominence of the greater tuberosity
  Abnormally inferior position of a humeral head prosthesis producing relative prominence of the greater tuberosity

Functional

Scapula
  Abnormal position
    Thoracic kyphosis
    Acromioclavicular separation
  Abnormal motion
    Paralysis (e.g., of trapezius)
    Fascioscapulohumeral muscular dystrophy
    Restriction of motion at the scapulothoracic joint
  Loss of normal head depression mechanism
    Rotator cuff weakness (e.g., suprascapular nerve palsy or C5 or C6 radiculopathy)
    Rotator cuff tear (partial or full-thickness)
    Constitutional or posttraumatic rotator cuff laxity
    Rupture of long head of biceps
  Tightness of posterior shoulder capsule forcing the humeral head to rise up against the acromion during shoulder flexion
  Capsular laxity

From Rockwell CA Jr, Matsen FA III, eds. The Shoulder. *Philadelphia: Saunders; 1990. With permission.*

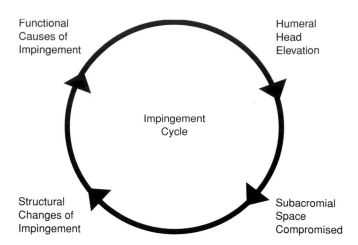

Figure 9–16. Impingement cycle. *(From Kevins MA. Conservative management of shoulder impingement. In: Andrews JR, Wilk KE, eds.* The Athlete's Shoulder. *New York: Churchill Livingstone; 1994:608. With permission.)*

beneath the acromion, whether due to congenital abnormalities or degenerative changes, increases the likelihood that resultant damage to the rotator cuff tendons will occur. Usually, shoulder impingement effectuated by congenital factors is but a precursor to degenerative changes of the underlying structures. For example, impingement caused by a "hooked" acromion may lead to scarring of the rotator cuff tendons, and ultimately a pronounced decrease in subacromial space.

Glenohumeral hypermobility, whether developed from disruption of the static stabilizers (ligament, labrum, capsule) or fatigue or weakness of the dynamic stabilizers (muscle), may provide predisposition to secondary impingement via excessive humeral head excursion. Even subtle instabilities may allow enough superior humeral head translation to initiate the impingement process. Clinical overlap between impingement syndrome and anterior shoulder instability, as well as a relative weakness of the internal rotators of the shoulder, is often seen. Glenohumeral hypomobility, most commonly posterior glenohumeral capsule stiffness, may also lead to shoulder impingement. Stiffness in the posterior capsule may aggravate the impingement process by forcing the humeral head upward against the anteroinferior acromion as the shoulder is flexed. Posterior capsule tightness is most often associated with a relative weakness of the external rotators of the shoulder.

Abnormal scapular position and motion leading to poor scapular stabilization may cause secondary impingement by diminishing scapula humeral rhythm and hindering the correct relationship of the acromion and the humeral head at the subacromial opening. Factors such as a postural dysfunction or nerve root entrapment for the scapula stabilizers may influence the function of the scapula.

The rotator cuff mechanism provides normal humeral head depression coupled with arm elevation. Rotator cuff weakness from disuse, cervical radiculopathy, suprascapular neuropathy, or cuff fiber failure will weaken the humeral head depressor mechanism, thereby rendering the rotator cuff incapable of stabilizing the shoulder against the actions of the deltoid and pectoralis major muscles. Contraction of the deltoid, in the presence of a weakened rotator cuff mechanism, causes superior displacement of the humeral head and ultimately, entrapment of the rotator cuff beneath the coracoacromial arch.

Clinical Presentation

Patients with shoulder impingement syndrome most often do not present to a physician with an acute shoulder impingement. Patients typically present after their shoulder symptoms have failed to subside with self-prescribed time, rest, or exercise. The patient's chief complaints are usually pain, stiffness, weakness, and often, "catching" when the arm is used in a flexed and internally rotated position. Associated symptoms may include difficulties sleeping, particularly on the affected side, performance of routine activities of daily living (ADLs), and overhead activity. Pain is often felt down the lateral aspect of the arm near the deltoid insertion, over the antero-proximal humerus, or in the periacromial region.

Physical examination and inspection of the shoulder may reveal atrophy of the deltoid or rotator cuff muscles, particularly if the condition has been chronic. Little to no point tenderness to palpation may be revealed. Range-of-motion (ROM) deficits are noted, most frequently limited in internal rotation and cross-body horizontal adduction, indicating posterior capsule tightness. A painful arc, noted by pain and crepitus, is found between the 60 and 90-degree arc of both passive and active flexion and is typically reported as more painful when elicited actively. Pain is usually noted with maximum forward flexion, as well. Muscle weakness may be noted in flexion, external rotation, and less frequently, internal rotation, as a result of disuse or tendon damage. Compromised integrity of the rotator cuff tendons may be indicated by pain or resisted abduction, flexion, external rotation, and again, less frequently, internal rotation.

Differential diagnosis is imperative in distinguishing among the signs of subacromial impingement (subacromial crepitus on flexion and rotation), signs of tightness (limited ROM), and signs of tendon involvement (atrophy, weakness, and pain on resisted motion).

The clinical presentation of the impingement syndrome may be altered by the presence of any associated conditions, such as cervical radiculopathy, acromioclavicular joint arthritis, partial and full-thickness rotator cuff tears, and acute or chronic adhesive capsulitis.

Conservative Management

Conservative nonoperative treatment of shoulder impingement syndrome has proven to be very effective and is considered the treatment of choice. Nonoperative treatment programs typically consist of rest, non-steroidal anti-inflammatory medications, and general shoulder rehabilitation. Nevaiser and co-workers recommend a conservative program consisting of moist heat, anti-inflammatory medication, restricted exercise, and avoidance of the overhead position. Matsen and Arntz advocate stretching, strengthening, and technique or job modification for management of the patient with impingement syndrome. Numerous comprehensive rehabilitation programs have been described in the recent past for conservative management of throwers and other overhead athletes with shoulder impingement syndrome. In accordance with Keirns, it appears that the common denominator in these programs is "allowing adequate rest and promoting rotator cuff strengthening." Hence, the goal of conservative management of shoulder impingement syndrome is selective strengthening of those muscles that are weak, with associated posterior capsule stretching, to reestablish the normal arthrokinematics of the humeral head depressor mechanism and subsequently, restore normal glenohumeral scapulothoracic function. The program should be a scientifically backed, physiologically based, comprehensive approach that consists of criteria, rather than time-based objectives to determine progression, and should include activity modification. The rehabilitation program proposed in this chapter consists of four stages or phases through which the patient must pass before completion. Adherance to the guidelines set forth in these phases will ensure thorough, systematic reevaluations, that the patient is progressed based on criteria, not time, and ultimately will guarantee the individuality of the program. Each phase has goals that are established and criteria that must be achieved before proceeding to the next phase. As advocated by Keirns, the primary focus of the program must be on "facilitating subacromial tissue healing and diminishing humeral head elevation." Although many programs include intensive modality prescription, exercise is the mainstay of nonoperative conservative management of shoulder impingement and should be the cornerstone of all rehabilitation programs.

Phase I: Acute Inflammatory Phase

During the initial acute inflammatory phase, an inflammatory process exists within the shoulder creating a stiff, painful shoulder. Impaired tissue healing is present due to bleeding into the tissue as a result of increased capillary pressure on the damaged tissue. The primary goal of this phase is to ease the patient's discomfort while maintaining or restoring range of motion. Maintaining joint mobility by addressing posterior capsule tightness is tantamount. Other goals include preventing muscular atrophy, as well as patient education on activity modification. It should be underscored during this phase that the inflammatory process must be arrested, therefore the impingement symptoms must not be exacerbated.

Easing Discomfort/Reducing Symptoms. Symptom reduction is synonymous with halting the acute inflammatory process. Proven adjuncts to achieving this are the initiation of nonsteroidal anti-inflammatories, rest, and therapeutic modalities. Accompanying the retardation of inflammation is an associated reduction in swelling, and undoubtedly a decrease in symptoms and discomfort. The modalities of choice in the management of acute inflammation are cryotherapy and low-frequency transcutaneous electrical nerve stimulation (TENS) application. Iontophoresis, phonophorcsis, and therapeutic ultrasound may be utilized in this stage to aid in inflammation reduction, but appear to have little effect on the natural history of rotator cuff problems, and would not ordinarily be used.

Physiologically, cryotherapy hinders the inflammatory process by acting as a vasoconstrictor and slowing metabolic activity. Cold application also eases discomfort by inducing analgesia and by elevating the pain threshold. Low-frequency TENS alleviates pain by increasing microcirculation and facilitating the absorption of calcific deposits in contractile tissue. Clinically, cryotherapy in conjunction with TENS reduccs the patient's symptoms and eases the discomfort associated with acute shoulder impingement.

Maintaining Joint Mobility. Inflammation associated with acute shoulder impingement may act as a precursor to increased scar tissue formation and subsequent joint capsule immobility. This, in conjunction with likely preexisting posterior capsule tightness, can significantly decrease glenohumeral capsular mobility and seriously alter arthrokinematics. Therefore, in the initial phases of rehabilitation, it is essential to restore and maintain normal joint mobility in the glenohumeral and associated joints, including the scapulothoracic, acromioclavicular, and sternoclavicular joints.

Glenohumeral joint mobility restoration and maintenance is critical to successful management of shoulder impingement. Mobilization of the glenohumeral joint should consist of grades I and II inferior and posterior glides to restore adequate capsular mobility, and thus normal arthrokinematics of the humeral head depressor mechanism (see Fig. 9–17).

Maintaining adequate scapulothoracic, acromioclavicular, and sternoclavicular joint mobility is equally as important as maintaining glenohumeral joint mobility, and often overlooked. A skilled manual therapist can

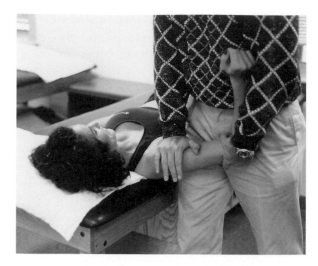

Figure 9–17. Posterior glenohumeral joint mobilization.

evaluate shoulder girdle arthrokinematics and appropriately treat any deficit through proper joint mobilization. Restoring and maintaining associated joint mobility must be performed without facilitating the inflammatory process.

In conjunction with joint mobilization, active assisted range-of-motion exercises should be initiated to increase and maintain shoulder range of motion and soft tissue flexibility. Activities to promote this include the pendulum activity, the rope and pulley exercise, and the wand exercises. The pendulum activity is performed standing in a bent over position, allowing the involved arm to hang freely from the body (see Fig. 9–18). Body movement in all planes causes the arm to swing freely, producing a sense of decreased apprehension while facilitating range of motion. The rope and pulley exercise is designed to facilitate active assisted shoulder flexion

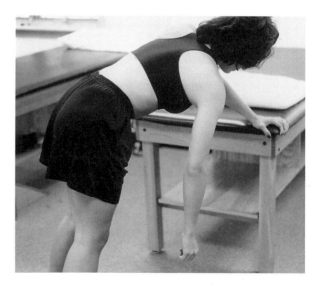

Figure 9–18. Pendulum exercise.

by using the contralateral extremity, and should be performed with the palm supinated and the humerus externally rotated, allowing the greater tuberosity to glide laterally off the anterior acromion, thereby lessening the chance of subacromial impingement (see Fig. 9–19). Additionally, the rope and pulley exercise creates gravity-assisted humeral head depression while the arm is elevated and is therefore an excellent maneuver. The wand exercises provide a method of increasing shoulder external rotation and yet another method of increasing shoulder flexion. The wand exercise for external rotation should be performed with the shoulder in the plane of the scapula and the arm in less than 90 degrees of abduction (see Fig. 9–20). Flexion with the wand should be performed with the arm maximally externally rotated and supinated, using the uninvolved extremity for assistance (see Fig. 9–21). During all active assisted range-of-motion exercises, it is critical to avoid any discomfort associated with the movement.

Preventing Muscular Atrophy. Shoulder musculature atrophy associated with injury should be prevented during the initial phase of rehabilitation as well. Emphasis should be placed on the rotator cuff muscles and the

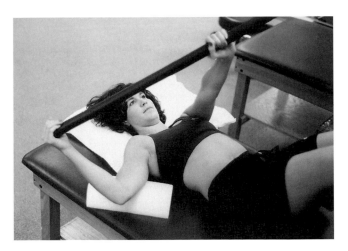

Figure 9–20. Active assisted external rotation with wand.

scapular stabilizer muscles. Submaximal shoulder isometric exercises should be utilized to preserve rotator cuff strength and endurance. Active postural exercises and active scapula muscle exercises may be beneficial in retarding atrophy associated with the scapular stabilizers. These include active scapular elevation, retraction, and "shoulder circles," but not the more advanced core scapular exercises described by Moseley and associates due to the advanced nature of such exercises. These will be incorporated in later rehabilitation phases. Active use of the arm below 90 degrees abduction and flexion in a pain-free motion during activities of daily living is also advocated to minimize muscular atrophy.

Patient Education. Patient education is likely the most important goal in rehabilitation of any pathology. Patient education consists of instruction on the pathogenesis of the injury, description of the rehabilitation program and its goals, and outlining the activities that are considered "dos and don'ts." Patient education should promote patient compliance and ensure a more timely recovery.

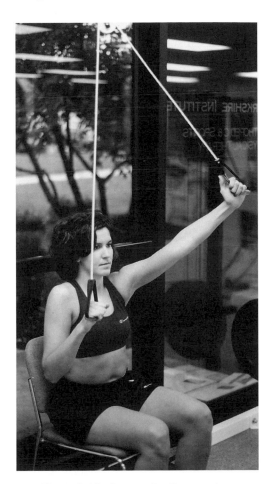

Figure 9–19. Rope and pulley exercise.

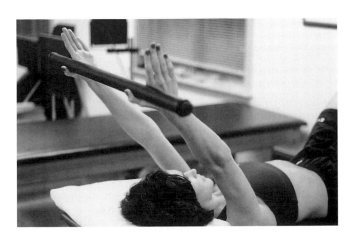

Figure 9–21. Active assisted flexion with wand.

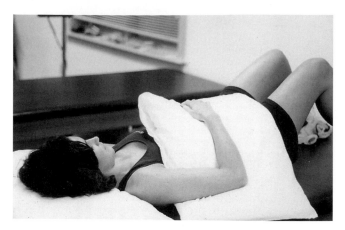

Figure 9–22. Recommended sleeping position.

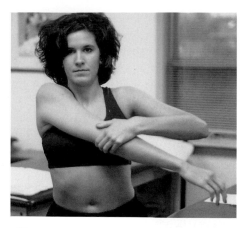

Figure 9–23. Posterior capsule self-stretch.

Specific activities to refrain from include shoulder activities where the humerus is elevated above the horizontal, as well as reaching and lifting activities, due to the likelihood of encroachment of the humeral head on the undersurface of the acromion. Any activity causing pain should be avoided.

Patient education on methods of protection for the arm is essential. Instruction on proper sleeping techniques and performance of activities of daily living should be provided. The recommended sleeping position is lying on the uninvolved side with a pillow under the arm for support (see Fig. 9–22). During activities of daily living, the time that the arm is resting at the side should be minimized, due to decreased subacromial vascularity while in this position.

Relative rest is yet another essential element in the initial phase of rehabilitation. Relative rest refers to avoidance of aggravating factors while maintaining strict compliance to the prescribed rehabilitation program. Patient education should include instruction on activities not included in the rehabilitation program that may be beneficial, such as aerobic nonweight-bearing arm activities. This will improve shoulder vascularity and may promote the healing process and facilitate progression through the rehabilitation phases.

Phase II: Subacute Phase

The subacute phase of rehabilitation generally coincides with tissue repair and remodeling, as described by Reed and Zarro. Inflammation has been retarded, and the period of scar tissue maturation has begun. The subjective criteria for progression into this phase are no discomfort at rest, no warmth noted with palpation of the joint, and good tolerance of the rehabilitation program thus far.

Physiologic changes in status are noted from the initiation of rehabilitation, but the program is modified in this stage only minimally. The goals of phase II remain the same as in the previous phase. The dissimilarity of

the two phases lies in the progression and advancement of the activities.

Joint mobility is maintained by the addition of the following: (1) active assisted abduction with the rope and pulley; (2) self-stretching for the posterior (see Fig. 9–23), inferior, and anterior capsule; and (3) progressive, aggressive joint mobilization. Muscular atrophy prevention is advanced with the addition of (1) progressive resistance exercises for strengthening of the muscles surrounding the joints above and below the shoulder, including biceps, triceps, and forearm and wrist muscles; and (2) advancement of scapular muscle strengthening with scapular proprioceptive neuromuscular facilitation (see Figs. 9–24 to 9–27). These exercises may be performed with dumbbells, various equipment, and with manual resistance applied by the skilled manual thera-

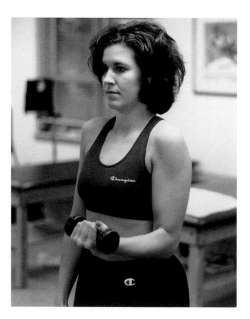

Figure 9–24. Biceps curl

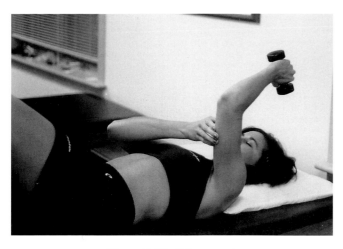

Figure 9–25. Triceps curl.

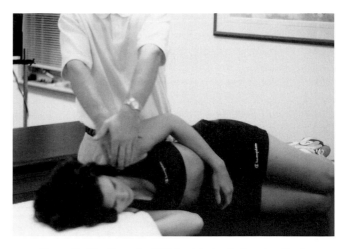

Figure 9–27. Scapular PNF (resisted anterior elevation).

pist. However, strict emphasis must be placed on avoidance of positional impingement.

Phase III: Selective Strengthening Phase

The criteria for advancement into this phase of rehabilitation include full normal passive shoulder range of motion, improved scapular and rotator cuff muscular performance, and the ability to perform activities of daily living pain-free. It is often beneficial to delay advancement into this phase due to the time constraints of tissue healing. Too rapid a progression into this aggressive strengthening phase may aggravate the patient's condition and cause a setback or even a failed rehabilitation program.

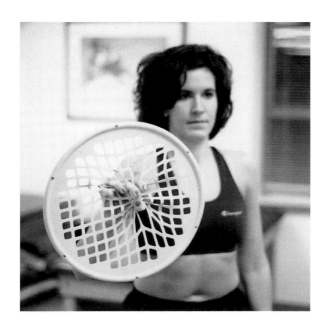

Figure 9–26. Wrist/hand strengthening with the Powerweb.

The goals in this phase are to normalize the arthro-kinematics of the shoulder complex while maintaining normal range of motion, thereby reestablishing the proper humeral head depressor mechanism, as well as to regain and improve shoulder muscle strength and improve neuromuscular control of the shoulder. Dynamic control of the humeral head must be achieved in this phase.

The concept of proximal stability for distal mobility is emphasized in this phase. Proximal stability through restoration of normal coordinated scapula thoracic motion and dynamic scapular stabilization accomplishes several things. First, it provides a stable base for the humerus to act upon. Second, it maintains the glenoid in a position that allows maximal congruency with the humeral head, allowing total arm strengthening without exacerbation of the shoulder impingement symptoms.

Exercise performance in the scapular plane is indicated in the treatment of many shoulder pathologies, including impingement. The scapular plane is 30 to 45 degrees anterior to the coronal plane. The scientific rationale for exercise performance in this plane is that it is believed to be a position of optimal length to tension relationships for the deltoid and rotator cuff musculature. It provides a more direct line of pull for the deltoid and the supraspinatus muscles, thereby avoiding subacromial impingement as the arm is abducted.

Normalizing Shoulder Arthrokinematics.
Shoulder complex arthrokinematics are restored through aggressive joint mobilization and performance of capsule self-stretching and active assisted range-of-motion exercises. Joint mobilization will address any limitation apparent upon evaluation, and may include mobilization of any of the previously mentioned joints of the shoulder complex, but likely will address the glenohumeral joint solely. The mobilization

techniques necessary are not unlike the ones previously described, but are more aggressive in nature, utilizing grades II and III primarily. The self-stretching and range-of-motion exercises from the previous phase should be continued, if indicated by any range-of-motion limitations.

Restoration of Strength and Neuromuscular Control. Regaining and improving strength and neuromuscular control of the shoulder is contingent on appropriate exercise prescription. The main emphasis in this phase should be increasing rotator cuff, scapular musculature, and total arm strength. Exercise prescription in this phase should at some point include the following specific core rotator cuff exercises: (1) prone horizontal abduction; (2) prone extension; (3) prone scapular retraction; (4) prone external rotation at 90 degrees of abduction; (5) supine scapular protraction; (6) supine upper extremity diagonal 1 pattern (proprioceptive neuromuscular facilitation), modified to avoid cross-body adduction; (7) supine upper extremity diagonal 2 pattern (proprioceptive neuromuscular facilitation); (8) standing shoulder elevation (shrugs); (9) standing flexion in the plane of the scapula with relative shoulder internal rotation and forearm pronation (supraspinatus), not to exceed 80 degrees; and (10) seated press-ups (see Figs. 9-28 to 9-37). Core scapular strengthening exercises, as indicated by Mosely and colleagues, should be incorporated, and include the following: (1) rowing; (2) elevation of the arm in the scapular plane with the humerus externally rotated, termed scaption; and (3) push-ups followed by scapular protraction when elbows are extended, termed "push-ups with a plus" (see Figs. 9-38 to 9-40). Recently, the addition of shoulder flexion in the plane of the scapula with neutral rotation in the range of 0 to 120 degrees has been shown to be beneficial for the recruitment of the scapular stabilizer muscles, while not increasing the likelihood of impingement. Upper arm ergometry (see Fig. 9-41) should be incorporated, and the previous upper extremity exercises should be continued.

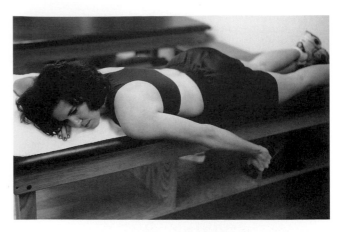

Figure 9–29. Prone extension.

With the introduction of the ever-evolving pieces of rehabilitation equipment, comes the responsibility of the rehabilitation provider to provide an appropriate method for exercise performance. If accessible, devices such as cable systems or isokinetic dynamometers are often effective in progressing the shoulder strengthening program, as well as aiding in patient compliance. However, many of these types of equipment are costly. Surgical tubing is often an inexpensive yet appropriate adjunct to exercise program performance, but caution must be used during performance due to the typically unquantified level of resistance provided by most tubing. Manual therapy techniques, including proprioceptive neuromuscular facilitation, are recommended and perhaps considered most appropriate for establishing an optimally individualized rehabilitation program.

As the rehabilitation program is accelerated, the concept of specificity of training should be addressed. When strength and level of neuromuscular control permit, functional activities should begin to dominate the program, including overhead activity, both open and

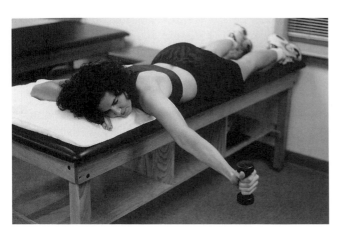

Figure 9–28. Prone horizontal abduction.

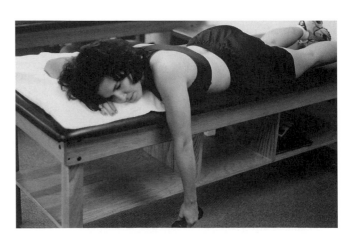

Figure 9–30. Prone scapular retraction.

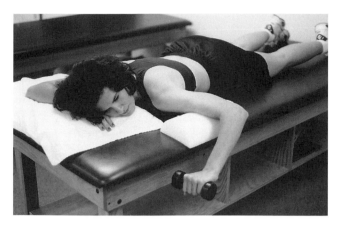

Figure 9–31. Prone external rotation at 90 degrees abduction.

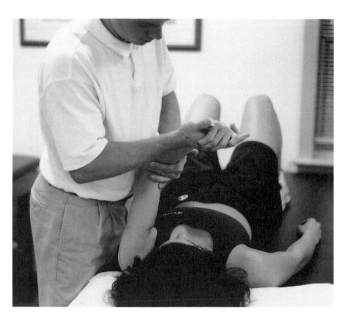

Figure 9–33. Upper extremity PNF (D1).

closed kinetic chain exercises, and plyometrics. Activities should attempt to duplicate the dynamics of overhead activity, whether athletic or occupational.

Although restoration of normal shoulder muscle strength and power should be addressed throughout this phase, endurance of the rotator cuff is of equal importance. Clinical rehabilitation protocols should emphasize increasing rotator cuff muscle endurance to produce a more fatigue resistant muscle group, thereby maintaining normal shoulder proprioception, yet another aspect of normal shoulder function.

Phase IV: Return to Function

This phase is characterized by a gradual return to normal function, including overhead activities of daily living, occupational activities, and athletic activities. The guidelines for progression into this phase include full pain-free range of motion, satisfactory strength, satisfactory neuromuscular control, and satisfactory clinical evaluation, including no pain or tenderness to palpation. The sole focus of this phase is resumption of unrestricted, symptom-free activity.

Activity and job modification may be appropriate to minimize the chance for reoccurrence of shoulder im-

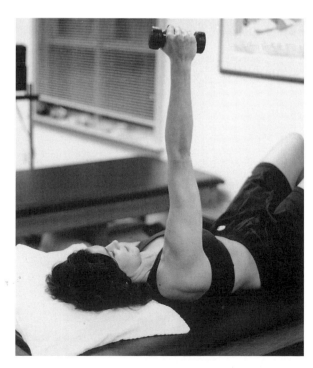

Figure 9–32. Supine scapular protraction.

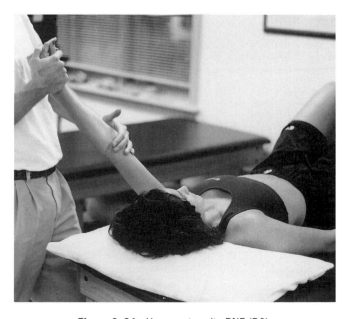

Figure 9–34. Upper extremity PNF (D2).

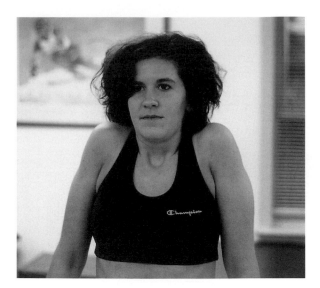

Figure 9–35. Shoulder elevation (shrugs).

pingement syndrome. A maintenance home exercise program should be initiated with an exercise prescription consisting of flexibility exercises, rotator cuff and scapular muscle strengthening exercises, and total arm strengthening exercises.

REHABILITATION PHASES FOR ROTATOR CUFF INJURIES

The aggressive treatment of athletic injuries is based not on arbitrary time frames but on an athlete's ability to perform certain activities based on what activities were done

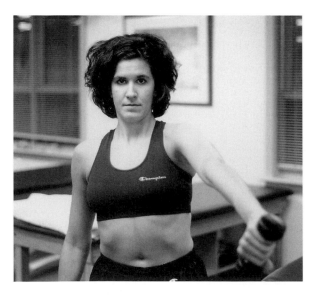

Figure 9–36. Flexion in plane of scapula, pronated, below 80 degrees ("empty can").

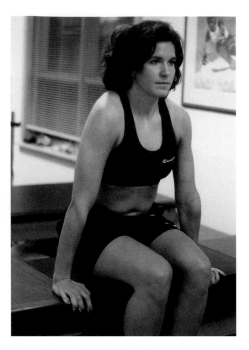

Figure 9–37. Seated press-up.

before as a foundation. Once preselected criteria are met, the athlete can advance to the next level of activity. This is performance-based rehabilitation or criteria-based rehabilitation.

The logic in this program is not to base advance of an athlete's progress on time only (healing time is the only reason this would be done), but to base it on a step-by-step progression based on range of motion, strength, endurance, neuromuscular coordination, and the tissue's ability to handle the stresses caused by these activities.

For example, passive range of motion must be established before active range of motion is effective.

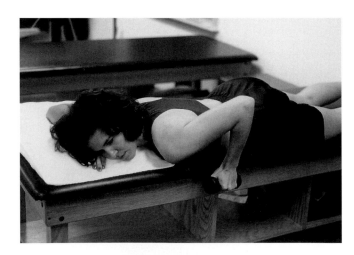

Figure 9–38. Prone row.

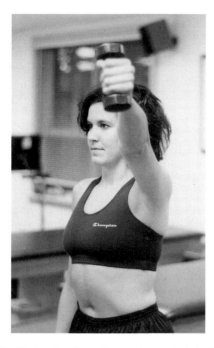

Figure 9–39. Flexion in plane of scapula, neutral, to 120 degrees ("scaption").

Gravity-assisted or gravity-eliminated exercises must be established if the patient is too weak to lift against gravity. Scapular stability and at least 4 plus out of 5 rotator cuff strength must be available before functional training begins. External rotation strength at the side should be established before working to the 90-degree position. Pain should be eliminated in active lifting against gravity before standing exercises are done. If lifting against gravity is contraindicated because of healing restraints, submaximal exercise is indicated. If range-of-motion exercises don't place undue stress or strain on the repair, they should be initiated as soon as comfortable for the patient.

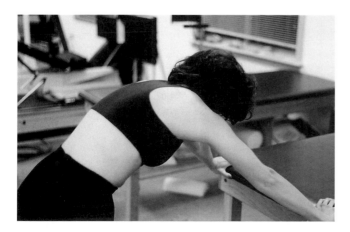

Figure 9–40. Push-up with scapular protraction ("push-up with a plus").

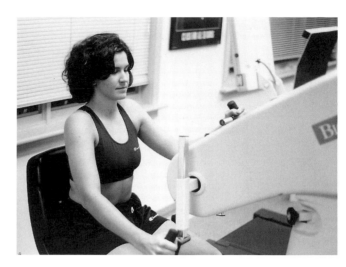

Figure 9–41. Upper body ergometer.

All shoulder soft-tissue rehabilitation can be divided into four healing phases based on the symptoms and healing activity as described earlier in this chapter. In postoperative situations, the acute phase (1 to 2 weeks) is the time that careful attention should be given to making certain that the sutured tissues are not overstressed. In the subacute or fibroblastic stage (1 to 3 weeks), more stress can be added to the tissues in the form of gravity-eliminated exercises and submaximal isometrics. In the selective strengthening phase, when tissue maturation and remodeling occurs (3 to 8 weeks), the patient will progress toward exercise against gravity. The final phase is that of final maturation that may take up to a year. After 8 to 12 weeks, the sutured material will take gradual passive stretching. Generally, soft tissue will be remodeled by 14 or 15 weeks and will be able to take normal stresses.

INTRODUCTION TO ROTATOR CUFF REHABILITATION

In previous pages of this chapter, the basic exercises for addressing scapular and rotator cuff musculature have been spelled out. Each pathology requires different application and timing of the exercises for strength and range of motion. Healing soft tissue must be respected. Surgical techniques also require special attention as to what tissues are split, released, taken down, and fixed. The type of fixation is important because it affects the aggressiveness of the rehabilitation.

The rehabilitation protocols for rotator cuff lesions can be divided into separate categories based on the type of lesion, size of the lesion, the surgical procedure, and how long it takes the lesion to heal. Impingement pathology and partial-thickness tears, the small tear, the medium to large tear, and the massive and redo tears divide the categories as to the timing of the application of the exercises.

Rotator Cuff Tears

Partial or split-thickness lesions of the rotator cuff that occur in overuse situations perhaps due to instability, are treated with arthroscopic debridement. The stresses put on the rotator cuff when lifting the arm overhead after this surgery will not damage the tendon. The rehabilitation program may progress symptomatically.

Tears of any size can occur in the athlete depending on the trauma. Routinely, small tears occur in the "younger" middle-aged patient. These 1-cm or smaller tears are usually along the lines of the fibers of the rotator cuff. The surgical approach does not require a large exposure, so that fiber splitting of the deltoid is all that is required. The tear can be sutured together in such a manner that the lines of pull of rotator cuff muscle contraction will not pull it apart. Anytime the fibers of the deltoid can be split rather than taken down from its origin, rehabilitation time can be accelerated, because fear of deltoid rupture has been lessened. Ultimately, healing time will be shortened.

The medium to large tear (1 to 5 mm) may require a larger exposure for the repair. This may require that the deltoid be taken down. This type of rotator cuff tear can be more perpendicular to the line of pull of the contraction of the rotator cuff and will need more protection during the healing phase. Generally, 3 weeks is needed for soft tissue to heal enough to take much stress and approximately 6 weeks of maturation for the deltoid and rotator cuff to withstand lifting the arm against gravity.

Massive tears (5 mm or more) and redos require even more time for healing. Approximately 6 weeks should be allowed before moderate stress is applied to the repaired structures and 12 weeks before lifting the arm against gravity.

The progression of an exercise program for the rotator cuff must take into consideration healing times and the biomechanics of movement as it relates to the lesion or the surgery to that lesion. When lifting the arm overhead, the scapula must be rotated into position so that the glenohumeral joint is in a functional position. Then the scapula must be stabilized to allow the upper arm to be utilized. Proximal to distal stabilization will occur.

In order for the arm to be elevated, the short rotators of the rotator cuff stabilize the humeral head on the glenoid so that the deltoid may lift the arm overhead, establishing the humeral head depressor mechanism. The simple movement of elevating the arm puts much stress on the deltoid and rotator cuff structures. In the postsur-

gical situation, this stress must be recognized and reduced until the tissues have healed enough to take the stress. This time frame is the only time-based reason for applying various exercises at certain times.

When designing a rehabilitation program for rotator cuff injuries, the vascular anatomy of the rotator cuff should be considered. Codman's critical portion of the cuff on a cadaveric study showed decreased vascularity within the tendinous portion of the supraspinatus tendon. Most rotator cuff tears occur in this zone. Rathburn and MacNab suggested that with the arm in adduction, this particular area is wrung out by the pressure between the humerus and the tendon and therefore, exercise should be avoided in 0 degrees of adduction. Lohr's microvascular studies disagree with this theory. Sigholm found that vascularity to the critical zone decreased when a 1-kg weight was lifted above shoulder level and promoted the theory that hypovascularity may be dynamic. But Swiontkowski and associates demonstrated, in microvascular studies using laser Doppler flowometry in living patients with intact rotator cuffs and clinical signs of impingement, that there was hypervascularity in the area of greatest mechanical impingement of the critical zone. So it's obvious that this issue isn't settled. The safest bet is to monitor symptoms and not increase them with the exercise program.

There are pretty good reasons to treat rotator cuffs conservatively. McLaughlin pointed out that at least 25 percent of cadavers have rotator cuff tears and 50 percent of patients with some degree of rupture recover spontaneously. An accurate diagnosis is hard to make when the shoulder is acutely painful and early surgery versus delayed repairs are substantially the same. It makes no sense to take a shoulder that is acutely painful, lacking range of motion and strength, operate on it, and expect the patient to do well after surgery. Many recommend 6 to 12 weeks of conservative therapy or at least until all symptoms have resolved.

Postoperative Management of Partial Rotator Cuff Tear and Decompression

Phase I: Acute Inflammatory Phase

The acute inflammatory phase is the time that an inflammatory process exists within the shoulder. Goals of this phase should include full range of motion (ROM) with no restriction, pain and inflammation reduction during the first 2 weeks, fair (3 of 5) strength as graded by manual muscle test evaluation, resumption of normal activities of daily living (ADL), and maintenance of total body fitness.

The rehabilitation program should consist of modalities for pain relief; exercises to achieve passive ROM in all directions, with the emphasis on external rotation; ac-

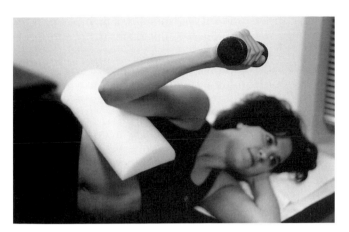

Figure 9–42. Sidelying external rotation with dumbbell.

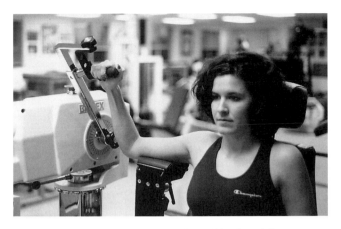

Figure 9–44. Upper extremity isokinetic training.

tive strengthening against gravity utilizing rotator cuff and scapula routines; joint mobilization for all restrictions; and cardiovascular (CV) fitness and conditioning and strengthening for noninjured body parts.

Phase II: Subacute Phase

The subacute phase includes the fibroblastic phase as well as the advancement of tissue maturation and remodeling. Goals of this phase are scar tissue remodeling (fibroblastic phase 1 to 4 or 6 weeks), achievement of 4 plus to 5 of 5 rotator cuff and scapula strength, full pain-free ROM, particularly external rotation in the overhead or throwing athletes, maintenance of CV fitness and strength of noninjured body parts, and adequate joint stabilization and neuromuscular coordination.

Rehabilitation should include the following: (1) continued phase one exercise program, (2) progression to resistance exercises with tubing or weights up to 5 lb for rotator cuff program, (3) isokinetic training as tolerated,

(4) proprioceptive neuromuscular facilitation (PNF), (5) modified weight-bearing stabilization drills, and (6) addition of functional activities and neuromuscular drills utilizing the Plyoback, Body Blade, Joystick, Right Weigh by BTE, and various other neuromuscular training devices (see Fig. 9-42 to 9-51).

Phase III: Selective Strengthening

The previous two phases have outlined the rehabilitation program and progression for the athletic population. It is likely that in sedentary or nonathletic individuals, the progression may be slower and the training techniques mentioned in those phases may not be utilized until later phases of rehabilitation. The experienced clinician must determine the rate of progression while considering all factors, as well as expected functional outcome. The following recommendations are directed towards the athletic population. Goals in this phase are advanced strength training, progression to 50 percent of functional activity for

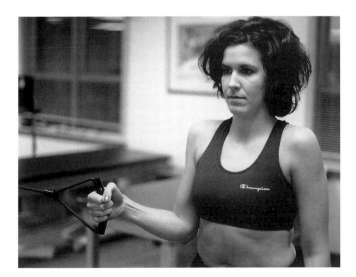

Figure 9–43. Standing internal rotation with tubing resistance.

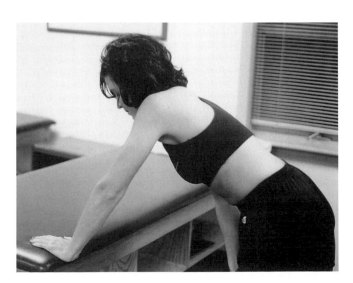

Figure 9–45. Modified upper extremity stabilization, weight bearing.

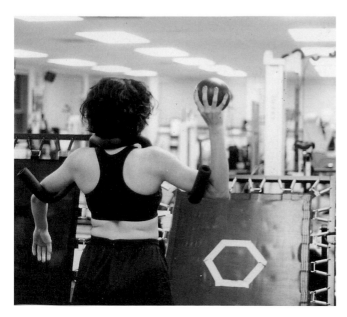

Figure 9–46. Plyoback ball toss.

overhead athlete, and soft-tissue early maturation (14 to 15 weeks).

The prescribed program should follow these guidelines: (1) continuation of the previous program for rotator cuff and scapula strengthening, (2) initiation of general upper extremity weight training, and (3) initiation of the return to throwing program (see Table 9–3.)

Phase IV: Return to Function
Goals in this phase are return to competition at full speed, normal (5 of 5) strength in all shoulder muscles, and mature soft tissue that can take the stress of activity without irritation. The program recommended to achieve these goals includes (1) advanced functional activities with continued progression, (2) advanced weight training, and (3) continued rotator cuff and scapula strengthening program.

Rehabilitation of Postoperative Small Rotator Cuff Tears

Phase I: Acute Inflammatory Phase
An associated increase in the duration of each rehabilitation phase will likely accompany an increase in relative size of a rotator cuff tear. Goals of this phase are gradual return of full passive ROM without restrictions, ability to perform gravity-eliminated active ROM, avoidance of irritation during acute phase (1 to 2 weeks), reduction of pain and inflammation, exercise activities for the uninvolved areas of the upper quarter, total body conditioning, and discontinuance of sling when tolerated.

The rehabilitation program will consist of (1) modalities for reduction of pain and inflammation; (2)

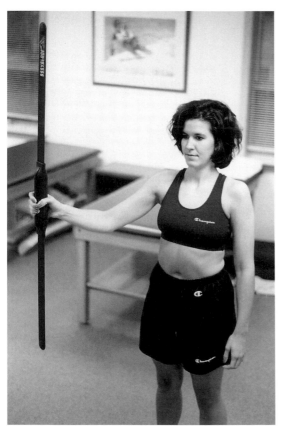

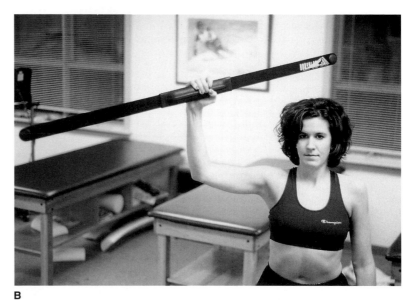

Figure 9–47. A. Body blade in plane of scapula. **B.** Body blade at 90 degrees of abduction and elbow flexion.

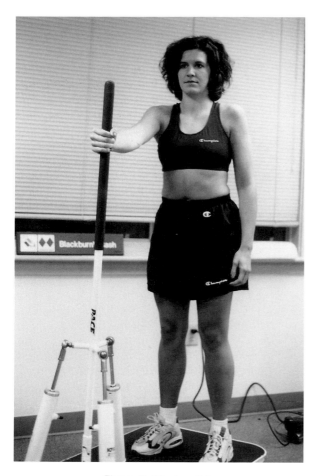

Figure 9–48. Joystick.

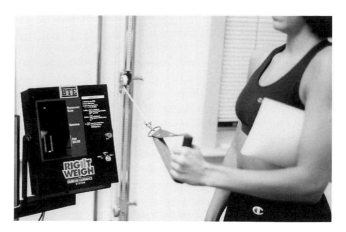

Figure 9–49. Standing external rotation with weighted pulley and Right Weigh (BTE).

ROM with wand and pulley for all motions with deemphasized internal rotation; (7) gravity-eliminated external rotation, internal rotation, abduction, and flexion active ROM; and (8) bike or other CV activities and entire body activities.

Phase II: Subacute Phase

Goals of the subacute phase for treatment of small rotator cuff tears are to remodel soft tissue and prevent inflammation (1 to 4 or 6 weeks), achieve full nonpainful passive ROM, perform ADLs, progress to 3 of 5 rotator cuff strength, and activate joint stabilization and neuromuscular training.

Program prescription includes (1) previous program continuation, (2) progressive rotator cuff and scapula routine, and (3) incorporation of PNF and Baltimore therapeutic exercise (BTE) programs for neuromuscular coordination and reflexive stabilization (see Figs. 9–51 and 9–52).

elbow, wrist, and hand stretching and strengthening; (3) scapular strengthening program including shoulder shrugs with scapula retraction and nonweight-bearing shoulder depression; (4) submaximal isometrics for all shoulder motions; (5) pendulum exercise; (6) passive

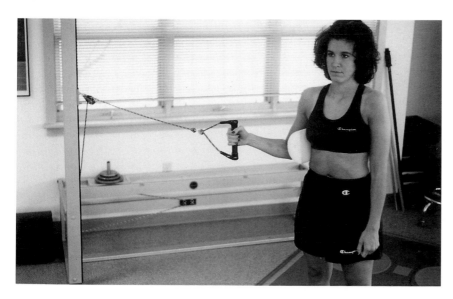

Figure 9–50. Impulse inertial trainer.

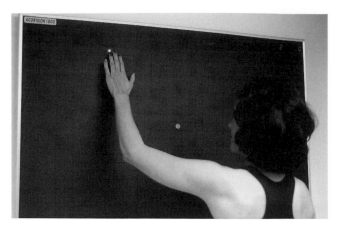

Figure 9–51. Upper extremity neuromuscular coordination with Acuvision 1000.

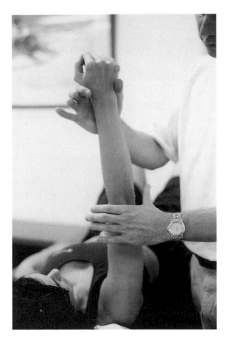

Figure 9–52. Supine upper extremity rhythmic stabilization.

TABLE 9–3. INTERVAL THROWING PROGRAM

Each phase consists of several throwing sessions. The athlete should work up to the parameters within each phase. Generally, the athlete throws daily. However, if soreness or stiffness develops after a throwing session and persists, then the next session should be reduced or skipped. Progression to the subsequent phase is based on achieving the phase goals without any symptoms.

Session Sequence
- Warm up (break sweat, stretch, "soft-toss" 10 to 15 feet until loose, work to long-toss distance)
- Long-toss interval
- Short-toss interval
- Rest 10–30 minutes
- Repeat warm-up
- Long-toss interval
- Short-toss interval
- Cool down (stretch, ice, monitor symptoms)

| Phase | Long-toss Interval | | Short-toss Interval | | Speed: Pitch Type/Surface |
	Distance (feet)	No. Throws[a]	Distance (feet)	No. Throws[a]	
1	90	25	30	50	½, straight, flat
2	120	25	60	50	½, straight, flat
3	150	25	60	50	¾, straight, flat
4	180	25	60	50	¾, straight, mound
5	210	25	60	50	½–¾, breaking, mound
6	240	25	60+	50	¾–full, all, mound
7	Work to game situations; number of pitches in game situation should be increased as able; monitor mechanics and accuracy (85 percent of pitches should be strikes).				

[a] In each phase, prescribed number of throws should be completed within a 5-minute time period.
From Blackburn TA Jr. Baseball and softball. In: Mellion MB, Walsh WM, Shelton GL, eds. The Team Physicians Handbook. *2nd ed. Philadelphia: Hanley & Belfus; 1997: 578. With permission.*

Phase III: Selective Strengthening Phase

Phase three goals consist of: early soft-tissue maturation (14 to 15 weeks) and 4 plus to 5 of 5 rotator cuff strength. The rehabilitation program should incorporate the following: (1) continuation of previous program when appropriate, (2) progressive resistance for rotator cuff and scapular muscles, (3) isokinetics as tolerated, and (4) advanced stabilization and reactive neuromuscular training program.

Phase IV: Return to Function

Goals outlined for the return to activity include: full return to all activities, normal (5 of 5) strength in all shoulder musculature, and full ROM. The program should include (1) advanced strengthening for upper body, (2) continued rotator cuff strengthening program, (3) maintenance of full ranges of motion, and (4) progression through functional activities for the particular sport or activity.

Rehabilitation of Postoperative Medium to Large Rotator Cuff Tears

Phase I: Acute Inflammatory Phase

Medium to large rotator cuff tears require increasing attention to activity modification and strict adherence to guidelines of healing. Healing time limitation in tears of this size is approximately 3 weeks. Goals of this phase in treatment are gradual return of full passive ROM excluding internal rotation, initiation of contraction of rotator cuff, scapular muscles and deltoid, avoidance of irritation during acute phase (1 to 2 weeks), reduction of pain and inflammation, exercise activities for the uninvolved areas of the upper quarter, and total body conditioning.

The program should include (1) modalities for reduction of pain and inflammation; (2) compliance to sling for healing time frame; (3) elbow, wrist, and hand stretching and strengthening; (4) scapular strengthening program including shoulder shrugs with scapula retraction and nonweight-bearing shoulder depression; (5) submaximal isometrics for all shoulder motions; (6) pendulum exercise; (7) passive ROM with wand and pulley for all motions with deemphasized internal rotation; (8) performance of gravity-eliminated external rotation, internal rotation, abduction, and flexion active ROM; and (9) bike or other CV activities and entire body activities.

Phase II: Subacute Phase

Goals of the subacute phase for medium to large rotator cuff tears are: remodeling soft tissue and prevention of inflammation (1 to 4 or 6 weeks), progression towards full nonpainful passive ROM, performance of ADLs with arm at side, and progression to gravity-eliminated active rotator cuff and deltoid strengthening. The outlined program is as follows: (1) continued previous program,

(2) work out of sling as is comfortable, and (3) gentle joint mobilization and stabilization drills.

Phase III: Selective Strengthening Phase

Goals during this phase include the early maturation of healing tissue (14 to 15 weeks SPO [status postoperation]), rotator cuff and deltoid strength greater than fair (3 to 3 plus of 5), and full pain-free passive ROM. The rehabilitation program should include (1) continuation of previous appropriate programs, (2) progression to against gravity rotator cuff and scapula exercises, (3) progression to stabilization drills, PNF, and modified weight-bearing activities.

Phase IV: Return to Function

Goals of this phase are normal (4 plus to 5 of 5) shoulder muscle strength, full active and passive pain-free ROM, resumption of pain-free ADLs, and resumption of sport-specific training. Program prescription should include (1) advanced strengthening for upper body, (2) continuation of rotator cuff strengthening program, (3) maintenance of normal ROM, and (4) progression through functional activities for the particular sport or activity.

Rehabilitation After Postoperative Massive Rotator Cuff Tears

Phase I: Acute Inflammatory Phase

Massive or redo rotator cuff tears require a prolonged duration of protection, usually up to 6 weeks. The goals of this initial phase include gradual return of full passive ROM excluding internal rotation; initiation of contraction of rotator cuff, scapular muscles, and deltoid; avoidance of irritation during the acute phase (1 to 2 weeks); pain and inflammation reduction; performance of exercise activities for the uninvolved areas of the upper quarter; and maintenance of total body conditioning.

The program consists of (1) modalities for relief of pain and inflammation; (2) maintenance of a sling for healing time frame; (3) elbow, wrist, and hand stretching and strengthening; (4) scapular muscle strengthening program including shoulder shrugs with scapula retraction and nonweight-bearing shoulder depression; (5) submaximal isometrics for all shoulder motions; (6) pendulum exercise; (7) passive ROM with wand and pulley for all motions with deemphasized internal rotation; (8) gravity-eliminated external rotation, internal rotation, abduction, and flexion active ROM toward the end of 6 weeks; and (9) bike or other CV activities and entire body activities.

Phase II: Subacute Phase

The subacute phase may last from weeks 6 to 12. Goals in this phase include remodeling of soft tissue and prevention of inflammation, progression towards full nonpainful passive ROM, performance of ADLs with the arm at the side, and progression to gravity-eliminated active rotator cuff and deltoid exercises. The program should consist of (1) continuation of previous program, (2) work out of sling as is comfortable, and (3) gentle joint mobilization and stabilization drills.

Phase III: Selective Strengthening Phase

Goals of this phase are early maturation of healing tissue (14 to 15 weeks SPO), greater than fair rotator cuff and deltoid strength (3 to 3 plus of 5), and full pain-free passive ROM. The program should include (1) continuation of previous appropriate programs, (2) progression to against-gravity rotator cuff and scapular muscle strengthening exercises, and (3) progression of stabilization drills, PNF, and modified weight bearing.

Phase IV: Return to Function

Goals in this phase include normal (4 plus to 5 of 5), shoulder muscle strength, full active and passive pain-free ROM, performance of ADLs, and initiation of sports-specific training. The program should incorporate (1) advanced strengthening for upper body, (2) continuation of rotator cuff strengthening program, (3) maintenance of normal ROM, and (4) progression through functional activities for the particular sport or activity.

REHABILITATION OF THE UNSTABLE SHOULDER

Stability of the glenohumeral joint (GH) is truly a wondrous happening. The joint allows almost a universal joint type of movement, yet it does not usually disarticulate. Because of the capsule and other mechanisms, the humerus stays within a centimeter of the center of the glenoid when the arm is moved. When lifting the arm overhead, the deltoid and rotator cuff force couple keeps the humeral head centered. When the arm is brought into abduction and external rotation, the glenohumeral ligaments tighten and translate the humeral head to its center point or even a bit posterior. The same process happens when the arm is brought into internal rotation and adduction with the posterior capsule tightening up to push the humeral head forward.

It is very important for the rehabilitation specialist to recognize that when the humerus is brought forward or backward out of the plane of the scapula, stress is put on the capsule in the opposite direction. If it is desired to protect the anterior capsule, then exercises done in the plane of the scapula or forward will not stress the capsule and vice versa for the posterior.

Exercises in different positions also put stress on different structures of the capsule. Internal rotation at 0 degrees of abduction stresses the upper portion of the posterior capsule. As the arm is raised overhead, this stress transfers more inferiorly. By the time the arm is overhead, the inferior capsule is taking the stress. External rotation of the arm at 0 degrees stresses the superior glenohumeral ligament; at 45 degrees the middle glenohumeral ligament is stressed; at 90 degrees the inferior glenohumeral ligament is stressed; as the arm moves further up into abduction, the inferior capsule becomes more taut. It is important to know what tissues were damaged or what have been repaired so that appropriate stress can be applied during the healing phases.

The rehabilitation specialist must also consider all the different ways the shoulder stays stable, even when there is such an extensive range of motion. The bony support cannot be considered very important in stability of the GH. By adding the glenoid labrum, the fossa is deepened. The labrum provides not only a ridge around the fossa that requires the humeral head to move away from the fossa tightening the capsule when it slides to the edge of the fossa, but it also allows for a suction-like effect that provides more stability. The wet surfaces of the joint also allow for adhesive and cohesive bonding to the humeral head and the glenoid. There is a vacuum in the joint that assists in keeping the joint articulated. All the passive mechanisms are important, as the capsule itself is not taut, except when the arm moves to extremes of motion. Active stability arises from tone in the rotator cuff that causes the joint to be compressed. All active movement causes joint compression and therefore stability.

Knowing the basic classifications of instability of the shoulder can help in understanding the prognosis for each type of instability, which will affect the rehabilitation program. There are several classification systems described in the literature, although none are used exclusively.

An acute dislocation will demand different treatment than a chronic or recurrent dislocation. The acute dislocator will have many more symptoms of pain, spasm, and swelling. There will also be healing time necessary for the soft tissue. This healing time is not completely agreed upon. The literature supports that if the patient is less than 20 years old and receives an acute anterior dislocation and attempts to return to the activity that caused the dislocation, he or she has an 80 to 90 percent chance of a second dislocation. The recurrent dislocator will have much fewer symptoms and may reduce the shoulder by his or her self. This athlete may return to activity immediately.

The direction of the instability is another way to classify it. Anterior, posterior, and inferior are different classifications. Some physicians believe that if the rotator cuff is torn, there is even a superior instability. Multidirectional instability (MDI) indicates a very loose capsule with excessive translation in all directions.

The amount of instability aids in describing the classification. This calls for several definitions to achieve common understanding of these classifications. Translation is the amount of passive movement that occurs across the GH joint. Instability is uncontrolled translation of the GH joint that causes pain and dysfunction. Disability is when the instability causes the patient to change wanted activities.

The traditional instability translation measurement is defined as a dislocation, that is, the humeral head is out of the confines of the glenoid fossa. A 50 percent translation is defined as a subluxation. Some describe a subluxation as a dislocation that patients reduce themselves. There are a number of different ways to describe the amount of translation such as the Hospital for Special Surgery's 0 through 3 scale. In this scale, 0 is a shoulder with normal translation of about a centimeter in any direction. A 1 is translation of the humeral head to the labrum. A 2 is when the humeral head is on top of the labrum (50 percent translation) and a 3 is a complete dislocation.

The cause of the instability is another way to classify shoulder instability. Macrotrauma causes most of the frank dislocations. Microtrauma may be the cause of secondary impingement and is the "silent subluxor" brought on by overuse and repetitive activities. The third type of instability is thought to be congenital by cause and is a result of hypoelastic connective tissue. Each of these types should be handled differently when it comes to rehabilitation.

The "torn loose" versus "born loose" classification results from the way these injuries are handled. The torn loose or patient with a *t*raumatic injury, *u*nidirectional, suffers a *B*ankart lesion, and usually doesn't respond to rehabilitation but to *s*urgery (TUBS). The "born loose" or patient with an *a*traumatic origin, is *m*ultidirectional, occurs *b*ilaterally, and does respond to *r*ehabilitation and if surgery is necessary it will involve an *i*nferior capsule shift (AMBRI). Determining this classification will help determine the best rehabilitation course.

Rehabilitation of Acute Dislocations

The classic external rotation and abduction position of anterior dislocation was traditionally treated with rest and attention to the internal rotators of the shoulder. This approach neglected the importance of a balanced muscular treatment. It is very important to have a posterior rotator cuff input to actively stabilize the humeral head. This balanced approach is used because of the need to protect the anterior capsule when the arm is forced into external rotation but also, to keep the humeral head centered. This balanced approach also works in the face of the "circle concept" of instability, where it is surmised that when the shoulder dislocates anteriorly and damages the anterior capsule, the posterior capsule would also have to be damaged for the head to escape the confines of the capsule thus, causing posterior instability.

There is some debate over how long the acute dislocation should be immobilized. Soft-tissue healing theories support as much as 6 weeks of immobilization and at least 3 weeks for the collagen tissue to stick down. Since the outlook is so poor for young people with acute anterior dislocations when they return to the same sport that they were injured in, the idea of treating the shoulder symptomatically may be best. The older the patient is, the more physicians worry about movement contractures. Earlier mobilization is probably indicated. It is possible that the hypoelastic patient will not suffer as much soft tissue damage because the capsule will give. The stiff-jointed individual may have more damage with the dislocation and therefore more symptoms.

Two things are certain. The scapular and rotator cuff musculature must be addressed as soon as possible, and the exercise application must be biomechanically sound so as not to have deleterious effects on the healing soft tissue. The key is keeping the arm in the plane of the scapula or more forward. Even though the plan may be to immobilize the shoulder, some rotator cuff and scapular exercises can be done during this time through judicious use of isometrics and limited arc exercises with the arm close to the side. The same concept of exercise is utilized as described in depth previously. If the athlete wishes to return to an activity that requires full ROM into the injury position, care must be taken to develop strength and coordination into this motion. If the dislocation is posterior in nature, this exercise rule is reversed. The arm will be immobilized at the side in neutral rotation. Exercises will be prescribed to be performed in the plane of the scapula and more posterior.

Phase I: Maximum Protection Phase

Goals during the initial postinjury phase include reduction of pain, spasm, and swelling; activation of scapular and rotator cuff musculature; allowing the soft tissue to calm down (1 to 2 weeks); and maintenance of total body fitness. The rehabilitation program should consist of the following: (1) immobilization in a sling; (2) modalities to treat acute symptoms; (3) shoulder shrugs with scapular retraction; (4) shoulder depressions performed non-weight bearing; (5) isometrics performed on all shoulder motions, as comfort allows, with the arm at the side; (6) elbow, wrist, and hand strengthening; and (7) strengthening and conditioning of the entire body (see Figs. 9–53 to 9–55).

Phase II: Tissue Maturation Phase

Tissue healing and maturation occurs predominantly in this phase. Goals of this phase are allowing soft-tissue remodeling (3 to 4 weeks); movement of the arm away from the side but maintaining the relative plane of scapula position, or forward towards 90 degrees, for performance of isometric and short arc exercises and 45 degrees of external rotation; lifting against gravity as tolerated; maintenance of fitness training; and stabiliza-

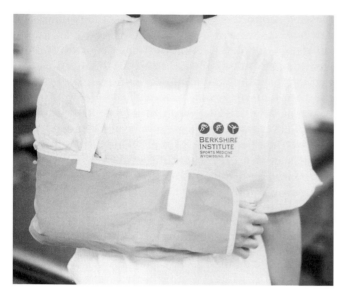

Figure 9–53. Upper extremity immobilization in arm sling.

tion development. The rehabilitation prescription should incorporate the following: (1) scapular and rotator cuff routines performed in 90 degrees of abduction in the scapular plane with 45 degrees of external rotation, as symptoms allow; exercise progression from gravity-eliminated to against gravity, with light resistance as tolerated; continued appropriate fitness training; and PNF and other stabilization drills including modified weight bearing.

Phase III: Selective Strengthening Phase
Goals during the progressive strengthening phase consist of gradual application of stress to soft tissue for early

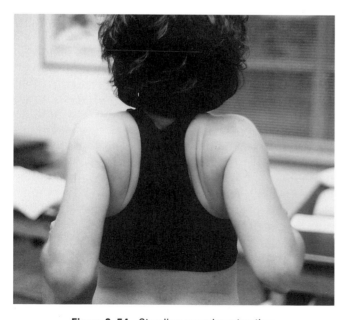

Figure 9–54. Standing scapular retraction.

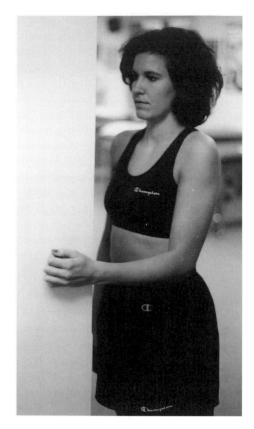

Figure 9–55. Standing isometric internal rotation.

maturation (14 to 15 weeks), progression overhead with AROM, gradual active external rotation to comfort, progression of scapular and rotator cuff routines to moderate to maximal resistance as tolerated, return to weight training following protective guidelines for soft tissue when rotator cuff muscle strength is normal (5 of 5), and continued stabilization training.

Rehabilitation should emphasize (1) scapular and rotator cuff routines in protected ROM; (2) no excessive and passive ROM training; (3) positional avoidance of full external rotation or horizontally abducted position during performance of dips, bench press (see Fig. 9–56), pec deck, and push-ups (achieved by maintaining a narrower grip on the bar); and (4) PNF and other stabilization training.

Phase IV: Return to Function
Goals established for return to activity should include: development of ROM necessary for sports-specific activity, normal strength (5 of 5) in all shoulder musculature, normal proprioception, progressive return to sport-specific training, and protection.

The final phase of rehabilitation should focus on the following: (1) continued strength and conditioning of upper extremity, (2) gradual performance of strength and neuromuscular control enhancing activities in the extremes of motion, as indicated by specific sports,

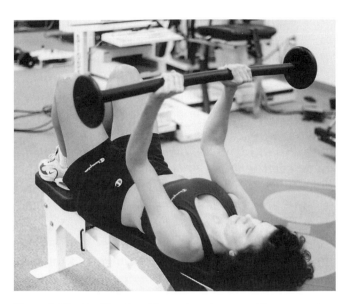

Figure 9–56. Positional avoidance, bench press with narrow grip.

(3) use of a brace or strap to prevent dislocation, and (4) return to sport activities when no apprehension is present in extremes of ROM.

CONSERVATIVE MANAGEMENT OF SHOULDER INSTABILITY

Proper treatment of shoulder instability requires an understanding of the pathophysiology and the classification system, described in this chapter. The appropriate treatment plan and prognosis cannot be defined without such understanding. The success of any rehabilitation program is ultimately dependent upon the ability to correct or control a variety of causal anatomic factors.

Chronic Shoulder Instability

Chronic shoulder instability typically carries an atraumatic etiology, and may present in a volitional or non-volitional manner. Repetitive microtrauma, leading to anterior instability, is commonly seen in the overhead athlete or worker that is younger than 35 years of age. Atraumatic etiology may be the result of congenital anomalies of the glenohumeral joint, systemic disorders, or generalized ligamentous hyperlaxity. This may present as unidirectional, but is most commonly associated with multidirectional instability.

The goal of any rehabilitation program designed to combat shoulder instability is, simply, to optimize shoulder stability. A conservative nonoperative program must attempt to maximize the function of the dynamic stabilizing mechanism. Therefore, the goal of this program is to create increased dynamic stability through a more efficient neuromuscular system to overcome a loss of static shoulder restraints. The functional needs of the patient

must be addressed when designing a treatment plan, however, because the plan will vary significantly between an overhead athlete, who needs normal mobility, and a sedentary elderly individual, who may sacrifice normal mobility for increased stability.

Rehabilitation Principles

Individualized rehabilitation programs differ based on the direction of the chronic instability. Situational avoidance is an essential element in any program, and will differ for each direction of instability. The patient must be well educated to avoid the apprehension position or any position of compromise with activities of daily living, exercise machines, and any and all events that may place undue forces on the restraining structures. Education consists of explaining not only the nature of the problem but also, and more importantly, identifying activities that aggravate symptoms. Unrecognized repetitive microtrauma is often experienced in performance of simple activities of daily living.

In chronic instability cases in which acute symptoms are present, treatment should include general parameters consisting of protected restoration of normal range of motion, submaximal shoulder strengthening to prevent muscle atrophy, and diminution of symptomatic apprehension. Treatment may include rest, anti-inflammatory medication, modality application such as cryotherapy and TENS, active assisted range-of-motion exercises, if indicated, rotator cuff isometrics, and scapular stabilization exercises. Initial treatment may also include brief upper extremity immobilization, which will be symptomatically dictated, but should be avoided if possible.

The prevailing commonality in the management of shoulder instability is the intention of creating adequate strength to aid in dynamic stability. This is achieved through an exercise prescription emphasizing strengthening of the scapular stabilizer muscles, rotator cuff muscles, and the muscles of the total arm. This is not unlike the exercise prescription in the management of shoulder impingement syndrome that was outlined in detail in this chapter. The core rotator cuff and scapular strengthening exercises described previously should be initiated as tolerated. Of utmost importance in the management of instability, is the incorporation of extensive upper extremity stabilization exercises to ensure restoration of neuromuscular control and subsequent stability. Proprioceptive training techniques through reactive neuromuscular training of the upper extremity will aid in dynamic stability of the shoulder. Closed kinetic chain exercises should comprise a strong portion of the program throughout progression, and will provide several advantages in treatment of shoulder instability. First, fixation of the distal end of the extremity creates an axial load and provides a compressive force to the joint, enhancing joint stability and decreasing the tensile stresses to the capsule.

Second, a cocontraction of the scapular stabilizing muscles is created, which further enhances joint stability. The emphasis of the selective rotator cuff strengthening exercises should be placed on endurance training. Creating a more fatigue-resistant group of shoulder muscles is necessary for maintenance of normal shoulder proprioception, which is essential in eliciting muscular reflexes that aid in shoulder joint protection and stabilization.

Rehabilitation for Anterior Glenohumeral Instability

Treatment for anterior instability, as with all shoulder instabilities, should emphasize the rehabilitation principles. Precautions must be taken not to place undesired stress on the static stabilizing structures, in this case, the anterior capsule. Positional avoidance for anterior instability includes excessive external rotation, particularly when the arm is abducted, and positioning of the humerus beyond the plane of the scapula, which may place tension on the anterior capsular structures, and ultimately complicate soft-tissue healing.

Specific joint and soft-tissue mobilization may be indicated to aid in the restoration of normal arthrokinematics. Posterior capsular mobilization should be performed if posterior capsule immobility is present, as this may contribute to anterior instability.

Rehabilitation for Posterior Glenohumeral Instability

Posterior glenohumeral instability is seen less frequently than other shoulder instabilities. It is typically characterized by subjective pain with a follow-through type of motion involving shoulder internal rotation and flexion or horizontal adduction. Subsequently, this is the position of avoidance. In contrast to anterior instability, most weight-bearing exercises must be modified or avoided. Attention must also be given to providing adequate humeral head support when positioned in the supine by using towels or bolsters to prevent posterior humeral head translation. Modification of activities of daily living are necessary as well, including restriction from reaching across the body and weight bearing through the arms.

Rehabilitation for Multidirectional Instability

Multidirectional instability is a condition in which an inferior component of instability will be seen in conjunction with either anterior or posterior instability, or both. Multidirectional instability was thought to have been primarily comprised of the inferior component, and was classified as such by a positive sulcus sign. Multidirectional instability is often associated with generalized ligamentous hyperlaxity.

Components of rehabilitation include those described for anterior and posterior instabilities. Adaptation of the program relates specifically to the inferior component of the instability. Positional avoidance for patients with multidirectional instability include proper support of the arms in a sitting position and avoidance of the arms in the dependent position or overhead with a significant amount of weight in the hands. This minimizes inferior humeral head translation. Multidirectional instability often requires more extensive activity and lifestyle modifications than the other shoulder instabilities.

Exercises emphasizing restoration of dynamic stability are emphasized in the multidirectionally unstable shoulder. All the muscles about the shoulder joint should be addressed, both anteriorly and posteriorly. Utilizing force couples as essential stabilizers will aid in promoting dynamic stability of the shoulder.

General Considerations

Although patients with any form of shoulder instability may benefit from this rehabilitation, it is particularly indicated in patients with the AMBRI syndrome. This rehabilitation program is designed for the chronically unstable shoulder, but may be appropriate for treatment of recurrent shoulder instability as the frequency of primary instability increases. A period of immobilization is more likely to be required in this population, however, than in that with the chronically unstable shoulder. Recurrent instability is the most common complication after primary glenohumeral instability or shoulder dislocation. The recurrence rate is directly related to the pathophysiologic mechanism of injury and to the age of the patient when the primary dislocation occurred. A conservative, nonoperative rehabilitation program may be indicated in such patients.

Operative Management of Shoulder Instability

Surgical stabilization of the glenohumeral joint is considered if instability or apprehension repeatedly compromises shoulder comfort or function, and participation in a well-designed conservative rehabilitation program has failed to diminish symptoms or restore function. In other words, surgery is indicated when instability becomes disability. However, participation in a poorly designed conservative program, or lack of patient compliance to an adequate program, does not qualify a patient as a surgical candidate. Similarly, surgical intervention is not indicated in patients with a desire to voluntarily subluxate or dislocate their shoulder.

Many surgical techniques have been described for the treatment of glenohumeral instability. The operative approach depends on the direction of the instability. Choice of surgical procedure also is dependent on the patient's diagnosis, the extent of pathology present, the surgeon's experience, and the patient's individual activities, expectations, and goals. Regardless of the procedure performed, the goals of each are universal, and include (1) restoration of static glenohumeral stability,

(2) elimination of pain, (3) restoration of adequate range of motion and normal strength, (4) restoration of function, and (5) ability to participate in an aggressive postoperative rehabilitation program.

Overview of Surgical Procedures

Many operative procedures have been described to correct glenohumeral instability. It is beyond the scope of this chapter, however, to explain in detail each of these procedures. Rather, several procedures will be briefly described.

The concept of repairing the capsular and periosteal separation at the anterior glenoid neck, referred to as the Bankart procedure, is directed at reconstitution of the primary static stabilizer of the shoulder, the inferior glenohumeral ligament complex (IGHLC). A Bankart repair is an open surgical procedure for correction of anterior instability that is designed to address the pathologic anatomy of the glenohumeral joint. The Putti-Platt, the Magnuson-Stack, and the Bristow procedures are techniques for restoration of anterior stability, but are designed to create functional restraints that would limit excessive humeral head translation. The Putti-Platt procedure involves division of the subscapularis tendon and capsule medial to the bony insertion. The lateral edge of the tendon and capsule are sutured to the tissue and the labrum at the glenoid rim, while the medial edge is pulled laterally and sutured to the rotator cuff at the greater tuberosity. In the Magnuson-Stack procedure, the subscapularis tendon and lateral capsule is transferred downward and outward to a position lateral to the bicipital groove, just below the greater tuberosity. The Bristow procedure involves transfer of the tip of the coracoid with the conjoined tendon to the inferior aspect of the glenoid rim, creating a bone block to restrict translation.

Arthroscopic techniques offer the advantage of less perioperative pain and morbidity, but have a higher risk of recurrence than open procedures. Methods of arthroscopic stabilization employ either sutures that are passed through drill holes in the glenoid neck and tied posteriorly, or the use of a biodegradable tac, to anatomically repair the anterior band of the IGHLC by advancing the anterior band superiorly, thereby removing any laxity from the axillary pouch.

A common surgical technique for correction of posterior instability is the posterior capsular shift. The open procedure is performed through a posterior approach involving detachment of the deltoid and infraspinatus muscles. The capsular shift employs anchor sutures that are passed through drill holes in the humerus, then through the capsule for attachment. The superior part of the capsule is shifted inferiorly.

Multidirectional instability is corrected similarly, with a capsular shift designed to reduce the volume of the glenohumeral joint anteriorly, posteriorly, and inferi-

orly by equalizing capsular tightness on all three sides. It is the decision of the surgeon whether an anterior or posterior approach should be taken, but is most often on the side with the greatest instability. The inferior capsular shift procedure is performed by pulling the inferior capsular flap upward to eliminate the inferior redundancy of the capsule and reattaching it to the soft tissue on the lesser tuberosity. The upper flap is then pulled downward and sutured to the humerus.

Postoperative Rehabilitation of Shoulder Instability

The guidelines of a postoperative rehabilitation program are dictated by the time constraints of tissue healing. Communication between the surgeon and the therapist is essential for appropriate postoperative management. Healing constraints must be backed by scientific, physiologic rationale, and may vary by several weeks or months. Additionally, detail must be given to the biomechanical analysis of each activity in an exercise prescription so as not to create unwanted tension on and risk compromise of the surgical repair.

The postoperative rehabilitation program should be a comprehensive approach that, like other programs outlined in this chapter, consists four phases, each of which consists of criteria-based objectives to determine rate of progression. The dissimilarity of this program from previous programs is that the rehabilitation program's progression is initially time-based in principle to allow adequate tissue healing, and ultimately adequate glenohumeral stability.

Phase I: Maximum Protection Phase
Based on physiological healing principles, the initial phase of rehabilitation is dictated by the properties of the specific tissue involved. During this phase, which may last several months depending on the procedure performed, the goals of rehabilitation include easing discomfort and symptom reduction, maintaining joint mobility within prescribed limitations, preventing muscular atrophy, and patient education on activity modification. Treatment techniques of choice include those previously outlined, but must not in any way compromise the integrity of the surgical repair. Active assisted range-of-motion techniques must incorporate positional avoidance. Grade I joint mobilization may be indicated for pain relief, but must be performed within the limitations of range of motion. Submaximal rotator cuff and scapular muscle isometric exercises should be initiated to combat muscular atrophy. A prescription of rest and anti-inflammatory medication should be initiated immediately postoperative.

Phase II: Tissue Maturation Phase
As the surgical repair continues to heal and maturation occurs, the postoperative program should progress ac-

cordingly. Progression into this phase is dictated by tissue healing properties, but certain criteria should be met prior to this time. Improvements in level of pain, range of motion, and shoulder muscle strength should be noted. Goals of this phase include restoration of normal range of motion if appropriate, improvements in strength, and diminution of pain. Normal glenohumeral arthrokinematics should be restored. An improved ability to perform routine activities of daily living should accompany the achievement of these goals.

In this phase, range-of-motion exercises will be advanced from gentle to aggressive as tolerated, as will strengthening exercises for the rotator cuff, scapular stabilizers, and the muscles of the total arm.

Phase III: Selective Strengthening Phase

Progression into this phase indicates the structural integrity of the surgical repair is adequate, pain is indistinguishable, and range of motion has normalized (or functionalized). Core rotator cuff and scapular stabilizer exercises should be initiated to patient tolerance, just as indicated in conservative management. Postoperative rehabilitation during this phase should incorporate the principles described previously, including muscle endurance training, the recruitment of force couples, the performance of closed kinetic chain exercises, as well as reactive neuromuscular training and proprioceptive training to aid in glenohumeral joint stability.

Phase IV: Return to Function

The patient's ultimate return to function is dependent on achievement of goal-related performance criteria. Restoration of functional range of motion, strength, endurance, and neuromuscular control are precursors to the patient's return to function. The criteria must be specific to include activities in which the patient will participate, whether activities of daily living, occupational, or athletic.

General Considerations

The length of the rehabilitation program is dictated by the degree of instability. The course of recovery is directly related to the severity of the instability. Other factors that influence recovery and return to function are the type of instability, acute versus chronic, the patient's range of motion and strength status, and the specific performance and activity demands of the patient, not to mention the level of patient compliance.

SUGGESTED READING

Bankart ASB. Recurrent or habitual dislocation of the shoulder joint. *Br Med J*. 1923;2:1132.

Bigliani LU. Anterior and posterior capsular shift for multidirectional instability. In: *Techniques in Orthopaedics*. Rockville, MD: Aspen; 1989.

Bigliani LU, Kimmel J, McCann PD, Wolf I. Repair of rotator cuff tears in tennis players. *Am J Sports Med*. 1992;20:112.

Bigliani LU, Morrison DS, April EW. The morphology of the acromion and its relationship to rotator cuff tears. *Orthop Trans*. 1986;10:216.

Brown LP, Niehues SL, Harrah A, et al. Upper extremity range of motion and isokinetic strength of the internal and external shoulder rotators in major league baseball players. *Am J Sports Med*. 1988;16:577.

Caspari R, Savoie F. Arthroscopic reconstruction of the shoulder: The Bankart repair. In: McGinty J, et al., eds. *Operative Arthroscopy*. New York: Raven; 1991.

Cofield RH. Current concepts review: Rotator cuff disease of the shoulder. *J Bone Joint Surg*. 1985;67A:974.

Cofield RH, Simonet WT. Symposium on sports medicine. Part 2, the shoulder in sports. *Mayo Clin Proc*. 1984;59:157.

Dines DM, Levinson M. The conservative management of the unstable shoulder including rehabilitation. *Clin Sports Med*. 1995;14:797.

Emery RJH, Mullaji AB. Glenohumeral joint instability in normal adolescents: Incidence and significance. *J Bone Joint Surg*. 1991;73B:406.

Engle RP, Canner GC. Posterior shoulder instability: Approach to rehabilitation. *J Orthop Sports Phys Ther*. 1989;10:488.

Fowler P. Swimmer problems. *Am J Sports Med*. 1979;7:141.

Fu HF, Harner CD, Klein AH. Shoulder impingement syndrome: A critical review. *Clin Orthop*. 1991;269:162.

Harryman DT, Sidles JA, Clark JM, McQuade KJ. Translation of the humeral head on the glenoid with passive glenohumeral motion. *J Bone Joint Surg*. 1990;72A:1334.

Harryman DT, Sidles JA, Harris SL, Matsen FA. Role of the rotator interval capsule in passive motion and stability of the shoulder. *J Bone Joint Surg*. 1990;72A:53.

Hawkins RJ. Surgical management of rotator cuff tears. In: Bateman JE, Welsh RP, eds. *Surgery of the Shoulder*. Philadelphia: Dekker; 1984.

Hawkins RJ, Kennedy JC. Impingement syndrome in athletes. *Am J Sports Med*. 1980;8:151.

Helfet AJ. Coracoid transplantation for recurring dislocation of the shoulder. *J Bone Joint Surg*. 1948;40B:198.

Jobe FW, Giangarra CE, Kvitne RS, et al. Anterior capsulolabral reconstruction of the shoulder in athletes in overhand sports. *Am J Sports Med*. 1991;19:428.

Jobe FW, Moynes DR. Delineation of diagnostic criteria and a rehabilitation program for rotator cuff injuries. *Am J Sports Med*. 1982;10:336.

Jobe FW, Moynes DR, Brewster CE. Rehabilitation of shoulder joint instabilities. *Orthop Clin North Am*. 1987;18:473.

Johnston TB. The movements of the shoulder joint. A plea for the use of the "plane of the scapula" as the plane of reference for movements occurring at the humeri-scapular joint. *Br J Surg*. 1937;25:252.

Kaada B. Vasolidation induced by transcutaneous nerve stimulation in peripheral ischemia. *Eur Heart J*. 1983;3:303.

Keirns MA. Conservative management of shoulder impingement. In: Andrews JR, Wilk KE, eds. *The Athlete's Shoulder*. New York: Churchill Livingstone; 1994.

Kerlan RK, Jobe FW, Blazina ME, et al. Throwing injuries of the shoulder and elbow in adults. In: Ahrstrom JP Jr, ed. *Current Practice in Orthopedic Surgery*. St. Louis: Mosby; 1975.

Matsen FA, Arntz CT. Subacromial impingement. In: Rockwood CA, Matsen FA, eds. *The Shoulder*. Philadelphia: Saunders; 1990.

Matsen FA, Thomas SC, Rockwood CA. Anterior glenohumeral instability: In: Rockwood CA, Matsen FA, eds. *The Shoulder*. Philadelphia: Saunders; 1990.

Michlovitz SL. Cryotherapy: The use of cold as a therapeutic agent. In: Michlovitz SI, ed. *Thermal Agents in Rehabilitation*. Philadelphia: Davis; 1990.

Morgan CD. Arthroscopic transglenoid Bankart suture repair. *Operative Tech Orthop*. 1991;1:171.

Morrison DS. Conservative management of partial-thickness rotator cuff lesions. In: Burkhead WZ, ed. *Rotator Cuff Disorders*. Baltimore: Williams & Wilkins; 1996.

Mosely JB, Jobe FW, Pink M, et al. EMG analysis of the scapular muscles during a shoulder rehabilitation program. *Am J Sports Med*. 1992;20:220.

Neer CS. *Shoulder Reconstruction*. Philadelphia: Saunders; 1990.

Neer CS. Impingement lesions. *Clin Orthop*. 1983;173:70.

Neer CS. Anterior acromioplasty for the chronic impingement syndrome in the shoulder. A preliminary report. *J Bone Joint Surg*. 1972;54A:41.

Neer CS, Welsh RP. The shoulder in sports. *Orthop Clin North Am*. 1977;8:583.

Neviaser TJ, Nevaiser RJ, Nevaiser JS, Nevaiser JS. The four-in-one arthroplasty for the painful arc syndrome. *Clin Orthop*. 1982;163:107.

Norwood LA, Terry GC. Shoulder posterior subluxation. *Am J Sports Med*. 1984;12:25.

O'Brien SJ, Pagnani MJ, et al. Anterior instability of the shoulder. In: Andrews JR, Wilk KE, eds. *The Athlete's Shoulder*. New York: Churchill Livingstone; 1994.

Pappas AM, Zawacki RM, McCarthy CF. Rehabilitation of the pitching shoulder. *Am J Sports Med*. 1985;13:223.

Pappas AM, Zawacki RM, Sullivan TJ. Biochemanics of baseball pitching. A preliminary report. *Am J Sports Med*. 1985;13:216.

Peterson L, Renstrom P. *Sports Injuries: Their Prevention and Treatment*. Chicago: Year Book; 1986.

Reed B, Zarro V. Inflammation and repair and the use of thermal agents. In: Michlovitz SL, ed. *Thermal Agents in Rehabilitation*. Philadelphia: Davis; 1990.

Regan WD, Webster-Bogaert S, Hawkins RJ, Fowler PJ. Comparative functional analysis of the Bristow, Magnuson-Stack, and Putti-Platt procedures for recurrent dislocation of the shoulder. *Am J Sports Med*. 1989;17:42.

Richardson AB, Jobe FW, Collins HR. The shoulder in competitive swimming. *Am J Sports Med*. 1980;8:159.

Rowe CR, Patel D, Southmayd WW. The Bankart procedure: A long term end-result study. *J Bone Joint Surg*. 1978;60A:1.

Sutter JS. Conservative treatment of shoulder instability. In: Andrews JR, Wilk KE, eds. *The Athlete's Shoulder*. New York: Churchill Livingstone; 1994.

Swiontkowski M, Ionnotti JP, Bolts JH, et al. Inappropriate assessment of rotator cuff vascularity using laser Doppler flowmetry. In: Post M, Morrey B, Hawkins RJ, eds. *Surgery of the Shoulder*. St. Louis: Mosley-Year Book; 1990:208–212.

Townsend H, Jobe FW, Pink M, Perry J. EMG analysis of the glenohumeral muscles during a baseball rehabilitation program. *Am J Sports Med*. 1991;19:264.

Voight ML, Hardin JA, Blackburn TA, et al. The effects of muscle fatigue on and the relationship of arm dominance to shoulder proprioception. *J Orthop Sports Phys Ther*. 1996;23:348.

Warner JJP, Lyle JM. Flexibility, laxity, and strength in normal shoulders and shoulders with instability and impingement. *Am J Sports Med*. 1990;18:366.

Wilk KE, Andrews JR. Rehabilitation following arthroscopic shoulder subacromial decompression. *Orthopedics*. 1993;16:349.

Yahiro MA, Matthews LA. Arthroscopic stabilization procedures for recurrent anterior shoulder instability. *Orthop Rev*. 1989;11:1161.

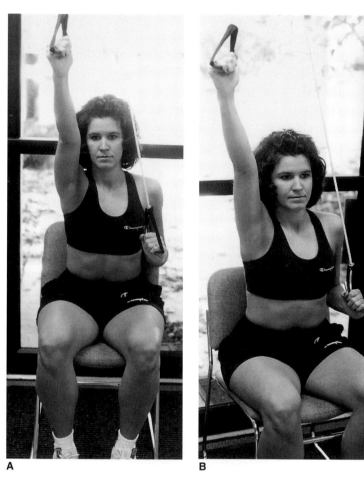
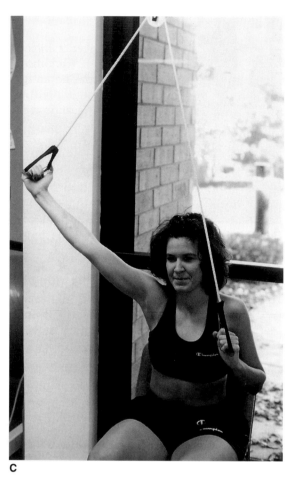

Figure 9–62. Rope and pulley exercise. **A**. Flexion. **B**. Abduction in POS. **C**. Abduction.

middle trapezius muscle (see Fig. 9-67). Rowing is performed by both arms pulling against resistance towards the body while simultaneously pinching the shoulder blades together in order to work the rhomboid muscles (see Fig. 9-68). The seated press-up or sitting dip exercises the pectoralis minor muscle (see Fig. 9-69).

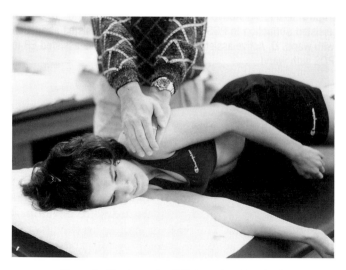

Figure 9–63. Scapular PNF (anterior elevation).

Blackburn described the core exercises for the rotator cuff musculature. Prone horizontal abduction is the strongest EMG position for the supraspinatus muscle (see Fig. 9-70). Prone external rotation at 90 degrees of abduction was the strongest EMG position for the infraspinatus muscle (see Fig. 9-71). Prone extension works the teres major muscle (see Fig. 9-72).

There are many options available to the athletic trainer or physical therapist for resistive exercise training: manual resistance, water, rubber tubing, weights, and isokinetics. While there is no right method to strength training, any one form may be wrong for a specific patient. The key to the selection process is the experience of the clinician and constant reevaluation of the patient.

All resistance exercises are progressed at the patient's own rate. Initially, the resistance program begins with no resistance until proper technique has been achieved. Following this, incremental loading is used to progressively load the healing tissues. For most of the exercises, resistance is kept low (1 to 3 pounds) to prevent substitution of the larger muscles for the commonly involved rotator cuff muscles. Any exercise that seems to aggravate the shoulder should be modified or discontinued.

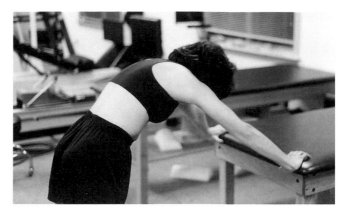

Figure 9–66. Push-up with scapular protraction ("push-up with a plus").

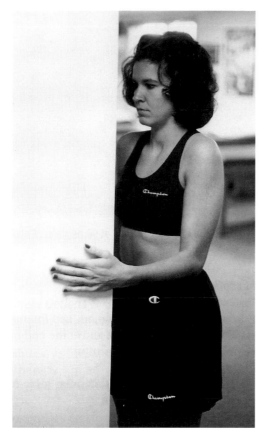

Figure 9–64. Isometric internal rotation.

Goals

- Decrease pain and inflammation.
- Increase shoulder flexibility—full pain-free AROM.
- Proprioception deficit less than 30 percent (shoulder ER) by end of phase.

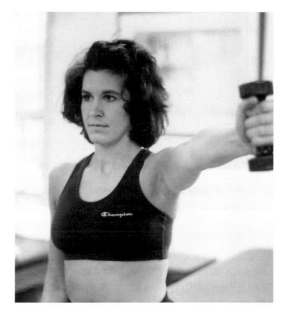

Figure 9–67. Scaption.

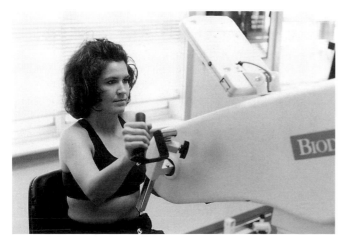

Figure 9–65. Upper body ergometer.

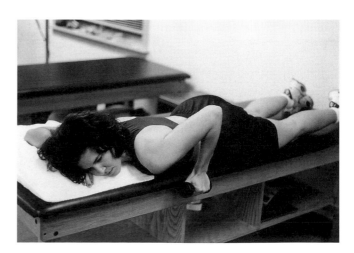

Figure 9–68. Rowing.

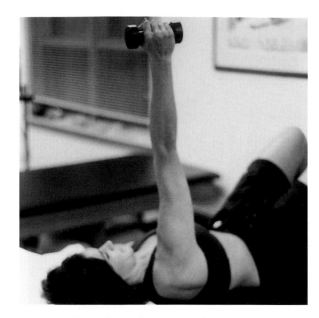

Figure 9–77. Supine scapular rotation.

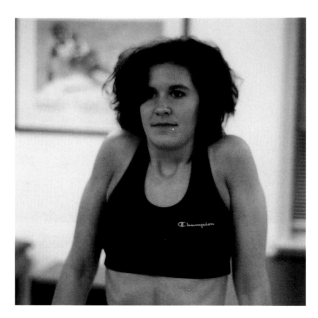

Figure 9–79. Standing scapular elevation ("shrugs").

- BTE Right Weigh deficit less than 30 percent
- Isokinetic strength deficit below 30 percent

Phase Three (Advanced Strengthening Phase)

The main goal of phase III rehabilitation is to prepare the shoulder for high-velocity ballistic concentric and eccentric stresses encountered in the return to activity phase. Once the patient is able to contract and control the synchrony of all glenohumeral and scapulothoracic musculature, has demonstrated complete flexibility, and has full range of motion, an activity specific strengthening program may begin. The basic cornerstone of this phase is the law of specificity, or the principle of specific adaptions to imposed demands (SAID). This requires that the treating therapist or trainer have a good understanding of the biomechanics of the sport and be creative with the rehabilitation program to help patients achieve their ultimate goal.

Remember that many of the injuries commonly seen about the shoulder are caused by excessive loads on the musculotendinous junctions and ligamentous tissues. After the tissue is repaired or healed, which usually occurs during phases I and II, the capacity for these tissues to handle high-velocity loads must be regained during phase III. Therefore, the focus of this phase's exercises are to progressively increase the eccentric and concentric capacity of the shoulder.

Goals

- Pain: No complaint of pain throughout ROM.
- No effusion present.
- Full pain-free ROM (both active and passive).
- Proprioceptive deficit less than 20 percent by end of phase.
- BTE motor control deficit less than 20 percent by end of phase.
- Acuvision 1000 hand–eye coordination deficit less than 20 percent by end of phase.
- Strength deficits less than 20 percent by end of phase.
- No complaints of palpable tenderness.

Clinical Examination

- Visual analog pain scale
- Pain: Location, quality, duration, and intensity. Evaluate pain throughout ROM and at the end ranges
- General history and observation
  Muscle hypertrophy
  Scapular winging (lateral scapular glide test)
  Scapular/humeral rhythm
- Range of motion: Should have full AROM and PROM
- Strength testing: Bilateral isokinetic comparison 180 and 300 degrees (IR/ER)

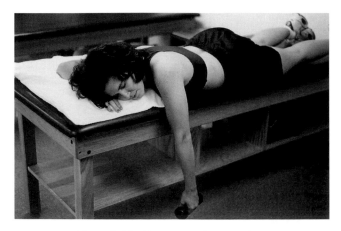

Figure 9–78. Prone scapular retraction.

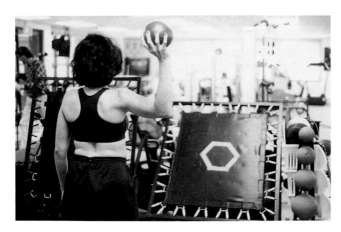

Figure 9–80. Plyoback testing.

- Proprioception testing: ER reposition sense (both active and passive)
- BTE Right Weigh motor control test: ER/IR, PNF D2 diagonal
- Acuvision 1000 hand-eye coordination test: Bilateral comparison of tracking and reaction/transit times
- Plyoback test: Determine accuracy of upper quarter motion. Patient stands back from wall/plyoback 2 1/2 times arm length. Plyoball (1#) is tossed at a 6-inch target for a 30-second time period. At the end of 30 seconds the number of repetitions in the circle will be counted. (Index = number thrown/number in circle × 100; see Fig. 9–80.)

Clinical Treatment Options
- Reduce pain, edema/inflammation, and muscle spasm

Modalities, as indicated
  Cryotherapy
  Joint mobilization: Grade I oscillations
  NSAIDs
- ROM exercises: Self-stretching to maintain shoulder mobility
- Strengthening exercises
  Scapulothoracic neuromuscular control exercises: Protraction/retraction and elevation/depression
  Isotonic prime mover strengthening: Military press, bench press, lateral raises
  Tubing drills: IR/ER, scapular exercises, diagonals
  Impulse inertial exercise program (see Fig. 9–81)
  Acuvision 1000 hand-eye coordination training program (see Fig. 9–82)
  Isokinetic glenohumeral strengthening (IR/ER): Velocity spectrum training (180 by 300 degrees/second)
  Manual resistance exercises—magic three program (three positions, three exercises, three sets): Supine = D1, D2, scapular protraction; prone = scapular retraction, hori abduction, ER; and seated = scaption, shrug, press-up
  Plyometric program (see Fig. 9–83)
    Wall push-ups
    Underhand throws
    Chest throws
  Elbow/wrist isotonic strengthening
- Cocontraction stabilization exercises
  Body blade (see Fig. 9–84)
  Floor exercises (begin with feet on the floor and progress to an unstable surface)

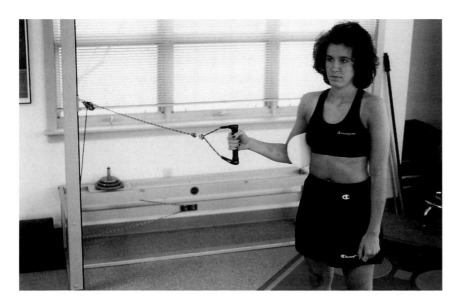

Figure 9–81. Impulse initial training.

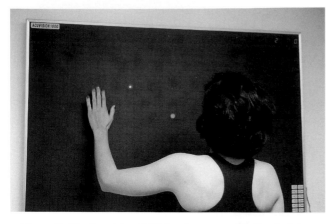

Figure 9–82. Acuvision 1000 hand–eye coordination training.

Gymnastic ball (see Fig. 9–85)
- Proprioceptive exercises: Joint repositioning drills
- Cardiovascular training
  Upper body ergometry
  Bicycling
  Stairmaster/treadmill

Criteria to Progress to Phase IV
- No pain on visual analog scale
- No increased complaint of pain with activity
- Strength deficit less than 20 percent
- BTE motor control deficit less than 20 percent
- Acuvision 1000 hand–eye coordination deficit less than 20 percent
- Proprioception deficit less than 20 percent

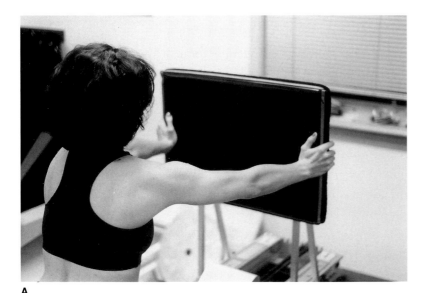

A

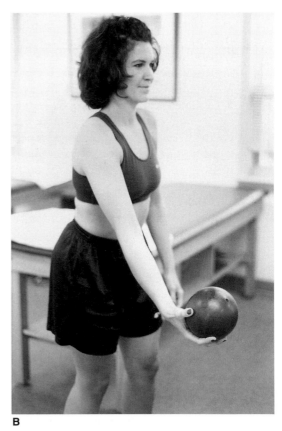

B

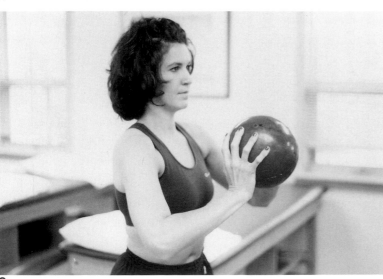

C

Figure 9–83. A. Plyometric wall push-up. **B**. Plyometric underhand throws. **C**. Plyometric chest throws.

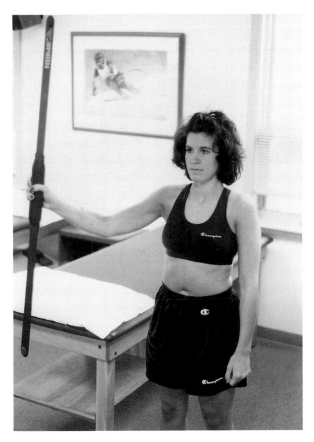

Figure 9–84. Body blade exercise.

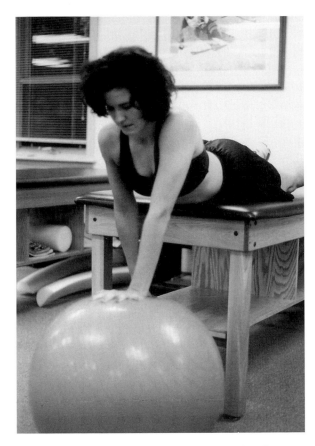

Figure 9–85. Stabilization with gymnastic ball.

Phase Four (Return to Activity Phase)

The main focus of phase IV rehabilitation is preparation of the patient to return to activity. The most important aspect of phase IV rehabilitation is the progressive return to ADL and sports. The critical step from rehabilitation to normal performance should be closely supervised.

Goals (for Return to Full Activity)

- No complaint of pain throughout the ROM.
- No effusion present.
- Full pain-free functional activity-specific ROM.
- Strength equal bilaterally (note: strength levels are dependent upon ADL).
- BTE motor control deficit less than 10 percent.
- Acuvision 1000 hand–eye coordination deficit less than 10 percent.
- Proprioception deficit less than 10 percent.
- Activity-specific tests WNL (within normal limits).

Clinical Examination

- Visual analog pain scale
- Pain: Location, quality, duration, and intensity. Evaluate pain throughout ROM and at the end ranges
- General history and observation
  Muscle hypertrophy
  Scapular winging (lateral scapular glide test)
  Scapular humeral rhythm
- Range of motion: Should have full AROM and PROM. Perform functional ROM tests to ensure that the patient can go through the entire ROM that will be utilized during activity.
- Strength testing: Bilateral isokinetic comparison 180 by 300 degrees (ER/IR)
- Proprioception testing: ER reposition sense (both active and passive)
- BTE Right Weigh motor control test: ER/IR, PNF D2 diagonal
- Acuvision 1000 hand–eye coordination test
- Plyoback test

Clinical Treatment Options

- Reduce pain, edema/inflammation, and muscle spasm
    - None should be noted during this phase
    - May need to control postexercise PRN
- ROM exercises: The patient should have full pain-free ROM at this time
- Strengthening exercises
    - Scapulothoracic neuromuscular control exercises: Protraction/retraction and elevation/depression
    - Isotonic prime mover strengthening: military press, bench press, lateral raises
    - Tubing drills: IR/ER, scapular exercises, diagonals
    - Acuvision 1000 hand–eye coordination training program
    - Impulse inertial exercise program
    - Isokinetic strengthening: IR/ER and PNF D2 diagonal, velocity spectrum training (180 by 300)
    - Manual resistance exercises—magic three program (three positions, three exercises, three sets): Supine = D1, D2, scapular protraction; prone = scapular retraction, hori abduction, ER; and seated = scaption, shrug, press-up
    - Plyometric program: Push-ups, plyoback exercises
    - Elbow/wrist isotonic strengthening
- Cocontraction stabilization exercises
    - Body blade
    - Floor exercises (begin with feet on the floor and progress to an unstable surface)
    - Gymnastic ball
- Proprioceptive exercises: Joint repositioning drills
- Cardiovascular training
    - Upper body ergometry
    - Bicycling
    - Stairmaster/treadmill
- Initiate interval return to sports/ADL program. Activity-specific exercises should be initiated as well as tested throughout this phase. The patient should have no difficulty or increased complaints of pain following these exercises

Criteria to Return to ADL

- No pain on visual analog scale
- No increased complaint of pain with activity
- Strength deficits WNL bilaterally
- BTE motor control deficits WNL bilaterally
- Acuvision 1000 hand–eye coordination deficit WNL bilaterally
- Proprioception deficits WNL bilaterally

CONCLUSION

The unique demands placed upon the shoulder put it at a high risk for both overuse and overloading of the soft tissues of the shoulder girdle. Tremendous stresses and angular velocities are generated about the shoulder girdle. The rehabilitation provider must have knowledge of these increased stresses and strains. This increased knowledge will aid in the recognition, prevention, and treatment of injury. In the past several years, the knowledge base has been increased, thereby changing the treatment of shoulder injuries dramatically.

This chapter discussed the basic principles of shoulder rehabilitation. The rehabilitation of the shoulder should begin with a thorough evaluation of the entire shoulder girdle followed by an eclectic approach to the treatment plan. The rehabilitation process must have a basic and clinical science basis for the application.

SUGGESTED READING

Albert M. *Eccentric Muscle Training in Sports and Orthopaedics.* New York: Churchill Livingstone; 1991.

Andrews JR, Wilk KE, eds. *The Athlete's Shoulder.* New York: Churchill Livingstone; 1994.

Blackburn TA, McLeod WD, White B, Wofford L. EMG analysis of posterior rotator cuff exercises. *Athletic Training.* 1990;25:41.

Burkhead WZ, ed. *Rotator Cuff Disorders.* Baltimore: Williams & Wilkins; 1996.

Burkhead WZ Jr, Rockwood CA Jr. Treatment of instability of the shoulder with an exercise program. *J Bone Joint Surg.* 1992;74A:890.

Davies GJ. *A Compendium of Isokinetics in Clinical Usage and Rehabilitation Techniques.* 4th ed. Onalaska, WI: S&S Publishers; 1992.

Davies GJ, Dickoff-Hoffman S. Neuromuscular testing and rehabilitation of the shoulder complex. *J Orthop Sports Phys Ther.* 1993;18:449.

Dillman CJ, Fleisig GS, Werner SL, Andrews JR. Biomechanics of the shoulder in sports-throwing activities. *Forum Med.* 1991;4:1–9.

Donatelli RA, Wooden MJ. Mobilization of the shoulder. In: Donatelli RA, ed. *Physical Therapy of the Shoulder.* 2nd ed. New York: Churchill Livingstone; 1991.

Greenfield BH, Donatelli RA, Wooden MJ, Wilkens J. Isokinetic evaluation of shoulder rotational strength between plane of scapula and functional plane. *Am J Sports Med.* 1990; 18:124.

Harryman DT, Sidles JA, Clark JM, McQuade KJ. Translation of the humeral head on the glenoid with passive glenohumeral motion. *J Bone Joint Surg.* 1990;72A:1334.

Harryman DT, Sidles JA, Harris SL, Matsen FA. Role of the rotator interval capsule in passive motion and stability of the shoulder. *J Bone Joint Surg.* 1990;72A:53.

Hawkins RJ. Basic science and clinical application in the athlete's shoulder. *Clin Sports Med.* 1991;10:4.

Hawkins RJ, Kennedy JC. Impingement syndrome in athletes. *Am J Sports Med*. 1990;8:151.

Howell SM, Inobersteg AM, Seger OH, et al. Clarification of the role of the supraspinatus muscle in shoulder function. *J Bone Joint Surg*. 1986;68A:398.

Jobe FW, Mones DR, Tibone JE, Perry J. An EMG analysis of the shoulder in pitching: A second report. *Am J Sports Med*. 1984;12:218.

Keirns MA. Conservative management of shoulder impingement. In: Andrews JR, Wilk KE, eds. *The Athlete's Shoulder*. New York: Churchill Livingstone; 1994.

Kibler BW. Role of the scapula in the overhead throwing motion. *Contemp Orthop*. 1991;22:525.

Matsen FA, Harryman DI, Sildes JA. Mechanics of glenohumeral instability. *Clin Sports Med*. 1991;10:786.

Mosely JB, Jobe FW, Pink M, et al. EMG analysis of the scapular muscles during a shoulder rehabilitation program. *Am J Sports Med*. 1992;20:220.

Paine RM, Voight M. The role of the scapula. *J Orthop Sports Phys Ther*. 1993;18:386.

Palmittier RA, An KN, Scott SG, et al. Kinetic chain exercise in knee rehabilitation. *Sports Med*. 1991;11:402.

Rockwood CA, Matsen FA, eds. *The Shoulder*. Philadelphia: Saunders; 1990.

Saha AK. Mechanics of elevation of glenohumeral joint: Its application in rehabilitation of flail shoulder in upper brachial plexus injuries and poliomyelitis and in replacement of the upper humerus by prosthesis. *Acta Orthop Scand*. 1973; 44:668.

Saha AK. Dynamic stability of the glenohumeral joint. *Acta Orthop Scand*. 1971;42:491.

Steindler A. *Kinesiology of the Human Body Under Normal and Pathological Conditions*. Springfield, IL: Thomas; 1955.

Tippett SR. Closed chain exercises. *Orthop Phys Ther Clin North Am*. 1992;1:253.

Townsend H, Jobe FW, Pink M, Perry J. EMG analysis of the glenohumeral muscles during a baseball rehabilitation program. *Am J Sports Med*. 1991;19:264.

Voight ML, Hardin JA, Blackburn TA, et al. The effects of muscle fatigue on and the relationship of arm dominance to shoulder proprioception. *J Orthop Sports Phys Ther*. 1996; 23:348.

Wilk KE. Current concepts in the rehabilitation of athletic shoulder injuries. In: Andrews JR, Wilk KE, eds. *The Athlete's Shoulder*. New York: Churchill Livingstone; 1994.

Wilk KE, Arrigo CA. An integrated approach to upper extremity exercises. In: Timm KE, ed. *Orthop Clin North Am*. 1992;9:337.

Wilk KE, Arrigo CA, Andrews JR. Standardized isokinetic testing protocol for the throwing shoulder. The thrower's series. *Isokin Exerc Sci*. 1991;1:63.

Wilk KE, Voight ML, Keirns, et al. Stretch-shortening drills for the upper extremities: Theory and clinical application. *J Orthop Sports Phys Ther*. 1993;17:225.

Wyke B. Articular neurology—a review. *Physiotherapy*. 1972;58:94.

Chapter 10

The Elbow

Athletic Injuries of the Elbow

Pietro M. Tonino

Injuries of the elbow are common in both young and old athletes. Most injuries are due to repetitive microtrauma and are often amenable to conservative treatment. Acute injuries, such as fractures and dislocations, occur most frequently in certain sports such as a gymnastics and wrestling.[1] These injuries can cause permanent damage in young patients and proper initial treatment is critical.

ANATOMY

The elbow is a hinge joint, and unlike the shoulder, has a bony architecture that makes instability problems relatively uncommon. Anatomic studies of the elbow have shown that in extension the bony anatomy is responsible for most of the stability of the elbow. This consists of the distal humerus, the proximal ulna, and the proximal radius.

The function of the ligaments, particularly the medial collateral ligament, is to provide stability when the elbow is in the flexed position. The medial (ulnar) collateral is the primary ligamentous stabilizer of the elbow.[2] The medial ligament consists of an anterior and posterior portion. The anterior component of the ligament is responsible for most of the ability of this ligament to resist valgus stress (see Fig. 10-1).[3]

The medial and lateral epicondyle are the sites of origin of the flexors and extensors of the forearm. The origin of the flexor pronator mass at the medial epicondyle is closely related to the humeral attachment of the ulnar collateral ligament. The medial muscles, by virtue of their location, protect the ulnar collateral during activities that stress this ligament, such as valgus stress.[4]

The elbow neurovascular anatomy consists of numerous nerves and blood vessels that supply the forearm and the hand. Injuries of the elbow may cause injuries to these structures, particularly the ulnar and median nerves, and may cause permanent damage to the arm (see Fig. 10-2).

MECHANISM OF INJURY

Most injuries of the elbow are due to repetitive microtrauma. Overuse can cause tendinitis or may eventually lead to ligamentous injuries of the elbow.

The throwing motion places the elbow in a valgus position that tenses the medial collateral ligament and causes compression of the radiocapitellar joint (see Fig. 10-3). Overuse may cause rupture of the medial collateral ligament and osteochondral injuries of the capitellum.

Tendinitis occurs from repetitive use of the elbow and occurs most often on the lateral side of the elbow. Tennis players are particularly prone to lateral epicondylitis, while medial epicondylitis is more common in golfers.

Acute injuries of the elbow are less common but can be quite serious. Fractures, particularly in young patients with open growth plates, can cause permanent problems

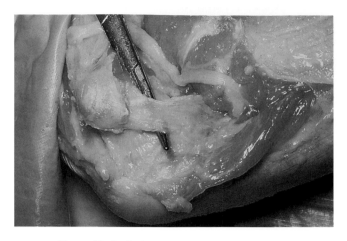

Figure 10–1. Cadaveric ulnar collateral ligament.

such as growth deformities. The numerous nerves and blood vessels of the elbow region can potentially be damaged by fractures of the elbow.

Dislocations of the elbow are uncommon but not rare. These types of injuries occur most in gymnastics and wrestling, and require immediate medical attention.

LATERAL EPICONDYLITIS

Lateral epicondylitis (tennis elbow) is a common source of elbow pain.[5-7] The name itself is really a misnomer since the condition involves a tendinitis of the forearm extensors. This condition presents with pain and tenderness along the lateral aspect of the elbow, centered at the lateral epicondyle. Patients may complain that the pain radiates upward toward the shoulder and distally into the forearm. This condition may initially be present during or after athletic activities such as tennis, but as the tendinitis worsens, pain can be felt during activities of daily living. Simple tasks such as lifting a gallon of milk or turning a doorknob may become difficult. Lateral epicondylitis can also occur from repetitive activities at home or work and is common in women between 40 and 50 years of age.[8,9]

Tennis elbow results from repetitive microtrauma at the site of origin of the forearm extensors. The extensor carpi radialis brevis origin is the most common tendon involved. The tennis grip and stroke require extensive use of the forearm extensors. These muscles function to grasp the racquet and hold it firmly during the tennis stroke. The extensors become injured as the muscles fatigue due to repetitive activity.

Improper technique is also a common cause of lateral epicondylitis. Patients who develop a tennis elbow typically hit their backhand shots with a "leading elbow" and do not follow through with their backhand stroke (see Fig. 10-4). This is thought to cause excessive stress

at the lateral epicondyle and abnormal activity of the forearm musculature.[10,11]

Lateral epicondylitis may occur due to improper equipment. The size of the grip of the racquet should be chosen carefully and should be customized to the size of the athlete's hand. The tension of the racquet strings should also be measured to ensure that it is appropriate for the athlete.

Patients with lateral epicondylitis have point tenderness at the lateral epicondyle. Athletes with this condition point to this area as the area of maximal discomfort (see Fig. 10-5). This must be distinguished from posterior interosseous nerve entrapment syndrome that presents with tenderness distal to the lateral epicondyle (see Fig. 10-6). Pain is elicited by having the patient attempt to elevate the arm while grasping the examiner's fingers with the elbow fully extended and the forearm in maxi-

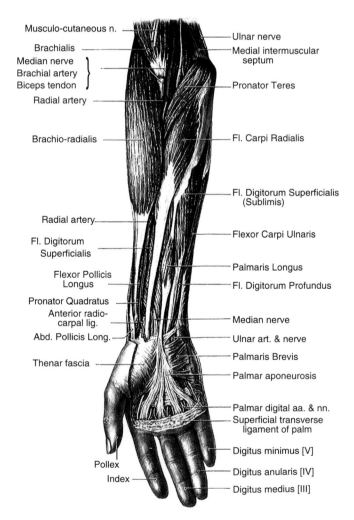

Figure 10–2. Drawing showing the ulnar and median nerves and the superficial muscles of the front of the forearm. *(From Anderson JE. Grant's Atlas of Anatomy. 7th ed. Baltimore: Williams & Wilkins; 1978. With permission.)*

Patients with this syndrome may present with moderately severe pain that is chronic and has not responded to oral medication. Injections are very helpful in this group of patients and provide dramatic relief of pain. Local anesthetic is combined with an injectable anti-inflammatory agent. It is injected at the point of maximal tenderness (see Fig. 10-8).[12] Patients who have received injections may experience severe pain within a few hours following their injection. This occurs when the local anesthetic loses its effectiveness. Patients who are injected should be forewarned that this may occur and should be instructed to apply ice to the affected area. Physicians may routinely provide patients with prescriptions for oral analgesics following injections for lateral epicondylitis.

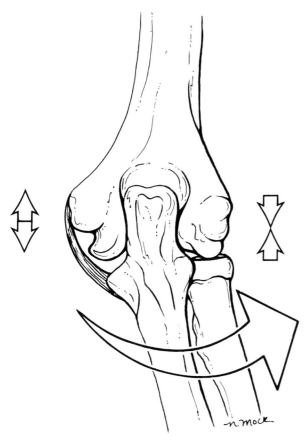

Figure 10–3. Traction of the median collateral ligament and compression of the radiocapitellar joint during the throwing motion.

mal pronation (see Fig. 10-7). The examiner attempts to resist the elevation of the forearm. This pain is differentiated from that in patients with posterior interosseous syndrome, where pain is elicited by attempting to resist extension of the long finger.

Initial treatment of tennis elbow involves reducing pain. This can be accomplished by aspirin, acetaminophen, or nonsteroidal anti-inflammatory agents. There have been no studies that show that nonsteroidal anti-inflammatory drugs are more effective in reducing inflammation than aspirin. These medications reduce the pain of tennis elbow due to their anti-inflammatory effect.

Flexibility and strengthening exercises are instituted as soon as the patient's pain allows. The forearm extensors are typically weak, and the rehabilitation program should include strengthening exercises that increase endurance and strength. Endurance can be improved by performing high-repetition exercises with low weights.

Flexibility is also important and involves stretching exercises for the forearm extensors. This should be incorporated into any rehabilitation program for lateral epicondylitis.

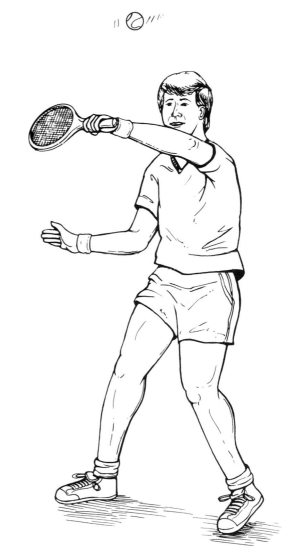

Figure 10–4. Tennis backhand that may produce microtrauma to the lateral epicondylar region.

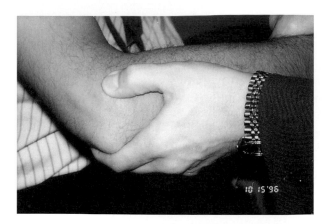

Figure 10–5. Palpation over the lateral epicondyle.

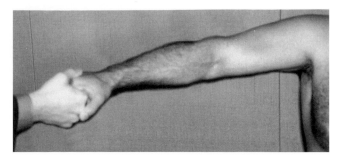

Figure 10–7. Resisted forearm pronation with the elbow extended and the shoulder in the elevated position.

Injections are not without their side effects. Patients with dark skin may experience lightening of skin color following the injection. This should be told to patients. Injections may also cause thinning of the subcutaneous fat, which can be quite disfiguring in some patients.

Patients with symptoms severe enough to require injections should be sent to physical therapy. Modalities such as iontophoresis relieve pain and allow the therapist to increase the flexibility of the forearm musculature, which is typically reduced in patients with tennis elbow. Patients with lateral epicondylitis also have weak forearm muscles. These muscles can be strengthened by the therapist once pain is reduced by medication and therapy.

Counterforce bracing can also be helpful in patients with lateral epicondylitis. A variety of braces are available but there are no studies that show that any one brace is the most effective.

Surgical intervention for lateral epicondylitis is normally not needed and is reserved for patients who have failed to improve with conservative treatment, including

therapy.[13] There are several procedures that have been described for tennis elbow. All involve resection of pathologic tissue from the tendon of the extensor radialis brevis near its origin at the lateral epicondyle. MRI studies have been used by some to demonstrate the abnormal tissue that occurs with lateral epicondylitis.[14,15] Surgical treatment involves debridement of the epicondyle. The tendons are then reattached to the epicondyle. Two to three months may be required for full recovery. Patients with work-related lateral epicondylitis should have their occupations analyzed to help reduce the repetitive activity that caused the injury.

MEDIAL EPICONDYLITIS

Medial epicondylitis occurs much less frequently than lateral epicondylitis. It is an overuse injury of the flexor pronator musculature and causes pain along the medial side of the elbow. This injury can occur frequently in throwing athletes and may be difficult to distinguish from

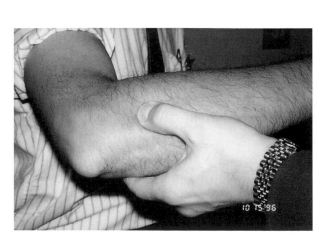

Figure 10–6. Palpation distal to the lateral epicondyle.

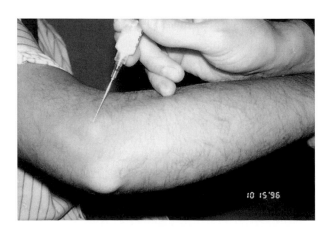

Figure 10–8. Injection of anesthetic with an anti-inflammatory agent in the lateral epicondylar region.

injuries of the ulnar collateral ligament. This is due to the fact that the flexor pronator musculature lies adjacent to the ulnar collateral ligament. Therefore, tenderness at the medial epicondyle may be due to tendinitis of the medial musculature or may indicate a sprain of the ulnar collateral ligament. The close association of the flexor pronator musculature and the ulnar collateral ligament has a protective effect on the ligament. EMG studies have shown that the activity of the medial musculature is at its highest level when the stress on the ulnar collateral ligament is at its highest.[15]

Overuse injuries in throwing athletes may be associated with tendinitis of the flexor pronator muscles or may cause injuries to the ulnar collateral ligament. Ligamentous injuries are associated with pain with valgus stressing of the elbow, whereas tendinitis causes pain with resisted elevation of the arm with the elbow fully extended and fully supinated (see Fig. 10-9). Physical examination of patients with medial epicondylitis reveals tenderness at the medial epicondyle without pain or instability with valgus stressing (see Fig. 10-10).

Radiographs may be useful in young patients who have persistent medial epicondylitis. These studies often show widening of the medial epicondylar apophysis. Comparison views of the contralateral elbow are needed to make this diagnosis since it is difficult to determine if radiographic findings represent an abnormal finding or are normal for that patient. Widening of the apophysis represents a stress reaction due to repetitive traction on the medial epicondyle by overuse of the elbow (see Figs. 10-11 and 10-12).

Medial epicondylitis is also a common overuse injury in golfers. "Golfer's elbow" can be seen in golfers at all levels and can be debilitating. Unlike throwing athletes, injuries in this group of athletes are commonly due to muscular fatigue and tendinitis, rather than an injury of the ulnar collateral.

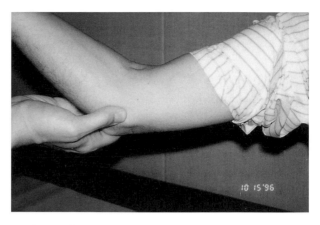

Figure 10–10. Palpation over the median epicondyle.

Treatment of medial epicondylitis is relative rest and avoidance of activities that can exacerbate the tendinitis. This may involve temporary cessation of throwing until the tendinitis has resolved or a decrease in the amount of golfing in that group of athletes.[16] Evaluation and treatment by a licensed physical therapist or certified athletic trainer are helpful along with the short-term use of non-steroidal anti-inflammatory medicines. Injections to this area may be useful, but should be done carefully to avoid injury to the ulnar nerve (see Fig. 10-13). Therapists and trainers can help the patient recover from injury and can also instruct the patient in an exercise program that can prevent the condition from recurring. Surgery may be necessary in rare cases for patients who have not responded

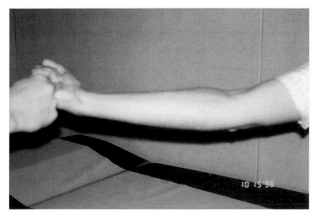

Figure 10–9. Resisted elevation of the arm with the elbow extended and the forearm fully supinated.

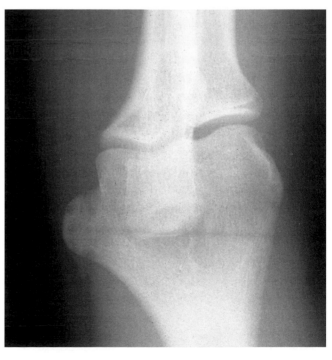

Figure 10–11. Radiograph of a normal elbow joint.

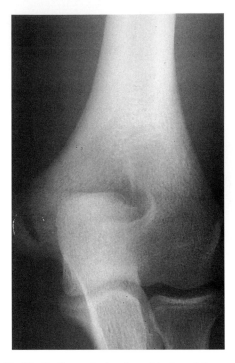

Figure 10–12. Radiograph showing widening of the apophysis.

to conservative treatment. These procedures involve excising the chronic inflammatory tissue. They produce good results in most patients.[17]

TRICEPS AND BICIPITAL TENDINITIS

Tendinitis also can affect the triceps and the biceps tendons, although these injuries are much less common than medial and lateral epicondylitis. Tendinitis at both of these sites can often be treated by rest and avoidance of activities that aggravate the athlete's symptoms. Inflammation of these tendons is often due to overuse and does not cause persistent symptoms.

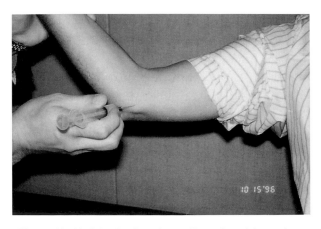

Figure 10–13. Injection into the median epicondylar region.

Rupture of the bicipital tendon is difficult to diagnose and may often be confused with a strain of the elbow or forearm. This injury commonly presents as an acutely painful condition of the elbow. It is common in weight-lifters. Pain, tenderness, and ecchymosis are often present in the cubital fossa of the elbow. Weakness may be difficult to demonstrate since other intact muscles, such as the brachialis, can adequately flex the elbow without an intact biceps. Athletes with this injury may have experienced bicipital tendinitis prior to rupture. This condition may be a precursor to complete rupture.

Treatment of this injury is surgical. Repair should be performed within 7 to 10 days of rupture. Appropriate referral to an orthopedic surgeon is necessary. Athletes are normally able to resume sports without residual weakness following surgical repair.

ULNAR NEURITIS

Ulnar neuritis can also cause medial elbow pain. Neuritis may be due to an incompetent ulnar collateral ligament, which allows tension on the nerve. This tension will not resolve until the ulnar collateral is surgically reconstructed. Injury to this nerve may also be due to subluxation of the nerve from the cubital tunnel or compression of the nerve along the medial side of the elbow. EMG and nerve conduction studies may be helpful, but may not always be positive in patients with compression or subluxation of the ulnar nerve.

Treatment of ulnar neuritis is relative rest and avoidance of activities that stress the nerve. This involves cessation of throwing in patients who have unstable elbows. Surgical treatment is reserved for those patients who do not respond to rest and conservative treatment. Compression of the ulnar nerve at the level of the elbow can be surgically treated by decompression of the nerve and submuscular or subcutaneous transposition of the nerve. Some surgeons prefer medial epicondylectomy in patients with ulnar nerve compression at the elbow.[18] This surgery is performed so as not to violate the origin of the ulnar collateral ligament.[19]

ULNAR COLLATERAL LIGAMENT INJURIES

Ulnar collateral ligament injuries can occur in throwing athletes and may be partial or complete tears. Throwing causes stress on the ulnar collateral ligament due to the valgus position that the elbow assumes during throwing activity. This can cause the ligament to tear (see Fig. 10–14). This injury can also occur in patients who dislocate their elbows in sports such as wrestling or gymnastics, where forces can reach several times body weight.[20]

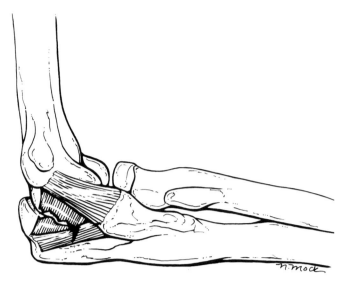

Figure 10–14. Medial collateral ligament sprain.

Diagnosis of ulnar collateral ligament tears can be made by clinical examination of the elbow. The most consistent finding is pain with valgus stress of the elbow. This test should be performed with the elbow at 20 to 30 degrees of flexion, since stability of the elbow in this partially flexed position to valgus stress is dependent on a competent ulnar collateral ligament (see Fig. 10–15).

Diagnostic tests can be helpful when clinical signs of a ligament tear are equivocal. Valgus stress radiographs have been used by some to diagnose tears of this ligament.[21] Magnetic resonance imaging is becoming the diagnostic test of choice for these tears. This test allows visualization of ligamentous fibers and can help determine if the tear is partial or complete.[22,23]

Partial tears of the ulnar collateral ligament can be successfully treated conservatively with rest and avoidance of throwing activity. Rest is continued until valgus stress of the elbow is painless. Range-of-motion and strengthening exercises are performed while the ligament

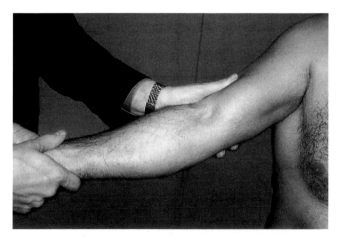

Figure 10–15. Valgus stress with elbow flexed 20 degrees.

is healing. Athletes can return to throwing as soon as the ligament has healed fully.

Surgical treatment of the ulnar collateral ligament is necessary only in athletes who are involved in throwing activities. Other athletes who tear this ligament can be treated successfully with nonoperative treatment. Throwers require surgical treatment due to the extensive valgus forces that the elbow sustains during the throwing motion. These forces require that the medial collateral be fully functional.

Reconstruction of the ulnar collateral requires use of a substitute for the ligament. Jobe popularized use of the palmaris graft for reconstruction of this ligament. Recent modification of this procedure allows it to be performed without transposition of the ulnar nerve. This was not possible with the earlier procedure.

OSTEOCHONDRITIS DESSICANS

Osteochondritis dessicans occurs most commonly in throwing athletes and in athletes who sustain repetitive trauma to the elbow, such as gymnasts. The elbow assumes a valgus position in the throwing motion. This causes tension in the medial collateral ligament and compresses the lateral elbow joint. Repetitive throwing can cause undue stress on the radiocapitellar joint, particularly in those who have mild or significant laxity of the medial collateral ligament. The etiology of osteochondritis dessicans is uncertain but repetitive stress, with resultant injury to the articular surfaces of the capitellum, is probably responsible for the majority of cases of this syndrome.

Osteochondritis dessicans most commonly presents with pain and tenderness along the lateral aspect of the elbow due to the involvement of the capitellum. Motion of the elbow may be diminished and the elbow may assume a flexed position.

Treatment for this condition is rest and therapy. The prognosis for patients with open physes is good. Athletes with loose bodies and closed physes do not fare well and may require surgical intervention.

FRACTURES AND DISLOCATIONS

Fractures and dislocations of the elbow are the result of severe trauma to the elbow. These injuries can be devastating in the young athlete with open growth plates who may experience permanent growth deformities as a result of their injuries. These types of injuries require consultation with an orthopedic surgeon on a timely basis to prevent long-term injuries to the elbow.

Dislocations are common, particularly in sports such as gymnastics. Conservative treatment is the treatment of choice in this group of athletes,[24] and consists of immediate reduction of the dislocation and short-term immobilization.

SUMMARY

Injuries of the elbow are common in athletes of all ages. Most of these injuries are the result of overuse and can be effectively treated with a reduction of activity, physical therapy, and the use of oral anti-inflammatory medicines.[25] Young athletes are not immune to serious elbow injuries. Fortunately, most athletic injuries of the elbow have an excellent prognosis for full return to sports.[26]

REFERENCES

1. Chan D, Aldridge MJ, Maffulli N, Davies AM. Chronic stress injuries of the elbow in young gymnasts. *Br J Radiol.* 1991;64:1113-1118.
2. Regan WD, Korinek SL, Morrey BF, An KN. Biomechanical study of ligaments around the elbow joint. *Clin Orthop.* 1991;271:170-179.
3. Timmerman LA, Andrews JR. Histology and arthroscopic anatomy of the ulnar collateral ligament of the elbow. *Am J Sports Med.* 1994;22:667-673.
4. Werner FW, An KN. Biomechanics of the elbow and forearm. *Hand Clin.* 1994;10:357-373. Review.
5. Noteboom T, Cruver R, Keller J, et al. Tennis elbow: A review. *J Orthop Sports Phys Ther.* 1994;19:357-366.
6. Bennett JB. Lateral and medial epicondylitis. *Hand Clin.* 1994;10:157-163. Review.
7. Gellman H. Tennis elbow (lateral epicondylitis). *Orthop Clin North Am.* 1992;23:75-82. Review.
8. Verhaar JA. Tennis elbow. Anatomical, epidemiological and therapeutic aspects. *Int Orthopaed.* 1994;18:263-267. Review.
9. Foley AE. Tennis elbow. *Am Fam Physician.* 1993;48:281-288. Review.
10. Kelley JD, Lombardo SJ, Pink M, et al. Electromyographic and cinematographic analysis of elbow function in tennis players with lateral epicondylitis. *Am J Sports Med.* 1994;22:359-363.
11. Ilfeld FW. Can stroke modification relieve tennis elbow? *Clin Orthop.* 1992;276:182-186.
12. Price R, Sinclair H, Heinrich I, Gibson T. Local injection treatment of tennis elbow—hydrocortisone, triamcinolone and lignocaine compared. *Br J Rheumatol.* 1991;30:39-44.
13. Verhaar J, Walenkamp G, Kester A, et al. Lateral extensor release for tennis elbow. A prospective long-term follow-up study. *J Bone Joint Surg.* 1993;75A:1034-1043.
14. Nirschl RP. Elbow tendinosis/tennis elbow. *Clin Sports Med.* 1992;851-870. Review.
15. Regan W, Wold LE, Coonrad R, Morrey BF. Microscopic histopathology of chronic refractory lateral epicondylitis. *Am J Sports Med.* 1992;20:746-749.
16. Glazebrook MA, Curwin S, Islam MN, et al. Medial epicondylitis. An electromyographic analysis and an investigation of intervention strategies. *Am J Sports Med.* 1994;22:674-679.
17. Vangsness CT Jr, Jobe FW. Surgical treatment of medial epicondylitis. Results in 35 elbows. *J Bone Joint Surg.* 1991;73B:409-411.
18. Froimson AI, Anouchi YS, Seitz WH Jr, Winsberg DD. Ulnar nerve decompression with medial epicondylectomy for neuropathy at the elbow. *Clin Orthop.* 1991;265:200-206. Review.
19. O'Driscoll SW, Jaloszynski R, Morrey BF, An KN. Origin of the medial ulnar collateral ligament. *J Hand Surg.* 1992;17:164-168.
20. Werner SL, Fleisig GS, Dillman CJ. Biomechanics of the elbow during baseball pitching. *J Orthop Sports Phys Ther.* 1993;17:274-278.
21. Rijke AM, Goitz HT, McCue FC, et al. Stress radiography of the medial elbow ligaments. *Radiology.* 1994;19:213-216.
22. Huynh PT, Kaplan PA, Dussault RG. Magnetic resonance imaging of the elbow. *Orthopedics.* 1994;17:1029-1035.
23. Murphy BJ. MR imaging of the elbow. *Radiology.* 1992;184:525-529.
24. Habernack H, Ortner F. The influence of anatomic factors in elbow joint dislocation. *Clin Orthop.* 1992;274:226-230.
25. Wilk KE, Arrigo C, Andrews JR. Rehabilitation of the elbow in the throwing athlete. *J Orthop Sports Phys Ther.* 1993;17:305-317.
26. Nicola TL. Elbow injuries in athletes. *Prim Care.* 1992;19:283-302.

Rehabilitation of the Elbow

Kevin E. Wilk and Terri Chmielewski

Injuries to the elbow joint complex are common in athletes. These injuries may be significant injuries with pronounced tissue damage, as seen in a fracture, dislocation, or ligamentous rupture. Conversely, other injuries may be due to less significant forces and may represent microtraumatic injuries or repetitive overuse syndromes such as tendinitis, valgus extension overload syndrome, or mild ulnar collateral ligament sprains. This section will discuss the nonoperative and postoperative rehabilitation programs for numerous elbow injuries commonly seen in the athlete.

The rehabilitation of various elbow injuries often represents a significant challenge to the rehabilitation specialist due to the unique configuration of the elbow joint complex, its functional interaction with the other joints in the kinetic chain such as the shoulder joint and wrist and hand, and the potential for an adverse healing response. The rehabilitation specialist must be aware of the common complications encountered following specific elbow injuries.

Rehabilitation following an elbow injury progresses through a systematic multiphased treatment program. Each phase of the rehabilitation program expands on the previous phase with specific goals that introduce more challenging exercises and drills. Treatment progression only occurs when the patient meets specific criteria, thus ensuring rate of progression based on the patient's individual rate of healing.

Most rehabilitation programs encompass three to four phases of rehabilitation, depending on the activity level and goals of the patient. The phases include the acute, intermediate, advanced, and return-to-activity phases. In the acute phase, the goals are to reduce inflammation and pain, gradually restore motion, and prevent muscular atrophy. Thus, in the first phase, the goals address preventing the negative effects of immobilization. In the intermediate phase, the goals are to improve muscular strength, increase endurance, and enhance neuromuscular control of the joint. During this phase, the exercises are designed to address the deficits that may have contributed to the current condition, correct any muscular imbalances, and promote dynamic joint stability. The advanced phase is designed to enhance muscular strength, power and endurance, improve neuromuscular joint control, and

to utilize higher speed, functional exercises. During this phase, the athletic patient will perform sport-specific simulated exercises. The final phase is the return-to-activity phase. In this phase the patient will continue to perform functional exercises. Additionally, the recreational or competitive athlete will be placed on an interval sport program to gradually return the athlete back to sports.

Before the patient is initiated on an interval sport program, the patient must exhibit specific criteria. These criteria include full, nonpainful range of motion, satisfactory clinical muscular strength, and a satisfactory clinical examination. Isokinetic testing is often utilized to objectively quantify muscular strength. The results are used to determine whether an athlete is ready to begin strenuous sports participation.

NONOPERATIVE REHABILITATION

Frequently, the clinician is required to design and implement a nonoperative treatment program for an injury to the elbow joint complex. Often the rehabilitation program is for a minor but persistent injury, such as overuse tendinitis (medial and lateral epicondylitis or flexor pronator tendinitis). The injury may be due to a single traumatic event often affecting the ligamentous or osseous structures. In either case, the nonoperative treatment program must be a well designed rehabilitation program that addresses the patient's primary and secondary problems and progresses to the patient's ultimate goals.

The clinician must possess a thorough understanding of the anatomy and biomechanics of the elbow joint complex. This is especially true when treating the athlete. An understanding of the elbow joint biomechanics during the specific demands of the sport will assist the clinician in designing a rehabilitation program. In the following rehabilitation programs we will discuss the specific rehabilitation guidelines for various elbow injuries.

ULNAR NEUROPATHY

Ulnar neuropathy can result from various mechanisms of trauma.[1] Tensile force, in the form of valgus stress, is one common mechanism seen in the overhead athlete. Often valgus stress is coupled with an external rotation and supination overload. Medial elbow instability from an ulnar collateral ligament tear can further increase valgus stress and injury to the ulnar nerve. This is commonly seen in the overhead thrower, during the acceleration phase of the throw.[2] A second mechanism of trauma is from compressive force. The soft tissue surrounding the ulnar nerve may hypertrophy or scar tissue may be present, both can compress the ulnar nerve.[2] Compression can also result if the nerve is entrapped between the two heads of the flexor carpi ulnaris. Finally, ulnar nerve instability can lead to neuropathy. Repetitive flexion and extension of the elbow with an unstable ulnar nerve can cause irritation and inflammation of the nerve. It has been reported that 16 percent of patients with ulnar neuropathy have exhibited this mechanism.[3] Two types of instability may be present. If the nerve subluxes or rests on the medial epicondyle (type A) direct trauma may result. Complete dislocation anteriorly (type B) can lead to a friction neuritis. Any of these mechanisms alone or a combination of them can be responsible for causing ulnar neuropathy.

Ulnar neuropathy can present in three stages.[4] The first stage is the acute onset of radicular symptoms. The second stage involves the recurrence of symptoms as the athlete attempts to return to throwing or other sports. In the third stage, persistent motor weakness and sensory changes have evolved. Once the third stage is reached, it is often difficult to reverse the symptoms through conservative measures such as rehabilitation, and often surgery is required.

The primary goal of conservative treatment is to decrease nerve irritation. Since medial joint instability resulting from ulnar collateral insufficiency is often responsible for nerve irritation, the other primary treatment goal is to improve the dynamic medial elbow joint stability. The ultimate goal is to safely return the athlete to his or her sport without a recurrence of symptoms.

Once the athlete has been diagnosed with ulnar neuritis, the patient is instructed to discontinue participation in the irritating sport for 4 to 5 weeks. The rehabilitation program can be found in Table 10-1.

The acute phase usually lasts approximately 2 weeks, or until the neuritis symptoms abate. In this phase, the athlete performs a strengthening program consisting of isometrics for the wrist and forearm musculature, as well as shoulder strengthening exercises. Flexibility exercises are also begun to prevent muscular tightness and restore normal motion. Modalities such as warm whirlpool, cryotherapy, and high-voltage galvanic stimulation are used to help control pain and inflammation.

In the second phase, or advanced strengthening phase, the goals are to improve strength, power, and endurance; enhance dynamic joint stability; and begin high-speed training. Strengthening exercises for the

TABLE 10–1. NONOPERATIVE TREATMENT FOR ULNAR NEURITIS

Acute Phase
  Goals
    Diminish ulnar nerve inflammation
    Restore normal motion
    Maintain/improve muscular strength
- Brace: Optional, only used if patient is externally inflamed
- Range of motion: Restore full nonpainful ROM as soon as possible
    Initiate stretching exercises for wrist, forearm, and elbow musculature
- Strengthening exercises: If patient is extremely painful/inflamed, utilize isometrics for approximately 1 week
    Initiate isotonic strengthening
      Wrist flex/ext
      Forearm supination/pronation
      Elbow flex/ext
      Shoulder program
- Pain control/inflammation control
    Warm whirlpool
    Cryotherapy
    High-voltage galvanic stimulation

Advanced Strengthening Phase (weeks 3 to 6)
  Goals
    Improve strength, power, endurance
    Enhance dynamic joint stability
    Initiate high-speed training
- Exercise: Throwers ten program
    Eccentrics wrist/forearm muscles
    Rhythmic stabilization drills for elbow joint
    Isokinetics for elbow flex/ext
    Plyometric exercise drills
- Continue stretching exercises

Return to activity phase (weeks 4 to 6)
  Goals
    Gradual return to functional activities
    Enhance muscular performance
  Criteria to begin throwing
    Full nonpainful
    Satisfactory clinical exam
    Satisfactory muscular performance
- Initiate interval sport program
- Continue thrower's ten program
- Continue all stretching exercises

wrist, forearm, and shoulder are continued with an emphasis on eccentric muscle contractions. Dynamic stability drills are initiated for the elbow stabilizers, specifically the pronator teres and wrist flexor musculature. These muscle groups assist the ulnar collateral ligament in stabilizing the medial side of the elbow, especially during the cocking and acceleration phases of throwing.[5,6] During this phase, rhythmic stabilization drills can be performed to enhance dynamic stability (see Fig. 10-16).

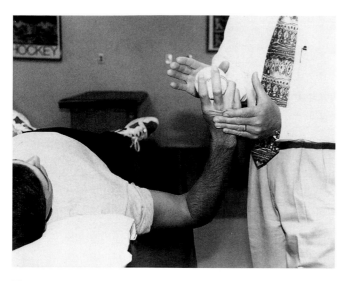

Figure 10–16. Rhythmic stabilization drills performed in the throwing position.

Plyometrics are initiated to further train the dynamic stabilizers and to help prepare the athlete for sport activities. Stretching exercises are still performed in this phase. This phase usually lasts approximately 2 to 4 weeks.

The final phase is the return to activity phase, in which the goal is to gradually return the athlete to throwing or other sports activities. The criteria that must be met before throwing is initiated include full, nonpainful range of motion; satisfactory clinical exam with no neurologic symptoms and adequate medial elbow stability; and satisfactory strength based on isokinetic assessment. The isokinetic test criteria used by the authors can be found in Table 10-2. Once the athlete meets these criteria, the interval throwing program can be initiated. All throwers start on the long toss program, beginning with light tossing from 45 feet. In the interval throwing program, the distance, intensity, and number of throws are gradually increased. When the thrower successfully completes step 8 (phase I), then pitchers can initiate phase II, which is throwing from the mound. The entire interval throwing program is outlined in Tables 10-3 and 10-4. Strengthening exercises are performed and progressed during this phase as well. After the thrower successfully completes the throwing program, a gradual return to play is allowed.

TABLE 10–2. ISOKINETIC ASSESSMENT

Bilateral comparison	Elbow flexor	180/sec	300/sec
	Elbow extensor	110–120%	105–115%
		105–115%	100–110%
Flex/ext ratio		70–80%	63–69%

TABLE 10–3. INTERVAL THROWING PROGRAM, PHASE I

45-Feet Phase

Step 1
a. Warm-up throwing
b. 45 feet (25 throws)
c. Rest 15 minutes
d. Warm-up throwing
e. 45 feet (25 throws)

Step 2
a. Warm-up throwing
b. 45 feet (25 throws)
c. Rest 10 minutes
d. Warm-up throwing
e. 45 feet (25 throws)
f. Rest 10 minutes
g. Warm-up throwing
h. 45 feet (25 throws)

60-Feet Phase

Step 3
a. Warm-up throwing
b. 60 feet (25 throws)
c. Rest 15 minutes
d. Warm-up throwing
e. 60 feet (25 throws)

Step 4
a. Warm-up throwing
b. 60 feet (25 throws)
c. Rest 10 minutes
d. Warm-up throwing
e. 60 feet (25 throws)
f. Rest 10 minutes
g. Warm-up throwing
h. 60 feet (25 throws)

90-Feet Phase

Step 5
a. Warm-up throwing
b. 90 feet (25 throws)
c. Rest 15 minutes
d. Warm-up throwing
e. 90 feet (25 throws)

Step 6
a. Warm-up throwing
b. 90 feet (25 throws)
c. Rest 10 minutes
d. Warm-up throwing
e. 90 feet (25 throws)
f. Rest 10 minutes
g. Warm-up throwing
h. 90 feet (25 throws)

120-Feet Phase

Step 7
a. Warm-up throwing
b. 120 feet (25 throws)
c. Rest 15 minutes
d. Warm-up throwing
e. 120 feet (25 throws)

Step 8
a. Warm-up throwing
b. 120 feet (25 throws)
c. Rest 10 minutes
d. Warm-up throwing
e. 120 feet (25 throws)
f. Rest 10 minutes
g. Warm-up throwing
h. 120 feet (25 throws)

150-Feet Phase

Step 9
a. Warm-up throwing
b. 150 feet (25 throws)
c. Rest 15 minutes
d. Warm-up throwing
e. 150 feet (25 throws)

Step 10
a. Warm-up throwing
b. 150 feet (25 throws)
c. Rest 10 minutes
d. Warm-up throwing
e. 150 feet (25 throws)
f. Rest 10 minutes
g. Warm-up throwing
h. 150 feet (25 throws)

180-Feet Phase

Step 11
a. Warm-up throwing
b. 180 feet (25 throws)
c. Rest 15 minutes
d. Warm-up throwing
e. 180 feet (25 throws)

Step 12
a. Warm-up throwing
b. 180 feet (25 throws)
c. Rest 10 minutes
d. Warm-up throwing
e. 180 feet (25 throws)
f. Rest 10 minutes
g. Warm-up throwing
h. 180 feet (25 throws)

Step 13
a. Warm-up throwing
b. 180 feet (25 throws)
c. Rest 10 minutes
d. Warm-up throwing
e. 180 feet (25 throws)
f. Rest 10 minutes
g. Warm-up throwing
h. 180 feet (25 throws)

Step 14
Begin throwing off the mound
  or return to respective position

TABLE 10–4. INTERVAL THROWING PROGRAM, PHASE II

Stage One: Fastball Only

Step 1:   Interval throwing
           15 throws off mound 50%

Step 2:   Interval throwing
           30 throws off mound 50%

Step 3:   Interval throwing
           45 throws off mound 50%

Step 4:   Interval throwing
           60 throws off mound 50%

Step 5:   Interval throwing
           30 throws off mound 75%

Step 6:   30 throws off mound 75%
           45 throws off mound 50%

Step 7.   45 throws off mound 75%
           15 throws off mound 50%

Step 8:   60 throws off mound 75%

Stage Two: Fastball Only

Step 9:   45 throws off mound 75%
           15 throws in batting practice

Step 10:   45 throws off mound 75%
           30 throws in batting practice

Step 11:   45 throws off mound 75%
           45 throws in batting practice

Stage Three

Step 12:   30 throws off mound,
              75% warm-up
           15 throws off mound,
              50% breaking balls
           45–60 throws in batting practice
              (fastball only)

Step 13:   30 throws off mound 75%
           30 breaking balls 75%
           30 throws in batting practice

Step 14:   30 throws off mound 75%
           60–90 throws in batting practice,
              25% breaking balls

Step 15:   SIMULATED GAME:
           PROGRESSING BY 15
           THROWS PER WORKOUT

Use interval throwing to 120 feet phase as warm-up.

ALL THROWING OFF THE MOUND SHOULD BE DONE IN THE PRESENCE OF YOUR PITCHING COACH TO STRESS PROPER THROWING MECHANICS.

Use speed gun to aid in effort control.

Medial and Lateral Epicondylitis

Rehabilitation for medial and lateral epicondylitis is similar for both conditions, although they are distinct pathologies. Medial epicondylitis, often referred to as golfer's elbow, involves microscopic or macroscopic disruption within the flexor carpi radialis or pronator teres near the origin on the medial epicondyle.[2] In the thrower, this condition can result secondarily to a partial tear or sprain of the ulnar collateral ligament. In the adolescent athlete, chronic medial elbow pain is often referred to a "little leaguer's elbow," which includes the diagnosis of medial epicondylitis.[7] Lateral epicondylitis, on the other hand, involves disruption of the extensor mass, usually the extensor carpi radialis brevis.[8] This condition is often called tennis elbow, although it is estimated that approximately 5 percent of all cases actually result from playing tennis.[9,10] In both medial and lateral epicondylitis, palpation over the site of pathology and resisted muscle contraction of the involved muscle group will cause pain. The differential diagnosis is critical to the nonoperative success rate. Often the patient exhibits associated disorders, such as cervical disorders or radial head pathologies. In addition, the duration of the symptoms will provide some information on the rate of recovery.

Table 10–5 outlines the rehabilitation program for medial and lateral epicondylitis. The goals in the acute phase are to diminish inflammation and pain, promote tissue healing, and retard muscle atrophy. Modalities can help achieve the first goal. Useful modalities include cryotherapy, high-voltage galvanic stimulation, iontophoresis, phonophoresis, and whirlpool. Stretching of the involved muscles is beneficial during the healing process. Gentle strengthening exercises should be performed isometrically initially, and then progressed to isotonics. Strengthening should focus on the involved muscle group. Friction massage has been advocated during this phase to assist in the healing response of the tendon.[11] It is the authors' opinion that cross-friction massage is not beneficial to tendinitis patients and often exacerbates the patient's symptoms. It is important that the patient be given education in avoiding activities and movements that aggravate the condition; specifically, patients with lateral epicondylitis should be advised to use caution with gripping activities. A counterforce brace may be issued as an adjunct to treatment. It has been found that the use of these braces stimulates skin receptors with subsequent facilitation of muscle contraction.[12]

After pain has decreased and range of motion is normalized, the patient may begin phase II, the subacute phase. In this phase the goals are to improve flexibility, improve muscular strength and endurance, and increase functional activities. Strengthening exercises are progressed and should emphasize eccentric contractions. The patient is placed on a strengthening program for the entire upper extremity. In addition, flexibility exercises are continued. As the patient's symptoms diminish, more stressful activities may be attempted with caution. Cryotherapy should be used after exercise and activity to minimize pain and inflammation.

The goals of the final phase remain the same as in the previous phase, with the addition of gradually returning the athlete to sport activities. All strengthening and stretching activities are continued and possibly pro-

TABLE 10–5. EPICONDYLITIS REHABILITATION PROTOCOL

Phase I. Acute Phase
  Goals
    Decrease inflammation/pain
    Promote tissue healing
    Retard muscular atrophy
  • Cryotherapy
  • Whirlpool
  • Stretching to increase flexibility
    Wrist extension/flexion
    Elbow extension/flexion
    Forearm supination/pronation
  • Isometrics
    Wrist extension/flexion
    Elbow extension/flexion
    Forearm supination/pronation
  • HVGS
  • Phonophoresis
  • Friction massage
  • Iontophoresis (with anti-inflammatory, e.g., dexamethsone)
  • Avoid painful movements (e.g., gripping)

Phase II. Subacute Phase
  Goals
    Improve flexibility
    Increase muscular strength/endurance
    Increase functional activities/return to function
  Exercises
  • Emphasize concentric/eccentric strengthening
    Concentration on *involved* muscle group(s)
    Wrist extension/flexion

    Forearm pronation/supination
    Elbow flexion/extension
  • Initiate shoulder strengthening (if deficiencies are noted)
  • Continue flexibility exercises
  • May utilize counterforce brace
  • Continue use of cryotherapy after exercise/function
  • Gradual return to stressful activities
  • Gradually reinitiate once-painful movements

Phase III. Chronic Phase
  Goals
    Improve muscular strength and endurance
    Maintain/enhance flexibility
    Gradual return to sport/high-level activities
  Exercises
  • Continue strengthening exercises (emphasize eccentric/concentric)
  • Continue to emphasize deficiencies in shoulder and elbow strength
  • Continue flexibility exercises
  • Gradually diminish use of counterforce brace
  • Use of cryotherapy as needed
  • Gradual return to sport activity
  • Equipment modification (grip size, string tension, playing surface)
  • Emphasize maintenance program

---

gressed as the athlete prepares for the stresses of his or her sport. Plyometrics are an example of an advanced strengthening exercise. Equipment modifications and alterations in biomechanics may need to be made to minimize the stresses experienced at the elbow. Tennis players are often encouraged to increase the racquet grip size, reduce the string tension, and play with new tennis balls as often as possible. The patient is encouraged to continue a maintenance program after formal rehabilitation is completed.

Ulnar Collateral Ligament Sprains

Sprains or partial tears of the ulnar collateral ligament (UCL) can result in throwing athletes as a sequelae to the repetitive valgus forces applied across the elbow. An in vitro study by Morrey and An[13] showed that the UCL contributes approximately 54 percent of the resistance to valgus stress. The anterior band of the UCL is the main stabilizing structure in the elbow, and it is the structure most commonly affected.[14] Since other structures can give rise to medial elbow pain, such as the flexor and

pronator mass and the ulnar nerve, a careful examination is pertinent.

The goals in the acute phase for UCL sprains are similar to other protocols, including decreasing pain and inflammation, increasing range of motion, retarding muscle atrophy, and promoting healing. Controversy exists about whether immobilization or immediate motion is the best way to achieve these goals. We recommend restricting elbow motion from 20 to 90 degrees initially to allow the injured tissues to calm down and allow scar formation. Often a range-of-motion brace is issued to prevent valgus stress to the joint. Strengthening exercises consist of isometrics for the elbow and wrist musculature. Cryotherapy should be used 4 to 6 times per day to control inflammation and pain. Table 10-6 describes the entire rehabilitation program.

In the second phase, the goals are to gradually restore full range of motion and increase strength and endurance. Motion is increased in both flexion and extension by 5 to 10 degrees each week until full motion is achieved, usually by 4 to 6 weeks. Isometric exercises are progressed to isotonic exercises, addressing musculature of the entire

TABLE 10–6. CONSERVATIVE TREATMENT FOLLOWING ULNAR COLLATERAL SPRAINS OF THE ELBOW

Immediate Motion Phase (weeks 0 to 2)
  Goals
    Increase range of motion
    Promote healing of ulnar collateral ligament
    Retard muscular atrophy
    Decrease pain and inflammation
  • ROM: Brace (optional), nonpainful ROM (20–90 degrees)
    AAROM, PROM elbow and wrist (nonpainful range)
  • Exercises: Isometrics—wrist and elbow musculature
    Shoulder strengthening (no ext. rotation strengthening)
  • Ice and compression

Intermediate Phase (weeks 3 to 6)
  Goals
    Increase range of motion
    Improve strength/endurance
    Decrease pain and inflammation
    Promote stability
  • ROM: Gradually increase motion 0–135 degrees
    (increase 10 degrees per week)
  • Exercises: Initiate isotonic exercises
    Wrist curls
    Wrist extensions
    Pronation/supination
    Biceps/triceps
    Dumbbells: external rotation, deltoid, supraspinatus,
      rhomboids, internal rotation
    Initial rhythmic stabilization drills
  • Ice and compression

Advanced Phase (weeks 6/7 to 12/14)
  Criteria to progress
  • Full range of motion
  • No pain or tenderness
  • No increase in laxity
  • Strength $4/5$ of elbow flex extensor

  Goals
    Increase strength, power, and endurance
    Improve neuromuscular control
    Initiate high-speed exercise drills
  • Exercises: Initiate exercise tubing, shoulder program
    Throwers ten program
    Biceps/triceps programs
    Supination/pronation
    Wrist extension/flexion
    Plyometrics throwing drills

Return to Activity Phase (week 12/14)
  Criteria to progress to return to throwing:
  • Full nonpainful ROM
  • No increase in laxity
  • Isokinetic test fulfills criteria
  • Satisfactory clinical exam

  Exercises: Initiate interval throwing
    Continue throwers ten program
    Continue plyometrics

shoulder girdle, in addition to the elbow and wrist. Rhythmic stabilization drills are also initiated to enhance neuromuscular control and dynamic stability of the medial elbow (see Fig. 10-16). Strengthening exercises that emphasize the elbow flexors, flexor carpi ulnaris, flexor carpi radialis, and pronator teres are performed to enhance dynamic stabilization.[15]

The advanced strengthening phase is initiated approximately 6 to 7 weeks after injury. This phase builds upon the strength foundation formed in the second phase with an emphasis on power and endurance. The thrower's ten isotonic program[15] is performed and modified, if needed, based on the patient's individual muscular deficiencies. The thrower's ten program includes exercises to specifically strengthen scapular and rotator cuff musculature. Table 10-7 outlines this program. Higher-speed drills in the throwing position and plyometrics are gradually initiated as the athlete prepares to return to throwing. Recommended plyometric drills include the two-hand overhead soccer throw, two-hand chest pass, two-hand side-to-side throw, two-hand overhead side throw, and one-hand baseball throw (see Figs. 10–17 to 10–22).

Once the patient is able to meet the criteria to return to throwing, the interval throwing program is initiated and then progresses to off the mound throwing. In general, it may take the athlete 3 to 4 months to return to throwing. As soon as the throwing program is completed, the athlete may return to competition. The athlete is strongly encouraged to continue the prescribed exercise program.

Osteochondritis Dissecans

The etiology of osteochondritis dissecans (OCD) is unclear. It has been theorized that vascular compromise or repetitive trauma is responsible for this condition.[16] In the thrower, repetitive extension coupled with forceful pronation causes stress to be transmitted from the radius to the capitellum, thus, the capitellum is the most common site for OCD to develop in the elbow.[17] Gymnasts frequently develop this lesion due to excessive loading on the lateral side of the elbow joint.[18] In addition, end arteries terminate in the subchondral plate of the capitellum, which are at risk for disruption.[2]

TABLE 10–7. THROWERS TEN EXERCISE PROGRAM

The throwers ten program is designed to exercise the major muscles necessary for throwing. The program's goal is to be an organized and concise exercise program. In addition, all exercises included are specific to the thrower and are designed to improve strength, power, and endurance of the shoulder complex musculature.

1. a. Diagonal Pattern D2 Extension

Involved hand will grip tubing handle overhead and out to the side. Pull tubing down and across your body to the opposite side of leg. During the motion lead with your thumb. Perform__sets of__repetitions__times daily.

b. Diagonal Pattern D2 Flexion

Gripping tubing handle in hand of involved arm, begin with arm out from side 45° and palm facing backward. After turning palm forward, proceed to flex elbow and bring arm up and over uninvolved shoulder. Turn palm down and reverse to take arm to starting position. Exercise should be performed in controlled manner. Perform__sets of__repetitions__times daily.

2. a. External Rotation at 0° Abduction

Standing with involved elbow fixed at side, elbow at 90° and involved arm across front of body. Grip tubing handle while the other end of tubing is fixed. Pull out with arm, keeping elbow at side. Return tubing slowly and controlled. Perform__sets of__repetitions__times daily.

b. Internal Rotation at 0° Abduction

Standing with elbow at side fixed at 90° and shoulder rotated out. Grip tubing handle while other end of tubing is fixed. Pull arm across body keeping elbow at side. Return tubing slowly and controlled. Perform__sets of__repetitions__times daily.

c. External Rotation at 90° Abduction

Stand with shoulder abducted 90° and elbow flexed 90°. Grip tubing handle while the other end is fixed straight ahead, slightly lower than the shoulder. Keeping shoulder abducted, rotate shoulder back keeping elbow at 90°. Return tubing and hand to start position.

I. *Slow Speed Sets* (slow and controlled): Perform__sets of__ repetitions__times daily.

II. *Fast Speed Sets:* Perform__sets of__repetitions/seconds__ times daily.

d. Internal Rotation at 90° Abduction

Stand with shoulder abducted to 90°, externally rotated 90° and elbow bent to 90°. Keeping shoulder abducted, rotate shoulder forward, keeping elbow bent at 90°. Return tubing and hand to start position.

I. *Slow Speed Sets* (slow and controlled): Perform__sets of__repetitions__times daily.

II. *Fast Speed Sets:* Perform__sets of__repetitions/seconds__ times daily.

3. Shoulder Abduction to 90°

Stand with arm at side, elbow straight, and palm against side. Raise arm to the side, palm down, until arm reaches 90° (shoulder level). Hold 2 seconds and lower slowly. Perform__sets of__repetitions__times daily.

4. Scaption, Internal Rotation

Stand with elbow straight and thumb down. Raise arm to shoulder level at 30° angle in front of body. Do not go above shoulder height. Hold 2 seconds and lower slowly. Perform__sets of__repetitions__times daily.

5. a. Prone Horizontal Abduction

(Neutral): Lie on table, face down, with involved arm hanging straight to the floor, and palm facing down. Raise arm out to the side, parallel to the floor. Hold 2 seconds and lower slowly. Perform__sets of__repetitions__times daily.

b. Prone Horizontal Abduction (Full ER, 100° Abd.)

Lie on table, face down, with involved arm hanging straight to the floor, and thumb rotated up (hitchhiker). Raise arm out to the side with arm slightly in front of shoulder, parallel to the floor. Hold 2 seconds and lower slowly. Perform__sets of__repetitions__times daily.

6. Press-ups

Seated on a chair or on a table, place both hands firmly on the sides of the chair or table, palm down and fingers pointed outward. Hands should be placed equal with shoulders. Slowly push downward through the hands to elevate your body. Hold the elevated position for 2 seconds and lower body slowly. Perform__sets of__repetitions__times daily.

7. Prone Rowing

Lying on your stomach with your involved arm hanging over the side of the table, dumbbell in hand and elbow straight. Slowly raise arm, bending elbow, and bring dumbbell as high as possible. Hold at the top for 2 seconds, then slowly lower. Perform__sets of__repetitions__times daily.

8. Push-ups

Start in the down position with arms in a comfortable position. Place hands no more than shoulder width apart. Push up as high as possible, rolling shoulders forward after elbows are straight. Start with a push-up into wall. Gradually progress to table top and eventually to floor as tolerable. Perform__sets of__repetitions__times daily.

9. a. Elbow Flexion

Standing with arm against side and palm facing inward, bend elbow upward turning palm up as you progress. Hold 2 seconds and lower slowly. Perform__sets of__repetitions__times daily.

b. Elbow Extension

Raise involved arm overhead. Provide support at elbow from uninvolved hand. Straighten arm overhead. Hold 2 seconds and lower slowly. Perform__sets of__repetitions__times daily.

10. a. Wrist Extension

Supporting the forearm and with palm facing downward, raise weight in hand as far as possible. Hold 2 seconds and lower slowly. Perform__sets of__repetitions__times daily.

(continued)

TABLE 10–7. (*Continued*)

b. Wrist Flexion

Supporting the forearm and with palm facing upward, lower a weight in hand as far as possible and then curl it up as high as possible. Hold for 2 seconds and lower slowly. Perform__sets of __repetitions__times daily.

c. Supination

Forearm supported on table with wrist in neutral position. Using a weight or hammer, roll wrist taking palm up. Hold for a 2 count

and return to starting position. Perform__sets of__repetitions__ times daily.

d. Pronation

Forearm should be supported on a table with wrist in neutral position. Using a weight or hammer, roll wrist taking palm down. Hold for a 2 count and return to starting position. Perform__sets of__repetitions__times daily.

Osteochondritis dissecans has been classified into three stages.[19] Stage 1 lesions are those with no radiographic evidence of subchondral displacement or fracture. Stage 2 lesions are those that show evidence of subchondral detachment or articular cartilage fracture. Stage 3 lesions occur when chondral or osteochondral fragments become detached and result in intra-articular loose body or bodies. Treatment is dependent on the clinical and radiographic findings. Conservative treatment is indicated for stage 1 or 2 lesions when the subchondral bone or articular cartilage have not become detached fragments.

The acute phase begins with a period of relative immobilization of the elbow at 90 degrees of flexion for 3 to 6 weeks (usually 3 to 4 weeks). This allows the irritability of the lesion site to diminish. The patient is instructed to perform gentle range-of-motion exercises in a nonpainful arc of motion 3 to 4 times each day. Strengthening exercises are started when the symptoms resolve. Isometrics are performed initially, usually for the

first week; then the patient is allowed to progress to isotonic exercise. In addition, flexibility exercises are performed for the entire upper extremity.

Once the patient is pain free and the range of motion is normalized, the advanced strengthening phase can be started. Plyometric and high-speed drills can be added, as well as aggressive eccentric strengthening. When the patient meets the criteria to return to throwing, the athlete may initiate a gradual return to sports.

Valgus Extension Overload

Valgus extension overload occurs during the acceleration and deceleration phases of throwing.[14] Valgus forces produce medial elbow stress that causes the olecranon to compress against the medial wall of the olecranon fossa.[20-22] In addition, forceful extension, caused by contraction of the triceps, contributes to this pathology. Eventually an osteophyte may form posteriorly on the olecranon process. This formation may be accelerated if

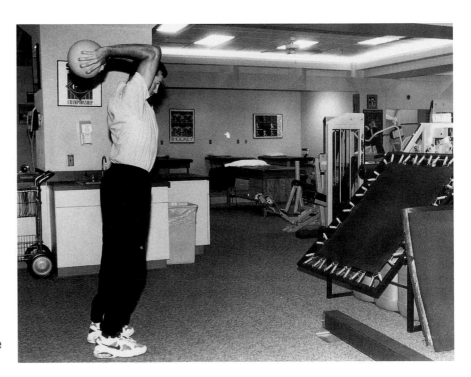

Figure 10–17. A plyometric exercise drill: the two-hand overhead soccer throw.

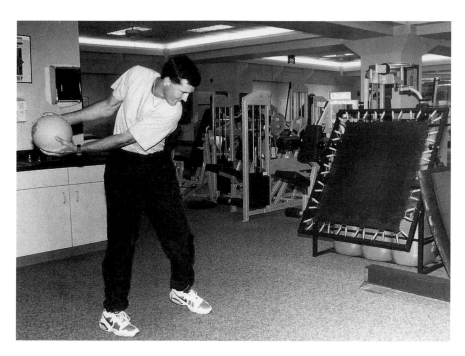

Figure 10–18. A plyometric exercise drill: the two-hand side throw (underhand).

medial elbow instability is present, since valgus forces would be increased. Through repetitive impact of the olecranon in the olecranon fossa, the spur may become fragmented with subsequent loose body formation.

The acute phase of conservative treatment is aimed at decreasing posterior elbow pain. Modalities such as warm whirlpool, high-voltage galvanic stimulation, and cryotherapy may assist in reducing the patient's symptoms. Isometrics are performed for the shoulder, elbow, and wrist musculature. Stretching exercises are also performed to help regain full range of motion.

Strengthening exercises in the advanced phase should concentrate on those muscle groups that counteract the stresses that led to the condition. Specifically,

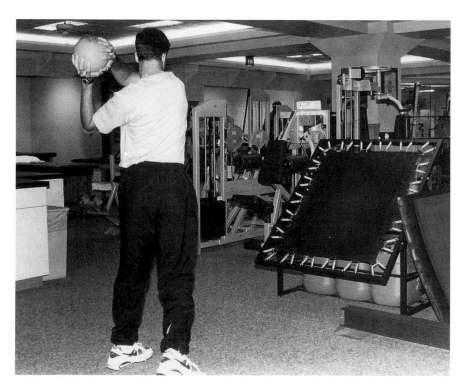

Figure 10–19. A plyometric exercise drill: the side-to-side throw.

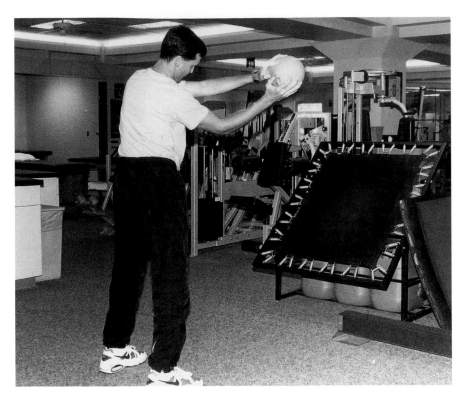

Figure 10–20. A plyometric exercise drill: the two-hand side throw (overhand).

eccentric strength of the biceps, brachioradialis, and brachialis should be emphasized since these muscles control elbow extension during the deceleration phase.[15,23] Strength of the flexor and pronator muscles should also be emphasized, since they are responsible for stabilizing the medial elbow against the valgus forces during acceleration. Rhythmic stabilization drills are added to improve neuromuscular control and dynamic stability of the medial joint (see Fig. 10–16). Plyometric drills can also be added gradually.

The patient progresses to the return to activity phase once the patient meets the criteria to begin throwing or to return to the specific sport, and the physician has determined that such activity is safe. Progression through the interval sport program will lead to return to competition.

Degenerative Joint Disease

Early wear of the articular surface and osteophyte formation may occur in the elbow of overhead throwers, tennis players, gymnasts, and other athletes secondary to the repetitive stresses experienced during stressful sport movement.[24-27] Often the resulting pain and loss of motion do not interfere with daily activities, but can restrict participation in sports. As with conservative treatment for other conditions, rehabilitation attempts to decrease pain, improve range of motion and flexibility, and enhance strength and endurance.

The initial phase of treatment often focuses on improving capsular extensibility. By normalizing motion, stresses during sport participation can be dissipated normally, rather than concentrated on a small area.[20] This will aid in slowing down the degenerative process. Useful techniques to improve range of motion include gentle stretching, joint mobilizations, low-load long-duration stretching, contract and relax techniques, and proprioceptive neuromuscular facilitation stretching. Warm whirlpool and an active warm-up, such as with the upper body ergometer, can increase soft-tissue extensibility prior to stretching. The authors recommend low-load, long-duration stretching (see Fig. 10–23) to gradually change the resting length of soft tissue without causing significant pain or greater contracture.

Strengthening exercises for the entire upper extremity are also performed, but certain exercises may need to be modified. In general, lighter weight and higher repetitions are encouraged, particularly for those exercises that place high compressive and shear forces on the humeroulnar joint. Exercises that may require modification include bench press, triceps push-down, French curls, push-ups, and press-ups.

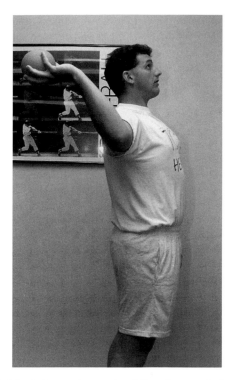

Figure 10–21. A plyometric exercise drill against a wall: the one-hand overhead baseball throw.

Increasing the strength and endurance of the muscles surrounding the elbow will help protect the joint by lessening the forces experienced during sports. With improved muscular strength and capsular flexibility, the patient may be able to increase his or her ability to remain competitive.

POSTOPERATIVE REHABILITATION

The rehabilitation program following elbow surgery is similar to most of the nonoperative programs with several important exceptions. The rehabilitation specialist must carefully consider the type of surgery performed, the integrity of the structures, and most significantly, the healing constraints of the procedure. Several basic principles inherent to any rehabilitation program must be considered when treating the postoperative elbow patient. First, the effects of immobilization must be minimized. Second, healing tissue must never be over stressed. Third, the patient must fulfill specific criteria to progress from one phase to the next during the rehabilitation process. Fourth, the rehabilitation program must be based on current clinical and basic science research. Finally, the program must be adaptable to the patient and his or her goals.

Rehabilitation after operative procedures to the elbow follows a progressive, multiphased program designed to address the potential complications that may arise during the course of rehabilitation. Regaining full extension is the most challenging and important aspect of postoperative rehabilitation secondary to the unique anatomic features of the elbow joint. Not only is the humeroulnar joint highly congruent, but the elbow joint capsule is a tight structure, and the anterior capsule has a tendency to scar. The combination of these factors predisposes the patient to develop a flexion contracture postsurgically.[8] The following programs emphasize immediate, controlled motion within the healing constraints of the involved tissue. Regardless of which

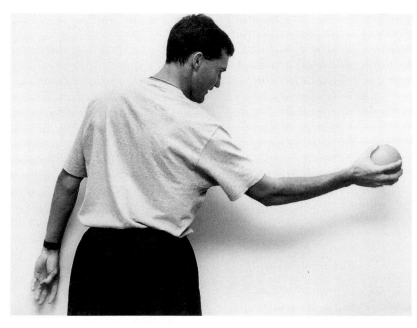
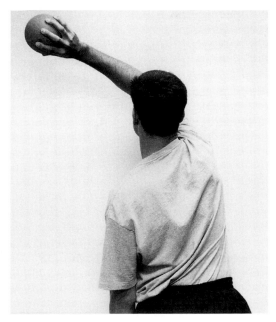

Figure 10–22. A plyometric exercise drill, referred to as wall dribbling. The athlete uses a 2 to 6-pound plyoball and dribbles it against the wall in a half-circle radius. This exercise drill promotes shoulder muscle endurance.

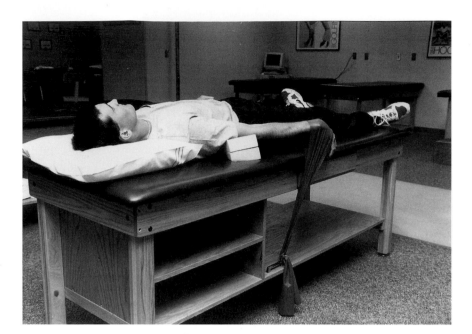

Figure 10–23. A low-load, long-duration stretch is performed to improve elbow extension. A low-resistance theraband is secured at one end and wrapped around the patient's distal forearm. The stretch should be mild in intensity and sustained for a long duration (8 to 12 minutes).

protocol is being followed, regaining full extension by 6 to 8 weeks postoperative is imperative, since collagen will begin to mature after this time frame and obtaining full range of motion will be extremely difficult.

Ulnar Collateral Ligament Reconstruction

Rehabilitation following UCL reconstruction should be based on the type of surgery performed, the method of transposition of the ulnar nerve, and the extent of injury within the elbow joint. The following rehabilitation program is based on the surgical technique described by Andrews and colleagues.[28] This surgical technique uses an autogenous palmaris longus tendon, when available, to reconstruct the ulnar collateral ligament. When the palmaris longus is not available, a toe extensor tendon is utilized. The graft is woven through the medial epicondyle of the humerus and medial ulna in a figure-eight fashion. The ulnar nerve is simultaneously transposed anteriorly and superficially beneath fascial slings, referred to as a subcutaneous nerve transfer. This type of reconstructive surgery attempts to recreate the anterior oblique portion of the UCL, which provides the primary restraint to valgus stress during throwing.[14,26] The rehabilitation program is thoroughly outlined in Table 10–8.

Immediately following surgery, the patient's elbow is immobilized in a posterior splint at 90 degrees of flexion. Immobilization allows initial soft-tissue healing of the fascial slings.[15] The patient's wrist is free to move in the splint, which permits wrist ROM exercises and submaximal isometrics for the elbow and wrist. Gripping exercises are also performed. A bulky compression dressing and cryotherapy are utilized for swelling control.

The patient is progressed to a range-of-motion brace 7 days postsurgery. Initially, motion is allowed from 30 to 100 degrees of flexion. The brace is readjusted during the third week to allow motion from 15 to 110 degrees. Each week thereafter, elbow ROM and the brace settings are increased by 5 degrees of extension and 10 degrees of flexion. Thus, the patient should achieve full elbow range of motion by the end of the sixth week. This allows a gradual restoration of elbow range of motion.

It is important to monitor the neurovascular status of the patient during the first few weeks after surgery. Ulnar neuropathy has been noted to occur at an incidence of 22 to 31 percent after UCL reconstruction with intramuscular ulnar nerve transposition.[29-30] We have noted only an 8 to 10 percent incidence of ulnar neuropathy with the subcutaneous nerve transposition method, with less than 2 percent of patients exhibiting symptoms longer than 8 weeks.[31] Sensory changes can occur in the little finger and ulnar side of the ring finger. Motor weakness may also be present, with the patient exhibiting difficulty performing thumb abduction, finger abduction and adduction, little finger abduction, or ulnar flexion of the wrist. All of these symptoms suggest possible ulnar nerve injury. Most commonly, decreased sensation along the ulnar side of the hand is the symptom experienced. Usually this symptom is transient, resolving within 7 days. If any of these symptoms are expressed, the compressive dressing should be assessed for tightness and loosened if needed to alleviate the symptoms.

Cryotherapy is another potential cause for ulnar nerve symptoms. Temporary nerve palsies at the elbow and knee resulting after the use of cryotherapy have been reported in the literature.[32,33] These nerve palsies were

TABLE 10–8. POSTOPERATIVE REHABILITATION FOLLOWING CHRONIC ULNAR COLLATERAL LIGAMENT RECONSTRUCTION USING AUTOGENOUS GRAFT

Phase I. Immediate Postoperative Phase (weeks 0 to 3)
 Goals
  Protect healing tissue
  Decrease pain/inflammation
  Retard muscular atrophy
 • Postoperative Week 1
  Posterior splint at 90 degrees elbow flexion
  Wrist AROM ext/flexion
  Elbow compression dressing (2 to 3 days)
  Exercises: Gripping exercises, wrist ROM, shoulder isometrics (except shoulder ER), biceps isometrics
  Cryotherapy
 • Postoperative Week 2
  Application of functional brace 30 to 100 degrees
  Initiate wrist isometrics
  Initiate elbow flex/ext isometrics
  Continue all exercises listed above
 • Postoperative Week 3
  Advance brace 15 to 110 degrees (gradually increase ROM; 5 degrees extension/10 degrees flexion per week)

Phase II. Intermediate Phase (weeks 4 to 8)
 Goals
  Gradual increase in range of motion
  Promote healing of repaired tissue
  Regain and improve muscular strength
 • Week 4
  Functional brace set (10 to 120 degrees)
  Begin light resistance exercises for arm (1 lb) wrist curls, extensions pronation/supination elbow ext/flexion
  Progress shoulder program emphasize rotator cuff strengthening (avoid ER until 6th week)

 • Week 6
  Functional brace set (0 to 130 degrees); AROM 0 to 145 degrees (without brace)
  Progress elbow strengthening exercises
  Initiate shoulder external rotation strengthening
  Progress shoulder program

Phase III. Advanced Strengthening Phase (weeks 9 to 13)
 Goals
  Increase strength, power, endurance
  Maintain full elbow ROM
  Gradually initiate sporting activities
 • Week 9
  Initiate eccentric elbow flexion/extension
  Continue isotonic program: Forearm and wrist
  Continue shoulder program: Throwers ten program
  Manual resistance diagonal patterns
  Initiate plyometric exercise program
 • Week 11
  Continue all exercises listed above
  May begin light sport activities (golf, swimming)

Phase IV. Return to Activity Phase (weeks 14 to 26)
 Goals
  Continue to increase strength, power, and endurance of upper extremity musculature
  Gradual return to sport activities
 • Week 14
  Initiate interval throwing program (phase I)
  Continue strengthening program
  Emphasis on elbow and wrist strengthening and flexibility exercises
 • Weeks 22 to 26
  Return to competitive throwing

attributed to the use of cryotherapy for longer than 30 minutes or the use of cryotherapy over superficial nerves, such as the ulnar nerve or common peroneal nerve. Protecting superficial nerves during the application of cryotherapy or limiting the application of cryotherapy to 20 minutes was suggested as a means to avoid complications.[32]

Progression to the intermediate phase occurs around week 4. Goals in this phase are to gradually increase ROM, promote healing of the repaired tissue, and improve muscular strength. Isotonics are performed for wrist flexion and extension, elbow flexion and extension, and elbow pronation and supination. Isotonic strengthening may be started for the shoulder, too, but it is important to avoid external rotation strengthening until the sixth week because of the valgus stress it imparts across the elbow. All isotonics can be advanced during the sixth week, with the addition of external rotation strengthening. Neuromuscular control drills including rhythmic stabilizations should also be added to address dynamic control of the medial elbow.

It is important to assess the progress with ROM during the sixth week. Attention should be paid to elbow extension since the formation of a flexion contracture is a common postoperative occurrence.[8,34,35] If tightness is noted at end range extension, aggressive techniques are necessary to avoid flexion contracture formation. Starting these techniques in a timely fashion is critical as mature collagen is more difficult to stretch. Several techniques have been found to be useful in improving flexibility. Joint mobilizations for the humeroulnar and humeroradial joints are also beneficial.[36] A posterior glide of the ulna on the humerus can assist in regaining elbow extension (see Fig. 10–24). During the intermediate phase, grade III oscillations can be performed to produce a slight stretch on the anterior capsule. In later phases of the rehabilitation program, grade IV oscillations can be performed to produce a greater stretch on the anterior capsule. This type of aggressive mobilization is not performed until pain has been eliminated.

Low-load, long-duration stretching is also effective in helping to regain full extension (see Fig. 10–23). This

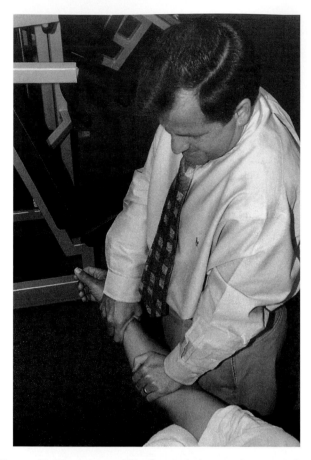

Figure 10–24. Joint mobilization technique to increase elbow extension: a posterior glide of the ulna.

type of stretching is usually performed with a towel roll placed posterior to the elbow joint to create a fulcrum. Then, theraband is applied at the wrist and tensioned to create a stretch. The stretch is low intensity, barely perceivable by the patient, so that pain and a protective muscular response are not elicited. The stretch should last 10 to 15 minutes. The combination of a low intensity and long duration has been reported in the literature to produce a plastic response of the collagen tissue, resulting in permanent elongation.[36,38-40] Utilizing heat in conjunction with this type of stretch has been found to produce a greater response.[41] Therefore, the application of a hot pack or use of ultrasound while stretching can be beneficial.

A final option for increasing range of motion is the application of a splint, either static or dynamic. A static splint holds the joint in a constant position. A dynamic splint uses a spring to exert a force, and the spring can be tightened to create a progressive stretch. The patient is encouraged to remove the brace for motion and strengthening exercises 2 to 3 times daily.

When treating the patient with a stiff elbow both a passive (warm whirlpool) and an active (upper body ergometer) warm-up are utilized to increase tissue extensibility prior to stretching. Joint mobilizations, as previously described, are then performed. Low-load, long-duration stretching is performed next. Proprioceptive neuromuscular facilitation stretching utilizing the contract and relax technique helps the clinician stretch to end range when muscle guarding is present. This stretching program is repeated during the treatment session for maximum benefit. Table 10–9 outlines the stretching program in detail.

The advanced strengthening phase is usually initiated at week 9, as long as the patient can meet the criteria documented in Table 10-8. Strengthening is performed aggressively with a focus on eccentrics, plyometrics, and neuromuscular control drills. Specifically, the thrower's ten program (see Table 10-7) should be used for strengthening, as it is directed at strengthening those muscle groups most active during throwing. Numerous plyometric drills can be performed, depending on whether the goal is to replicate the throwing motion, improve flexibility, or teach weight transferring and the use of the legs to accelerate the arm. Figures 10-17 to 10-22 are examples of various plyometric drills. For a more complete description, a wide variety of upper extremity plyometric techniques can be found in an article by Wilk and colleagues.[42] Neuromuscular control drills should emphasize the pronator and wrist flexor muscle groups since these muscles contribute to medial elbow stability. Muscle endurance is also enhanced in this phase. This is to maintain dynamic joint stability.

The patient can begin the interval throwing program approximately 4 months after surgery. In most cases, the patient can throw from the mound once the long toss program has been completed. A return to competitive throwing can take place at approximately 6 to 7 months following surgery.

Although returning an athlete to throwing is a significant challenge to the rehabilitation team, Jobe has reported that 63 percent of patients return to the previous level of throwing.[24] A retrospective study by Conway showed that 72 percent of athletes with UCL reconstructions returned to their previous level of throwing.[29] Recently, we have conducted retrospectively studies of results of UCL reconstruction in the overhead athlete. In our series of 86 throwers, 92 percent returned to throwing, with 82 to 86 percent returning to preinjury level.[31] Appropriate rehabilitation that prevents early motion complications, addresses strength deficits, and emphasizes dynamic stability of the medial elbow is paramount for a successful outcome following UCL reconstructive surgery.

TABLE 10–9. PROGRAM TO INCREASE ELBOW EXTENSION

- Passive warm-up (warm whirlpool) 7 to 10 minutes
- Active warm-up (upper body ergometer) 10 minutes

- Joint mobilization
  Distraction glides
  Posterior ulna glide for upward elbow extension
  Mobilization of radial head
- Low head long duration stretching (12 to 15 minutes)
- Manual PNF stretches contract relax technique
- Passive stretching
- Repeat process twice
- Evaluate for static or dynamic splint

Arthroscopy (Debridement, Loose Body Removal, Synovectomy)

Rehabilitation progresses rapidly and aggressively following diagnostic arthroscopy or arthroscopy for debridement, loose body removal, or synovectomy because postoperative pain and stiffness are minimal compared to open procedures. Phase I usually lasts 7 to 10 days and concentrates on regaining full range of motion, decreasing pain and inflammation, and retarding muscle atrophy. Active and active-assisted motion exercises are initiated and performed to tolerance during the first few days after surgery. Stretching exercises are utilized to help increase flexibility. Gripping exercises are included to maintain grip strength and help reduce edema formation in the hand. Submaximal isometrics are performed for the elbow and wrist musculature for approximately 3 days after surgery, then an isotonic program is initiated, usually at 10 to 14 days. The entire rehabilitation program can be found in Table 10-10.

The intermediate phase usually begins the second postoperative week. Criteria to move into this phase include full ROM, minimal pain and tenderness, and at least a good grade on manual muscle testing of the elbow flexors and extensors. The goals are to improve the patient's strength and endurance, as well as enhance neuromuscular control. Isotonic exercises for the elbow and wrist musculature are progressed with an emphasis on eccentric contractions. It is important to also include isotonics for the shoulder girdle, since proximal stability is necessary for distal mobility. Neuromuscular control drills can also be performed to increase dynamic stability of the shoulder and elbow.

The patient is progressed to the advanced strengthening phase when the following criteria are fulfilled: full, nonpainful ROM; no pain or tenderness; and strength that is 70 percent of the contralateral side. Usually, this criteria can be met around 4 weeks after surgery. The advanced strengthening phase focuses on increasing strength, power, and endurance of the entire arm. Advanced

TABLE 10–10. POSTOPERATIVE REHABILITATIVE PROTOCOL FOR ELBOW ARTHROSCOPY

Initial Phase (week 1)
  Goal
    Full wrist and elbow ROM, decrease swelling, decrease pain, retardation of muscle atrophy
- Day of Surgery
    Begin gently moving elbow in bulky dressing
- Postop Days 1 to 2
    Remove bulky dressing; replace with elastic bandages
    Immediate postop hand, wrist, and elbow exercises
      Putty/grip strengthening
      Wrist flexor stretching
      Wrist extensor stretching
      Wrist curls
      Reverse wrist curls
      Neutral wrist curls
      Pronation/supination
      A/AAROM elbow ext/flex
- Postop Days 3 to 7
    PROM elbow ext/flex (motion to tolerance)
    Begin PRE exercises with 1 lb weight
      Wrist curls
      Reverse wrist curls
      Neutral wrist curls
      Pronation/supination
      Broomstick roll-up

Intermediate Phase (weeks 2 to 4)
  Goal
    Improve muscular strength and endurance, normalize joint arthrokinematics
- Week 2. Range of Motion Exercises (overpressure into extension)
    Addition of biceps curl and triceps extension
    Continue to progress PRE weight and repetitions as tolerable
- Week 3
    Initiate biceps and triceps eccentric exercise program
    Initiate rotator cuff exercise program
      External rotators
      Internal rotators
      Deltoid
      Supraspinatus
      Scapulothoracic strengthening

Advanced Phase (weeks 4 to 8)
  Goal
    Preparation of athlete for return to functional activities

  Criteria to progress to advanced phase:
    Full nonpainful ROM
    No pain or tenderness
    Isokinetic test that fulfills criteria to throw
    Satisfactory clinical exam
- 3 to 6 Weeks
    Continue maintenance program, emphasizing muscular strength, endurance, and flexibility
    Initiate interval throwing program, phase I

nally rotated to relieve pressure within the hip. There may also be a "snapping" sensation of the iliopsoas tendon over the iliopectineal eminence.[14]

Physical exam reveals the enlarged bursae as palpable masses in the groin area. These soft-tissue masses can be distinguished from tumors by MRI. Extension of the hip, placing tension on the iliopsoas tendon, exacerbates the patient's discomfort.

Initial treatment is nonoperative, consisting of relative rest and nonsteroidal anti-inflammatory medication. Physical therapy modalities as well as iliopsoas stretching are also helpful.

Rarely, surgical release of the iliopsoas tendon at its insertion into the lesser trochanter is required for chronic cases refractory to nonoperative management.[10]

Snapping Hip Syndrome

Snapping hip syndrome is a clinical entity that causes pain and snapping in the hip joint. There are several known causes, the most common being the iliotibial band snapping over the greater trochanter.[10,13] It can also be caused by snapping of the iliopsoas tendon over the iliopectineal line, the iliofemoral ligaments over the femoral head, the long head of the biceps femoris tendon over the ischial tuberosity, as well as by certain intra-articular pathology.

Snapping of the Iliotibial Band

Snapping of the iliotibial band causes friction over the trochanteric bursa that can create a bursitis. Pain may or may not be present. Athletes will complain of snapping within the hip as the hip goes from flexion to extension. If the athlete remains asymptomatic, treatment of the snapping alone is not necessary. With painful snapping, treatment is directed toward the bursitis and includes relative rest, nonsteroidal anti-inflammatory medication, and a physical therapy program to include modalities and iliotibial band therapy.

Injection of corticosteroids into the bursa can be helpful. In most cases, the painful snapping is relieved by these measures. In certain cases refractory to nonoperative treatment, surgery may be indicated. Several procedures have been described with good results.[16,17]

Snapping of the Iliopsoas Muscle

This syndrome is due to snapping of the iliopsoas tendon over the iliopectineal eminence. The snapping can be painful as a result of a secondary bursitis that may develop following repetitive friction to the bursa as the hip goes from flexion, adduction, and external rotation to full extension.

Treatment generally consists of relative rest, non-steroidal anti-inflammatory medication, and a physical therapy program for stretching of the hip flexors and modalities as indicated. Surgery, including iliopsoas tendon lengthening, is rarely indicated.

Osteitis Pubis

Osteitis pubis is a rare cause of pelvic pain in the athlete. More commonly, osteitis pubis is a complication following bladder and prostate surgery.[17-19] There have been cases of osteitis pubis related to athletic activity reported in the literature.[19-21] Long-distance runners, weight lifters, soccer players, and football players are most commonly affected.[19,22]

The exact cause of osteitis pubis in athletes is unknown, but there is evidence to support repeated microtrauma as a cause. Other theories suggest muscle strain, avascular necrosis, and osteochondritis desiccans as possible causes.

The underlying etiology is thought to be overuse of the adductors, gracilis muscles, or rectus abdominis muscles with degenerative changes at their bony attachments.

Athletes experiencing this entity often complain of gradual onset of pain in the pelvic area that may extend to the groin or the abdomen. Stretching exercises can exacerbate their pain.

Physical examination typically reveals pain with palpation along the subcutaneous border of the pubic symphysis. Other characteristic signs include pain in full flexion of either leg, on passive abduction of the hips, and on resisted adduction of the hips. In severe cases, the athlete may present with an antalgic or waddling gait due to spasm of the adductors.

Radiographic changes can lag behind the clinical picture for 3 or 4 weeks. Specific radiographic changes have been reported by Harris and Murray.[20] Characteristic features described by them include symmetric bone resorption at the medial ends of the pelvic bones, widening of the symphysis, and sclerosis along the pubic rami.

When evaluating an athlete with pain in the pubic or groin area, the physician must consider more serious causes, such as infection, ankylosing spondylitis, or hernia.

This disorder is self-limiting, usually lasting several months. Initial treatment is focused around relative rest and nonsteroidal anti-inflammatory medication. Exercises that stretch the adductor muscles should be avoided and will worsen these symptoms. Most athletes respond to nonoperative treatment within 2 to 3 months, when light jogging may begin. A progressive exercise program should be followed, with the athlete returning to full activities in approximately 3 months.

In rare cases refractory to conservative treatment, surgery is indicated. Surgical procedures that have been described in the treatment of osteitis pubis include debridement[19] and pubic symphysis arthrodesis.[23,24]

Muscle Strains

The hip and pelvis region is a very common location for muscular and musculotendinous injuries in the athlete. Many major muscle groups either insert or originate from the pelvic ring and proximal femur. The abdominal and gluteal muscles attach to the iliac wing, while the hamstrings attach to the ischium. The adductors originate from the pubis and the iliopsoas inserts on the lesser trochanter.

In the adult, the most common site for musculotendinous injuries is at the musculotendinous junction. These injuries usually occur as acute muscle strains or pulls.[25] Among the adolescent population, avulsion injuries of the tendon-cartilaginous insertion is most common. Muscle strains and tears are classified as partial or complete and usually result from stretching the muscle against a forceful contraction.[25]

External Oblique Strains

Strains of the aponeurosis of the external oblique muscle are often caused by forceful contraction of the abdominal muscles while the trunk is forced to the contralateral side. The aponeurosis may be partially or completely torn from the iliac crest. This injury is commonly seen among football and hockey players.

The athlete typically presents with severe pain, difficulty in straightening the upper torso, and localized tenderness along the iliac crest. A defect may sometimes be palpable just above the iliac crest. A useful examining maneuver is to have the patient lie on the contralateral side and actively abduct or extend the involved thigh. Pain with this maneuver indicates injury to the gluteal attachments or the tensor fasciae lata and lateral abdominals.

Treatment of these injuries consists of rest, ice, compression, and restriction of vigorous activities. Abdominal binders and taping may aid in reducing pain and increase muscular support until symptoms resolve.

Physical therapy should be initiated when the acute pain has diminished. Protective devices, such as taping and padding, should be worn for early return to sports. In rare cases, surgical intervention to repair the injured tissues is indicated.[9,26]

Iliopsoas Injury

Iliopsoas tendon strains occur by forceful contraction of the iliopsoas tendon with the thigh fixed or forced into extension. This produces deep discomfort and tenderness in the groin that may extend into the lower abdomen. Passive external rotation of the extended hip, or resisted hip flexion, exacerbates the pain. In the younger population, this injury can create an avulsion fracture from the lesser trochanter. Treatment is focused on relative rest, with an early physical therapy program when the acute episode resolves. Most patients return to sports by 4 to 6 weeks.

Adductor Injuries

Strains of the adductor muscle group, commonly known as pulled groin is very frequent among athletes in the older population. It has been reported by Merifield and Cowan[27] that a difference in strength between both hip adductor muscle groups may be a predisposing factor in this injury. Ice hockey players are most susceptible due to the forceful hip adduction motion required for push-off. Groin injuries are also common among football, soccer, and rugby players and are caused by forceful external rotation of the abducted leg. Patients experience pain in the groin area. Passive abduction of the thigh and resisted active adduction exacerbate this pain. Tenderness occurs as the subcutaneous border of the pelvic ramus is palpated. In certain cases, a defect may be palpable when a complete avulsion of an adductor muscle occurs.

Treatment of these injuries occurs in several stages and depends on the severity of the injury. Initially, relative rest, ice, protection, and nonsteroidal anti-inflammatory medication is used. A useful way to protect the adductors is to strap the hip in a spica wrap with the thigh flexed and externally rotated. Approximately 48 hours after the acute pain resolves, stretching and range-of-motion exercises are initiated within the patient's comfort zone. Active resisted exercises are usually begun at 4 to 6 weeks. The athlete should be instructed in a home therapy program to prevent recurrence.

In most instances, athletes are able to return to full activities following a therapy program. These injuries can lead to chronic tendonitis or recurrent strains of the adductors. In certain chronic cases, where nonoperative management has not been successful, release of the adductors from the pelvic ring may be necessary as described by Martens and associates.[28]

The gracilis muscle crosses both the hip and knee and functions similar to the adductors. It is both a hip adductor and medial rotator. If the knee is extended, the gracilis functions as an active hip flexor, but becomes inactive with increasing knee flexion. It is often strained in association with the hip adductors and is treated similarly.

Hamstring Strains

Strains of the hamstring muscles most commonly occur at the proximal muscle tendinous junction. They usually occur with the hip maximally flexed while the knee is extended, such as occurs while hurdling an object or in forceful straight leg raising. Injury is associated with poor flexibility, failure to stretch prior to strenuous exercise, muscle strength imbalance between quadriceps and hamstrings, and poor coordination. On physical examination, hamstring strains typically cause localized tenderness over the ischial tuberosity. Straight leg raising and active resisted extension of the hip exacerbate the pain.

Treatment of these various muscle and tendon injuries of the hip and pelvis is centered around a staged, progressive, well-defined protocol in most instances. It is essential that these injuries are addressed immediately following the acute event. The vast majority of these injuries are first- or second-degree strains according to the American Medical Association classification of athletic injuries. The treatment plan outlined for management of these injuries consists of four stages.

Stage I

Treatment during the first stage is focused on limiting pain, bleeding, swelling, and inflammation. This typically is done with rest, ice, compression, and elevation in the acute phase. Cryotherapy, or cold packs, compressively wrapped into place for 20 minutes every hour is very effective to control pain, swelling, and inflammation. Also nonsteroidal anti-inflammatory medication can be initiated to help in decreasing the inflammation. Resting the injured muscles is crucial at this stage. The involved area should be elevated and positioned to avoid stressing injured tissues. Protective devices such as crutches, taping, and orthotic devices can also be useful. Hip spiker wraps for groin injuries or abdominal corsets for oblique muscle strains provide both compression and protection and help reduce pain. Stage I lasts approximately 48 to 72 hours, when the acute symptoms resolve.

Stage II

The object of stage II treatment is to regain normal range of motion, prevent joint contracture and muscle atrophy, limit muscle spasm, and reduce stiffness. Modalities such as contrast heat and cold treatments can be helpful. Ultrasound and high-intensity muscle stimulation may be added to the program. Hydrotherapy using warm water in a whirlpool tank often reduces muscle spasms and stiffness in hip and pelvic injuries. Active and gentle passive assisted range-of-motion exercises are begun within a pain-free range of motion. Neuromuscular reeducation exercises are emphasized if there is evidence of muscular incoordination. Protected weight-bearing using a crutch or cane for ambulation may be necessary until strength and coordination return.

Stage III

The third stage is centered around regaining normal strength, flexibility, and endurance. During this stage, muscle spasms should have resolved and a pain-free state of range of motion is achieved. Exercises should be started with isometrics followed by dynamic exercises with the aid of machines. Concentric and eccentric exercises are both utilized.

Stage IV

The final stage is aimed at the athlete returning to preinjury status with full range of motion, strength, and mobility. Exercises are focused on improving strength, flexibility, endurance, and coordination. Sport-specific activities, such as agility training, are resumed. Heat and ultrasound are useful before stretching exercises are performed. Cryotherapy is continued following exercises to prevent further inflammation and muscle spasm. When the athlete has regained normal strength, range of motion, and mobility, and can perform specific skills required by his or her particular sport, he or she can be allowed to return to full activities.

Sacroiliac Sprains

The sacroiliac joint consists of the sacrum and ilia and is lined by articular cartilage. This joint is supported by major ligamentous structures that allow it to withstand major forces. These ligaments include the anterior and posterior sacroiliac, the interosseous sacroiliac, and the sacrotuberous ligaments. All of these ligaments can be injured when exposed to the tremendous forces created by athletic activities. These forces are basically generated via two mechanisms. Superior forces are produced from above the sacroiliac joint through the lumbar spine. These forces tend to move the upper portion of the sacrum forward and downward with the coccyx moving upward and backward. The other major forces are produced from below the sacroiliac joint, acting through the hip joint and into the ilium, forcing the ilia upward and posterior. These two major forces oppose one another and create great shear forces at the sacroiliac joint during athletic competition.

Specific activities known to result in sacroiliac joint sprains include sudden, forceful contraction of the hamstrings or the abdominal muscles, sudden twisting motions of the torso, a forceful blow to the buttocks, or forceful straightening from a bent position. The patient usually experiences pain immediately or the following day. The pain in the region of the sacroiliac joint may radiate to the lumbar region, thigh, or groin. The athlete with an injury to one sacroiliac joint ambulates with a limp, avoiding weight bearing on the affected limb.

Physical examination reveals tenderness over the sacroiliac joint. Range of motion of the lumbar spine and pelvis is often limited secondary to pain. Specific diagnostic maneuvers should include testing for Lasegue's sign, which is usually present, and Gaenslen's test. Gaenslen's test is performed by having the patient lie on the unaffected side while hyperflexing the lower hip and hyperextending the upper hip. A positive test reproduces the pain over the sacroiliac joint. Lateral compression of both iliac wings should be performed manually and may also produce similar pain over the sacroiliac joint. Rectal examination should not be neglected and may reveal swelling and tenderness over the sacroiliac joint.

Treatment of sacroiliac sprains include bedrest, heat, and pain management. An exercise program can be initiated when the pain level is tolerable. These should include flexion and extension exercises of the lower back, along with abdominal strengthening exercises. A constricting elastic bandage or belt can help provide pain relief by stabilizing the sacroiliac joint. Injections of steroids into the sacroiliac joint has been described, but its value is not well defined. Most patients require 4 to 6 weeks of protected motion while the inflammation and pain subsides, and healing is sufficient to return to previous activities.

Fractures

Fractures of the pelvis are very serious and are often associated with other injuries. These can be relatively minor avulsion fractures, or more serious open, unstable fractures. Minor avulsion fractures are relatively straightforward, whereas more complex fracture patterns may require life-saving external and possibly internal fixation devices.

When evaluating a patient with a pelvic fracture, one must be aware of the possible life-threatening injuries associated with these fractures. These include injuries to the genitourinary and gastrointestinal systems, and most importantly, retroperitoneal vascular injuries. An assessment of a pelvic fracture begins with a general examination and overall assessment of the patient. A careful history is obtained, which may provide information as to the mechanism of injury and the degree of energy absorbed during the injury.

On physical examination, swelling, lacerations, abrasions, contusions, or ecchymoses may be indicative of serious injuries and must be evaluated carefully.

There are many classification systems for pelvic fractures reported in the literature. One that helps classify the fracture pattern based on the mechanism of injury and stability is the Tile classification.[29]

Once a patient is suspected of having sustained a fracture of the pelvis, the pelvis should be stabilized and the patient immobilized. The athlete should be transferred emergently to a proper medical facility where he or she can be evaluated thoroughly and definitive treatment begun.

Fractures of the Pelvic Ring

Pelvic ring fractures are rare among athletic injuries. When they do occur, it is important to recognize them quickly because of the possibility of associated injuries.

These injuries are caused by great forces that are transmitted through the pelvis and abdomen, resulting in visceral damage, soft tissue injury, and major vascular injuries that can be life-threatening.

These types of injuries have been reported to occur in horseback riding, hang-gliding, football, hockey, cycling, and snowmobiling. The mechanism of injury is usually a direct blow, but may be associated with rotational forces. They are best classified as either stable or unstable injuries. Stable fractures involve individual bones in the pelvis without disruption in the integrity of the pelvic ring. Treatment of these fractures remains symptomatic.

Unstable fractures are more severe injuries. Various unstable fracture patterns have been described elsewhere.[30]

When treating unstable fractures of the pelvic ring, the physician should strive for anatomic reduction and maintenance to prevent subsequent and chronic sacroiliac pain. Once stability is maintained, the patient may begin protected weight bearing.

The principles of surgical intervention for these injuries is beyond the scope of this textbook and is covered in detail elsewhere.[31-33]

Avulsion Fractures

Avulsion fractures frequently occur at the various apotheoses located in the pelvis. These fractures can affect all age groups, but are most common among adolescents. The mechanism is usually a violent contraction or a sudden passive stretch of the muscles that insert along the pelvis. The areas most commonly affected are the anterior and superior iliac spine (ASIS), the anterior and inferior iliac spine (AIIS), the insertion of the sartorius, the insertion of the superior head of the rectus femoris, the ischial tuberosities, and the insertion of the hamstrings. Patients with pelvic avulsions will generally complain of a popping sensation and immediate severe pain at the time of injury. There is often no recall of significant trauma. Hip flexion may often be present with ASIS or AIIS avulsions. Knee flexion may be present with ischial tuberosity avulsions. Radiographs are useful in confirming the diagnosis. Comparison views of the contralateral side may be required to determine the degree of skeletal maturity.

Treatment of these injuries is usually straightforward. Initial treatment generally consists of relative rest, while placing the extremity in a comfortable position. Crutches for assistance in ambulation can be helpful. When the pain is tolerable, a progressive physical therapy program should be instituted as described by Metzmaker and Pappas.[34] The vast majority of these injuries can be treated nonoperatively. In high demand athletes, ischial tuberosity fractures may be treated operatively when there is greater than 1 or 2 cm of displacement. Displaced fractures treated nonoperatively may cause a painful prominence while sitting, groin and buttock pain, and muscle weakness.

In rare cases, excision of the fragment and reattachment of the muscles to the bone is indicated. In most cases of avulsion fractures, following completion of a physical therapy program, the athlete can return to sports in approximately 2 to 3 months.

Lesser Trochanteric Avulsion Fractures

These injuries occur mainly in the adolescent age group. The mechanism is believed to be a sudden forceful contracture of the iliopsoas muscle. Most athletes give a history of severe anteromedial hip pain while running. Physical examination reveals pain with resisted hip flexion. Radiograms confirm the diagnosis.

Treatment consists of bedrest, until the acute pain resolves, followed by a progressive physical therapy program with protected weight bearing. Controversy surrounds the treatment of displaced fractures of the lesser trochanter. Some authors suggest surgery to reduce and fix the fracture fragment,[35,36] while others favor nonoperative management.[38] With a typical avulsion fracture, most athletes return to sports within 2 months after injury.

Stress Fractures

Stress fractures of the proximal femur are relatively rare. Stress fractures result from cumulative, repetitive stresses applied to bone over a period of time. During this time of repetitive stress, bone resorption is greater than bone deposition. When these cumulative forces exceed the structural strength of bone, stress fractures can occur.

Stress fractures of the femoral neck have been reported to occur in military recruits and runners.[38,39] Factors such as muscle fatigue, training errors, improper footwear, and poor surfaces can predispose an athlete to the development of stress fractures. Most patients with femoral neck stress fractures present with pain in the hip, groin, thigh, or knee. Pain may often be exacerbated with exercise and is relieved by rest.

Physical examination reveals painful, limited range of motion of the hip, especially with internal rotation, antalgic gait, and tenderness to palpation over the femoral neck. If a femoral neck stress fracture is suspected, it must be ruled out. Serious complications of untreated stress fractures include complete displaced femoral neck fractures, avascular necrosis, nonunion, and varus deformity.

Radiograms may lag behind the clinical picture for 2 to 4 weeks.[5,38,39] Bone scan has proven to be a very sensitive diagnostic tool in the detection of femoral neck stress fractures. A negative bone scan virtually excludes the diagnosis of stress fracture.

Treatment of femoral neck stress fractures depends upon the location of the fracture and the results of diagnostic testing. Initially, if a stress fracture is suspected and radiograms are negative, the athlete should be placed on strict, nonweight-bearing status for 7 to 10 days, after which repeat radiograms and bone scan are performed. If both studies remain negative, they should be repeated after another week. After that, if the bone scan is positive with negative radiograms, the athlete is kept on bedrest until he or she is free of pain. At this point, the athlete may gradually increase his or her activity level until he or she returns to preinjury level of activity. Weekly x-rays should be obtained to monitor the status of the fracture. When the repeat bone scan is negative, fracture healing is complete and the athlete may return to full activities.

Fractures on the medial side of the femoral neck, or compression stress fractures, are treated with bedrest until the pain resolves. Nonweight-bearing ambulation with crutches is continued until there is radiographic evidence of fracture healing. If any changes, such as displacement, occur in the fracture status, as seen in periodic x-rays, internal fixation is recommended. Also, in cases where nonoperative management fails to relieve the patient's symptoms, internal fixation is indicated.

Fractures that occur on the lateral or tension side are more likely to displace if not treated aggressively. Due to the serious complications that may result from fracture displacement, once this type of fracture is diagnosed, internal fixation should be performed immediately. If the fracture is already displaced, closed reduction and internal fixation is performed urgently.

Transient Synovitis

Transient synovitis is a nonspecific inflammatory condition and is the most common cause of hip pain in the young athlete.[40] Its etiology remains unknown; however, trauma and viral infection appear to be possible causes. This is a self-limiting condition that usually resolves within several weeks. The athlete usually presents with an antalgic gait. The child may also complain of acute or gradual onset of thigh or hip pain.

Physical examination typically reveals localized tenderness and painful range of motion of the hip. Laboratory studies and radiograms are usually negative.

Other causes of hip pain in a young person must be considered. These include infection, rheumatoid disease, and slipped capital femoral epiphysis. Treatment includes bedrest in a comfortable position, skin traction for immobilization, and nonsteroidal anti-inflammatory medication. Significant improvement in symptoms is noted within 1 to 2 days. Crutches are used for assistance in ambulation during the early stages. When the acute pain has resolved, the athlete may gradually return to his or her previous activities over a 2-week period. Early return to full activities before the pain has resolved can lead to early recurrence of the patient's symptoms.

REFERENCES

1. Sashin D. A critical analysis of the anatomy and the pathologic changes of the sacroiliac joints. *J Bone Joint Surg.* 1930;12:891.
2. Hollishead WH. *Anatomy for Surgeons*, vol. 3. *The Back and Limbs*. Philadelphia: Harper & Row; 1958.
3. Gardener E, Gray DJ, O'Rahilly R. *Anatomy, A Regional Study of Human Structure*. Philadelphia: Saunders; 1975.
4. Rydell N. Biomechanics of the hip joint. *Clin Orthop.* 1973;92:6.
5. Morris JM. Biomechanical aspects of the hip joint. *Orthop Clin North Am.* 1971;2:33.
6. Nordin M, Frankel VH. Biomechanics of the hip. In: Frankel VH, Burstein AH, eds. *Orthopaedic Biomechanics*. Philadelphia: Lea & Febiger; 1970.
7. American Medical Association, Subcommittee on Classification of Sports Injuries. *Standard Nomenclature of Athletic Injuries*. Chicago: American Medical Association; 1966.
8. Kulund DN. *The Injured Athlete*. Philadelphia: Lippincott; 1982.
9. O'Donoghe DH. *Treatment of Injuries to Athletes*. Philadelphia: Saunders; 1970.
10. Waters PM, Millis MB. Hip and pelvic injuries in the young athletc. *Clin Sports Med.* 1988;7:513.
11. Jeffreys TE. Pseudomalignant osseous tumor of soft tissue. *J Bone Joint Surg.* 1966;48B:488.
12. Antao NA. Myositis ossificans of the hip in a professional soccer player. *Am J Sports Med.* 1988;16:82.
13. Zoltan DJ, Clancy WG, Keene JS. A new operative approach to snapping hip and refractory trochanteric bursitis in athletes. *Am J Sports Med.* 1986;14:201.
14. Scharberg JE, Harper MC, Allen WC. The snapping hip syndrome. *Am J Sports Med.* 1984;12:361.
15. Brignall CG, Stainsby GD. The snapping hip: Treatment by Z-plasty. *J Bone Joint Surg.* 1991;73B:253.
16. Bruckl R, Rosemeyer B, Schmidt JM, Froschl M. Zur operativen Behandlung der schnappenden Hufte. *Z Orthop.* 1984;122:308.
17. Beach EW. Osteitis pubis. *Urol Cutan Rev.* 1949;53:577.
18. Beer E. Periostitis and osteitis of the symphysis pubis following suprapubic cystotomies. *J Urol.* 1928;20:233.
19. Wiley JJ. Traumatic osteitis pubis: The gracilis syndrome. *Am J Sports Med.* 1983;11:360.
20. Harris NH, Murray RO. Lesions of the symphysis in athletes. *Br Med J.* 1974;4:211.
21. Rosenthal RE, Spickard WA, Markham RD, Rhamy RK. Osteomyelitis of the symphysis pubis. *J Bone Joint Surg.* 1982;64A:123.
22. Koch R, Jackson D. Pubic symphysitis in runners. *Am J Sports Med.* 1981;9:62.
23. Adams RJ, Chandler FA. Osteitis pubis of traumatic etiology. *J Bone Joint Surg.* 1953;35A:685.
24. Olerud S, Gerusten S. Chronic pubic symphysiolysis. *J Bone Joint Surg.* 1974;56A:799.
25. Garrett WE, Safran MR, Seaber AV, et al. Biomechanical comparison of stimulated and nonstimulated muscle pulled to failure. *Am J Sports Med.* 1987;15:448.
26. Sim FH, Scott HG. Injuries of the pelvis and hip in athletes. In: Nicholas JA, Hershmann EB, eds. *The Lower Extremity and Spine in Sports Medicine*. St. Louis: Mosby; 1986.
27. Merrifield HH, Cowan RF. Groin strain injuries in ice hockey. *Am J Sports Med.* 1973;1:41.
28. Martens MA, Hansen L, Mulier JC. Adductor tendinitis and musculus rectus abdominis tendopathy. *Am J Sports Med.* 1987;15:353.
29. Tile M. Pelvic ring fractures. Should they be fixed? *J Bone Joint Surg.* 1988;70B:1–12.
30. Judet R, Judet J, Letournel E. Fractures of the acetabulum: Classification and surgical approaches for open reduction. *J Bone Joint Surg.* 1964;46A:1615.
31. Canale ST, King RE. Pelvic and hip fractures. In Rockwood CA Jr, Wilkins KE, King RE, eds. *Fractures in Children*. Philadelphia: Lippincott; 1984.
32. Kane WJ. Fractures of the pelvis. In: Rockwood CA Jr, Green DP, eds. *Fractures in Adults*. Philadelphia: Lippincott; 1984.
33. Milch H, Milch RA. *Fracture Surgery*. New York: Paul B. Hoeber; 1959.
34. Metzmaker JN, Pappas AM. Avulsion fractures of the pelvis. *Am J Sports Med.* 1985;13:349.
35. Delee JC. Fractures and dislocations of the hip. In Rockwood CA Jr, Green DP, eds. *Fractures in Adults*. Philadelphia: Lippincott; 1984.
36. Poston H. Traction fracture of the lesser trochanter of the femur. *J Bone Surg.* 1921;9:256.
37. Dimon JH III. Isolated fractures of the lesser trochanter of the femur. *Clin Orthop.* 1972;82:144.
38. Fullerton LR, Snowdy HA. Femoral neck stress fractures. *Am J Sports Med.* 1988;16:365.
39. Hajek MR, Noble HB. Stress fractures of the femoral neck in runners. *Am J Sports Med.* 1982;10:112.
40. MacEwen GD, Bunnell WP, Ramsey PL. The hip. In: Lovell WW, Winter RB, eds. *Pediatric Orthopaedics*. Philadelphia: Lippincott; 1986.

Management of Hip and Pelvic Injuries

Robert G. Kelly

Although they occur less frequently than those of the knee and lower leg,[1] hip and pelvic injuries are most often encountered in sports requiring running or jumping, and in sports with frequent collisions. When involved in the treatment of athletes with hip and pelvic injuries, the athletic trainer and physical therapist must have a thorough understanding of the anatomy and biomechanics of the hip, pelvis, and surrounding soft tissue, as well as the specific athletic demands placed on the athlete upon a return to his or her specific sport. The physical therapist or athletic trainer must also address the predisposing factors that contribute to a variety of overuse and traumatic hip and pelvic injuries. As with all injuries, a thorough evaluation of the athlete's injury is necessary to formulate an appropriate individualized treatment plan. Most hip and pelvic injuries encountered in sports are caused by overuse.[1] The hallmark of treatment is relative rest from aggravating activities and specific therapeutic intervention to address limitations in flexibility, strength, and endurance. Counseling is indicated to prevent recurrence of symptoms. Effective management of acute hip and pelvic injuries requires a systematic approach to treatment with a criteria-based advancement through the phases of rehabilitation, from initial first aid to the eventual return to sporting activities (Table 11-1). With timely, appropriate management of the injury, the athlete's down-time will be reduced, and the risk of the reinjury will be minimized.

TABLE 11-1. REHABILITATION PHASE PROGRESSION: A CRITERIA-BASED APPROACH

Present Phase	Criteria for Phase Progression
I	Athlete experiences decreased pain, spasm, and swelling.
II	Full AROM, isometrics are pain free.
III	PREs are pain free.
IV	Running, eccentric exercises are pain free.
V	Agility drills at 100 percent intensity are pain free.
Return to sport!	

As with many injuries, the most effective form of treatment is prevention. Athletes and coaches must be educated on the importance of principles such as a proper warm-up prior to strenuous exercise, a year-round conditioning program to improve flexibility, strength, and fitness level, and the use of proper equipment to prevent overuse and traumatic hip and pelvic injuries.

TREATMENT OF SPECIFIC INJURIES

Greater Trochanteric Bursitis

Athough the onset of trochanteric bursitis may be traumatic resulting from a direct blow to the lateral hip, the most common presentation is a gradual, insidious, onset of pain along the lateral aspect of the hip. The cause of trochanteric bursitis is thought to be repetitive friction of the bursa from the overlying iliotibial band.[2] Because trochanteric bursitis is most commonly considered an overuse injury, the main emphasis of treatment is relative rest from aggravating activities. The athlete is, however, encouraged to maintain an upper body conditioning program and to incorporate activities such as a swimming to maintain cardiovascular fitness while not increasing hip pain. Rehabilitation of trochanteric bursitis begins with a comprehensive evaluation of the athlete's lower extremities including, but not limited to, hip range of motion, strength and flexibility, limb length, foot biomechanics, footwear, and a lumbar spine evaluation. An understanding of the athlete's running habits and sporting activity is also important. Goals of treatment for trochanteric bursitis include pain relief, the correction of causative factors such as limited iliotibial band flexibility, weak gluteals, excessive foot pronation or poor running form, and a pain-free return to sporting activities. Initial treatment of trochanteric bursitis depends on the severity of symptoms.

If pain is constant and not proportional to the degree of activity, possibly indicating an acute inflammatory process, modalities such as ice and electrical stimulation (TENS) are effective in reducing pain. Ice bags or commercial cold packs may be applied over the greater trochanter simultaneously with electrical stimulation. Interferential electrical current is also an effective analgesic. Because the electrodes are not placed directly over the injury but rather surrounding it, such treatment provides the added benefit of maintaining the exposure of the inflamed area to direct contact with ice. Nonsteroidal anti-inflammatory medications are also prescribed by the physician to reduce inflammation.

The main emphasis in the treatment of trochanteric bursitis is on tensor fasciae latae and iliotibial band stretching to improve flexibility and reduce friction on the underlying bursa. Because the tensor fascia latae is a hip flexor and abductor, as well as a weak hip internal rotator, the most effective way of stretching it is to combine the motions of hip extension, adduction, and external rotation (see Fig. 11–3). Also included in the stretching program is gluteus medius, gluteus maximus, and hip flexor stretching. It has been shown that stretching to increase tissue extensibility and flexibility is most effective immediately following a warm-up period.[3,4] Superficial heat modalities such as moist heat to the hip and warm whirlpool; and deep heat such as continuous ultrasound, can be used prior to stretching to improve effectiveness. Phonophoresis in the continuous mode will also increase tissue temperature prior to stretching, but its anti-inflammatory effects are largely unproven. Passive modalities have inherent disadvantages. Superficial heating agents fail to increase tissue temperature deeply enough, therefore limiting their effectiveness. Deep heating modalities, such as ultrasound, effectively raise tissue temperature to therapeutic levels at depths as great as 5 cm.[5,6] However, attempting to heat large areas with ultrasound can cause inadequate temperature changes. Therefore, when tolerated by the athlete, the preferred method to increase tissue temperature prior to stretching is by active warm-up. Hip stretching is performed following an aquatic program or low-intensity, pain-free lower extremity exercise such as brisk walking for 5 to 10 minutes. The athlete is then instructed in the principles of pain-free stretching using a static technique. Stretches are held for 15 to 30 seconds, and each stretch is performed five times. The athlete is instructed to repeat the stretching routine two to three times per day. If gluteal muscle weakness is present, the athlete is begun on strengthening exercises such as bridging, as well as hip abductor strengthening (for example, abduction straight leg raises) or resistive exercises using a hip machine or surgical tubing, as they become pain free. Exercises are performed using appropriate resistance for 3 sets of 8 to 15 repetitions. Should a true leg length discrepancy or poor foot biomechanics, such as hyperpronation, be present, the athlete is evaluated for and fitted with orthotics with the appropriate accommodations.

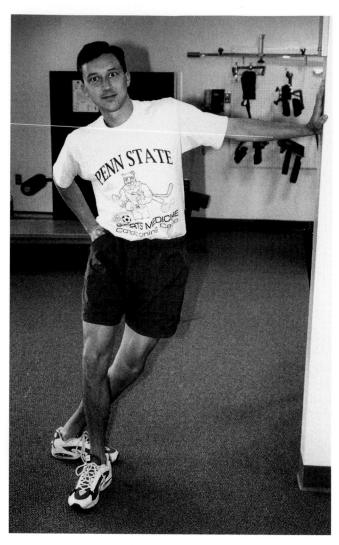

Figure 11–3. Standing iliotibial band stretching. Motions of hip adduction, extension, and external rotation are combined for the most effective stretch.

The main goal of rehabilitation is to return the athlete to prior levels of functioning. Therefore, functional training designed to simulate functional and recreational activities that were once painful should begin as early as safely tolerated. This can be done early in the rehabilitation process by "unweighting" the athlete to a degree necessary to perform the activity without pain. Also known as assisted exercise, examples of unweighting activities include aquatic walking, running, agility drills such as jumping, hopping, and side-to-side movements, and similar activities on unweighting devices such as those manufactured by Vigor (Stevensville, MI) or SOMA (Austin, TX) (see Fig. 11–4). The goal of functional training is to duplicate, as closely as possible, necessary functional and sporting activities that were once painful,

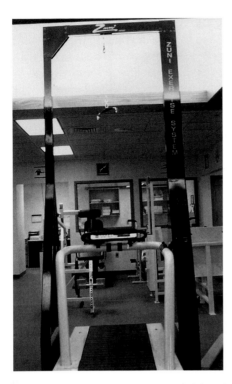

Figure 11–4. Assisted exercise using an unweighting device (Zuni: Soma Inc., Austin). Pain-free running is made possible by decreasing weight-bearing forces while maintaining normal speed of movement.

without increasing pain. This includes normal movement patterns as well as the appropriate speed of movement. Therefore, unweighting devices that allow for normal speed of exercise may be more beneficial than aquatic activities, which limit the speed of exercise. Ultimately, the athlete can benefit from either form of treatment, and the decision often comes down to the availability of equipment. Functional training using assisted exercise is progressed with decreasing amounts of unweighting until the athlete is full weight bearing (on land if aquatic therapy was chosen). Duration and intensity of functional training, beginning with straight-line jogging, and progressing to agility exercises and finally to sports-specific activities, is progressed according to patient tolerance. Throughout the rehabilitation, as well as following a return to sports, proper warm-up and adequate stretching is continued prior to activity, followed by stretching and ice for 15 to 20 minutes after activity. A full return to sports is permitted when the athlete demonstrates a full hip range of motion and strength and is pain free during and after sports activities. The athlete is advised to continue a regular hip stretching program to increase or maintain iliotibial band flexibility. Appropriate suggestions should be made, such as changing shoes every 300 to 500 miles of running, varying running courses, and cross-training to avoid recurrence of overuse symptoms.

Hip Pointer

The term "hip pointer" refers to an injury sustained from a direct blow to the iliac crest and surrounding abdominal musculature.[7,8] A contusion to the inadequately protected iliac crest can result in bleeding within the subperiosteum and into the surrounding soft tissue. Hip pointers are most common in collision sports such as football and ice hockey. Common mechanisms include a hard blow to the player's side or a hockey player being checked into the boards. Contusions to the iliac crest and adjoining abdominal musculature can be very painful and temporarily debilitating. Treatment of a hip pointer should be initiated immediately to minimize the amount of bleeding and swelling at the injury site. Initial management of a hip pointer involves applying ice and compression to the contusion for 15 to 20 minutes. This is to be repeated every 2 to 3 hours for 24 to 48 hours, depending on the clinician's judgment as to the severity of the injury. When not using ice, a wrap and padding combination should be used to further minimize the amount of bleeding. A one-half inch thick pad made of orthopedic felt or foam rubber cut to a size slightly larger than the area of swelling, in conjunction with an elastic bandage, is effective in providing added compression to the pelvic contusion (see Fig. 11–5). Treatment consisting of ice and compression should be continued as long as signs of bleeding are present, usually at least 48 hours following the injury. The use of electrical stimulation during the acute phase of injury management may also be effective in reducing pain and swelling.

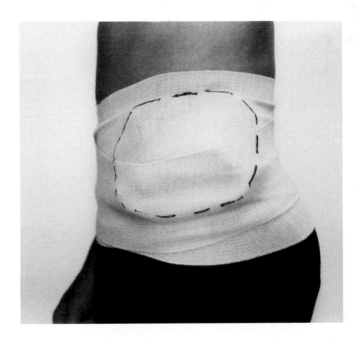

Figure 11–5. A compressive dressing, using ½-inch foam rubber and a 6-inch elastic bandage, is applied immediately following a hip pointer to minimize swelling and bleeding at the injury site.

Transcutaneous electrical nerve stimulation (TENS) is effective in reducing pain. Direct current electrical stimulation such as high voltage pulsed galvanic stimulation (HVPGS), has been shown to be effective in reducing swelling due to injury when the cathode is over the injury site.[9-11]

HVPGS can be used simultaneously with ice, provided that the electrodes do not insulate the injured area from the ice application. Treatment is carried out for 20 to 30 minutes per session on a daily basis. For athletes with severe pain, home TENS units are available for the athlete to use. The athlete is instructed on the use of TENS including electrode placement, current intensity, and treatment duration. Home TENS treatments may last up to 60 minutes and may be safely used as often as necessary to control pain.[12]

Beginning on the third or fourth day, trunk and lower extremity stretching exercises are begun to restore lost flexibility. Specific exercises are chosen based on motions limited due to the injury. Generally, trunk exercises such as lateral side bends, trunk extensions, and trunk rotations are necessary to restore full trunk range of motion (see Fig. 11-6). These exercises, as well as hip stretching, are done within the athlete's pain-free limits. Hip exercises such as hip flexor and tensor fasciae latae stretches are incorporated as needed based on the athlete's symptoms. Superficial and deep heating modalities should be used with caution. Premature use of these modalities may cause increased bleeding and swelling, adding to the athlete's recovery time.

A return to more strenuous exercises such as conditioning and sporting activities, is done as symptoms subside and trunk range of motion and flexibility return. As pain diminishes and range of motion nears normal, the athlete advances through progressively more demanding functional activities, incorporating sport-specific activities and playing surfaces into his or her training. Upon a return to full activity, including contact

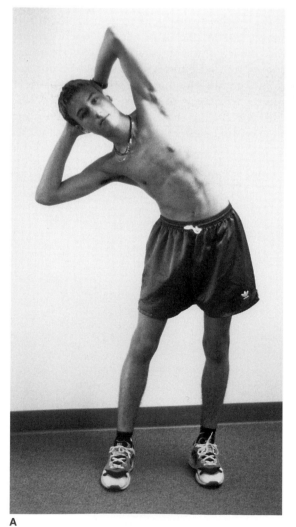

A

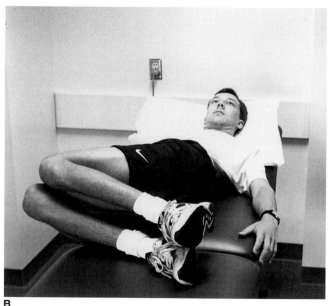

B

Figure 11–6. Exercises to restore trunk range of motion. **A.** Lateral side bends. **B.** Hooklying trunk twists.

drills and activity, the athlete is fitted with added rigid support over the injured area to protect against reinjury. This can be done using a rigid thermoplastic material and foam "donut" combination used to relieve the contusion from further direct trauma (see Fig. 11-7). The rigid padding should be worn until all signs of the injury have resolved.

Osteitis Pubis

Osteitis pubis is described as a chronic inflammatory condition of the pubic symphysis.[13,14] It is an overuse injury that most commonly presents as a gradual onset of pain in the pubic region that may radiate into the groin and lower abdomen.[2,15,16] Osteitis pubis is a rarely diagnosed condition in athletes, but has been reported in distance runners,[1,13,17] soccer players,[18] ice hockey players,[19] and football players.[20] The management of osteitis pubis in the injured athlete can be difficult for the health care team, as well as for the frustrated athlete. Often, an initial diagnosis of a groin or lower abdominal strain is made because of prevailing symptoms, as well as pain-provoking activities such as adductor pain at the end range of hip abduction, with resisted hip adduction or with trunk flexion against gravity. By the time an accurate diagnosis of osteitis pubis is made and confirmed via radiographs and bone scans, conventional treatment including therapeutic modalities, such as heat, ultrasound, and phonophoresis to the groin, as well as adductor stretching and strengthening, have failed to provide

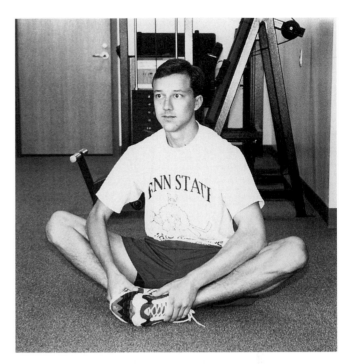

Figure 11–8. "Butterfly" groin stretching. Stretches must be done in static fashion within pain-free limits.

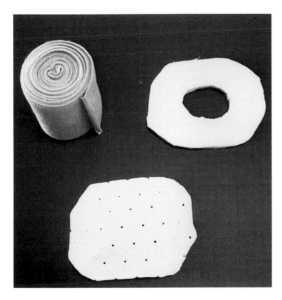

Figure 11–7. Protective padding materials. A rigid thermoplastic shell over a ½-inch foam "donut" pad, secured with an elastic wrap, is used for added protection against reinjury upon a return to contact activities.

pain relief and attempts at a return to activity have been unsuccessful. The most effective treatment of an athlete with a diagnosis of osteitis pubis involves rest from physical activity, the use of nonsteroidal anti-inflammatory medications, and pain-free hip adductor stretching.[15,16] Although variable, 3 to 6 months of physical inactivity may be necessary for symptoms to subside.[15,20] Aside from rest, there seems to be no universally preferred treatment for this disorder. During this time of inactivity, the athlete begins hip adductor stretching within pain-free limits (see Fig. 11-8). Stretches are done in a static fashion with each stretch held for 15 to 30 seconds. Each stretch is repeated 3 to 5 times, and the stretching session is repeated 2 to 3 times per day.

It has been suggested that the etiology of osteitis pubis is overuse and repetitive microtrauma to the pubic symphysis through running, kicking, and activities requiring forceful hip adductor activity such as ice hockey.[15,16] Because of their origins on the pubic rami, repetitive adductor muscle contractions may cause shear forces at the pubic symphysis.[16,21] Another suggested factor contributing to osteitis pubis in runners is excessive up and down pelvic motion in the frontal plane or horizontal side-to-side sway of the pelvis.[1,22] Therefore, increasing adductor muscle flexibility and improving pelvic stability through gluteal strengthening should be the goals of treatment during the period of relative rest from activity. It has also been suggested that, whether a possible cause or effect of osteitis pubis, many patients have decreased hip range of motion.[20,23] Therefore, a comprehensive hip stretching program should be incorporated including hip flexor and hip rotator stretching. Throughout the healing process, ice is used liberally to decrease pain. Other local modalities such as phonophoresis may be used, but the therapeutic benefit is uncertain. Upper body and lower extremity strength training can continue with closed-chain lower extremity strengthening initially avoided to minimize stress at the pubic symphysis. Adductor and abdominal strengthening should also be avoided. Conditioning exercises, such as upper body ergometry and freestyle swimming, are continued throughout the course of treatment. As pain resolves with a full range of hip motion and with daily activities, a stationary biking program can be added, but care must be taken that symptoms are not exacerbated by prolonged pressure of the bicycle seat on the pubis. Seat height changes and a more upright cycling position may help control symptoms. Gradually, a walk and run program is established and progressed as per the athlete's tolerance. Agility training including plyometrics and lateral motions are added as straight-line running becomes pain free. Sports-specific activities such as skating and kicking are finally added as tolerated.

A return to sports is based on the athlete's ability to perform the necessary skills at full intensity without pain. Upon a return to activity, the athlete is instructed to maintain a pre- and postexercise stretching program to avoid recurrence of symptoms.

Hamstring Strains

Hamstring strains are the most common muscle strains in the thigh, and the second most common sports injury to the thigh.[7,24] Strains are created by a violent stretch or a rapid contraction of the hamstrings resulting in varying degrees of rupture within the musculotendinous unit.[25,26] Hamstring strains are common in sports requiring powerful movements such as sprinting and jumping.[27] Often, hamstring strains occur either following an inadequate warm-up or at the end of practice or athletic competition when the athlete is fatigued and the muscles are less capable of withstanding tensile forces.

Effective management of hamstring strains begins immediately following the injury. Initial management, including the immediate application of ice, is aimed at minimizing bleeding and swelling associated with the primary tissue damage, and reducing secondary hypoxic injury to surrounding tissue, as well as reducing pain and secondary muscle spasms that result from the injury.[28-30]

Phases of Rehabilitation

All phases of rehabilitation guidelines for hip and thigh muscle strains are summarized in Table 11-2.

Phase I. Initial treatment consists of icing, compression, and elevation (ICE), as well as the use of assistive devices such as crutches in cases of severe injuries. Icing the injured area begins immediately to decrease pain and minimize swelling and inflammation. The athlete receives ice in the form of ice bags or cold packs for 20 to 30 minutes in conjunction with compression from an elastic bandage. Following the removal of the ice, a foam pad measuring slightly larger than the painful area is held in place by an elastic wrap for added compression. The athlete should be advised to continue icing the

TABLE 11–2. REHABILITATION GUIDELINES FOR HIP AND THIGH MUSCLE STRAINS

Phase	Rehabilitation Emphasis	General Treatment Plan
I	Decrease pain, swelling, secondary muscle spasms	ICE Electrical stimulation Crutches, if necessary Compressive dressing
II	Decrease pain, swelling, secondary muscle spasms	Continue ice, electrical stimulation Superficial heat Active and passive ROM
	Increase range of motion Increase flexibility Maintain cardiovascular fitness	Stretching Nonaggravating fitness exercises Isometric exercises
III	Increase flexibility	Warm-up, stretching exercises (self, PNF stretching)
	Increase strength Increase endurance	PREs, isokinetic exercises Endurance exercise (stationary bike, stair-climber) High-repetition, low-resistance strength training
IV	Increase flexibility Increase strength Increase endurance	Warm-up, stretching PREs, eccentric exercises Continue endurance exercises Running rehabilitation
	Improve proprioception	Balance, coordination exercises
V	Maximize strength Maximize flexibility Maximize endurance	Continue PREs Continue stretching Continue endurance exercises
	Gradual return to sport	Agility drills Sports-specific drills

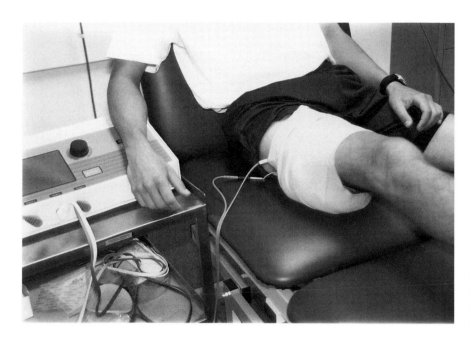

Figure 11–9. Initial management of hamstring strains includes the use of ice with electrical stimulation to decrease pain and secondary muscle spasms.

injured area every 2 to 3 hours for the first 24 to 48 hours to minimize pain and swelling. When not icing the injury, the athlete should use the compressive dressing and be advised to rest from painful activities. If daily activities, such as level walking, are painful and a normal gait is not possible, a cane or crutches can be used until gait is normal. The athletic trainer or physical therapist can also incorporate the use of modalities such as (TENS) or HVPGS to control pain. Initially, electrical stimulation can be used in conjunction with ice, pro-

vided that the injured tissue is able to be effectively cooled with electrical stimulation electrodes in place (see Fig. 11-9). Within 24 to 48 hours, active knee extension exercises are begun within the athlete's pain-free range of motion (see Fig. 11-10). The goal of early motion exercises is to minimize the formation of adhesions within the connective tissue[31] and to prevent the deleterious effects of immobilization. The athlete is advised to continue active knee extension exercises within his or her pain-free range for up to 5 minutes,

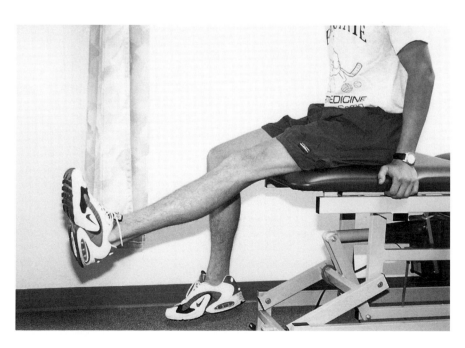

Figure 11–10. Active knee extensions are done within the athletes pain-free range of motion.

several times per day. Pain-free exercise must be stressed to the athlete. Light passive stretching is also begun within 24 to 48 hours of the injury, again with an emphasis on pain-free exercise. The athlete is instructed to maintain a gentle, static pain-free stretch to the hamstrings for 15 to 30 seconds and repeat the exercises 3 to 5 times (see Fig. 11–11). Exercises are also done independently 2 to 3 times throughout the day. Because much of the rehabilitation is done without supervision, it is important to educate the athlete on the importance of proper technique and pain-free exercise.

Phase II. As acute symptoms subside, walking becomes pain free, and the athlete demonstrates full, pain-free knee range of motion—generally within 2 to 4 days—light resistive exercises can be incorporated into the rehabilitation program. Submaximal isometric hamstring contractions are begun at various angles of knee flexion (e.g., angle increments of 15 to 20 degrees).[32] Isometric contractions must be pain free, and are held for 5 to 10 seconds, performing 10 repetitions at each of the various angles. Also, activities such as swimming and upper body ergometry can be started soon after injury to maintain the athlete's fitness level.

Phase III. As healing continues and stretching and isometrics are tolerated well, the emphasis of treatment is changed to address limitations in strength, muscular endurance, and flexibility. At this stage, treatment is usually begun with a form of heat such as moist heat, ultrasound, or hydrotherapy prior to exercise. Light exercise, such as stationary biking or treadmill walking for 5 to 10 minutes, is also an effective warm-up

prior to stretching to improve flexibility. Immediately following an adequate warm-up, passive hamstring stretching is performed to improve flexibility, apply controlled stress to the new collagen, and prepare the area for resistive exercises. As tolerated, isotonic progressive resistive exercises (PREs) are begun through a full range of knee motion. A progression from less stressful positions to more challenging positions is followed based on the athlete's tolerance. For example, hamstring curls are begun in a prone position to reduce the effect of gravity on knee flexion. As the athlete improves, he or she is progressed to a standing position using ankle weights and finally to traditional strength training equipment (see Fig. 11–12). Initially, weights are kept to a minimum and resistive exercises are done emphasizing more repetitions with low resistance to avoid placing excessive stress on the healing tissue. At this stage in the athlete's rehabilitation, hydrotherapy can play a beneficial role. By exercising in warm water, the athlete receives the effects of heat such as pain relief, spasm reduction,[33,34] and increased tissue extensibility.[4,32] An advantage of performing hamstring PREs in water is that it becomes a form of accommodative resistance concentric strength training. This is a safer form of a resistive exercise, and therefore can be begun earlier in the rehabilitation process. It is also important to incorporate cardiovascular exercises as soon as possible to limit the amount of deconditioning. This is especially important with in-season athletes hoping to return to physically demanding sports. Activities such as stationary biking can usually be started safely within the subacute stage of injury, and the athlete's cardiovascular exercise is progressed as he or she tolerates.

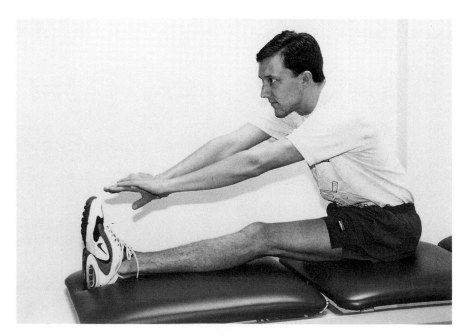

Figure 11–11. Self-hamstring stretching with the involved lower extremety in a nonweight-bearing position to ensure muscle relaxation.

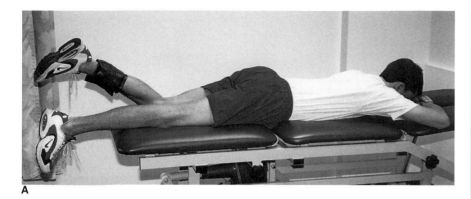

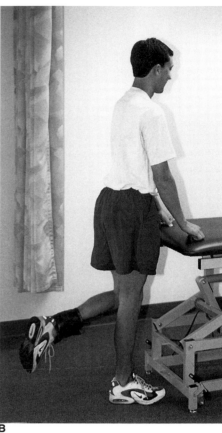

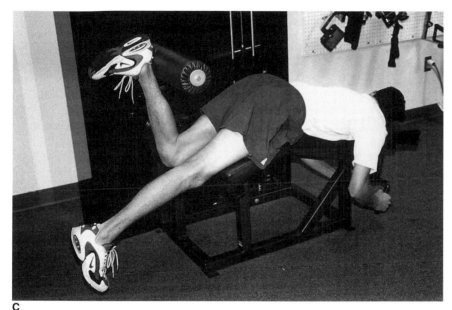

Figure 11-12. Hamstring progressive resistive exercises progressing from less stressful positions to more aggressive forms of exercise: **A.** Prone hamstring curls. **B.** Standing hamstring curls. **C.** Isotonic resistive exercise using traditional strength-training equipment.

Proprioceptive neuromuscular facilitation (PNF) using a contract and relax technique, is an effective form of stretching to maximize hamstring flexibility. At progressively increasing angles of hip flexion, the athlete performs 5 to 10-second submaximal isometric contractions of the hip extensors, followed by a 10-second passive stretch provided by the physical therapist or athletic trainer (see Fig. 11-13). PNF stretching must be pain-free to prevent reinjury and to maximize flexibility gains.

The use of high-speed isokinetic exercises has been suggested in the rehabilitation of hamstring strains.[35] The advantage of high-speed training is the high speed of movement that corresponds to lower rates of tension development in the contracting muscles. The contraction is concentric only, which also generates less tension than eccentric muscle contraction at a given speed and resistance. Therefore high-speed, low-tension isokinetic exercise can usually be started safely as a means of early strength training. Also,

because the hamstrings are composed largely of type II muscle fibers, they should be selectively trained at higher speeds.[24] Speed selection with isokinetic training is subjective. It is important to select speeds that the athlete can perform without pain for 20 to 30 repetitions. Two to four sets of high-speed exercises are done within the athlete's tolerance. Generally, speeds ranging from 180 to 450 degrees per second are used for high-speed isokinetic training.

Phase IV. Hamstring weakness has been described as a predisposing factor of hamstring strains.[32,36-38] Therefore, it is important to maximize strength to prevent reinjury. When high-speed isokinetic and low-resistance hamstring isotonic PREs are tolerated well, higher resistance isotonic PREs, such as hamstring curls, are incorporated. As resistance increases per patient tolerance, the number of repetitions decreases. Three sets of 8 to 15 repetitions are used as strength training parameters to progressively overload the hamstrings.

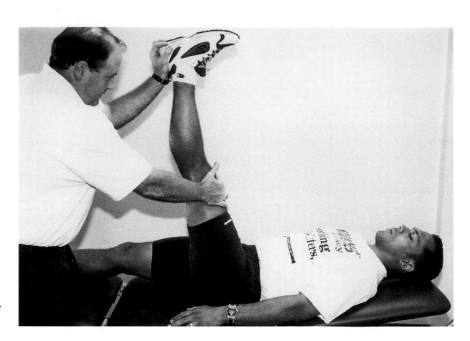

Figure 11–13. PNF contract and relax hamstring stretching.

Because most hamstring injuries occur eccentrically, it is important to incorporate eccentric hamstring strengthening into the athlete's program (see Fig. 11–14). Eccentric exercise can be performed on isokinetic devices, which have the advantage of a safety feature that automatically stops movement when resistance is discontinued. Eccentric exercises can also be done effectively using free weights or standard strength training machines. Exercises are initially done at low, controlled velocities with light weight to ensure safety. Caution should be exercised with eccentric training due to increased forces at the musculotendinous junction, where most injuries occur.[32,39] Gradually, the speed of training is increased at given amounts of resistance. Many hamstring strains occur with eccentric forces that are placed on an overstretched muscle, such as in the late swing phase of sprinting. Because the goal in the later stages of rehabilitation is specifity of training, the rehabilitation program should include exercises that simulate aspects such as limb position, speed of movement, and resistance encountered on the field and are areas of possible injury. Eccentric exercises, for example, can be done with the hips in a flexed position and the knee approaching full extension to mimic the eccentric loading of the hamstrings during the terminal swing phase of running. Again, resistance is initially low and velocity is slow to minimize risk of aggravating the injury. As the athlete adapts to low-speed, light-resistance eccentric exercise, speed is increased to the athlete's highest achievable speed. As maximum-velocity eccentric training becomes comfortable at a given resistance, weight is added and speed is reduced. Again, the athlete increases speed of exercise as he or she tolerates. The

passive mode on an isokinetic device can be used to introduce eccentric training by combining concentric and eccentric hamstring exercise. Initially, the athlete begins at a slow speed, approximately 30 degrees per second, at submaximal levels. He or she is instructed to pull with the machine into knee flexion with a submaximal effort and to resist the machine as it goes into knee extension. The advantage of this exercise is the safety associated with accommodative resistance and the ability to reproduce the speed of training. As the athlete accommodates to a given velocity, exercise speed is increased, eventually to the maximum limits of the isokinetic equipment.

Phase V. At this point in his or her rehabilitation, the athlete begins the exercise session with a proper warm-up, performs lower extremity stretching, and is comfortable performing concentric and eccentric strengthening exercises and endurance exercise. The athlete is now begun on functional exercises such as straight-line jogging at low, comfortable speeds. The goal of this final stage of rehabilitation is to progressively prepare the athlete for a return to competition. Functional exercises are introduced in predictable, straight-plane motions at low speeds (25 to 50 percent of the athlete's maximum speed), such as forward and backward running. These are progressed to include activities involving changes of direction. Initially, these activities such as "figure 8" and "circles" are done at low speeds with wide turns and are made more challenging by increasing speed and decreasing the turning radius as the athlete is able to perform the activities without a gait deviation or pain. Exercises are made increasingly challenging by incorpo-

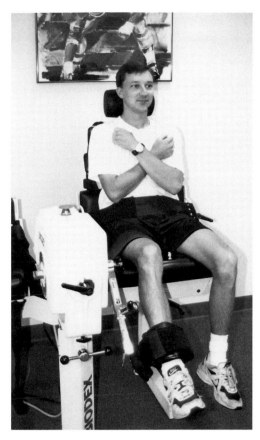

Figure 11–14. Eccentric hamstring strengthening exercises using isokinetic equipment.

rating sudden stops, starts, and "cutting" activities into the program. As with straight-line running, the speed at which an athlete performs agility drills is increased as pain and performance allow. Finally, sports-specific activities are introduced. Specific exercises and drills are based on the athlete's sport and position needs. Progressing an athlete through functional training may take from days to weeks, depending on the severity of injury.

For a safe return to the practice field, the athlete must demonstrate full, pain-free knee range of motion, nearly symmetrical hamstring flexibility, and pain-free, normal function at maximum speed functional training. If isokinetic testing is performed, a maximum side to side difference of 10 percent in hamstring peak torque and total work has been suggested as the criteria for return to full participation.[35] The athlete is given the option of using a neoprene sleeve or an elastic wrap for comfort upon his or her return to running activities and sports. Several etiologic factors may predispose the athlete to a hamstring strain; lack of hamstring flexibility,[32,38,40,41] low hamstring strength,[32,36-38] muscle fatigue,[32,38,42,43] and inadequate warm-up prior to strenuous activity.[3,4,32,38,42,44] The athlete's specific limitations must be identified, and the athlete must be counseled on the importance of a maintenance program to address limitations in strength, endurance, and flexibility, as well as proper warm-up techniques to reduce the risk of reinjury.

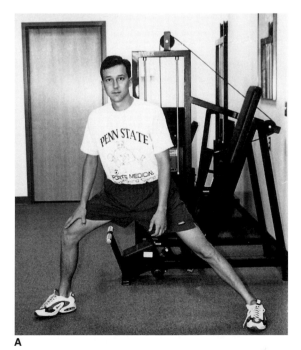

A

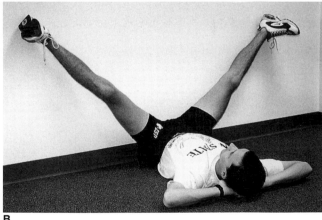

B

Figure 11–15. **A.** Standing adductor stretching. **B.** Supine adductor stretching.

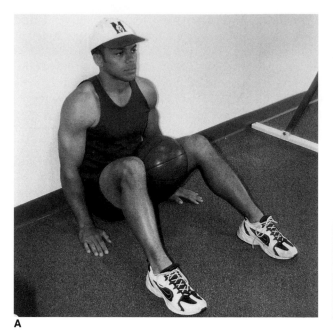

A

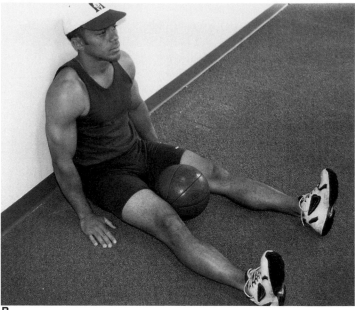

B

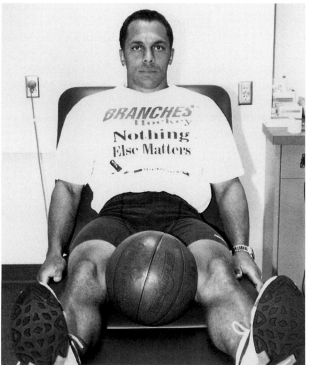

C

Figure 11–16. Hip adductor isometrics are done at several angles of hip and knee flexion.

Adductor Strains

Hip adductor muscle strains, commonly referred to as groin strains, occur in all sports, but most commonly in sports such as ice hockey[45] and soccer.[46,47] The most common mechanisms of injuries have been described as either a forceful abduction force during an intentional adduction motion or an overstretching of the adductors into hip abduction.[48] A soccer player, for example, may suffer an adductor strain when the leg is struck while kicking the ball. In most cases, the site of the injury is in the musculotendinous junction rather than the adductor tendon itself.[49] The most frequently injured of the hip adductors is the adductor longus.[45-50] Treatment of adductor strains is sometimes difficult, and rehabilitation must be progressed systematically from the acute phase of injury to the athlete's eventual return to full activity (see the case study later in the chapter).

Phases of Rehabilitation

Phase I. The primary goals of treatment immediately following an adductor strain are to minimize bleeding and swelling and to reduce pain. Acutely, adductor strains are treated with ice and compression to achieve these goals. Ideally, treatment begins at the time of injury. Using ice reduces hemorrhage and minimizes secondary hypoxic injury to surrounding tissue due to resulting inflammation and edema.[28-30,51] For the first 2 to 3 days following the injury, ice is used for 20 minutes every several hours. Between icing sessions, a groin spica may be applied using a double length, 6-inch, elastic wrap to provide compression, which reduces intramuscular bloodflow.[52] One-half inch foam or felt padding is held in place over the injured area with the elastic wrap for added compression to limit bleeding and swelling. Also, during the initial phase of injury management, crutches can be used, depending on the severity of injury. The injured tissue must be protected from further damage. Therefore, if walking is painful and a normal gait is difficult, crutches should be used to ambulate, applying weight bearing as tolerated. Electrical stimulation is also beneficial in the early management of adductor strains to reduce pain and secondary muscle spasms. Using a low pulse width to stimulate afferent neurons without causing muscle contraction is a safe, effective way of achieving pain relief.[53-55] Gentle, pain-free adductor stretching should be included during the early stages of rehabilitation. Although relative immobilization of the injured area is important to allow healing, light stress to the damaged tissue will stimulate the formation of more organized collagen scar tissue that is better able to withstand tensile forces.[56] Early, pain-free stretching, therefore, is needed to maximize tissue strength and to reduce the risk of reinjury upon a return to full sporting activities. The athlete is begun on early, pain-free static adductor stretching with instructions to maintain a stretch for 15 to 30 seconds and to repeat this procedure 5 times. The exercise is repeated several times per day. Light stretching can usually be tolerated within 48 to 72 hours following the injury.

Phase II. As pain decreases, the emphasis of treatment shifts to regaining hip range of motion and preventing atrophy. For minor strains, superficial heat may be added to the treatment prior to exercise to decrease pain and increase tissue extensibility. As with all acute injuries, caution should be exercised to avoid introducing heating

TABLE 11-3. SAMPLE WEEK OF ADDUCTOR STRAIN REHABILITATION: ADVANCED PHASES[a]

Day 1
1. 5 to 10-minute stationary bike warmup.
2. Ultrasound to groin.
3. Self-stretching: hip adductors (long and short), hip flexors, quadriceps, hamstrings.
4. Contract and relax stretching adductors (long and short), 6-second hold, 10-second relax, 5 repetitions,
5. PREs, surgical tubing vs. weights vs. pulleys; hip adductors, flexors; 3 sets of 8 to 15 repetitions.
6. Proprioceptive exercises: Biomechanical angle platform system (BAPS), unilateral balance activities, slide-board; 30-second bouts.
7. Cardiovascular exercise 20 to 30 minutes (bike, stair-climber).
8. Stretching (self).
9. Ice.
10. Home exercise program: stretching 3 to 4 times per day, ice as needed.

Day 2
1. Warm-up.
2. Ultrasound.
3. Continue stretching.
4. Jogging program: level surfaces, walk-jog intervals progressing to 20 to 30-minute jogging sessions.
5. Agility drills:
   Carioka, side-to-side shuffles; begin at 50 percent intensity, 10 yards, 30 seconds, and 4 to 6 repetitions.
   Forward, backward shuttle runs: 10 yards, 4 to 6 trials of 30-second bouts.
6. Stretching.
7. Ice.

Day 3
1. Warm-up.
2. Stretching.
3. Proprioceptive program per Day 1.
4. PREs per Day 1: decreased resistance, 2 sets, repetitions to fatigue—tubing vs. pulleys vs. weights.
5. Cardiovascular, muscular endurance training per Day 1.
6. Stretching.
7. Ice.

Day 4
1. Warm-up.
2. Stretching (self, contract and relax).
3. Jogging program per Day 2: increase jog: walk ratio as tolerated.
4. Agility drills: increase intensity, duration as tolerated.
5. Stretching.
6. Ice.

Day 5
1. Warm-up.
2. Stretching.
3. PREs per Day 1: 3 sets of 8 to 15 repetitions.
4. Proprioceptive program continued.
5. Cardiovascular, muscular endurance training continued.
6. Stretching.
7. Ice.

[a]Agility exercises: Incorporate activities specific to athlete's sport or position.

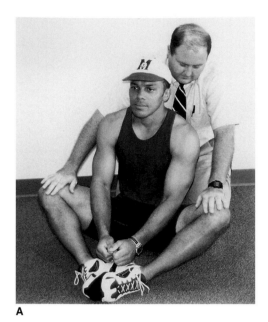

A

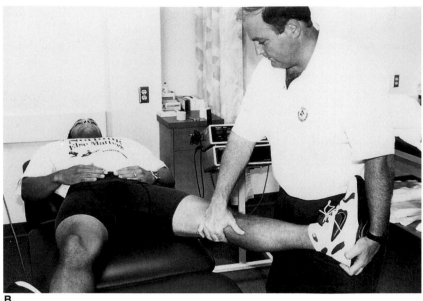

B

Figure 11–17. PNF contract-relax stretching. **A.** Groin. **B.** Long hip adductors.

modalities prematurely. These can contribute to bleeding and inflammation at the injury site if incorporated too early. As hip range of motion and flexibility are restored through passive range-of-motion exercises and light stretching, and full weight bearing is less painful, adductor isometrics are incorporated to prevent disuse atrophy and begin muscle reeducation. At this stage, usually within the first 3 to 7 days, a comprehensive stretching program is added to include hip flexor, quadriceps, and hamstring muscles, as well as the short and long hip adductors. Adductor stretching is begun in a nonweight-bearing position with the effects of gravity reduced, and progressed to more aggressive stretching techniques including standing and supine adductor stretching as the athlete tolerates (see Fig. 11-15). Hip adductor pillow squeezes are begun with submaximal contractions within the athlete's pain-free limits (see Fig. 11-16). Isometrics are done at various hip and knee angles from 90 degrees to full extension to maximize muscle recruitment. Exercises are performed for 5 to 10 seconds and repeated 10 times at each angle. As the athlete improves, adductor isometrics can also be done in greater degrees

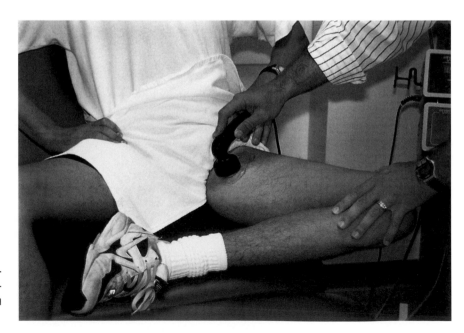

Figure 11–18. Ten-minute ultrasound treatment in the continuous mode to the hip adductors in conjunction with static passive groin stretch.

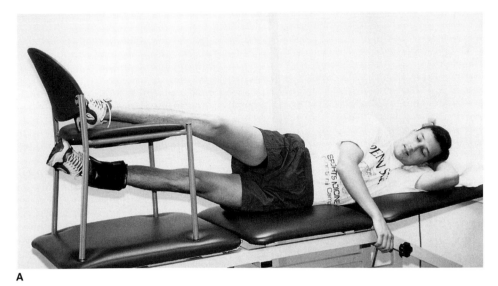

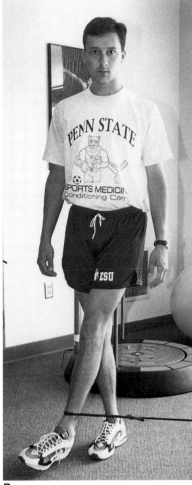

Figure 11-19. Examples of hip adductor PREs. **A.** Sidelying using ankle weights. **B.** Surgical tubing exercises.

of hip abduction, which places greater tension on the musculotendinous unit.

Phase III. As healing continues and pain with hip motion and weight-bearing has subsided, the goals of treatment change to emphasize flexibility and strength improvement. Table 11-3 summarizes a week of treatment in this advanced phase of rehabilitation. With significant adductor strains, this stage may be 1 to 2 weeks after the injury. Independent stretching is continued intermittently throughout the day, and PNF stretching is incorporated. A contract and relax technique, using 5 to 10-second submaximal isometric contractions of the hip adductors followed by a prolonged passive stretch done at progressively increasing degrees of hip abduction, is added to maximize flexibility (see Fig. 11-17). As with adductor isometrics, these are done with the involved hip and knee flexed, and then extended, to stretch the short and long hip adductors. The use of ultrasound in the continuous mode for 8 to 10 minutes immediately prior to or during adductor stretching can enhance the effectiveness of stretching (see Fig. 11-18). Light adductor PREs

are begun when active hip adduction is pain free. Conventional hip adductor resistive exercises using ankle weights are begun in a standing position to reduce the effect of gravity, and are progressed to performance while lying on the side as the athlete tolerates. Initially, resistance is low and a high number of repetitions are performed to avoid placing excessive stress on the healing tissue. Resistance is gradually increased as the athlete tolerates. Resistive equipment used for strength training include ankle weights, surgical tubing, pulleys, or commercial hip machines (see Fig. 11-19).

Aquatic therapy is a very valuable rehabilitation tool at this stage (see Fig. 11-20). Depending on the athlete's position in the water, the intensity of hip strengthening can range from assisted exercise to accommodative resistive exercises. Because of the principles of buoyancy, when the athlete lies on his or her involved side, hip adductor training is assisted by the upward force of the limb in water. Likewise, when the athlete lies on his or her uninvolved side, and performs active hip adduction exercises in a downward direction, resistance is greater due to the upward effect of buoyancy on the moving

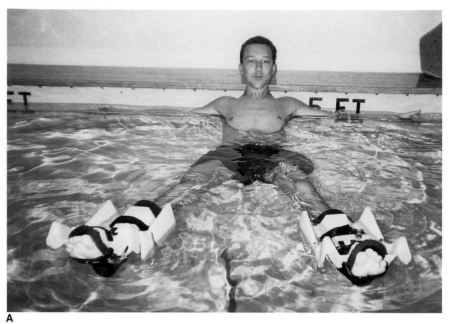

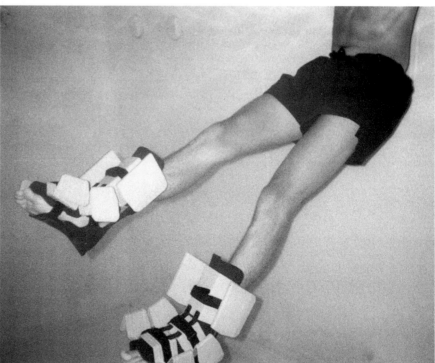

Figure 11–20. A. The use of aquatic therapy in hip adductor strength training. **B.** Aquatic aides may be used to provide added resistance.

limb. Commercial boots or surgical tubing can also be used to further challenge the athlete. If available, aquatic therapy is a safe, effective adjunct to traditional land rehabilitation.

Cardiovascular and muscular endurance exercises are also emphasized at this stage in the athlete's rehabilitation. Activities such as stationary biking, stair stepping on a stair climber, and swimming programs can be introduced as soon as they are tolerated.

Phase IV. Muscle strengthening emphasizing eccentric training is introduced when the athlete tolerates isotonic exercises well (see Table 11-3). The athlete initially begins eccentric exercise with low resistance at slow speeds. Gradually, the resistance and the speed of exercise are increased to simulate functional activities. It is important to incorporate eccentric training at the end ranges of motion, especially at the end range of hip abduction, as this places maximal stress on the muscle tendon unit in a position susceptible to reinjury. Resistive hip adductor exercises are initially done in the frontal plane, progressed to more functional patterns, including diagonals, and are done with various degrees of hip rotation. Resistive exercises are done by performing 3 sets of 8 to 15 repetitions. As resistance increases, frequency of resistive training is reduced to every other day to allow adequate recovery of the adductor muscles.

Phase V. Functional training is a crucial component of the rehabilitation program. As strength and flexibility improve, it is important to incorporate activities that improve kinesthetic awareness and proprioception in preparation for a return to sporting activities. In most cases, functional training begins with low-intensity, straight-plane movements. Progression and selection of activities depend on the individual athlete's needs, based on his or her particular sport or position. Typically, the athlete begins with light straight-line jogging and progresses in distance speed as tolerated. Lateral movements are incorporated beginning with low-intensity side-to-side movements on stable surfaces. Examples include shuffles and carioka exercises at low speed. Figure 8s and cutting activities are also introduced. Progression of these exercises is based on the athlete's pain and ability to function without favoring the injured limb. As tolerated, speed, length of stride, and time is increased to gradually simulate future demands on the adductor muscles. Athletes returning to activities such as ice skating, in-line skating, and skiing should also be trained on unstable surfaces such as a slide board or Fitter (Fitter International, Calgary, Canada) (see Fig. 11–21). Exercises are begun at low intensity with duration based on the athlete's tolerance. Gradually, exercise parameters are modified to meet the athlete's sporting needs. For example, an ice hockey player will eventually progress to high-speed slide board activities for 30 to 45-second bouts to simulate an ice hockey shift (see Fig. 11–22). As the athlete approaches full recovery from his or her adductor strain, sports-specific activities are added to the program.

A progressive return to sporting activity is begun when the athlete demonstrates full, pain-free, hip range of motion, symmetrical hip flexibility, full hip strength upon examination, and is pain free with functional training including sports-specific activities. Upon a return to sports, the athlete has the option of wearing an elastic groin spica or a commercial restraint as an added precaution (see Fig. 11–23). Finally, the athlete must be counseled on the importance of a maintenance program to prevent reinjury. Specifically, the importance of a proper warm-up, pre- and postexercise stretching, and a continued lower extremity conditioning program, including strength and endurance training, should be addressed.

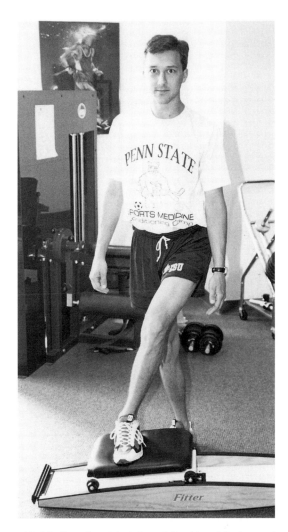

Figure 11–21. Functional training of the hip adductors using the Fitter; the exercise demonstrated is done using the uninvolved as well as involved lower extremity to improve dynamic stability at the hip and pelvis.

Iliopsoas Strains

As with adductor strains, the rehabilitation of iliopsoas strains, commonly referred to as hip flexor strains, is sometimes lengthy. Rehabilitation must be gradual and systematic from time of injury to a full return to sporting activities.

Phases of Rehabilitation

Phase I. Initial treatment of acute iliopsoas muscle strains involves rest from painful activities, ice, and compression for the first 48 to 72 hours. The initial goals of treatment are to permit tissue healing, minimize bleeding, and reduce pain and secondary muscle spasms. Often in the acute stage of an iliopsoas strain, level walking is painful and normal gait is impossible. If so, the use of axillary crutches as needed for pain relief is advisable until a normal gait is achieved. As with other acute mus-

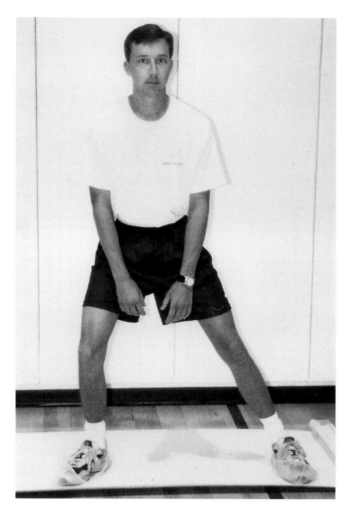

Figure 11–22. Functional training of the hip adductors using a slide-board.

cle strains, ice is used over the painful area for 15 to 20 minutes, and repeated every 2 to 3 hours for at least 24 to 48 hours. A groin spica wrap, applied with the athlete's hip in slight flexion, may also be used between icing sessions to provide gentle support, especially with walking activities, and for compression. Initial treatments may also consist of electrical stimulation to the painful area. TENS and high-voltage pulsed galvanic stimulation are forms of electrical stimulation that are effective in decreasing pain and secondary muscle spasms.

Phase II. Goals of phase II rehabilitation of iliopsoas strains include continuing to reduce pain and muscle spasms, restoring hip range of motion, promoting the organized formation of scar tissue, improving flexibility, and maintaining the athlete's fitness level. Phase II rehabilitation usually begins within 2 to 3 days of injury. With mild strains, treatment is begun with superficial heat, such as hydrotherapy or moist heat. Caution must be used to avoid using heating modalities prematurely as

this may cause increased bleeding at the injury site. Deep heating modalities, such as ultrasound, are also incorporated into treatment only when bleeding has stopped. Hip range of motion exercises should be instituted to restore range of motion. The athlete is initially instructed in standing active hip extension within pain-free limits. Hip adductor stretching is also begun, and an upper body conditioning program is also continued.

Phase III. When active hip range of motion, including hip extension, becomes less painful, hip flexor stretching is begun (see Fig. 11–24). The athlete is instructed to maintain a pain-free static stretch of the hip flexors for 15 to 30 seconds and repeat the exercise 5 times. Light stretching begins early in the rehabilitation to prevent the formation of disorganized collagen scar tissue.[57] Quadriceps stretching is also included to stretch the rectus femoris (see Fig. 11–25). As pain subsides with active hip flexion,

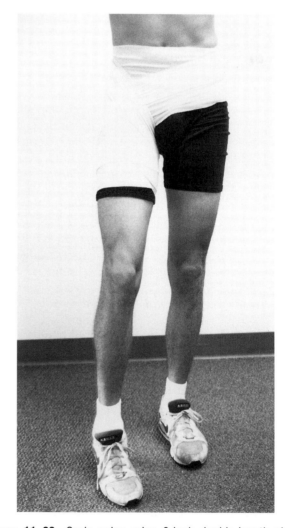

Figure 11–23. Groin spica using 6-inch double-length elastic bandage. The wrap should be applied with the athlete's hip slightly flexed and internally rotated.

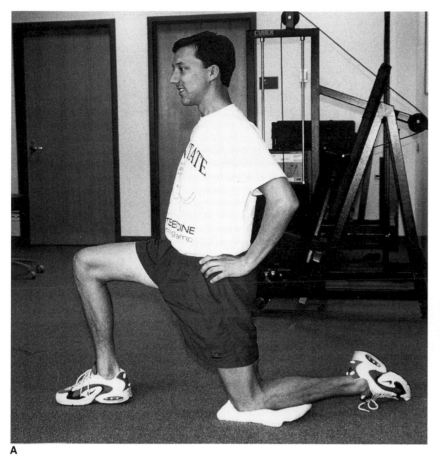

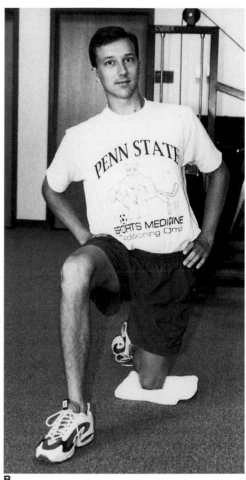

Figure 11–24. A. Hip flexor self-stretching. **B.** The athlete side-bends to the opposite side while performing the stretch to increase the intensity of the exercise.

and walking becomes pain free, light resistive exercises are incorporated into the athlete's rehabilitation. Initially, iliopsoas strengthening is done with the athlete in a short-sitting position on the edge of a treatment table. Hip flexion exercises are performed with the knee flexed, isolating the iliopsoas group (see Fig. 11-26). Initial resistance is the weight of the leg only, and the number of repetitions is increased as the athlete tolerates. When the athlete is able to perform 25 to 30 repetitions without pain, resistance is added at the ankle, and exercises using lengthened lever arms are incorporated. An example is straight-leg hip flexion exercises, progressing from standing to supine as tolerated.

Aquatic therapy can play a valuable role in strength training following muscle injury. Because it is a form of accommodative resistance, strengthening can be started safely early in the rehabilitation process. It can be made progressively more challenging by using resistance boots or tubing for aquatic PREs.

The athlete continues performing independent static stretching several times throughout the day to increase flexibility. Contract and relax PNF stretching, using 5 to 10-second submaximal isometric hip flexor contractions, followed by a 10 to 15-second passive stretch at progressively increasing angles of hip extension, is incorporated into the athlete's rehabilitation (see Fig. 11-27).

Phase IV. In the later phases of rehabilitation, the emphasis shifts from pain relief and restoring range of motion, to improving strength, flexibility, and muscular endurance. Flexibility exercises are continued, emphasizing hip flexor, adductor, and quadriceps stretching. Contract and relax PNF stretching is also continued to maximize hip flexor flexibility.

As strength improves, and the athlete is pain free with light resistive exercise, training is advanced to progressively overload tissues by increasing resistance or exercise repetitions. Advanced strength training is done using surgical tubing, ankle weights, commercial hip machines, or manual resistance (see Fig. 11-28). The athlete performs resistive exercises every other day to allow adequate recovery between training sessions. During each strengthening session, exercises are performed using 3 sets of 8 to 15 repetitions as training

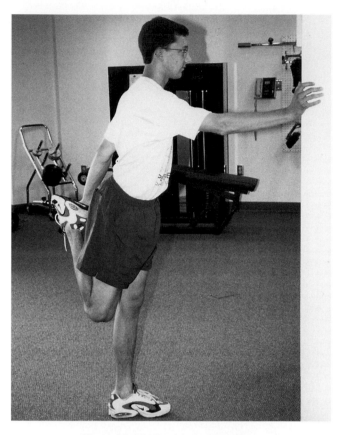

Figure 11–25. Quadriceps stretching.

iliopsoas strain are introduced at low speeds in straight planes. The speed and intensity of exercise are increased to provide progressively greater stress to the athlete. A typical functional progression of activities would include slow, straight-line jogging in forward and backward directions. Speed is progressively increased as pain permits, and the quality of exercise is not compromised. Also, the athlete incorporates a jogging program, gradually increasing duration as tolerated, to improve muscular as well as cardiovascular endurance. As the athlete progresses through functional training, exercises are made more challenging by incorporating change of direction into running activities. Initially, the athlete begins with figure 8s and circular running patterns and progresses to activities involving cutting, jumping, and side-to-side motions.

Eventually, activities specifically related to the athlete's sport and position must be incorporated into his or her program. Agility training is a vital component in the athlete's rehabilitation to fully prepare for the increased demands of a return to competitive sports. Agility and plyometric exercises are begun when the athlete tolerates straight-line jogging and gradual changes in direction well. Controlled agility and plyometric drills are introduced using stable, level surfaces with the intensity and duration of exercise at low

parameters. Proprioception and kinesthetic awareness exercises are also incorporated to improve coordination and dynamic stability at the hip and pelvis (see Fig. 11-29).

Whether in water or on land, hip strength training begins in the sagittal plane and progresses to more functional, combined motions, such as PNF diagonal patterns, as the athlete tolerates.

Phase V. Throughout the remainder of rehabilitation, the athlete continues with daily, frequent stretching, strengthening every other day, cardiovascular and muscular endurance exercises, and is introduced to functional exercises. Goals in the final stages of rehabilitation are to maximize strength, flexibility, and muscular endurance, and to improve power and coordination. The definitive goal is for the athlete to safely return to sports. Functional training is designed to improve strength, power, coordination, and endurance in specific movement patterns that progressively simulate future demands placed on the injured athlete. As hip flexor strength nears normal and the athlete is pain free upon resistance, functional, more sports-specific exercises are added to the rehabilitation program. As with other forms of functional training, exercises for the athlete with an

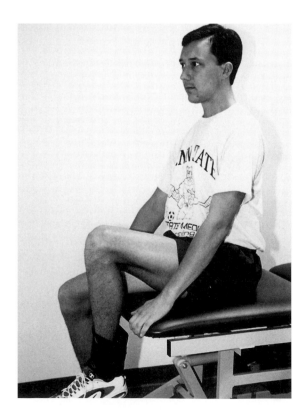

Figure 11–26. Iliopsoas strengthening exercises in the short sitting position.

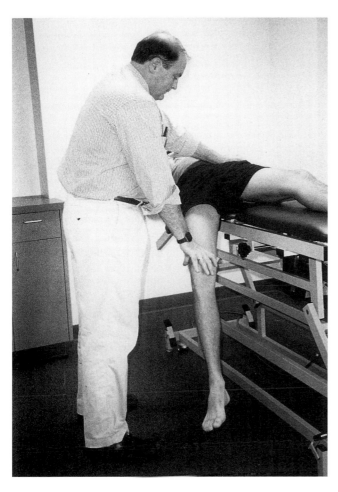

Figure 11–27. PNF contract and relax stretching for the hip flexors.

levels. As the athlete tolerates, agility training is progressed to include sudden changes of direction with speed and the duration of exercises is progressively increased (see Fig. 11–30).

A return to unrestricted sporting activities is permitted when the athlete demonstrates full, pain-free hip range of motion, near normal hip flexor strength, and symmetrical hip flexor flexibility. As an added safety measure, an elastic groin spica is applied upon the athlete's return to the practice field. Following a full return to sports, the athlete continues with a proper warm-up and stretching routine prior to activity, and stretching and icing following activity, to prevent reinjury.

Case Study. Adductor Strain in a Hockey Player

A 30-year-old professional ice hockey player was referred to physical therapy with a diagnosis of a left groin strain. The athlete reported suffering the injury earlier in the day while performing sprints at the end of practice. At the time of injury, the athlete felt a sudden pull with an immediate onset of left groin pain. He was unable to continue skating and was sent to the team physician. The physician immediately referred the patient to physical therapy. No diagnostic tests were performed.

Upon his arrival in physical therapy, the athlete was fully weight bearing and without gait deviation, although walking was described as painful. On physical examination, there was no apparent swelling or discoloration. Left hip range of motion was within normal limits actively and passively, except for a 15-degree loss of hip abduction with an empty end-feel. The athlete complained of pain approaching the end range of his available motion into

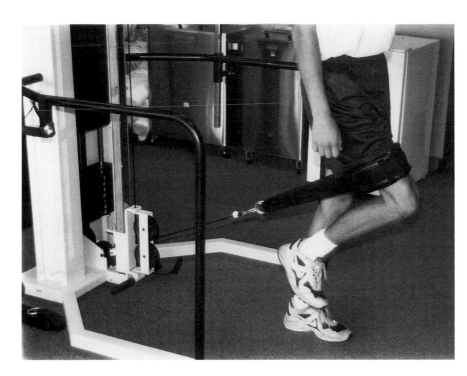

Figure 11–28. Hip flexor strength training using a pulley system.

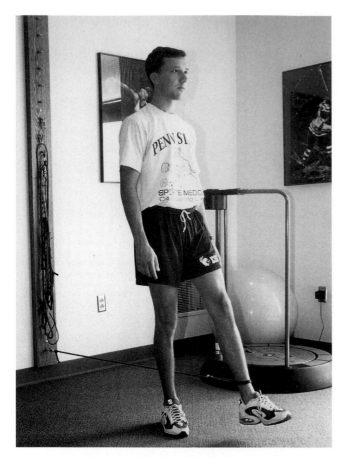

Figure 11–29. Dynamic stability functional training using surgical tubing. The athlete performs the exercise with the uninvolved lower extremity, while the involved lower extremity provides stability at the hip and pelvis.

abduction. Manual muscle testing of left hip adduction was four-fifths and painful. On palpation, the athlete was tender along the proximal adductor musculature, although no defect was felt. The athlete was nontender at the pubic symphysis.

Initial treatment consisted of ice in conjunction with high-voltage pulsed galvanic stimulation for 20 minutes using a high pulsed rate and negative polarity with sensory stimulation only. The athlete was instructed to rest and continue using ice frequently throughout the day. At 24 hours following his injury, the athlete was reevaluated. He reported a significant decrease in pain and demonstrated full hip range of motion and four-fifths hip adduction strength, with mild pain upon resistance. He received moist heat to the left medial thigh, and was begun on gentle independent stretching exercises for the hip adductors, hamstrings, hip flexors, and quadriceps. Treatment was concluded with ice and electrical stimulation. The athlete was instructed to continue gentle stretching 3 to 4 times per day.

Daily treatments were continued, and endurance training was incorporated on the fourth day following the injury. The athlete began a conditioning program on the

stair-climber and stationary bike to maintain his fitness level while not practicing ice hockey. Hip adductor PREs were begun by performing hip adduction straight leg raises for 3 sets of 10 repetitions.

On the seventh day following his groin strain, he received continuous ultrasound combined with a light stretch to the left hip adductors for 8 minutes prior to his exercise program.

On days 8 to 10, the athlete participated in an aquatic therapy program consisting of hip adductor and hip flexor PREs, lower extremity stretching, and functional exercises such as long-stride walking, lateral striding, and carioka walking. The above exercises were continued and dry land functional training was begun on days 9 to 10, consisting of 30-second bouts on the slideboard at a pain-free intensity level. The athlete resumed light ice skating on day 11, with no discomfort. He continued skating daily with a groin splica for added support. Moist heat, ultrasound, and stretching were continued prior to skating. He continued to use ice following skating.

The athlete then resumed ice hockey practice within his tolerance, and was discharged from physical therapy on day 17 with a pain-free return to unrestricted ice hockey activities. He finished the season with no future episodes of groin pain.

This case demonstrates a typical rehabilitation program for the athlete with a mild adductor strain. How rapidly

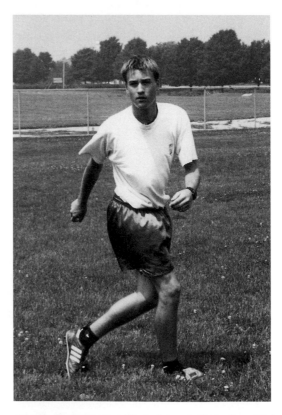

Figure 11–30. Example of agility training. Initially, the athlete performs agility drills at 25 to 50 percent intensity, and progresses to full speed as tolerated.

the athlete advances through the phases of rehabilitation is based on factors including the severity of injury and the athlete's response to treatment.

REFERENCES

1. Lloyd-Smith R, Clement DB, McKenzie DC, Taunton JE. A survey of overuse and traumatic hip and pelvic injuries in athletes. *Phys Sportsmed.* 1985;13:131-141.

2. Gross ML, Nasser S, Finerman GAM. Hip and pelvis. In: DeLee JC, Drez D Jr, eds. *Orthopaedic Sports Medicine: Principles and Practice.* Philadelphia: Saunders; 1994; 2:1063-1085.

3. Safran M, Garrett WE Jr, Seaber A, et al. The role of warm up in muscular injury prevention. *Am J Sports Med.* 1988;16:123-128.

4. Strickler T, Malone T, Garrett WE Jr. The effects of passive warming on muscle injury. *Am J Sports Med.* 1990; 18:141-145.

5. Spiker JC. Ultrasound. In: Prentice WE, ed. *Therapeutic Modalities in Sports Medicine.* 2nd ed. St. Louis: Mosby; 1990:129-147.

6. Ziskin MC, McDiarmid T, Michlovitz SL. Therapeutic ultrasound. In: Michlovitz SL, ed. *Thermal Agents in Rehabilitation.* 2nd ed. Philadelphia: Davis; 1990: 134-169.

7. Arnheim DD, Prentice WE. The thigh, hip, groin and pelvis. In: Arnheim DD, Prentice WE, eds. *Principles of Athletic Training.* 8th ed. St. Louis: Mosby; 1993: 585-617.

8. The pelvis. In: *Athletic Training and Sports Medicine.* 2nd ed. Park Ridge, IL: American Academy of Orthopedic Surgeons; 1991:295-300.

9. Taylor K, Fish DR, Mendel FC, Burton HW. Effect of a single 30 minute treatment of high voltage pulsed direct current on edema formation. *Phys Ther.* 1991;71:S117.

10. Karnes JL, Mendel FC, Fish DR. Effects of low voltage pulsed direct current on edema formation following impact injury. *Phys Ther.* 1991;71:S116.

11. Bettany JA, Fish DR, Mendel FC. Influence of high voltage pulsed direct current on edema formation following impact injury. *Phys Ther.* 1990;70:219-224.

12. Lampe GN, Mannheimer JS. The patient and TENS. In: Lampe GN, Mannheimer JS, eds. *Clinical Transcutaneous Electrical Nerve Stimulation.* Philadelphia: Davis; 1984:219-247.

13. Gamble JG, Simmons SC, Freedman M. The symphysis pubis: Anatomic and pathologic considerations. *Clin Orthop.* 1986;203:261-272.

14. Karpos PAG, Spindler KP, Pierce MA. Osteomyelitis of the pubic symphysis in athletes: A case report and literature review. *Med Sci Sports Exerc.* 1995;27:473-478.

15. Holt MA, Keene JS, Graf BK, Helwig DC. Treatment of osteitis pubis in athletes. *Am J Sports Med.* 1995;23:601-606.

16. Hanson PG, Angevine M, Juhl JH. Osteitis pubis in sports activities. *Phys Sportsmed.* 1978;6:111-114.

17. Rold JF, Rold BA. Pubic stress symphysitis in a female distance runner. *Phys Sportsmed.* 1986;14:61-65.

18. Harris NH, Murray RO. Lesions of the symphysis in athletes. *Br Med J.* 1974;4:211-214.

19. Briggs RC, Kollojornsen PH, Southall RC. Osteitis pubis, Tc-99m MDP, and professional hockey players. *Clin Nucl Med.* 1992;17:861-863.

20. Batt ME, McShane JM, Dillingham MF. Osteitis pubis in collegiate football players. *Med Sci Sports Exerc.* 1995; 27:629-633.

21. Bowerman JW. *Radiology and Injury in Sports.* New York: Appleton-Century Crofts; 1977:241-245.

22. Brodie DM. Running injuries. *CIBA Clinical Symposia.* 1980;32:5-7.

23. Williams JG. Limitation of hip joint movement as a factor in traumatic osteitis pubis. *Br J Sports Med.* 1978;12:129-133.

24. Coole WG, Gieck JH. An analysis of hamstring strains and their rehabilitation. *J Orthop Sports Phys Ther.* 1987;9:77-85.

25. Sutton G. Hamstring by hamstring strains: A review of the literature. *J Orthop Sports Phys Ther.* 1984;5:184-195.

26. Alexius R, chairman. American Medical Association, Subcommittee on Classification of Sports Injuries. *Standard Nomenclature of Athletic Injuries, 1966.* Chicago: AMA; 1966.

27. Stanton B, Purdam C. Hamstring injuries in sprinting—the role of eccentric exercise. *J Orthop Sports Phys Ther.* 1989;10:343-349.

28. Bell GW. Infrared modalities. In: Prentice WE, ed. *Therapeutic Modalities in Sports Medicine.* 2nd ed. St. Louis: Mosby; 1990:89-128.

29. McMaster WC. A literary review on ice therapy in injuries. *Am J Sports Med.* 1977;5:124-126.

30. Olson JE, Straveno V. A review of cryotherapy. *Phys Ther.* 1972;52:840-853.

31. Kisner C, Colby LA. The hip. In: Kisner C, Colby LA, eds. *Therapeutic Exercise: Foundations and Techniques.* 2nd ed. Philadelphia: Davis; 1990:317-335.

32. Worrell TW. Factors associated with hamstring injuries: An approach to treatment and preventative measures. *Sports Med.* 1994;17:338-345.

33. Michlovitz SL. Biophysical principles of heating and superficial heat agents. In: Michlovitz SL, ed. *Thermal Agents in Rehabilitation.* 2nd ed. Philadelphia: Davis; 1990:88-108.

34. Krumholz AL, Gelfand B, O'Connor PA. Therapeutic modalities. In: Nicholas JA, Herschman EB, eds. *The Lower Extremity and Spine in Sports Medicine.* 2nd ed. St. Louis: Mosby-Yearbook; 1995;1:207-234.

35. Brunet ME, Hontas RB. The thigh. In: DeLee JC, Drez D Jr, eds. *Orthopaedic Sports Medicine: Principles and Practice.* Philadelphia: Saunders; 1994;2:1086-1112.

36. Burkett LN. Causative factors in hamstring strains. *Med Sci Sports Exerc.* 1970;2:39-42.

37. Christensen CS, Wiseman DC. Strength. The common variable in hamstring strain. *Athletic Training.* 1972;7: 36-40.

38. Worrell TW, Perrin DH. Hamstring muscle injury: The influence of strength, flexibility, warm-up, and fatigue. *J Orthop Sports Phys Ther.* 1992;16:12-18.

39. Garrett WE Jr, Rich FR, Nikolaou PK, Vogler JB III. Computed tomography of hamstring muscle strains. *Med Sci Sports Exerc.* 1989;21:506-514.

40. Worrell TW, Perrin DH, Gansneder B, Gieck J. Comparison of isokinetic strength and flexibility measures between hamstring injured and non-injured athletes. *J Orthop Sports Phys Ther.* 1991;13:118-125.

41. Liemohn W. Factors related to hamstring strains. *J Sports Med Phys Fitness.* 1978;18:71-76.

42. Dornan P. A report on 140 hamstring injuries. *Aust J Sports Med.* 1971;4:30-36.

43. Glick JM. Muscle strains: Prevention and treatment. *Phys Sportsmed.* 1980;8:73-77.

44. Ekstrand J, Gillquist J, Moller M, et al. Incidence of soccer injuries and their relation to training and team success. *Am J Sports Med.* 1983;11:63-69.

45. Merrifield HH, Cowan RF. Groin strain injuries in ice hockey. *J Sports Med.* 1973;1:41-42.

46. Akermark C, Johansson C. Tenotomy of the adductor longus tendon in the treatment of chronic groin pain in athletes. *Am J Sports Med.* 1992;20:640-643.

47. Smodlaka VN. Groin pain in soccer players. *Phys Sportsmed.* 1980;8:57-61.

48. Hasselman CT, Best TM, Garrett WE Jr. When groin pain signals an adductor strain. *Phys Sportsmed.* 1995; 23:53-60.

49. Garrett WE Jr. Basic science of musculotendinous injuries. In: Nicholas JA, Herschman EB, eds. *The Lower Extremity and Spine in Sports Medicine.* 2nd ed. St. Louis: Mosby-Yearbook; 1995;1:39-51.

50. Symeonides PP. Isolated traumatic rupture of the adductor longus muscle of the thigh. *Clin Orthop.* 1972;88:64-66.

51. Michlovitz SL. Cryotherapy: The use of cold as a therapeutic agent. In: Michlovitz SL, ed. *Thermal Agents in Rehabilitation.* 2nd ed. Philadelphia: Davis; 1990:63-87.

52. Thorsson O, Hemdal B, Lilja B, Westlin N. The effect of external pressure on intramuscular bloodflow at rest and after running. *Med Sci Sports Exerc.* 1987;19:469-473.

53. Gersh MR. Applications of transcutaneous electrical nerve stimulation in the treatment of patients with musculoskeletal and neurologic disorders. In: Wolf SL, ed. *Electrotherapy.* New York: Churchill Livingstone; 1981: 155-177.

54. Hooker DN. Electrical stimulating currents. In: Prentice WE, ed. *Therapeutic Modalities in Sports Medicine.* 2nd ed. St. Louis: Mosby; 1990:51-88.

55. Starkey C. Electrical agents. In: Starkey C, ed. *Therapeutic Modalities for Athletic Trainers.* Philadelphia: Davis; 1993:97-172.

56. Padgett LR, Dahners LE. Rigid immobilization alters matrix organization in the injured rat medial collateral ligament. *J Orthop Res.* 1992;10:895-900.

57. Magnusson SP, McHugh MP. Current concepts on rehabilitation in sports medicine. In: Nicholas JA, Herschman EB, eds. *The Lower Extremity and Spine in Sports Medicine.* 2nd ed. St. Louis: Mosby-Yearbook; 1995; 1:177-206.

Chapter 12

The Knee

Medical Aspects of Athletic Knee Injuries

Robert D. Bronstein and Kenneth E. DeHaven

The knee is one of the most commonly injured joints in the athlete. This is due to its exposure, anatomy, and the functional demands placed upon it. Due to the significant morbidity resulting from an injury to the knee in an athlete, much emphasis has been placed on developing and refining methods of diagnosis and treatment of knee injuries.

This chapter reviews the functional anatomy of the knee, the diagnosis of knee injuries, and various treatment options and protocols in treating these injuries. With a thorough understanding of these principles, the sports medicine team of the physician, athletic trainer, and physical therapist can combine forces to most effectively treat the athlete with a knee injury.

ANATOMY

In order to evaluate and treat knee injuries, one must first have an understanding of the normal anatomy of the knee. The knee is a triaxial joint involving the femoraltibial, patellofemoral, and proximal tibialfibular articulations integrated with active and passive stabilizers. When all components are fully functional, it allows for activities ranging from normal ambulation to running and agility sports.

The bony architecture consists of the femur, tibia, patella, and proximal fibula. The femoral condyles project eccentrically from the distal femoral shaft. Anteriorly, the condyles are relatively flat and project only slightly from the femoral shaft. The groove between the condyles anteriorly articulates with the patella. Posteriorly, the condyles project markedly from the femoral shaft and are separated by the intercondylar notch. The anterior and posterior cruciate ligaments and the ligaments of Humphry and Wrisberg arise from this notch.

The patella is a triangular-shaped sesamoid bone of the quadriceps tendon. The articular surface of the patella is divided into seven facets.[1] The medial and lateral facets are each divided into thirds with the seventh facet being most medial and often called the odd or extreme medial facet. The patellofemoral articulation shows the most contact at approximately 45 degrees of knee flexion, with contact moving proximally on the patella as flexion is increased.[2] The odd facet articulates only in maximal knee flexion.

The proximal tibia has two incongruent surfaces to accept the femoral condyles. The medial plateau is relatively flat, whereas the lateral plateau is convex. The medial and lateral tibial spines project between the medial and lateral plateaus. The cruciate ligaments and menisci insert anterior and posterior to the tibial spine. The proximal fibula articulates with the proximal tibia and provides the attachment site for the lateral collateral ligament, biceps femoris, and poplitealfibular ligament.

The medial and lateral menisci improve the contact of the noncongruent femoral tibial articulation. The resultant congruent surface provides a degree of mechanical stability to the joint, and by increasing the contact area, decreases the contact stress at any one point. The congruent surface provided may also aid in the distribution of synovial fluid throughout the joint. The lateral meniscus is more C shaped than the medial meniscus, which is deficient anteriorly. Posteriorly, the lateral meniscus is attached to the femur via the ligament of Humphry (anterior meniscal femoral ligament) or the ligament of Wrisberg (posterior meniscal femoral ligament). The medial meniscus has peripheral attachments to the medial capsule. The lateral meniscus only has capsular attachments anterior to the popliteus tendon. Posterior to the popliteal hiatus, the lateral meniscus has attachments to the popliteus muscle and the meniscal femoral ligaments. The internal structure of the menisci is primarily collagen oriented in a circumferential pattern. Blood supply is from the superior and inferior medial and lateral talicenate arteries and enters the menisci peripherally.[3] These vessels are circumferential with radial projections into the meniscus.

The anterior cruciate ligament (ACL) originates in the intercondylar notch from the posteromedial aspect of the lateral femoral condyle and has a broad tibial insertion anterior and lateral to the tibial spine. The ACL is the primary restraint to anterior translation of the tibia on the femur and to internal rotation of the tibia on the femur and serves as a secondary restraint to varus or valgus knee instability.[4]

The posterior cruciate ligament (PCL) originates in the intercondylar notch from the anterior aspect of the lateral surface of the medial femoral condyle and inserts 1 cm distal to the joint line on the posterior aspect of the tibia. The PCL is the primary restraint for posterior tibial translation on the femur and acts to control tibial external rotation.[4] The meniscal femoral ligaments of Humphry and Wrisberg originate on the femur anterior to and posterior to the PCL and are believed to augment the PCL in restraining posterior tibial translation.

The medial complex consists of the superficial medial collateral ligament (MCL), the deep MCL, and the posterior capsule. The superficial and deep MCL originate at the medial femoral epicondyle. The deep MCL inserts on the tibia, just distal to the joint line, while the superficial MCL inserts more distally, deep to the pes ansurinus tendons. The semimembranosus has five medial attachments and is an important component of the medial complex. These attachments are to the MCL, the posterior tibia, the posterior oblique ligament (the posterior portion of the deep MCL), the oblique popliteal ligament (an expansion of the posterior capsule), and to the popliteus. Superficial to the medial complex are the pes tendons, which consist of the sartorius, gracilis, and semitendinosis.

The lateral complex consists of the lateral collateral ligament (LCL), the biceps femoris, and the posterolateral capsule. The lateral complex provides a restraint against varus stress and against posterolateral and anterolateral rotational stresses. The posterior third of the lateral capsule forms the arcuate ligament. The arcuate ligament, the popliteus tendon, and the LCL together make up the arcuate complex, an important posterolateral restraint.

BIOMECHANICS

The knee joint is not a simple hinge joint. Within normal activity there exists flexion and extension, medial to lateral, anterior to posterior, rotational, and axial motion. The combining of these motions is controlled by interplay between the osseous structures, menisci, ligaments, and muscles about the knee. Injury to any of these components can, therefore, affect normal knee function.

The medial femoral condyle projects further distally than the lateral femoral condyle and has a different curvature anteriorly than posteriorly. This causes the tibia to externally rotate as the knee is extended. This rotation or screw-home mechanism tightens the ligaments and results in an inherently stable articulation in extension. The menisci provides for low transmission and for congruency of the femoral tibial articulation. Working in conjunction with the cruciate ligaments, the menisci help control anteroposterior motion and rotation.

The biomechanics of the knee are important as the normal and abnormal coupled motions of the knee determines the stresses applied to the articular cartilage, menisci, and ligaments. The knee moves through 6 degrees of freedom with flexion and extension, translation (anterior to posterior, medial to lateral and axial), rotation, and adduction and abduction. Ligaments function best when loaded in the direction of their fibers. The bony architecture and menisci act in concert to apply the stresses along the paths of the ligaments. When the load overcomes the ultimate strength of the ligament, the ligament fails.

KNEE INJURIES

Tears of the Medial Collateral Ligament

The medial collateral ligament is the primary restraint to valgus stress across the knee.[5] Therefore, when sufficient valgus force is applied to the knee, such as from a direct lateral blow to the fixed knee in a contact sport, the MCL will tear. Due to the distraction force applied to the medial meniscus, it is usually spared injury with such a mechanism. The coronary, or meniscotibial ligament may tear, however, detaching the medial meniscus from the tibia and rendering it unstable.

On examination following an MCL injury, the athlete will present with swelling and tenderness along the

MCL. Careful palpation can elicit the point of maximal tenderness along the ligament to determine the level of the injury. Instability to valgus stress in full extension indicates tearing of the MCL, posteromedial capsule, and at least one cruciate ligament. Stability in extension with instability in 30 degrees of flexion indicates MCL injury. MCL laxity can be graded by the laxity presented in 30 degrees of knee flexion. In a first-degree sprain, the ligament is tender but has no instability to valgus stress. Laxity up to 5 mm with a firm end point indicates a grade II injury, whereas a grade III injury is present with laxity of greater than 5 mm with a soft end point. Radiographs should be obtained on any athlete that presents with an MCL sprain to rule out a fracture. In addition, any skeletally immature athlete with valgus laxity to examination should have stress radiographs taken to be certain that the medial opening is occurring through the joint and not through a nondisplaced (usually femoral) physeal fracture.

Isolated MCL injuries can be treated nonoperatively with bracing and early mobilization.[6,7] Return to sports is usually possible within 3 to 6 weeks depending on the extent of the tear.

Tears of the Anterior Cruciate Ligament

The anterior cruciate ligament (ACL) is the primary restraint to anterior tibial translation.[4] It also controls tibial internal rotation and is a secondary restraint to varus or valgus forces across the knee. The ACL has a fascicular makeup with a broad tibial attachment (see Fig. 12–1). This provides for a continuum of control throughout a range of motion that is probably not reproduced with current methods of ACL reconstruction.

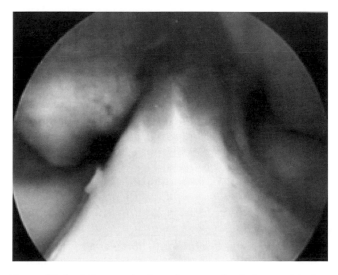

Figure 12–1. Arthroscopic view of a normal anterior cruciate ligament of a 17-year-old football player with an isolated meniscus tear. Note the broad flattened tibial insertion.

"Isolated" anterior cruciate ligament tears are usually caused by a sudden rotation on a planted foot. The injury may be a contact or noncontact stress. The athlete may describe hearing a pop or crunching noise, often loud enough for others to hear. An effusion is usually detectable within hours of the injury, indicating a hemarthrosis.

On physical examination, the athlete may have an effusion and may present with a limited range of motion, particularly in the acute setting. Lachman examination is the most sensitive test for ACL insufficiency.[8] Assuming a normal contralateral knee, the Lachman examination can be graded with a 1 plus Lachman showing up to 5 mm greater anterior tibial translation than the normal contralateral knee; a 2 plus 5 to 10 mm; and a 3 plus greater than 10 mm.

The Lachman examination is performed with the knee flexed approximately 20 to 30 degrees. The examiner stabilizes the femur laterally (right hand for left knee, left hand for right knee) and gently applies an anterior translation force to the tibia from the medial side. This allows the examiner to easily grasp the tibia in extremities of all sizes as the tibia is a subcutaneous bone medially. The amount of anterior translation is compared with the uninjured knee, and the quality of the end point is assessed. A soft end point is indicative of an ACL tear. The pivot shift test can be used to confirm the diagnosis of an ACL tear.[9] This test begins with the knee in extension. While maintaining internal rotation of the tibia, a valgus stress is applied and the knee is flexed. As flexion occurs the tibia can be felt to reduce from its anteriorly subluxed position. This reproduces the athlete's instability.

The treatment of the athlete with an isolated ACL tear is not always clear. Those athletes participating in high-risk sports involving agility running such as basketball, soccer, and football (corresponding to the International Knee Documentation Committees Level I and Level II sports), usually are candidates for surgical reconstruction, while those participating in lower level sports or no sports may do well without reconstruction. It is important to realize, however, that nonsurgical treatment does not mean no treatment. If surgical reconstruction is elected, it should not be performed until the athlete has regained all or nearly all of his or her range of motion. Although this is usually a 3-week process from the time of injury, the exact time frame is not as important as the clinical status of the knee.

Meniscal Tears

Meniscal tears are common sports injuries. The most frequent mechanism is a noncontact stress resulting from deceleration or acceleration coupled with the athlete changing direction, as occurs with a running and cutting maneuver. Meniscal tears may also result from contact stress or, in the older athlete, from a degenerative process.

Anatomically, meniscal tearing occurs with knee flexion and compression combined with femoral tibial rotation. This results in a sheer stress to the meniscus causing the meniscus to tear. As discussed in this chapter, the same mechanisms can produce ligament injuries as well. Therefore, the evaluation and treatment of meniscal lesions must include evaluation and treatment of any associated knee injury. The athlete with a torn meniscus will complain of pain or mechanical symptoms in the knee. A displaced or displaceable fragment can produce mechanical locking and symptoms of giving way. Displaced or nondisplaced tears can alter meniscus mobility, causing traction of the richly intervated capsule and synovium resulting in knee pain. A torn meniscus can also alter the instant center of rotation, change the contact area, and cause mechanical irritation, all of which can lead to secondary articular cartilage lesions.

The standard treatment for all meniscal tears used be total or near total meniscectomy. This removed all mechanical symptoms from the abnormal meniscus. Unfortunately, the long term results of the procedure were poor. Following meniscectomy, the contact stresses acting across the knee increase significantly, resulting in early degenerative arthritis.[10-14] It has been demonstrated in dogs that the degree of degenerative change is directly related to the amount of meniscus removed.[15] The knee menisci, therefore, once felt to be functional remnants of knee musculature, now are known to be integral components of normal knee function. Recent techniques, therefore, have concentrated on meniscal preservation over excision.

The development and subsequent refinements in arthroscopy of the knee have aided in meniscal preservation. Arthroscopy permits precise classification of the type, extent, and location of meniscal tears. Arthroscopic surgical techniques permit partial meniscectomies and meniscal repairs to be performed with little morbidity.

The athlete with a torn meniscus may complain of pain, locking, instability, and swelling. If the problem only presents with unusual activity or motions, the physician may be more inclined to attempt a more prolonged trial of conservative treatment than when symptoms occur daily. The athlete usually will describe a giving way at the moment of injury. The knee may instantaneously lock short of full extension with displacement of the meniscus. It is important to ask if the athlete was able to fully extend the knee immediately following the injury, since lack of full extension often develops gradually with increasing pain or effusion even in the absence of a major meniscal injury.

Edema should be distinguished from a true knee effusion. In a knee effusion, the fluid is contained within the capsule of the joints, whereas edema refers to fluid in the subcutaneous tissues. The athlete is usually able to make this distinction by the location and nature of the swelling.

An effusion that occurs within hours of the injury is a result of bleeding within the joint (hemarthrosis) and usually indicates rupture of the anterior cruciate or posterior cruciate ligament, or an osteochondral fracture. Although the typical effusion following a meniscal tear develops gradually over 1 to 3 days, a tear at the vascular periphery of the meniscus may cause an acute hemarthrosis as well.

Individuals with a chronic meniscal injury typically give the history of an acute episode, followed by gradual improvement but persistent disability. They may complain of medial or lateral pain, giving way, and perhaps, intermittent locking. The position of any locking is important. Athletes with medial meniscal locking will have their knee locked at approximately 10 to 30 degrees of flexion whereas, those with lateral meniscal tears tend to lock in greater degrees of flexion (70 degrees or more).

Degenerative meniscal tears are being encountered with increasing frequency as more people over the age of 40 are becoming or staying active in sports or fitness activities. The patient with a degenerative meniscus tear may or may not give a history of a specific injury episode, but the diagnosis should be suspected in an older individual with a history of pain, effusions, or mechanical knee symptoms in the absence of significant arthritic changes.

The athlete with knee pain requires a comprehensive examination of the lower extremity and knee. Specific findings for meniscal tears include pain or limitations at the extremes of motion and joint line tenderness. Numerous stress tests for meniscal injury have been described. All have in common the attempt to trap abnormally mobile fragments of meniscus between the femur and tibia.

Circumduction maneuvers such as those described by McMurray are accurate in diagnosing posterior horn meniscal lesions.[16] With the athlete in the supine position, the hip is flexed 90 degrees and the knee is fully flexed. The examiner places one hand over the joint line while securely holding the patient's foot with the other hand. The foot (and tibia) is then externally rotated to bring the posterior horn of the medial meniscus anterior, and the knee is slowly extended. As the femoral condyle moves over the torn meniscus, there may be a palpable click over the joint line. The reproduction of pain without a click may indicate a meniscus tear as well. The maneuver is then repeated in internal rotation of the foot to test the lateral meniscus.

Nonoperative management is frequently indicated for patients with symptoms suggestive of a meniscus tear. With time and therapy the athlete's symptoms often improve or may completely resolve. If the knee is locked, prompt, although not emergent, arthroscopic surgery is warranted. In making such a recommendation, however, it is important to distinguish true locking from hamstring spasm. Arthroscopy is also indicated in the absence of locking when the clinical picture suggests a major meniscal tear or when nonoperative treatment has not resolved the athlete's symptoms.

The arthroscopy should evaluate every tear to see if it meets the criteria for repair. We have found that approximately 30 percent of isolated meniscal tears and 60 percent of meniscal tears associated with ACL tears in athletes under 30 years of age are repairable (see Fig. 12-2). Lesions requiring treatment and unsuitable for repair are treated with removal of the unstable torn fragment, leaving behind a stable contoured rim (see Fig. 12-3).

Tears of the Posterior Cruciate Ligament

The posterior cruciate ligament (PCL) is the primary restraint for posterior tibial translation.[4] The PCL also provides a restraint to tibial external rotation and, with the ACL, a secondary restraint against varus or valgus stress. The PCL is often described as consisting of two bands that are named based on their relative positions at the femoral and tibial insertions. The anterolateral band, which makes up the bulk of the ligament, is the least isometric portion of the PCL while the smaller posteromedial portion is more isometric. This two component idea is actually an oversimplification of a ligament with a continuum of fibers. The concept, however, is useful in reconstructions, which attempt to replace the functionally and anatomically more robust anterolateral portion of the PCL.

A tear of the PCL can be caused by a blow to the anterior tibia, a hyperflexion injury, a hyperextension injury, or by cutting maneuvers. With a cutting maneuver, a PCL injury can occur as a player's body rotates on a planted foot and minimally flexed knee causing internal rotation and anterior translation of the femur on the tibia (a relative external rotation and posterior translation of the tibia on the femur).

On physical examination, the tibia will sag posteriorly when the knee is flexed 90 degrees eliminating the normally present anterior tibial shelf as the tibial plateau drops near or posterior to the femoral condyles. The

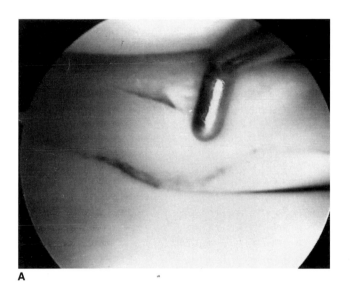

A

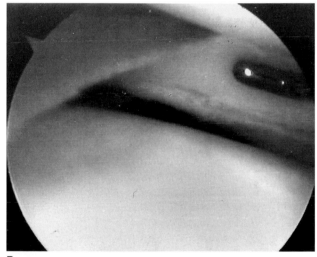

B

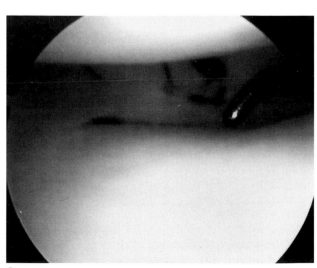

C

Figure 12-2. A, B. Peripheral lateral meniscus tear in a 16-year-old high school football player with an anterior cruciate ligament tear. **C.** The meniscus was repaired at the time of ACL reconstruction.

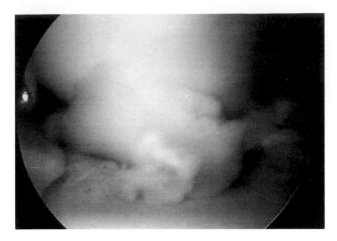

Figure 12–3. An irreparable deformed flap tear of the medial meniscus in a 17-year-old basketball player. The torn fragment was excised back to a stable border.

tibia can be seen to reduce anteriorly as the athlete contracts the quadriceps (quadriceps active test).

PCL tears are graded on physical examination based on the position of the anterior tibial plateau relative to the femoral condyle. In a grade I injury, the tibia remains anterior to the femoral condyles. In a grade II injury, the tibia is even with the femoral condyle, while the tibia drops posterior to the femur in a grade III injury. In contrast to the ACL, most athletes will do well with nonoperatively

treated PCL tears. There does seem to be a predisposition for degenerative changes of the medial compartment over time, although this does not correlate with functional outcome. Most surgeons, therefore, recommend nonoperative treatment for isolated (grades I or II) PCL tears with no abnormal external tibial rotation. Surgery is indicated in avulsion injuries, grade III tears, multiple ligament injuries, and in those athletes who develop chronic functional instability with nonoperative treatment.

Patellofemoral Pain

Symptoms related to the patellofemoral joint are common problems in the athletic population. Patellofemoral pain syndrome (PFPS) may occur as an isolated entity or in concert with other knee pathology. The disorder may be associated with a congenital or developmental predisposition and may or may not involve an acute injury. The result is an abnormality in patellofemoral tracking causing localized patellofemoral stress.

Patellar fracture is at the extreme end of patellofemoral disorders. Although sometimes the result of a direct blow to the patella, the more common mechanism is a violent quadriceps contraction with a flexed knee. This results in a disruption of the extensor mechanism of the knee. Treatment is open reduction and internal fixation with a tension band technique and repair of the medial and lateral retinaculum, allowing early motion (see Fig. 12–4). Patellectomy or partial patellectomy is rarely required.

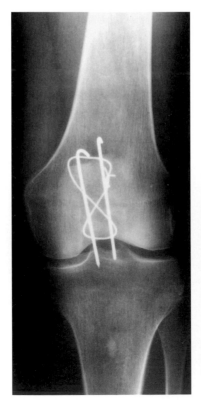
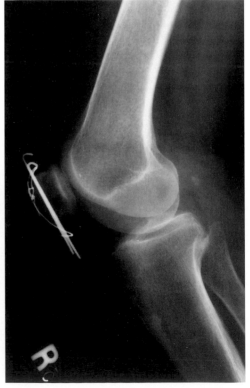

Figure 12–4. Open reduction and internal fixation of a patella fracture in a 55-year-old skier using a tension band technique.

Acute patellar dislocation can occur with a valgus blow to the knee with a concomitant quadriceps contraction. This is usually associated with a valgus predisposition to patellar dislocation or subluxation. Following reduction, a brief period of immobilization is warranted, followed by a full patellofemoral rehabilitation program. There is no evidence that prolonged immobilization decreases the risk of recurrence.

More commonly, patellofemoral pain is more insidious in onset. The pain is usually described as a vague, poorly localized anterior pain. The pain is generally increased with prolonged sitting ("movie sign") and with stairs. Mechanical symptoms may be present as well. On examination, one should look for excessive femoral anteversion resulting in an apparent internal femoral torsion (squinting patella), pes planus or cavus, and for an abnormal quadriceps angle. We prefer to measure the Q-angle in a supine position with the knee extended. The center of the goniometer is placed over the center of the reduced patella with the proximal limb pointed towards the anterior and superior iliac spine and the distal limb directed to the tibial tubercle. Normally, a male will have a Q-angle of less than 10 degrees while a female's Q-angle can normally be as high as 15 degrees. Higher Q-angles represent a relative risk for lateral patellar tracking, but do not make the diagnosis.

Quadriceps and hamstrings should be examined for atrophy and flexibility. Areas of tenderness about the patellofemoral joint should be elicited. Following an acute dislocation or subluxation episode, the athlete will often be tender over the medial femoral epicondyle, presumably secondary to tearing the patellofemoral ligament. Mobility of the patella should also be assessed and apprehension with lateral patellar glide should be sought.

The vast majority of patellofemoral pain responds to an exercise program. Although this is discussed in more detail in the rehabilitation section, the key principles are to avoid aggravating activities and to engage in a program that allows increased flexibility and strength in a pain-free manner.

Patellofemoral disorders occasionally do require surgical treatment. If surgery is warranted, it is imperative that the correct procedure is performed to prevent worsening of the problem. A lateral release, as an isolated procedure, is indicated only for patellofemoral pain syndrome with lateral tilt. It is contraindicated in athletes with anterior knee pain of adolescence, subluxation or dislocation, advanced patellofemoral arthrosis, or in knees without lateral patellar tilt. Realignment procedures (distal realignment with or without proximal realignment) may be indicated in athletes with recurrent patellar subluxation or dislocation with an abnormally high Q-angle. Distal realignment is contraindicated in athletes with open physes and in those with normal Q-angles. In other words, realignment is not indicated for an athlete with normal alignment.

Although patellofemoral disorders may be quite frustrating for the athlete, physician, trainer, and therapist, with proper treatment, good results can be obtained. If surgery is contemplated too soon, the wrong procedure is performed, or if the rehabilitation is not properly performed, the result can be disastrous.

REFERENCES

1. Insall JN. Anatomy of the knee. In: Insall JN, ed. *Surgery of the Knee.* New York: Churchill Livingstone; 1984.
2. Goodfellow J, Hungerford DS, Zindel M. Patellofemoral joint mechanism and pathology. *J Bone Joint Surg.* 1976;58B:287–290.
3. Arnoczky SP, Warren RF. Microvascular anatomy of the human meniscus. *Am J Sports Med.* 1982;10:90.
4. Butler DL, Noyes FR, Grood ES. Ligamentous restraints to anterior-posterior drawer in the human knee. *J Bone Joint Surg.* 1980;62A:259.
5. Warren RF, Marshall JL, Girgis F. The prime static stabilizer of the medial side of the knee. *J Bone Joint Surg.* 1974;56A:665.
6. Indelicato PA. Non-operative treatment of complete tears of the medial collateral ligament of the knee. *J Bone Joint Surg.* 1983,65A:323.
7. Indelicato PA, Hermansdorfer J, Huegel M. Non-operative management of complex tears of the medial collateral ligament of the knee in intercollegiate football players. *Clin Orthop.* 1990;256:174.
8. DeHaven KE. Diagnosis of acute knee injuries with hemarthrosis. *Am J Sports Med.* 1980;8:9–14.
9. Galway HR, MacIntosh DL. The lateral pivot shift as symptoms and sign of anterior cruciate ligament insufficiency. *Clin Orthop.* 1980;147:45–50.
10. Fairbank TJ. Knee joint changes after meniscectomy. *J Bone Joint Surg.* 1948;30B:664.
11. Huckell JR. Is meniscectomy a benign procedure? A long term follow-up study. *Can J Surg.* 1965;8:254.
12. Johnson R, et al. Factors affecting late results after meniscectomy. *J Bone Joint Surg.* 1974;56A:719.
13. Krause W, Pope MH, Johnson RJ, Wilder DG. Mechanical changes in the knee after meniscectomy. *J Bone Joint Surg.* 1976;58A:599.
14. Tapper E, Hoover N. Late results after meniscectomy. *J Bone Joint Surg.* 1969;51A:517.
15. Cox JS, Nye CE, Schafer WW, et al. The degenerative effects of partial and total resection of the medial meniscus in dog's knees. *Clin Orthop.* 1975;109:178.
16. McMurray TP. The semilunar cartilages. *Br J Surg.* 1941;29:407.

Knee Rehabilitation

Alan Peppard

Rehabilitation following knee injuries requires the physician, physical therapist, and athletic trainer to understand the forces in the knee with different exercises and the ability of the injured tissues to withstand stress. The rehabilitation program must be developed that follows the diagnosis of the tissue injured and the status of the injured tissue. Quadriceps, hamstrings, hip abduction, and adduction exercises are commonly used to improve knee function after injury. Understanding the forces imparted to the knee structures with these exercises is important (see Fig. 12-5). Quadriceps exercises extend the knee via the patella and patella tendon. The forces on the patella are defined in this chapter. Quadriceps exercises (knee extension) provide a posterior force on the proximal tibia when completed from full flexion to approximately 60 degrees, while anterior forces are produced from 60 degrees to 0 degree. Hamstring exercises (knee flexion) produce a posterior force throughout the range, with the maximum posterior force at 90 degrees. Hip abduction (with resistance below the knee) produces a varus force; hip adduction a valgus force at the knee joint. The same exercise on different equipment places varying stresses at the knee joint.

Isotonic equipment such as a free weight bench (see Fig. 12-6) will provide zero resistance at 90 degrees (the weight is maintained by the hinge on the bench) and maximum resistance at 0 degree of knee extension. Isotonic quadriceps and hamstring stations, such as a universal gym with a cable attaching the resistance arm to a weight that travels vertically (see Fig. 12-7), provides a resistance at 90 degrees equal to the weight selected and the weight of the bar. The weight will reduce slightly during extension to 0 degree. Weight training equipment such as Nautilus or Eagle provides variable resistance during the range provided by the CAM (see Fig. 12-8). These machines provide resistance that more closely matches the human torque capability of the joint to provide force during its range. Maximum resistance is provided at approximately 60 degrees for knee extension. The minimal resistance that can be selected also will vary with various weight training equipment and the clinician must ensure that the injured athlete can safely exercise with each machine selected.

Isokinetic exercise equipment provides different forces to the knee during exercise (see Figs. 12-9 to 12-11). During isokinetic exercise, the limb is accelerating at the beginning and decelerating at the end of the exercise; therefore, minimal forces are applied at these positions. Additionally, force generation ability of the muscle varies with speed.[1-3] The quadriceps possesses reduced force generation at faster speeds, and therefore reduced joint forces. The hamstrings maintain strength at faster speeds. Many isokinetic machines now provide eccentric exercise. The muscles can generate greater forces eccentrically,[3,4] and therefore greater joint forces. Many sport actions involve eccentric muscle contractions, hence eccentric strengthening exercises are needed in a strengthening program. But each professional must remain aware of the probability of increased delayed onset muscle soreness with eccentric exercise and carefully accommodate the athlete to the exercise.

"Closed-chain" exercises like the squat, leg press, and stair climbers produce different stresses for the knee.[5-7] Closed-chain exercise provides compression of the knee joint because most of the forces are generated by muscles from above the knee joint, and thereby increase joint stability due the structure of the joint. The quadriceps, hamstrings, and gluteal muscles are activated during the exercise and reduce the amount of anterior and posterior translation forces normally present with open-chain exercises.

When appropriate healing has occurred and strength and range of motion are adequate, the athlete must gradually be returned to full sports stress by completion of a functional rehabilitation program. The functional rehabilitation program must assess the present functional level of the athlete and the nature of stress present within the sport. If time goals are also present, they should be included when possible. A functional rehabilitation program for running and cutting follows. The program is modified to take into account the nature of the sport, present functioning level, and specific pathology.

Understanding the attitude of the athlete is important to motivate him or her to correctly and consistently complete the rehabilitation program. The knee has received much attention over the years because knee injuries have occurred to many successful athletes. Because of this publicity, many athletes that have sustained a knee injury have a hidden fear that they will be unable to recover and

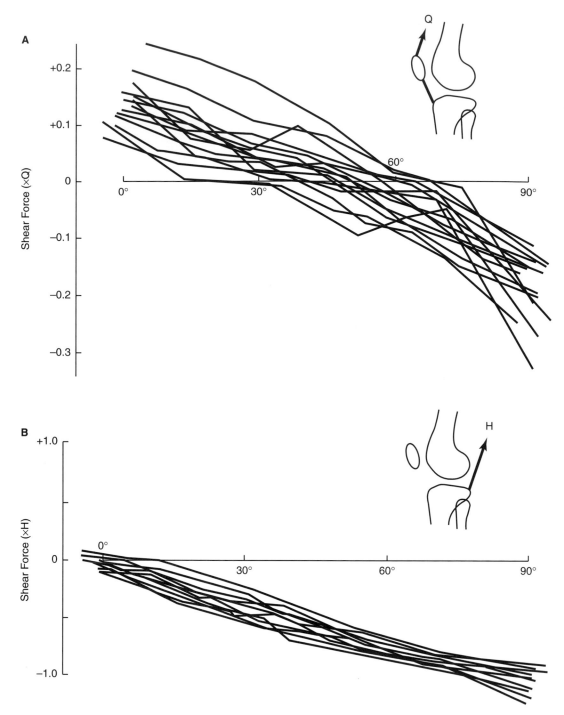

Figure 12–5. Shear force in isometric contraction of the quadriceps **(A)** or hamstrings **(B)** at various flexion angles of the knee. The abscissa shows the flexion angle of the knee, and the ordinate shows the coefficient of a linear function which gives the shear force in proportion to tension of the quadriceps **(A)** or the hamstrings **(B)**. Plus and minus values of the coefficient mean the anterior and posterior drawer force to the tibia. Each polygonal line shows a different subject. **(A)** The anterior drawer force is given in the area of large flexion angle. **(B)** The posterior drawer force is given to the tibia at every flexion angle of the knee. (*From Yasuda K, Sasaki T,[31] with permission.*)

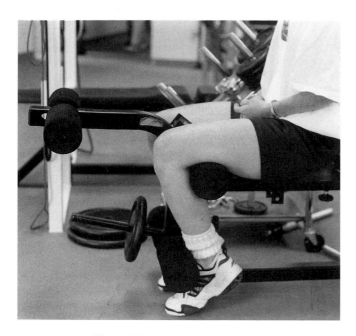

Figure 12–6. A free-weight bench.

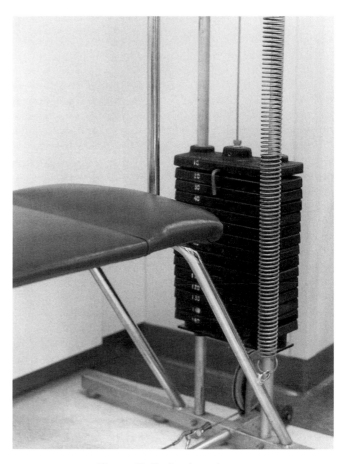

Figure 12–7. A universal gym.

return successfully to full athletic participation. The professional must be sensitive to the attitudes of the patient, and possibly his or her parents. Sometimes the athlete needs help to develop an optimistic attitude about his or her ability to successfully complete the rehabilitation. Also, athletes are familiar with the conditioning world and have been continuously instructed to give 100 percent to all conditioning and participation activities. But when injured, the athlete enters a new world, the reconditioning world.[8] Many athletes sustain an injury, seek medical care, and after a few weeks, the pain is gone. The athlete thereby fully returns to full sports participation, only to sustain a reinjury. The athlete returns to medical care and is provided an additional period of treatment and rest. The athlete rests for an additional 3 weeks, but sustains a reinjury with return to participation. This situation is very common. In fact, the high reinjury rate following a return to participation substantiates the rest and reinjury cycle. The athlete should be educated about the reconditioning process. The athlete is very familiar with the conditioning world. In conditioning, the athlete must give 100 percent and push through pain to maximize sports ability. But after an injury the athlete is in a different world. The reconditioning world differs from the conditioning world in two major aspects: the exercise tolerance window and exercise-associated versus postexercise pain.

The exercise tolerance window represents the level of exercise appropriate for any athlete. When he or she is not injured and is conditioning, the exercise tolerance window is very wide and can be pushed to the limits. But when injured, the exercise tolerance window narrows greatly and the athlete must carefully control his or her exercise level. If an athlete overexercises, a reinjury is sustained. However, inappropriate rest and underexercise leads to unrealized maximal gains. Therefore, there is a narrow window of exercise intensity and duration that must be adhered to if the athlete is to achieve a return to full participation. This will be frustrating because of prior experience with the conditioning world.

Exercise-associated pain is the pain encountered during exercise. This pain is produced by the accumulation of exercise metabolites and dissipates with rest after exercise. This is the pain that the athlete must learn to exercise with to maximize performance. "No pain, no gain" is accurate for many conditioning programs. But when an athlete has sustained an injury and pushes through the pain, he or she will find that the pain remains after exercise and recovery is delayed. Therefore, in the reconditioning world, an athlete must monitor his or her postexercise pain. If postexercise pain is minimal or relieved in 1 hour, the exercise intensity can be increased in the next exercise session. If postexercise pain is moderate, or swelling has developed, which is not reduced by the next day, the athlete has overexercised and should maintain or reduce exercise intensity or duration in the next session. With continued improvement, the exercise tolerance window

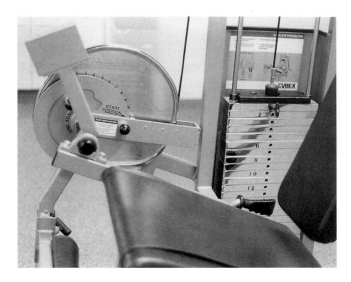

Figure 12–8. Weight-training equipment.

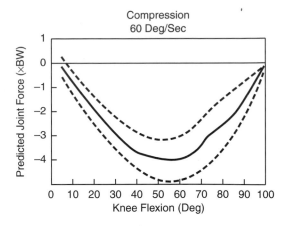

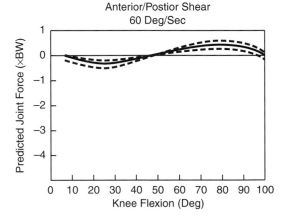

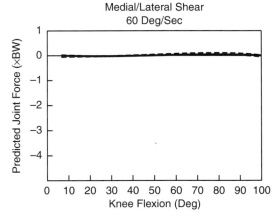

Figure 12–9. Tibiofemoral joint force during the extension portion of isokinetic exercise at 60 degrees/second. All forces are shown with respect to the tibia and have been normalized with respect to the subject's body weight. Posterior and lateral shear are positive. Solid line is average for five subjects. Dashed line indicates ± 1 SD. (*From Kaufman KR, et al.,[103] with permission.*)

will widen and he or she will be able gradually to return to the conditioning world using exercise-associated pain to control the level of exercise.

Reconditioning involves a program of gradually increasing stress. Reconditioning is initiated with exercises to increase range of motion (stretching), progressing to strength training exercises, and functional activities to prepare the athlete for successful return to his or her sport.

ANTERIOR CRUCIATE LIGAMENT REHABILITATION

Anterior cruciate ligament (ACL) rehabilitation requires restoration of normal range of motion (ROM), strength, and functional ability, while at the same time protecting the graft. The strength of the graft depends upon fixation strength during the first 4 to 6 weeks.[9] Studies indicate that the graft loses strength and is weakest during weeks 4 to 12.[10-12] The rehabilitation program must provide an appropriate level of stress to enhance healing and remolding without producing reinjury.[13-15] Reconstructions using patella tendon graft with bone plugs provide a strong graft with firm bone healing fixation, but the therapist and trainer should also be aware that hamstring or iliotibial tendon grafts can be done. These grafts provide differing strengths and fixation means and may require changes in timing and progression of the rehabilitation protocol.

Rehabilitation protocols also differ depending on the physician's experience and concerns. Therefore, it is important that the physical therapist and athletic trainer obtain and follow each surgeon's protocol. If the therapist or athletic trainer has a concern with the physician's protocol, they should review the literature and discuss it with the physician. Changes to the program can be made

to improve the patient's recovery based upon each individual's unique situation.

Anterior cruciate rehabilitation can involve different situations: ACL reconstruction, ACL reconstruction with meniscus repair, partial ACL sprain, ACL sprain and chronic ACL insufficiency, ACL with medical col-

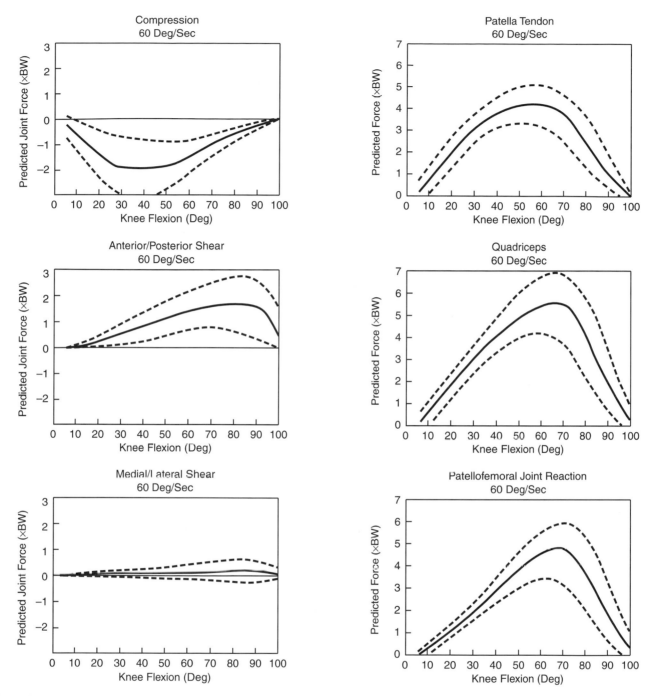

Figure 12–10. Tibiofemoral joint force during the flexion portion of isokinetic exercise at 60 degrees/second (see legend of Fig. 12–9 for detailed explanation). (*From Kaufman KR, et al.,[103] with permission.*)

Figure 12–11. Patellofemoral forces during isokinetic exercise at 60 degrees/second. All forces have been normalized with respect to the subject's body weight. Solid line is average for five subjects. Dashed line indicates ± 1 SD. (*From Kaufman K, et al.,[103] with permission.*)

lateral sprain, and ACL reconstruction with partial meniscectomy.

Anterior Cruciate Reconstruction

Surgeons will have different concerns and attitudes regarding rehabilitation procedures and techniques fol-

lowing ACL reconstruction. Therefore, it is important to obtain the surgeon's postoperative protocol to direct rehabilitation. Traditionally, rehabilitation has been staged to attempt to match the stress of rehabilitation exercise with the gains in strength of the graft. Protocols range from pages of description to a statement that the "patient may be progressed as tolerated." Most protocols provide a staged program of increasing stress that is both time dependent and provides criteria for advancement. Shelbourne[16] advocates an accelerated protocol that allows full weight-bearing at 2 days, agility at 5 weeks, and return to full sports at 4 months. DeHaven (personal communication) advocates a more conservative protocol that provides progression dependent on the time constraints evident within graft maturation and the athlete's progression in ROM, strength, and function. Shelbourne's accelerated protocol allows athletes with good motor control to protect the graft during the maturation process. But patients without good motor control will increase the possibility of reinjury.

Table 12–1 gives an overview of the ACL reconstruction process. A case study appears at the end of the chapter.

ACL Reconstruction With Meniscus Repair

Athletes with an ACL sprain also frequently sustain a meniscus injury.[17-19] Additionally, athletes participating in sports with chronic ACL insufficiency have an increased risk of meniscus injury.[20-23] Therefore, many athletes undergoing ACL reconstruction will also need meniscal surgery. Meniscus that cannot be repaired and undergoing a meniscectomy with ACL reconstruction, does not modify the ACL reconstruction protocol.

If the meniscus is repaired, the protocol is modified to protect the healing meniscus. Active ROM is completed from 90 to 20 degrees to protect the healing meniscus from the increased stress produced at full extension and flexion.[24] Passive range-of-motion exercise to obtain full extension is continued to prevent the development of posterior contracture and flexion contracture (DeHaven, personal communication). Progressive resistance exercise (PRE) is completed from 90 to 60 degrees for the quadriceps and 20 to 90 degrees for the hamstrings. Ambulation is initiated at 6 weeks, with 3-point crutch weight bearing and one-third body weight. This is progressed by one-third body weight every 5 days. Progression to full-range quadriceps strength training and running remain the same. During the rehabilitation process, the athlete is instructed to protect the meniscus by not completing a deep squat or twisting on a flexed knee. Because of the wide variation in surgeons' concerns for protecting the meniscus repair, each surgeon's protocol for ACL reconstruction with meniscus repair must be followed when rehabilitating the physician's patient.

Partial ACL Sprains

Because partial ACL sprains have little potential for healing[25,26] and clinical reports have demonstrated variable results,[27-29] partial ACL sprains are provided a rehabilita-

TABLE 12–1. ANTERIOR CRUCIATE LIGAMENT RECONSTRUCTION (PATELLAR TENDON: BONE-TENDON-BONE)[a]

0–4 weeks	Hinged splint with intermittent active assistive and passive ROM (ext, flex, patellar mobs); quad sets and SLR (without weights); isometric hams; ankle pumping; crutches-touch down; *Postop brace is locked at 0°* when not ranging; brace during sleep for 6 weeks.
5 days	Quad control: EMS and/or EMG biofeedback as needed with SLR; prone passive extension.
10–14 days	Hinges unlocked for active and passive ROM; quads and hams active within range against gravity; initiate weight bearing with one-third body weight (BW) with knee in extension with brace locked and increase by 1/3 BW every 3 days as tolerated; EMG biofeedback to hamstrings with gait (see Fig. 12–12) (and quads, if inadequate contraction).
2½ weeks	PRE (light weights with Q&H station) quads 90 to 60° and hams within available range, half squats, hip abduction and adduction (resistance above knees); continue SLR without weights; stationary bicycling when range is adequate. If able to SLR, ambulate FWB with brace locked in extension; intermittent ambulation 10% BW with normal gait pattern with brace unlocked; single leg balancing.
4–6 weeks	Ambulate with normal gait with brace unlocked: Level and smooth surface for 5 minutes 2 or 3 times/day. Increase each session by 5 minutes every other day. EMG biofeedback to hams with initial sessions; continue ambulation with brace locked in extension and ROM, PRE, and SLR as above. (*Brace locked at 0° for sleep* until 6 weeks.)
6–20 weeks	Ambulate FWB with ACL brace (brace with ambulation until 4 months) when comfort, size, and control allow (6–10 weeks) (EMG biofeedback to hams with initial sessions); ROM; SLR without weight; PRE quads 90 to 60° *only*, hams full range, squats, hip abduction and adduction (above knee); stationary bicycling; functional exercise: step-ups (StairMaster), rowing machine, swimming, sliding board.
5–7 months	ADD PRE: Begin quad PRE into full extension (gradual transition); initiate straight ahead jogging to ½ speed running, as tolerated, wearing ACL brace or custom brace (if ROM, strength, clinical status of knee are satisfactory).
7–8 months	ADD progress through graduated running program as tolerated (½, ¾, full speed), then agility (½, ¾, full), and then jumping.
8–9 months	ADD gradual increase in sport-specific activity.
9–12 months	Resume sports if all criteria met.

Physician Assessment: Day 1, 10–14 days, 4 weeks, 6 weeks, monthly until assured of adequate progression. Five, 7, 9 and 12 months. IKDC evaluation preop and 1 year postop; KT-1000 at preop, 5, 9, and 12 months.

Physical Therapy: Preop; postop; 5 days; 10–14 days; 2½, 4, 6 weeks; monthly, 5, 7, 9, and 12 months (as needs indicate). Strength testing: Prior to physician assessment after 5 weeks quads isometric at 60° (isokinetic dynamometer at 75°), hams isokinetic. Isokinetic Q & H after 5 months.

[a] Modifications may be made for each individual's unique situation.

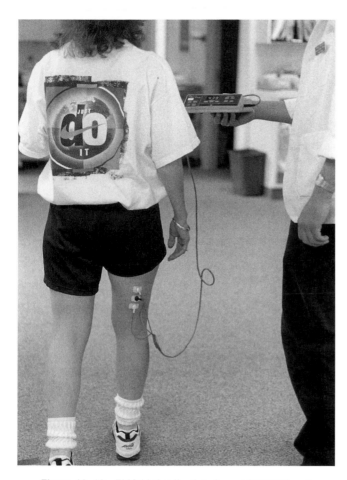

Figure 12–12. EMG biofeedback to hamstrings with gait.

Athletes who have sustained prior ACL injuries and have not selected surgical intervention as a treatment option, are provided care to enhance hamstring control[30] and to minimize situations where instability may occur. Athletes are educated regarding the nature of the injury and the importance of preventing additional injuries. The effect that quadriceps and hamstrings muscle activity have on the instability is reviewed, along with procedures to reduce stress to the anterior translation of the tibia. The athlete is educated to eliminate the "step-across cut" (see Fig. 12–13A) and instead, to use a "step-out cut" (see Fig. 12–13B). Sports that require jumping, cutting, and twisting should be eliminated or, minimally, modified to reduce stress. If the athlete is adamant about participating in a high-risk sport, the athlete is instructed about the hazards of such participation and sport techniques are modified, as much as possible, to reduce stress. Strength training involves emphasis upon hamstrings. Quadriceps exercises are completed from 90 to 60 degrees with light weights and gradual progression.[31] Hamstring PREs are completed full range with hip abduction and adduction completed with resistance above the knees. Closed-chain exercises (leg press) are also utilized. Electromyography (EMG) biofeedback is applied to the hamstrings during gait, stairs, and sports-specific movements to assist the athlete in learning hamstring dominance. In most cases, biofeedback is done for 2 to 3 sessions, or until the athlete has learned hamstring control during activity. The athlete is instructed to practice appropriate control intermittently during the day (at each meal time, before and after activity) for 20 to 30 steps to develop hamstring control. The athlete is continually reminded that the treatment involves learning control and even if the knee feels great, the knee has not been cured of ACL insufficiency. Control is continually necessary.

Table 12–2 summarizes the key points of nonsurgical acute ACL rehabilitation.

tion program that protects the injured ACL and secondary stabilizers, such as the medial and lateral capsular ligaments and the meniscus. The acute ACL protocol is initiated with continued protection provided by the chronic ACL protocol. The program is modified by the physician depending on the degree of injury to the ACL ligament.

Acute ACL Spain and Chronic ACL Insufficiency

The diagnosis of ACL sprain, with or without meniscus pathology, requires procedures that will reduce inflammation, swelling, return ROM, and protect the joint from additional injury. Many athletes, directly after injury, have not made a decision whether he or she will select reconstructive surgery or conservative care. Initial care involves the traditional RICE (rest, ice, compression, and elevation). All athletes are treated with the acute ACL protocol. To increase compliance, athletes who select surgery will be instructed in the purpose and techniques of the postoperative exercise program prior to surgery. Athletes selecting nonoperative treatment are counseled regarding the importance of not participating in high risk activities such as basketball and soccer, and maintaining motor control to prevent reinjuries.

ACL Reconstruction With Medial Collateral Ligament Sprain

Individuals who sprain the medial collateral ligament (MCL) recover effectively without surgical intervention.[18,32] Individuals who sprain their MCL and ACL have been treated with surgical repair. Some physicians repair both structures,[33] other physicians repair only the MCL,[34] and others surgically treat the ACL.[35] Daniel and Fritschy's preferred treatment is reconstruction of the ACL and allowing the MCL to heal.

Complications of ACL Reconstruction

ACL reconstruction is a major knee surgery and complications regarding ROM, pain, and motor control can occur. Loss of joint motion after surgery can produce disability. The shortening of the period of postoperative immobilization has reduced joint stiffness[36] and the use of immediate

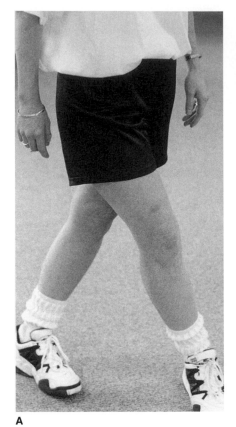
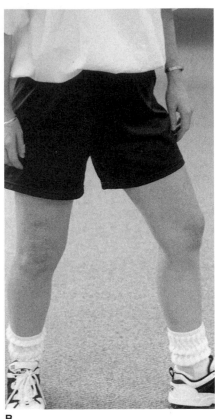

Figure 12–13. The athlete is taught to eliminate the "step-across cut" **(A)** and instead use a "step-out cut" **(B)** to reduce stress to the anterior translation of the tibia.

A

B

motion with active and passive ranging usually allows the athlete to obtain normal ROM. Delaying the reconstructive surgery 3 to 4 weeks after injury has been effective in reducing the incidence of ROM problems after surgery.[37] Continuous passive motion machines (CPM) are used by some physicians to enhance ROM. Other physicians have the opinion that early motion is important and that the use of CPMs, over other forms of motion, has not been supported by the literature. Preoperative evaluation, obtaining normal ROM, and instruction of the athlete in the postoperative rehabilitation program will increase the athlete's compliance in the exercise program. Athletes who are having difficulty obtaining ROM should be reinstructed in ROM exercises and treated more often. The use of a postoperative brace to maintain stretching should be considered. Additionally, proper pain control should be evaluated and treatment instituted if necessary. Constant stretch braces, such as DynaSplint or other similar ROM devices, could also be used.

Sapega[38] has also advocated the use of heat to the collagen tissue to enhance the elastic component of stretching while maintaining a light stretch. Ice is then applied to the collagen tissue while the stretch is maintained to enhance the plastic component of stretching. The addition of heat and cold to enhance ROM is incorporated in contrast stretching. Contrast stretching for extension is completed by placing the athlete prone at the end of a table and applying ultrasound or a hot hydrocollator to the posterior knee (see Fig. 12–14). The heat is applied for 20 minutes and then ice is applied for 15 minutes. As the athlete accommodates to the stretch, a 1-pound weight cuff is applied to the ankle during the contrast stretching. If discomfort develops, the athlete uses the other ankle to lift the injured leg to relieve the stretch for 30 to 60 seconds. If discomfort continues, the stretching force is reduced. The athlete maintains the stretch position for 1 to 2 hours after the treatment.

Contrast stretching for flexion is completed by sitting the athlete on the edge of a treatment table and attaching a cuff by twine to a weight pan to maintain a stretch (see Fig. 12–15). A felt pad is placed over the anterior patella to reduce heat buildup. The stretch can also be completed by placing the athlete supine with the foot on a wall (see Fig. 12–16), letting gravity flex the knee.

Measuring flexion contracture can be difficult when monitoring a postoperative ROM program and measuring prone heel height has been suggested.[39] The athlete is placed prone and flexion ROM is determined by measuring heel height difference (see Fig. 12–17). The use of a carpenter's square with extension assists with the measurement (see Fig. 12–18). The actual degrees of flexion contracture, as determined from heel height difference, is dependent on the athlete's leg length. The technique

TABLE 12–2. ACUTE ANTERIOR CRUCIATE LIGAMENT REHABILITATION (NONOPERATIVE/PRESURGICAL)

0–3 days	**Pain and Swelling Control** *Modalities*: Cryotherapy, trigger point stimulation, TENS, high-voltage/stimulation *ROM*: Knee splint in maximum comfortable extension, passive extension (gravity) stretching, patellar mobilizations QID (4 times/day)
	Strength: Quadriceps and hamstrings co-contractions in extension; electrical stimulation (EMS) and/or electromyography (EMG) biofeedback to medialis and/or quads and hams
	Weight Bearing: Touch down → partial weight bearing
3 days–1 week	Pain Control:
	Modalities: As above
	ROM: Splint in extension, ranging; extension each hour and flexion as tolerated to 120° four times each day; patellar mobs
	Strength: Q & H co-contractions at 45°, general for uninjured areas
	CV Conditioning: Upper extremity, single (uninjured) leg bike
	Weight Bearing: Partial → full weight bearing as tolerated
1–3 weeks	Pain Control: As necessary
	ROM: Gradual increase to full ROM for flex and ext
	Strength: PRE for quads from 90 to 60° and hams full range with light weights and gradual progress, general for uninjured areas
	CV Conditioning: Add involved leg with bicycle
	Weight Bearing: With adequate strength and ROM, gradual increase in WB; EMG biofeedback to hamstrings with initial ambulation sessions; instruct in eliminating "step-across turning"
3–6 weeks	Pain Control: As necessary
	ROM: Increase to full ROM
	Strength: PRF quads 90 to 60° and hams full range, ADD closed chain
	CV Conditioning: Add StairMaster; D/C hinged splint when ROM and quad control adequate
6–12 weeks	Strength: Continue as above
	CV Conditioning: Continue as above
	Brace: Fit for ACL brace
	Functional Rehabilitation: With full ROM and 60 percent strength,[a] slow, gradual increase in running from straight-ahead jogging to running and then sprinting. Progress to agility with reduced "step-across cutting"
3–4 months	Return to Sports: Gradual return to sports as tolerated after successful completion of functional rehabilitation with modification of techniques and activities as necessary to minimize risk of experiencing episodes of instability

[a] If episodes of instability occur, reduce functional level and return to physician for reevaluation.

has been very successful for following athletes to determine the status of the knee flexion ROM.

If gains are not obtained in the ranging program, the surgeon should be notified for consideration of additional procedures. Manipulation under anesthesia, arthroscopic, or open release may be necessary.[40-42] Paulos and associates[42] also reported the importance of patellar mobility following surgery and related patellar stiffness to reduced ROM.

Pain control is usually adequate with postoperative medication and physical therapy treatments. But reflex sympathetic dystrophy (RSD), a condition that presents with pain out of proportion to the pathology, cool mottled skin, atrophy, swelling, and reduced range of motion, will

increase pain.[43] RSD following ACL injury is rare. But because RSD responds more effectively with prompt care, professionals must continuously follow the athlete and if appropriate reduction in pain and progress is not evident, RSD should be considered and the treatment program modified. RSD treatment requires careful control of exercise and may also require sympathetic blocks and transcutaneous nerve stimulation for resolution.[44]

Anterior knee pain has been reported in approximately one third of ACL reconstruction patients.[39] Over the past several years, this may be due less to early ROM. A number of ACL reconstruction patients will present with quadriceps inhibition, producing inability to perform a quadriceps set or SLR after surgery. Prompt care

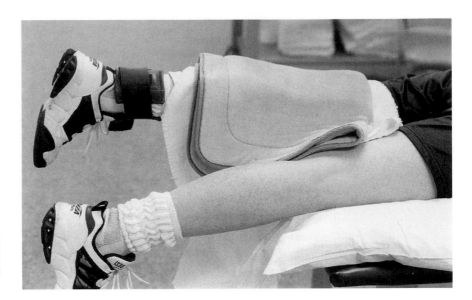

Figure 12–14. Contrast stretching completion for extension. With the athlete prone at the end of the table, a hot hydrocollator is applied to the posterior knee.

should resolve this. At the first postoperative therapy sessions, if quadriceps inhibition is present and the patient cannot complete (or weakly completes) a quadriceps set and straight leg raise, medium-frequency electrical muscle stimulation (ES-180) is applied to the quadriceps.[45] The patient contracts the quadriceps along with the muscle stimulation to relearn motor control, usually in one or two treatment sessions (see Fig. 12-19). EMG biofeedback is then applied to the quadriceps (see Fig. 12-20A) and to the vastus medialis (see Fig. 12-20B) to aid the patient in gaining self-control of the quadriceps.

Patellofemoral mobility and vastus medialis control are monitored during the rehabilitation program to ensure that the patient maintains appropriate patellofemoral control. Intermittent application of EMS or EMG biofeedback to the medialis may be necessary to maintain control. Intermittent increases in pain can be generally controlled with cryotherapy, TENS, or treatment to trigger points.

Evaluation of the ACL treatment program for an athlete requires an ongoing assessment of patient selection for different treatment programs, surgical techniques, documentation of associated injuries, rehabilitation specific for the pathology or surgery, and subjective, objective, and functional outcomes.

POSTERIOR CRUCIATE LIGAMENT

The treatment of isolated posterior cruciate ligament (PCL) instabilities range from surgical reconstruction to conservative management.[45a] A majority of physicians recommend an initial nonoperative approach, regardless of the degenerative changes that may occur over time. An important predictive factor of the success of conservative care is the strength of the quadriceps.[45a] The PCL deficit patient must increase quadriceps force, protect the patellofemoral joint, and become quadriceps dominant to compensate for the PCL deficiency. The nonoperative protocol for PCL sprains given in

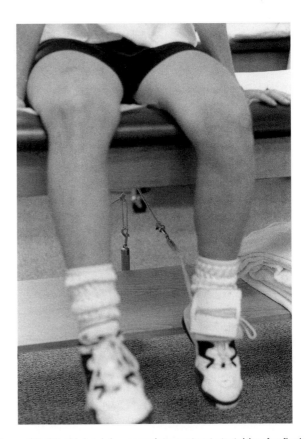

Figure 12–15. Maintaining complete contrast stretching for flexion. With the athlete sitting at the edge of the table, a cuff is held in place with twine to a weight pan, and a felt pad is placed over the anterior patella to reduce heat build-up.

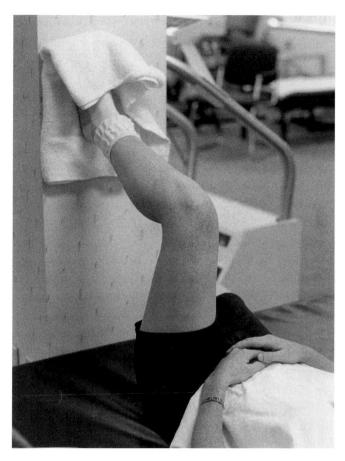

Figure 12–16. The stretch can also be completed by placing the athlete supine with the foot against a wall and letting gravity flex the knee.

Table 12-3 was developed by Dehaven and associates (personal communication).

Strength training for the quadriceps is usually completed with the athlete in a sitting position. Gravity, therefore, displaces the tibia in a posterior direction. To eliminate the shifting from the posterior position to a reduced position with the weight applied, the athlete is instructed to contract the quadriceps prior to lifting the weight. Hamstring PRE are completed with a limited range to protect the secondary stabilizers from additional injury. Most athletes with PCL injury will progress through the rehabilitation program without difficulty. If difficulties are encountered, the athlete should be reevaluated for appropriate motor control and completion of the exercise program. If modification of the program does not provide resolution of the problems, the athlete should be reevaluated by the physician to eliminate the possibility of additional pathology or to modify the rehabilitation program.

Chronic PCL instability that does not respond to conservative care is considered for PCL reconstruction. Limb alignment and additional pathologies must be considered and treatment planned prior to a reconstruction. Different techniques and graft materials can be used for

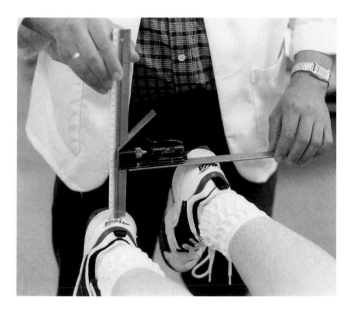

Figure 12–17. Determination of ROM flexion by measuring heel height difference in the prone athlete.

PCL reconstructions; therefore the rehabilitation program must be based on the specific surgical techniques used and the surgeon's experience. The PCL rehabilitation program given in Table 12-4 was developed by DeHaven and associates (personal communication).

MEDIAL COLLATERAL LIGAMENT

Medial collateral ligament sprains laxity-graded as 0 (normal), I (1 to 4 mm), and grade II (5 to 9 mm) with a

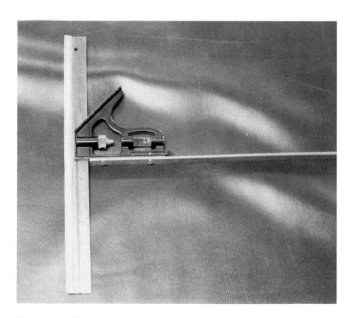

Figure 12–18. A carpenter's square with an extension is helpful in measuring heel height difference.

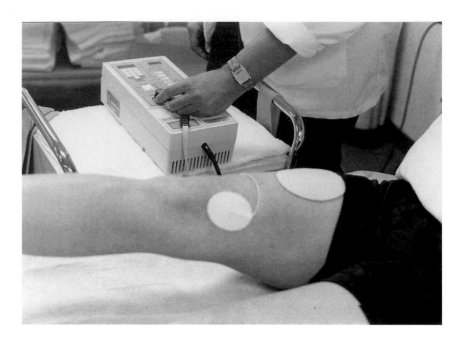

Figure 12–19. Contraction of the quadriceps alone with muscle stimulation (see Fig. 12–20) helps the patient relearn motor control.

definite end feel have been successfully treated with conservative procedures.[46,47] Some grade III sprains, without additional injuries, have been treated with surgery.[34] Recently, nonoperative treatment has been advocated by Indelicato[48] and Jones,[49] while Kannus did not find suc-

cess with nonoperative treatment of grade III MCL sprains.[50] Nonoperative treatment protocols have been provided by Steadman[51] and Bergfeld.[52]

DeHaven and colleagues have developed the nonoperative protocol for MCL sprains given in Table 12-5 (per-

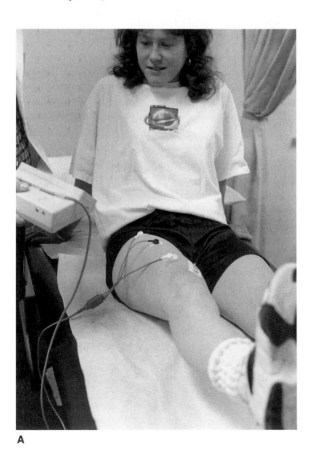

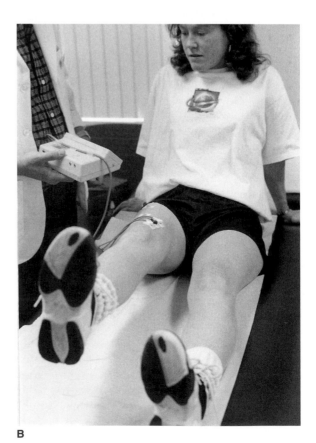

A   **B**

Figure 12–20. EMG biofeedback is applied to the quadriceps **(A)** and vastus medialis **(B)** to help the athlete learn self-control of these muscles.

TABLE 12–3. NONOPERATIVE PROTOCOL FOR POSTERIOR CRUCIATE SPRAIN

Stage I (1–3 days)
Rest, ice, compression, elevation; NWB-CWB; high-voltage, interferential stimulation for pain and swelling; hinged splint locked in full extension.

Stage II (2–4 days to 4–8 weeks)
Hinged splint to control ROM in comfortable range; AROM in brace within comfortable range; increase ROM daily to full ROM as tolerated; splint in full extension at night until 2 weeks; quad PREs from 30° to 0°; EMG biofeedback to vastus medialis with PRE and ambulation until appropriate control is demonstrated; possible use of EMS; ham PRE from 0° to 10° after full ROM is obtained. Closed-chain PRE and exercise; weight bearing as tolerated, use EMG biofeedback to quads until control is demonstrated. Hip abduction and adduction with resistance above knee; stationary bicycling and/or other cardiovascular conditioning; PREs for uninvolved body areas. Bracing if concerned with controlling valgus-varus and/or hyperextension forces.

Stage III (begins at end of stage II)
Functional rehabilitation, as well as gradual functional test, when quads equal 70 percent of contralateral and with physician's authorization. EMG biofeedback to quads with functional activities until control is demonstrated; gradual return to sports with completion of functional rehabilitation and physician's authorization. Continued strength and cardiovascular training.

sonal communication). Progress through the program is dependent upon the physician's determination of the severity of the sprain and the patient's response to the program.

The timing for return to sports is dependent upon the severity of injury and successful completion of the reconditioning program. Grade I injuries may only require a few days. Grade II injuries can vary from 2 weeks to a few months, and grade III injuries can require a few months for successful return to sport.

MENISCUS TEARS

Injuries to the meniscus can be left alone,[53,54] removed by meniscectomy,[55] or repaired.[56–58] The rehabilitation

for meniscus injuries will depend on the nature of the pathology and treatment provided.

Meniscectomies are treated with postsurgical pain and swelling control, active and passive ROM, and quadriceps and straight leg raises with progression to progressive resistance exercise, as tolerated by the athlete. Cardiovascular conditioning is maintained by exercise using the contralateral lower extremity and upper extremity, with progression to the involved lower extremity. With appropriate ROM and strength (generally 60 percent of contralateral), the athlete is progressed to functional rehabilitation and gradual return to sports.

Peripheral tears of the meniscus can be repaired and the repair should be protected until healing has occurred. The amount of protection required for meniscal

TABLE 12–4. POSTERIOR CRUCIATE LIGAMENT RECONSTRUCTION

0–4 weeks	Hinged splint is locked in full extension; pillow under calf with leg elevated; patellar mobs; quad sets and SLR; sidelying hip abd and add with knee in extension and resistance above knee; crutches-touch down; brace during sleep for 6 weeks.
5 days	Quad Control: EMS and/or EMG biofeedback as needed with SLR; with good quad control, ROM for flexion 0 to 45° in sitting with eccentric and concentric quads and avoiding contraction of hams; calf and hamstring stretching with knee in extension; resisted ankle plantarflexion with knee in extension with rubber tubing.
3 weeks start	ROM: Flexion, as above, increase to 0 to 90°; extension, in prone without active hams; PRE (light weights with Q&H station) quads 0 to 30°; *no* hams PRE; mini-squats (0 to 45°), hip abd and add (knee in ext and resistance above knees); stationary bicycling when range is adequate utilizing a high seat and foot forward on pedal (do not use toe clips).
4–6 weeks	Ambulate with normal gait with brace unlocked: 3-pt gait initiated with ⅓ BW and increased by ⅓ BW every 5 days. EMG biofeedback to quads with initial sessions; continue ROM and PRE, as above. (*Brace locked at 0° for sleep* until 6 weeks.)
6–20 weeks	ROM: Increase flexion to WNL; ambulate FWB with ACL-PCL brace (brace with ambulation until 4 months) when comfort, size, and control allow (6–10 weeks) (EMG biofeedback to quads with initial sessions); ROM; PRE quads 0 to 30° *only*, hams 0–10°; squats, hip abd and add (above knee); stationary bicycling; functional exercise: step-ups (StairMaster), rowing machine, swimming, sliding board.
5–7 months	ADD PRE: Begin quad and ham PRE into full range (gradual transition); initiate straight-ahead jogging to ½ speed running as tolerated wearing ACL-PCL brace (if ROM, strength, clinical status of knee are OK).
7–9 months	ADD progress through graduated running program as tolerated (½, ¾, full speed), then agility (½, ¾, full), and then jumping. Then add gradual increase in sport-specific activity.
9–12 months	Resume sports if criteria met and physician approval.

Physician Assessment: Day 1, 10–14 days, 4 weeks, 6 weeks, monthly until assured of adequate progression; five, 7, 9 and 12 months. IKDC evaluation preop and 1 year postop; KT-1000 at preop, 5, 9, and 12 months.

Physical Therapy: Preop; Postop; 5 days; 10–14 days; 3, 4, 6 weeks; monthly, 5, 7, 9, and 12 months (as needs indicate). Strength testing: Prior to physician assessment after 5 weeks quads isometric at 30° (isokinetic dynamometer at 45°), do not test hams. Isokinetic Q & H after 5 months.

TABLE 12–5. NONOPERATIVE PROTOCOL FOR MEDIAL COLLATERAL SPRAIN[a]

Stage I (1–3 days)
Rest, ice, compression, elevation; NWB-CWB; high-voltage, interferential stimulation for pain and swelling; hinged splint locked at midpoint of comfortable range.

Stage II (1–3 days)
Hinged splint to control ROM in comfortable range; AROM in brace within comfortable range; increase ROM weekly up to full ROM as tolerated; quad and hams isometrics at midpoint of comfortable range; possible use of EMS and/or EMG biofeedback for quad and/or ham control; touch-down weight bearing increased to 3 point and FWB as tolerated. Stationary bicycling (with appropriate ROM) and/or other cardiovascular conditioning; PRE for uninvolved body areas.

Stage III (begins at end of stage II)
Discontinue hinged splint, functional MCL brace; increase PREs with protection of PF joint (terminal knee extension and hams full range with gradual increase, closed-chain exercise); hip abduction and adduction with resistance above knee.

Stage IV (begins at end of Stage III)
Functional rehabilitation with brace when quad and hams equal 70 percent of contralateral and physician's authorization. Gradual return to sports with completion of functional rehabilitation and physician's authorization. Continued strength and cardiovascular training.

[a] MCL sprains vary in severity and response to treatment. The timing of progression through the stages of treatment for a specific injury will be determined both by the physician's determination of severity and the patient's response to treatment.

repairs can vary widely with surgical technique and the surgeon's experience. It is important that the physical therapist and athletic trainer obtain directions from the physician regarding the postoperative treatment plan. The postoperative protocol given in Table 12-6 was developed by DeHaven and associates (personal communication).

Rehabilitation after meniscus injury must be specifically designed based on the nature of the pathology, treatment provided, experiences of the physician, and progression of the athlete. The timing for return to sports is highly variable, and coordination of the treatment plan by the physician, therapist, athletic trainer, and athlete is needed to optimize care.

PATELLOFEMORAL REHABILITATION

The primary treatment for patellofemoral pain syndrome (PFPS) involves exercises to increase the flexibility of the quadriceps and hamstrings and to enhance control and strength of the vastus medialis obliquis to control positioning of the patella.[59] Busch and DeHaven[60] and Henry[60a] have reported success with nonoperative treatment for PFPS. The major concept of rehabilitation is to alter the static and dynamic forces to realign the patella to resolve the pain. Treatment procedures include flexibility, strengthening, braces or taping, foot orthotics, and, possibly, surgery for patients not responding to conservative care.

Flexibility

Reduced flexibility of the hamstrings and quadriceps, along with tightness of the lateral patellofemoral retinaculum, increases lateral compression pressures in the patellofemoral joint during activity. Flexibility exercises for the hamstring (see Fig. 12–21A), quadriceps (see Fig. 12–21B), and iliotibial band should be completed daily. The stretching exercises are performed 3 times daily, in addition to before and after exercise. The stretching posi-

TABLE 12–6. MENISCUS REPAIR PROTOCOL

0–2 weeks	Postop brace locked at 0°; patellar mobilizations; straight leg raises (SLR) without weights; touch-down weight bearing
2–4 weeks	Postop brace—hinges set to allow ROM 20 to 80°; add quad and hams isometrics at 45° with low resistance and gradual progression; SLR (with brace removed for exercise only) at 0° without weight
4–6 weeks	Graduated program of ROM for flex and extension; PREs (utilizing a Q & H machine with light weights and gradual progression) quads 90 to 20° and hams 20 to 90°; discontinue hinged brace
6 weeks	Initiate weight bearing with 1/3 body weight and increase by 1/3 body weight every 5 days. Full weight bearing requires quads strength equal to 10 percent of body weight
8 weeks	PREs for quads and hams completed with full range
3–6 months	Jogging to 1/2 speed running; bike riding, swimming
6 months	Running to full speed with agility
6–8 months	Return to sports

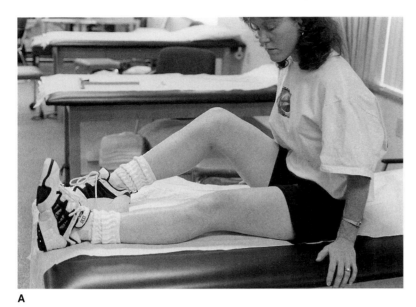

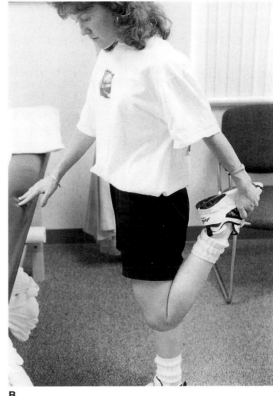

Figure 12–21. Flexibility exercises for the hamstring **(A)** and the quadriceps **(B)**.

tion is assumed and the stretch gradually increased until a stretching sensation is perceived just below pain. The stretch is held for 30 to 60 seconds, released for 5 to 10 seconds, and repeated 3 to 5 times. McConnell suggests that the physical therapist or athletic trainer stretch the lateral patellofemoral region (see Fig. 12-22).[61] The stretching force is applied for 30 seconds, rested for 5 seconds, and repeated 3 to 5 times. Certain athletes may be able to provide medial mobilization of the patella while sitting in a chair with the quadriceps relaxed (see Fig. 12-23).

Muscle Strength

Traditional strengthening exercises for PFPS include quadriceps strengthening in terminal position such as quad sets, straight leg raises, and terminal knee extension.[60] To enhance vastus medialis obliquis (VMO) control during quadriceps exercise, several approaches have been recommended. Some clinicians advocate the completion of quadriceps strengthening exercise from 90 to 60 degrees[62] as the patellofemoral joint has greater contact area from 90 to 60 degrees[63] and therefore reduces force to the patellofemoral joint when exercises are performed in that range. McConnell advocates leg press or squats[61] to improve strength without increasing patellofemoral pain.

Strength training must be completed pain free; therefore, modifications of traditional exercises may be necessary for specific patients. In general, quadriceps sets with progression to straight leg raises and terminal knee extension will be effective for many athletes. But specific athletes will require modification of the traditional exercises to provide pain-free exercise (DeHaven, personal communication). Leg press, squats, or quadriceps exercises from 90 degrees to 60 degrees with light weights and gradual progression may be effective.

Motor Control

Dynamic stabilization of the patellofemoral joint requires activation of the vastus medialis to counteract the forces produced by the Q-angle and the lateral forces of the vastus lateralis. Inappropriate motor schemas developed along with inhibition of the VMO will continue unless modified. Ingersoll has shown there is improved position of the patella when EMG biofeedback is used to enhance VMO control during quadriceps exercise.[64] McConnell has stressed the importance of the medialis contracting prior to the lateralis.[61] EMG biofeedback is used to evaluate and train the patient in the correct firing pattern. This hypothesis is substantiated by Voight and Wieder, who indicated that the firing pattern in PFPS patients was dysfunctional with an early firing of the vastus lateralis.[65]

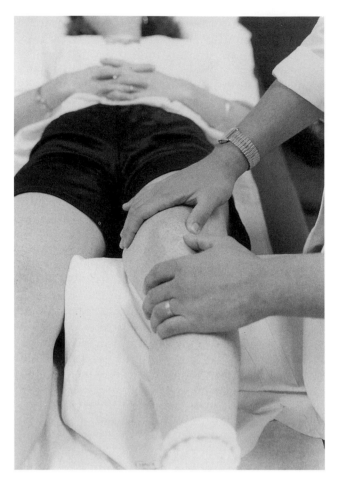

Figure 12–22. Lateral patellofemoral region being stretched.

Bracing and Taping

Patellofemoral braces of various styles have been used successfully for a number of years. Palumbo has presented his successful experience with the use of a brace.[66] McConnell advocates a specific taping technique to control glide, rotation, and tilt to control the patella[61] and many practitioners report success with the taping.

Foot Orthotics

Increased pronation of the foot during gait increases internal rotation of the tibia, thereby increasing patellofemoral stress. Foot orthotics can assist in controlling the pronation and decrease excessive forces during use of the extensor mechanism.[59] Individuals with abnormal foot mechanics should be evaluated, and minimally, provided a temporary orthotic, with probable development of a permanent foot orthotic.

Surgery

Patients who do not respond to conservative care may be treated with surgery. Surgical options include lateral release, proximal realignment, distal realignment, and proximal with distal realignment. Indicators for each surgical procedure and rehabilitation will be specific for each surgeon and his or her experience. Rehabilitation after surgery should follow the surgeon's protocol.

Author's Preference

Appropriate activation of the medial and lateral forces are necessary for exercises to provide resolution of PFPS. Most patients develop a dysfunction secondary to inadequate medialis activation. EMG biofeedback is used to evaluate and teach the patient enhanced medialis activation. Training with biofeedback is initiated with quads sets and straight leg raises, progressing to active knee extension in sitting. With improved activation, the patient is progressed to ambulation, running, and sport-specific movements. Generally, medialis control is obtained after 2 to 5 sessions, with intermittent biofeedback training after the development of control. Although most patients respond to medialis training, specific patients will continue to have difficulty. These patients may improve with the addition of biofeedback to the vastus lateralis to decrease activation level in comparison to medialis during a quadriceps contraction.

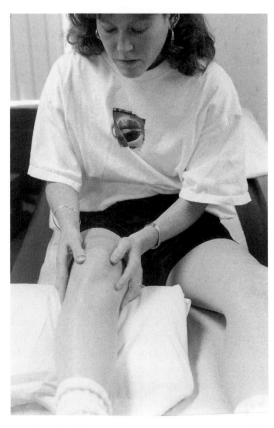

Figure 12–23. An athlete medially mobilizes the patella while sitting with the quadriceps relaxed.

Additionally, the medialis is trained to contract before the lateralis.[61] Specific patients may also become quadriceps dominant with emphasis on quadriceps function, and the addition of biofeedback to the hamstrings to improve use of the hamstrings during gait and sports activities will be assistive. The rehabilitation program must be specifically designed to the patient's unique anatomic, functional status. Careful control of all involved factors will allow most PFPS patients to respond successfully to conservative care.

BURSITIS

Swelling of the synovial-like sacs that act to reduce friction and protect structures from pressure is termed bursitis. Bursitis is usually produced by trauma or infection. Wrestlers and football players are at increased risk of developing bursitis.[67-69] Treatment of acute bursitis includes alleviating causative factors and controlling inflammation.[70] Compression wrap, taping, immobilization, anti-inflammatory medication, and ice should be used. Isometric exercise for the quadriceps, with or without electric muscle stimulation, will maintain strength. Aspiration is completed for extended inflammation. Cortisone injections have been advocated by some physicians, but the efficacy of cortisone has not been demonstrated.[67] Return to sports is allowed when swelling and pain have subsided, ROM is within normal limits, and protective padding is provided to lessen the effects of blows to the knee. Chronic bursitis may require surgical excision then rehabilitation.[67,71]

Septic bursitis should be managed by immediate aspiration and fluid analysis. Antibiotics and repeated aspirations or surgery may be necessary.[72-74] Isometric strength training may be utilized during the treatment phase with physician authorization.

Pes anserinus bursitis is usually caused by overuse or a contusion[75] and is difficult to differentiate from tendonitis. The treatment for bursitis and tendonitis is similar; therefore, determining the exact pathology is not usually necessary. Treatment should include heat, anti-inflammatory medication, and restricted activity.[70] Cortisone injection[69] and ultrasound[76] also have been successfully used for treatment. Stretching and isometric with progression to isotonic or isokinetic strength training should allow functional rehabilitation with return to sports.

MUSCLE STRAINS

Muscle strains, especially of the quadriceps and hamstrings, are common athletic injuries. Research[77-81] indicates that the lesion generally occurs at the musculotendenous junction. Strengthening and warm-up exercises have been used to prevent injuries.[78,81] The cellular injury

undergoes a typical inflammatory response[82] with RICE and anti-inflammatory medication used for control. NSAIDS are effective in controlling inflammation after stress.[83] Treatment of muscle injury involves RICE for the immediate postinjury period, with progression to ice and stretching, light isometric resistance exercise, and strength training progressive resistance exercise. When adequate strength (60 percent of the contralateral muscle) has been obtained, the athlete is progressed to functional rehabilitation and gradual return to sport. Physical therapy modalities such as ultrasound, TENS, cryotherapy, and EMS or high-voltage stimulation have been used to enhance recovery.

EMG indicates that during gait, the semimembranosus is active during the late swing phase to decelerate hip flexion. The semimembranosus, semitendinosus, and biceps femoris provide maximum activity during the take-off segment of the support phase.[84] The biceps femoris is the most commonly injured of the hamstring muscles.[85-87]

Causative factors for hamstring injuries include inadequate warm-up, inadequate stretching, poor technique, leg length inequalities, and muscle strength imbalances.[87-93] These factors should be eliminated, if possible, prior to a season. The athlete should be evaluated a minimum of 6 to 8 weeks prior to the start of the season to allow adequate time to eliminate causative factors.

Quadriceps strains can be produced by a strong contraction or forceful stretch of the muscle. The quadriceps is maximally active during the take-off phase of running, with the quadricep's primary function as a decelerator contracting with the hamstring during the support phase of running.[84,94] Injuries commonly occur in football, track and field, and basketball players.[95]

Treatment of muscle injuries involves an initial phase to control inflammation, with gradual increase in stress to the muscle as ROM, flexibility, and strength improve.[82] Initially, the muscle is treated with RICE for 2 to 3 days. The athlete is then progressed to mild stretching, NSAIDS, light isometric PRE, isotonic or isokinetic PRE, and functional rehabilitation, as signs and symptoms allow. General strength training and cardiovascular conditioning is maintained for uninvolved body areas. Electrical stimulation such as high volt, TENS, and interferential may be used to speed recovery. At times, medium-frequency electric muscle stimulation can aid recovery of muscle strength. Some clinicians have used heat modalities such as hot hydrocollator, whirlpool, and ultrasound, while other clinicians have not found heat to influence recovery. Complete tears may require surgical repair for recovery[96]; therefore, a physician should be consulted for major muscle injuries. After injury, prompt control of inflammation with progression to stretching, strengthening, and functional rehabilitation as symptoms indicate, will maximize return to athletic competition.

PATELLAR TENDON, QUADRICEPS, AND HAMSTRING TENDONITIS

With muscles, exercise can increase fiber size, number, and tensile strength of tendons.[97] Overuse of the musculotendinuous unit can cause inflammation or damage to the tendon. Tendons progress through a healing process of inflammation, fibroblastic deposit of collagen, and reorganization. Because of poor blood supply to the tendon, healing progresses slowly and may produce a chronic tendonitis. Symptoms usually occur gradually in phases.[98]

- Phase I. Pain after activity. No undue functional impairment.

- Phase II. Pain during and after activity. Patient is still able to perform at a satisfactory level.

- Phase III. More prolonged pain during and after activity. Patient has increasing difficulty performing at a satisfactory level.

Recognition of these phases for injury progression will allow modification of the athlete's conditioning intensity and duration to halt the progression.

Treatment of tendonitis depends upon the phase of healing.[98] First, inflammation is controlled with RICE and anti-inflammatory medication. Treatment is then progressed to therapeutic modalities, stretching and gradual strengthening. With improvement, the athlete is progressed to weight training and functional rehabilitation. Persistent symptoms may require surgery or the athlete modifying sport participation.

Therapeutic modalities for the treatment of tendonitis include ultrasound (with and without 10 percent hydrocortisone), ice, heat, and iontophoresis with hydrocortisone.[59] Rehabilitation exercises are initiated to restore hamstring, achilles, and quadriceps flexibility. The athlete is then progressed to a strengthening program of endurance training involving 10 to 30 repetitions increasing by 5 each day. (The athlete begins with 10 repetitions using light weights 3 times each day. If there is no increase in symptoms, repetitions are increased by 5 each day until the athlete can complete thirty repetitions. The repetitions are then reduced to 10 again and 1 pound weight is added.) This cycle is repeated until the athlete is lifting 3 to 5 pounds. The program is then progressed to traditional strength training completed 3 times per week, with gradually increasing resistance. With strength gains, the athlete progresses to functional rehabilitation and gradual return to sports participation.

Eccentric (lengthening) strengthening exercises have been advocated for tendonitis by Curwin and Stanish.[97] After a stretching warm-up, eccentric strengthening exercises are done, gradually increasing the speed. Treatment of patellofemoral pain and patellar tendonitis using a tap-ing procedure has been advocated by McConnell.[61] Additionally, various patellar tendon straps have been recommended (see Fig. 12–24). Reportedly, the straps alter mechanical stress. Levine and Splain have reported success with the strap for treating patellofemoral pain.[99] Results appear variable, with some athletes complaining of discomfort while using the strap, while others report a reduction in symptoms.

Blazina and associates have reported success with surgical treatment of chronic patellar tendonitis.[98] Debridement of granulated tissue, drilling of the infrapatellar pole, and incisions in the tendon were done to increase vascularity and produce a healing response. Others have not reported a high rate of effectiveness with surgery.[100,101]

Quadriceps tendonitis at the tendon's insertion into the proximal pole of the patella occurs much less frequently than patellar tendonitis.[59] Quadriceps tendonitis is generally treated nonsurgically, although surgical intervention is possible.[101] In the adolescent athlete, avulsion of the apophysis can also occur.[102] Treatment of quadriceps tendonitis is very similar to patellar tendonitis with modification of activity, flexibility exercises, endurance strength training with progression to strength training, and functional rehabilitation.

Hamstring tendonitis can occur medially at the pes anserinus (common tendon for the semitendoninus, gracilus, and sartorius) or laterally at the biceps femoris. The history will generally indicate that there has been a change in training (intensity, duration, or surface) with a gradual onset of symptoms. Treatment of hamstring tendonitis is similar to patellar tendonitis with control of in-

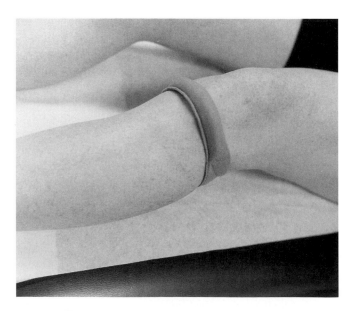

Figure 12–24. One type of patella tendon strap.

flammation, gradual progression to flexibility, endurance strength training, strength training, and functional rehabilitation.

SUMMARY

For knee injuries, prevention, treatment, and rehabilitation require a concentrated team approach by the physician, athletic trainer, physical therapist, coach, and athlete. Prevention of injuries is a major concern with the team assisting the coach in ensuring that appropriate flexibility, strengthening, and sport techniques are used to maximize performance while at the same time, minimizing the risk of injury or reinjury. When an injury occurs, after appropriate first aid, there is a progression of flexibility, strengthening, functional rehabilitation, and gradual return to sports participation. Specific care and rehabilitation is based on the diagnosis. Each athlete's treatment and rehabilitation program is closely monitored so that modifications can be made. If the athlete is not recovering satisfactorily, the team should evaluate and adjust the treatment plan as indicated. Successful prevention, care, and rehabilitation of knee injuries requires all members of the team, as well as the injured athlete, to be responsible for the outcomes.

Anterior Cruciate Ligament Reconstruction Case Study

1/22/96: 21 y/o male collegiate basketball player with weight of 170 pounds and height of 70 inches. His L knee was injured while landing from a jump. He felt a snap with the injury. He was treated by RICE and referred to a primary care sports medicine physician. Diagnosis of grade 3 ACL sprain was provided and the patient was referral to an orthopedist, who confirmed the diagnosis. The patient was referred to physical therapy for preoperative treatment.

1/28/96: Physical therapy/athletic training evaluation and treatment observation: nonweight bearing with locked brace. AROM: –15° from full extension (0°) to 105°; circumference: superior pole of patella: R-35.5 cm L-37.5 cm. Strength: isokinetic at 0°/sec and at 60° flexion; quads R-256 ft-lb, L-141; hams R-128, L-64. Special test: positive Lachman, negative valgus, varus, and posterior drawer. KT 1000: 15 lb L-4 mm R-5, 20 lb. L-4.5 R-7, 30 lb L-5 R-10, maximum L-5 R-11, quadriceps contraction L-3 R-7. Tx: instruct in postoperative exercise program. Self-ranging and pt to be treated by athletic trainer at college for ranging and electrical stimulation and cryotherapy for swelling.

2/21/96: ACL reconstruction on 2/15/96. Completing postoperative exercises. AROM: –20° to 80°. Strength: could not contract quadriceps. Tx: medium-frequency (ES-180) electrical stimulation to quadriceps completed along with straight leg raises. Electromyograpic biofeedback to quads and vastus medialis with straight leg raises. Review postoperative exercise program and instruct in home program of prone ranging for extension.

2/23/96: Subjective: still having difficulty with quadriceps contraction. Tx: medium-frequency electrical muscle stimulation to quadriceps and EMG biofeedback to quadriceps with straight leg raises. Review home exercise program.

2/26/96: Subjective: quad control is present. Tx: Hinges unlocked for AROM and PROM. Initiate weight bearing with 3-point crutch weight bearing with brace locked in extension with 60 pounds. EMG biofeedback to hams with weight bearing to enhance hamstring control. Pt is instructed to increase weight bearing by 60 pounds every 3 days as tolerated.

3/1/96: Orthopedist is concerned with ROM. Pt was ranged with prone contrast stretching for extension (i.e., prone position with pillow under thigh and patella beyond end of table). Pt is ranged and a 1-pound ankle weight is attached to leg with a hot hydrocollator applied to posterior knee for 20 minutes and then an ice pack is applied for 15 minutes. Stretching is maintained throughout the period. Postoperative brace is adjusted to maintain extension. Home exercise program is continued with emphasis upon ranging.

3/11/96: Orthopedist is satisfied with ROM gains. Pt to progress to 3-point crutch weight bearing on 3/15/96.

3/21/96: Subjective: no problems; ambulating without problems. Objective: AROM –10° to 130°. Tx: EMB biofeedback to hamstring with ambulation. Continue with home exercise program.

3/28/96: Tx: to normal ambulation with ACL brace. Add step-ups (StairMaster), rowing machine, swimming, and/or slide board.

4/16/96: Subjective: no problems. Objective: AROM: –5° to 140°. Tx: to continue with home exercise program.

5/28/96: Phone call from patient: increased pain with quadriceps PRE from 90 to 60°. Patient was instructed to place quadriceps PRE from 90 to 60 on hold. Complete straight leg raises without weights for 20 to 30 repetitions 2 to 3 times/day. With reduced pain to return PREs for quadriceps from 90 to 60° with light weight and gradual increase. To return for additional follow-up if pain does not resolve.

6/24/96: Subjective: no complaints. Doing quadriceps PRE from 90 to 60° without pain. Objective: AROM –5° to 140°. Tx: continue with home exercise program.

7/15/96: Subjective: no complaints. Tx: add gradual increase to full range quadriceps PRE and functional (running).

8/28/96: Subjective: no complaints. Running 1 mile at ½ speed. Objective: AROM +5 to 145°.

Strength	R	L	% Ratio
0°/sec and 60° flex			
Quadriceps	228 ft-lb	135	58
Hamstrings	100	102	102
60°/sec			
Quadriceps	211	114	54
Hamstrings	112	96	86
90°/sec			
Quadriceps	178	107	60
Hamstrings	98	93	95

9/20/96: Pt missed appointment.

10/11/96: Subjective: no complaints. Doing all running with agility. Objective: AROM +5 to 145°.

Strength	R	L	% Ratio
0°/sec and at 60° flex			
Quadriceps	218 ft-lb	216	99
Hamstrings	92	120	130
60°/sec			
Quadriceps	235	170	72
Hamstrings	111	123	111
90°/sec			
Quadriceps	194	142	73
Hamstrings	106	118	111
180°/sec			
Quadriceps	135	99	73
Hamstrings	92	95	105

11/11/96: Subjective: no problems. Objective: strength test only for appointment with physician.

Strength	R	L	% Ratio
0°/sec and at 60° flex			
Quadriceps	193 ft-lb	211	115
Hamstrings	112	122	109
60°/sec			
Quadriceps	201	177	88
Hamstrings	111	128	155
90°/sec			
Quadriceps	191	161	84
Hamstrings	105	116	110
180°/sec			
Quadriceps	140	110	79
Hamstrings	86	87	109

Tx: To continue with home exercise program.
Pt did not return for additional treatments or follow-ups.

Functional Rehabilitation

The progression is designed for a ¼-mile track (i.e., 110 yds to ¼ lap; 220 yds to ⅛ mile to ½ lap; 440-¼ mile-1 lap; 880-½ mile-2 laps; ¾ mile-3 laps; 1 mile-4 laps). If a ¼-mile track is not available, estimate distances as close as possible.

Stage 1
1. Walk 1 mile
2. Walk 110; jog 55; walk 110
3. Walk 110; jog 110; walk 110
4. Walk 220; jog 220; walk 220
5. Walk 220; jog 440; walk 220
6. Walk 220; jog 880; walk 220
7. Walk 220; jog ¾; walk 220
8. Walk 220; jog 1 mile; walk 220

Stage II
All running (compared to jogging) is completed at ¾ running speed (full speed for the mile).

9. Jog 110; run 110; jog 110; run 110; jog for completion of 1 mile. (If running area has curves, be sure to jog the curves)
10. Jog 110; run 110 for ½ mile; jog for ½ mile

11. Jog 110; run 110 for ¾ mile; jog for ¼ mile
12. Jog 110; run 110 for 1 mile
13. Jog 110; run 220; jog 110; run 220; jog for completion of 1 mile
14. Jog 110; run 440; jog 110; run 440; jog for completion of 1 mile
15. Jog 110; run 880; jog for completion of 1 mile
16. Jog 110; run ¾ mile; jog for completion of 1 mile
17. Jog 110; run 1 mile; jog 110

Distance runners: Continue to increase distance by 10%/week.

Stage III: Progression to Sprint Running
Distance running is completed as indicated in step 17. Walk for 440 and then complete the sprint running as indicated in step 18. Complete a cool-down jog for 440. Rest between intervals is completed by walking. Code: 220 (distance) × 2 (repeats) with 3 min (rest).

18. 110 × 2 with 5 min.
19. 110 × 4 with 5 min.
20. 40 × 6 with 3 min.
21. 40 × 10 with 2 min.

Stage IV: Agility Drills
Agility activities are utilized for the sports that involve jumping and cutting. Complete a warm-up jog of 440 and then initiate the agility with exercise 1. Complete one cycle of each exercise at 50% of full speed and then progress to one cycle at 75% and then one cycle at 100%. Distance and sprint running are then completed.

1. *Figure-eight running.* Run a figure-8 pattern 30 yds long (length and width of basketball court). Progress to 15 yds (length and width of ½ a basketball court) and then to 5 yds (length and width of the foul area and key). Complete each figure 8 three times.
2. *Carioca.* Run sideways crossing legs in front and then behind the lead leg for 10 yds; rest 5 sec and return in other direction. Repeat 5 × for each cycle.
3. *Backward running.* Run for 20 yds; rest 5 sec and repeat 3 × for each cycle.
4. *Box running.* Select an area and mark out a 5-yd box for the run. Initiate the run by running the box 5 times clockwise and then 5 times counterclockwise.
5. *Vertical jumping.* Jump with 50% effort and mark a spot on a wall. Repeat jumping to that mark 10 ×. Change the mark to 75% and jump 10 ×. Change the mark to 100% and jump 10 ×. If sport does not require jumping, do not include.

Stage V: Progression to Practice and Games
Practice sessions are not initiated until functional rehabilitation is successfully completed. All practice sessions are initiated with a warm-up that includes (1) light running and stretching, (2) gradual increase in speed to full-speed running, (3) completion of agility activities with gradual increase in intensity, and (4) gradual increase in speed and intensity of movements specific to the sport.

After practice complete a cool-down of running and stretching.

Practice is initiated by completing ¼ of practice activities. Progress to ½, ¾, and then full practice as benevolent pain allows. When three full practices are completed without difficulty, competition is initiated.

REFERENCES

1. Gregor R, Edgerton V, Perrine J, et al. Torque–velocity relationships and muscle fiber composition in elite female athletes. *J Appl Physiol.* 1979;47:388-396.

2. Hanten W, Ramberg C. Effect of stabilization on maximal isokinetic torque of the quadriceps femoris muscle during concentric and eccentric contractions. *Phys Ther.* 1988;68:219-222.

3. Thorstensson A, Grimby G, Karlsson J. Force-velocity relationships and fiber composition in human extensor muscles. *J Appl Physiol.* 1976;40:12-16.

4. Highgenboten C, Jackson A, Meske N. Concentric and eccentric torque comparisons for knee extension and flexion in young adult males and females using the kinetic communicator. *Am J Sports Med.* 1988;16: 234-237.

5. Henning C, Lynch M, Glick K. An in-vivo strain gauge study of elongation of the anterior cruciate ligament. *Am J Sports Med.* 1985;13:1322-1326.

6. Luta G, Palmetier R, An KN, Chao EY. Comparison of tibiofemoral joint forces during open kinetic chain and closed kinetic chain exercise. *J Bone Joint Surg.* 1993; 75A:732-739.

7. Palmitier R, An KN, Scott S, Chao EYS. Kinetric chain exercises in knee rehabilitation. *Sports Med.* 1991;11:402-413.

8. Peppard AP, Denegar CR. Pain and the rehabilitation of athletic injuries. *Orthop Phys Ther Clin North Am.* 1994;3:439-461.

9. Holden JP, Grood ES, Butler DL. Biomechanics of fascia data ligament replacements: Early postoperative changes in the goat. *J Orthop Res.* 1989;6:639-647.

10. Clancy WG Jr, Ray JM. Anterior cruciate ligament autografts. In: Jackson DW, Drez D Jr, eds. *The Anterior Cruciate Ligament Deficient Knee: New Concepts in Ligament Repair.* St. Louis: Mosby; 1987:193-210.

11. Kondo M. An experimental study on reconstructive surgery of the anterior cruciate ligament. *J Jpn Orthop Assoc.* 1979;53:521-533.

12. Newton PO, Horibe S, Woo S. Experimental studies on anterior cruciate ligament autografts and allografts. In: Daniel DM, Akeson WH, O'Connor JJ, eds. *Knee Ligaments: Structure, Function, Injury and Repair.* New York: Raven; 1990:389-399.

13. Akeson WH. The response of ligaments to stress modulation and overview of the ligament healing response. In: Daniel DM, Akeson WH, O'Connor JJ, eds. *Knee Ligaments: Structure, Function, Injury and Repair.* New York: Raven; 1990.

14. Amiel D, von Schroeder H, Akeson WH. The response of ligaments to stress deprivation and stress enhancement. In: Daniel DM, Akeson WH, O'Connor JJ, eds. *Knee Ligaments: Structure, Function, Injury and Repair.* New York: Raven; 1990.

15. Woo SLY, Wang CW, Newton PO, Lyon RM. The response of ligaments to stress deprivation and stress enhancement. In: Daniel DM, Akeson WH, O'Connon JJ, eds. *Knee Ligaments: Structure, Function, Injury, and Repair.* New York: Raven; 1990:337-350.

16. Shelbourne KD, Nitz PA. In: Reider B, ed. *Sports Medicine: The School Age Athlete.* Philadelphia: Saunders; 1990.

17. DeHaven KE. Diagnosis of acute knee injuries with hemarthrosis. *Am J Sports Med.* 1980;8:9-14.

18. Indelicato PA, Bittar ES. A perspective of lesions associated with ACL insufficiency of the knee. *Clin Orthop.* 1985; 198:77-80.

19. Noyes FR, Bassett RW, Grood FS, Butler DL. Arthroscopy in acute traumatic hemarthrosis of the knee. Incidence of anterior cruciate tears and other injuries. *J Bone Joint Surg.* 1980;62A:687-695.

20. Feagin JA Jr. Case study 1: Isolated anterior cruciate ligament injury. In: Feagin JA Jr, ed. *The Cruciate Ligament.* New York: Churchill Livingstone; 1988:15-25.

21. Feagin JA, Curl WW. Isolated tear of the anterior cruciate ligament: Five-year follow-up study. *Am J Sports Med.* 1976;4:95-100.

22. Hawkins RJ, Misamore GW, Merritt TR. Follow-up of the acute non-operative isolated anterior cruciate ligament tear. *Am J Sports Med.* 1986;14:205-210.

23. Satk K, Kudmar VP, Ngoi SS. Anterior cruciate ligament injuries. To counsel or to operate. *J Bone Joint Surg.* 1986;68B:458-461.

24. Thompson W, Thaete F, Fu F, Scott F. Tibial meniscal dynamics using three-dimensional reconstruction of magnetic resonance images. *Am J Sports Med.* 1991;3:210-216.

25. Amiel D, Kuiper S, Akeson WH. Cruciate ligament: Response to injury. In: Daniel DM, Akeson WH, O'Connor JJ, eds. *Knee Ligaments: Structure, Function, Injury and Repair.* New York: Raven; 1990.

26. Arnoczky SP, Rubin RM, Marshall JC. Microvasculature of the cruciate ligaments and its response to injury. *J Bone Joint Surg.* 1979;61A:1221-1229.

27. McDaniel WJ. Isolated partial tear of the anterior cruciate ligament. *Clin Orthop.* 1976;115:209-212.

28. Monaco BR, Noble HB, Bachman DC. Incomplete tears of the anterior cruciate ligaments and knee locking. *JAMA.* 1982;247:1582-1584.

29. Sandberg R, Balkford B. Partial rupture of the anterior cruciate ligament: Natural course. *Clin Orthop.* 1987;220: 176-178.

30. Walla DJ, Albright JP, McAuley E, et al. Hamstring control and the unstable anterior cruciate ligament deficient knee. *Am J Sports Med.* 1985;13:34-39.

31. Yasuda K, Sasaki T. Exercise after anterior cruciate ligament reconstruction: The force exerted on the tibia by the separate isometic contractions of the quadriceps or the hamstrings. *Clin Orthop.* 1987;220:275-283.

32. Fetto JF, Marshall JL. Medial collateral ligament injuries of the knee: A rationale for treatment. *Clin Orthop.* 1978; 132:206-218.

33. O'Donoghue DH. An analysis of end results of surgical treatment of major injuries of the knee. *J Bone Joint Surg.* 1955;37A:1.

34. Hughston JL, Barrett GR. Acute anteromedial rotatory instability: Long term results of surgical repair. *J Bone Joint Surg.* 1983;656A:145-153.

35. Daniel DM, Fritschy D. Anterior cruciate ligament injuries. In: DeLee JC, Drez D Jr, eds. *Orthopaedic Sports Medicine Principles and Practices.* Philadelphia: Saunders; 1994:1313-1361.

36. Arvidsson I, Eriksson F. Counteracting muscle atrophy after ACL injury: Scientific basis for a rehabilitation program. In: Feagin JA, ed. *The Cruciate Ligaments.* New York: Churchill Livingstone; 1988.

37. Shelbourne K, Wilckens J, Mollabashy A, DeCarlo M. Arethrofibrosis in acute ACL reconstruction. The effect of timing of reconstruction and rehabilitation. *J Bone Joint Surg.* 1991;19:332-336.

38. Sapega AA, Quedenfeld TC, Moyer R, Butler R. Biophysical factors in range-of-motion exercise. *Arch Phys Med Rehabil.* 1976;547:122-126.

39. Sachs RA, Daniel DM, Stone MC, Garfein RF. Patellofemoral problems after anterior cruciate ligament reconstruction. *Am J Sports Med.* 1989;17:760-765.

40. Parisien JS. The role of arthroscopy in the treatment of postoperative fibroarthosis of the knee joint. *Clin Orthop.* 1989;229:185-192.

41. Sprague NF III, O'Connor RL, Fox JM. Arthropscopic treatment of postoperative knee fibroarthrosis. *Clin Orthop.* 1982;166:165-172.

42. Paulos LE, Rosenberg TD, Drawbent J. Infrapatellar contracture syndrome. An unrecognized cause of knee stiffness with patella entrapment and patellar infera. *Am J Sports Med.* 1987;15:331-341.

43. Poplowski ZJ, Wiley AM, Murray JF. Post-traumatic dystrophy of the intramentia. *J Bone Joint Surg.* 1983;65A:642-655.

44. Sachs RA, Reznik A, Daniel DM, Stone MC. Complications of knee ligament surgery. In: Daniel DM, Akeson WH, O'Connor JJ, eds. *Knee Ligaments: Structure, Function, Injury, and Repair.* New York: Raven; 1990:505-520.

45. Reid DC. *Sports Injury Assessment and Rehabilitation.* New York: Churchill Livingstone; 1992;48-49.

45a. Parjolie JM, Bergfeld JA. Long term results of non-operative treatment of isolated posterior cruciate ligament injuries in the athlete. *Am J Sports Med.* 1986;14:35-38.

46. Hastings DE. The non-operative management of collateral ligament injuries of the knee joint. *Clin Orthop.* 1980;147:22-28.

47. Dersheid GL, Garrick JG. Medial collateral ligament injuries in football: Non-operative management of grade 1 and grade II sprains. *Am J Sports Med.* 1981;9:365-368.

48. Indelicato PA. Non-operative treatment of complete tears of the medical collateral ligament of the knee. *J Bone Joint Surg.* 1983;65A:323-329.

49. Jones RE, Henley MB, Francis P. Non-operative management of isolated grade III collateral ligament injuries in high school football players. *Clin Orthop.* 1986;213:137-140.

50. Kannus P. Long-term results of conservatively treated medial collateral ligament injuries of the knee joint. *Clin Orthop.* 1988;226:103-112.

51. Steadman J. Rehabilitation of first and second-degree sprains of the medial collateral ligament. *Am J Sports Med.* 1979;7:300-302.

52. Bergfeld J. Functional rehabilitation of isolated medial collateral ligaments sprains: First, second and third degree sprains. *Am J Sports Med.* 1979;7:207-209.

53. DeHaven KE. Decision making factors in the treatment of meniscus lesions. *Clin Orthop.* 1990;252:49-54.

54. Weiss LB, Lundberg M, Hamberg P, et al. Non-operative treatment of meniscal tears. *J Bone Joint Surg.* 1989;71A:811-822.

55. Northmore-Ball MD, Dandy DJ. Arthroscopic open partial and total meniscectomy. *J Bone Joint Surg.* 1983;65B:400-404.

56. Hendler RC. Arthroscopic meniscal repair. *Clin Orthop.* 1984;190:163-169.

57. Miller DB. Arthroscopic meniscus repair. *Am J Sports Med.* 1988;16:315-320.

58. DeHaven KE. Meniscus repair in the athlete. *Clin Orthop.* 1985;198:31-35.

59. Walsh WM. Patellofemoral joint. In: DeLee JC, Drez D Jr, eds. *Orthopaedic Sports Medicine: Principles and Practices.* Philadelphia: Saunders; 1994:1163-1248.

60. Busch MT, DeHaven KE. Pitfalls of the lateral retinacular release. *Clin Sports Med.* 1989;8:279-290.

61. McConnell J. The management of chondromalacia patellae. A long term solution. *Aust J Physiother.* 1986;2:215-223.

62. Irrgang J, Safran M, Fu F. The knee: Ligamentous and meniscal injuries. In: Zachazewski J, Magee D, Quillen W, eds. *Athletic Injuries and Rehabilitation.* Philadelphia: Sauders; 1996.

63. Goodfellow J, Hungerford DS, Zindel M. Patellofemoral joint mechanics and pathologies: Functional anatomy of the patellofemoral joint. *J Bone Joint Surg.* 1976;58B:287-290.

64. Ingersoll CD, Knight KL. Patellar location changes following EMG biofeedback and progressive resistive exercises. *Med Sci Sports Exerc.* 1991;23:1122-1127.

65. Voight ML, Wieder DL. Comparative reflex response times of vastus medialis obliquis and vastus lateralis in normal subjects and subjects with extensor mechanism dysfunction. *Am J Sports Med.* 1991;19:131-137.

66. Palumbo PM. Dynamic patellar brace: A new orthosis in the management of patellofemoral disorders. *Am J Sports Med.* 1981;9:45-49.

67. Mysnyk MC, Wroble BB, Foster BT, Albright JP. Prepatellar bursitis in wrestlers. *Am J Sports Med.* 1986;14:46-54.

68. Wroble RR, Mysnyk MC, Foster DI, et al. Patterns of knee injuries in wrestlers: A six year study. *Am J Sports Med.* 1986;14:55-66.

69. Larson RL, Osternig LR. Traumatic bursitis and artificial turf. *J Sports Med.* 1974;2:183-188.

70. Cox JS, Blanda JB. Peripatellar pathologies. In: DeLee JC, Drez D Jr, eds. *Orthopaedic Sports Medicine Principles and Practices.* Philadelphia: Saunders; 1994:1249-1260.

71. O'Donoghue DH. Reconstruction for medial instability of the knee: Technique and results: Sixty cases. *J Bone Joint Surg.* 1973;55A:941-955.

72. Ho G, Su EY. Antibiotic therapy of septic bursitis. *Arthritis Rheum.* 1981;24:905-911.

73. Ho G, Tice AD, Kaplan SR. Septic bursitis in the prepatellar and olecranon bursae. *Ann Intern Med.* 1978;88:21-27.

74. Wilson-MacDonald J. Management and outcome of infective bursitis. *Postgrad Med J.* 1987;63:851-853.

75. O'Donoghue DH. Injuries of the knee. In: O'Donoghue DH, ed. *Treatment of Injuries to Athletes.* 4th ed. Philadelphia: Saunders; 1987:470-471.

76. Ziskin MC, Michlovitz SL. Therapeutic ultrasound. In: Michlovitz SL, ed. *Thermal Agents in Rehabilitation.* Philadelphia: F.A. Davis Co.; 1986:159-160.

77. Garrett WE, Nikolaou PK, Rebveck BM, et al. The effect of muscle architecture on the biomechanical failure properties of skeletal muscle under passive extension. *Am J Sports Med.* 1988;16:7-12.

78. Garrett WE, Safran MR, Seaber AV, et al. Biomechanical comparison of stimulated and non-stimulated skeletal muscle pulled to failure. *Am J Sports Med.* 1987;15:448-454.

79. Nikolaou PK, MacDonald BL, Glisson RR, et al. The effect of architecture on the anatomic failure site of skeletal muscle. *Trans Orthop Res Soc.* 1986;11:228.

80. Nikolaou PK, Ribbeck BM, Glisson RR, et al. The effect of muscle architecture on the biomechanical failure properties of skeletal muscle under passive extension. *Am J Sports Med.* 1988;16:7-12.

81. Safran MR, Garrett WE, Seaber AV, et al. The role of warm-up in muscular injury prevention. *Am J Sports Med.* 1989;16:123-129.

82. Brunet ME, Hontas RB. The thigh. In: DeLee JC, Drez D Jr, eds. *Orthopaedic Sports Medicine Principles and Practices.* Philadelphia: Saunders; 1994:1091-1102.

83. Garrett WE, Lohnes J. Cellular and matrix response to mechanical injury at the myotendinous junction. In: *Sports Induced Inflammation.* Park Ridge, IL: American Orthopaedic Society for Sports Medicine; 1989: 215-224.

84. Elliott BC, Blanksy BA. The syncronization of muscle activity and body segment movements during a running cycle. *Med Sci Sports Exerc.* 1979;11:322-327.

85. Burkett LN. Investigation into hamstring stains: The case of the hybrid muscle. *J Sports Med.* 1976;3:228-231.

86. Heiser TM, Weber J, Sulllivan G, et al. Prophylaxis and management of hamstring muscle injuries in intercollegiate football. *Am J Sports Med.* 1984;12:368-370.

87. Kulund DN. *The Injured Athlete.* Philadelphia: Lippincott; 1982:72, 85, 356-359.

88. Basmajian JV. *Muscles Alive.* 3rd ed. Baltimore: Williams & Wilkins; 1974.

89. Burkett LN. Causation factors in hamstring strain. *Med Sci Sports Exerc.* 1970;2:39-42.

90. Casperson PC. Groin and hamstring injuries. *Athletic Training.* 1982;17:43-45.

91. Klafs CE, Arnheim DD. *Modern Principles of Athletic Training.* St. Louis: Mosby; 1977:370-372.

92. Liemohn W. Factors related to hamstring strains. *J Sports Med.* 1978;18:71-76.

93. Sutton G. Hamstring strains: A review of the literature. *J Orthop Sports Phys Ther.* 1984;5:184-195.

94. Slocum DB, James SC. Biomechanics of running. *JAMA.* 1968;205:721-728.

95. Garrett WE. Strains and sprains in athletics. *Postgrad Med.* 1983;73:200-214.

96. O'Donoghue DH. *Treatment of Injuries to Athletes.* Philadelphia: Saunders; 1984.

97. Curwin S, Stansish WD. *Tendonitis: Its Etilology and Treatment.* Lexington, MA: Health; 1984.

98. Blazina ME, Derlaqw RK, Jobe FW, et al. Jumper's knee. *Orthop Clin North Am.* 1973;4:665-678.

99. Levine J, Splain S. Use of the infrapatellar strap in the treatment of patellofemoral pain. *Clin Orthop.* 1979;139: 179-181.

100. Rocls J, Martens M, Mulier JJC, Burssens A. Patellar tendonitis (jumper's knee). *Am J Sports Med.* 1978;6:362-368.

101. Ferretti A, Ippolito E, Mariani P, Pudda G. Jumper's knee. *Am J Sports Med.* 1983;11:58-62.

102. Schmidt DR, Henry JH. Stress injuries of the adolescent extensor mechanism. *Clin Sports Med.* 1989; 8:343-355.

103. Kaufman KR, An K, Litchy WJ, et al. Dynamic joint forces during knee isokinetic exercises. *Am J Sports Med.* 1991;19:308-311.

Chapter 13

The Foot and Ankle

Shepard Hurwitz, Gregory P. Ernst, and Sok Yi

ANATOMY

Mechanical injuries to the foot and ankle are common from sports-related activities. The key to diagnosing and understanding the injury is the anatomy. This section is a general overview of the ankle and foot anatomy, with more detailed anatomy of the structures injured described in the following clinical sections (see Fig. 13-1).

Ankle

Bones

The distal tibia, distal fibula, and the body of the talus comprise the bones of the ankle (see Fig. 13-2). The distal tibia consists of a concave articular surface corresponding to the dome of the talus. The medial portion of the distal tibia forms the medial mallelus. The medial malleolus is the insertion site of the superficial and deep deltoid ligaments. It also articulates with the medial surface of the talus.[1] The posterior border of the medial malleolus contains a groove and gives attachment to the fibrous tunnel of the tibialis posterior tendon. The distal fibula forms the lateral malleolus and is positioned about 1 cm posterior to the medial malleolus.[2] The medial facet articulates with the lateral surface of the talus, and, just anterior and superior to this articular surface, contains a fossa for the syndesmosis between the tibia and fibula. The posterior border of the lateral malleolus contains a sulcus for the passage of the peroneal tendons. The medial and lateral malleolus and the distal tibia form a socket, holding the talus on three sides.[1] By all accounts, this provides the major stability of the ankle.

Ligaments

Additional stability of the ankle is provided by the ligaments (see Fig. 13-3). First, the anterior and posterior inferior tibiofibular ligaments, the transverse tibiofibular ligament, and the interosseous membrane help hold the fibula and tibia together. Next is the deltoid ligament, a very strong medial ligament comprised of two layers. The superficial layer originates on the tip of the medial malleolus and fans out in a triangular fashion to insert on the talus, while the deep layer of the deltoid originates on the undersurface of the medial malleolus and runs in a horizontal course within the ankle joint to the medial surface of the talus. Finally, the lateral ligament complex is composed of three ligaments: the anterior talofibular ligament, the calcaneofibular ligament, and the posterior talofibular ligaments. These ligaments are usually injured in an ankle sprain (see Fig. 13-4).

The ankle works as a single axis hinge oriented obliquely to the long axis of the leg, directed at an angle of 23 degrees with the transverse axis of the tibial plateaus.[1] The range of motion of the ankle is approximately 18 degrees of dorsiflexion and 48 degrees of plantar flexion.[3]

Foot

The talus and the calcaneus forms the subtalar joint. The subtalar joint consists of posterior, middle, and anterior articulating facets, with a strong interosseous ligament between the posterior and the middle facet. The subtalar joint is a single axis hinge-type joint with its axis offset 41 degrees from the horizontal axis and 23 degrees from the long axis of the foot.[4] The offset axis of the subtalar joint causes movement in three planes

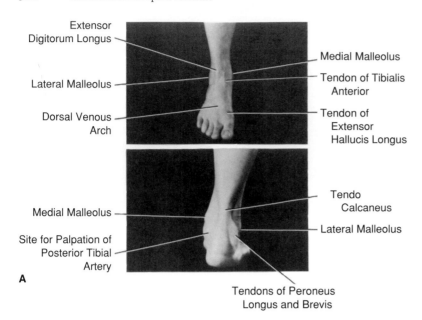

Extensor Digitorum Longus

Lateral Malleolus

Dorsal Venous Arch

Medial Malleolus

Tendon of Tibialis Anterior

Tendon of Extensor Hallucis Longus

Medial Malleolus

Site for Palpation of Posterior Tibial Artery

Tendo Calcaneus

Lateral Malleolus

A

Tendons of Peroneus Longus and Brevis

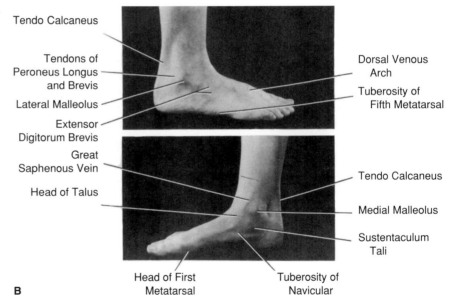

Tendo Calcaneus

Tendons of Peroneus Longus and Brevis

Lateral Malleolus

Extensor Digitorum Brevis

Great Saphenous Vein

Head of Talus

Dorsal Venous Arch

Tuberosity of Fifth Metatarsal

Tendo Calcaneus

Medial Malleolus

Sustentaculum Tali

Head of First Metatarsal

Tuberosity of Navicular

Figure 13–1. Topographic landmarks of the foot **(A)** and ankle **(B)**. *(From Snell RS.* Clinical Anatomy for Medical Students. *Boston: Little, Brown; 1992:576. With permission.)*   B

in two combinations: (1) pronation, abduction, and extension (eversion); and (2) supination, adduction, and flexion (inversion).[1] The range of motion of the subtalar joint is about 30 degrees of inversion and 10 degrees of eversion.[1]

Movement of the subtalar joint affects the rest of the joints of the foot through the longitudinal arches of the foot. The medial longitudinal arch consists of the calcaneus, talus, navicular, cuneiforms, and the first, second, and third metatarsals. The lateral longitudinal arch is made up of the calcaneus, cuboid, and the fourth and fifth metatarsals. When the subtalar joint everts, the calcaneus and the talus are relatively parallel, resulting in parallel medial and lateral longitudinal arches and a flexible forefoot. However, when the subtalar joint inverts, the calcaneus and the talus are divergent resulting in a rigid foot.

A transverse arch is formed by the cuneiforms, cuboid, and the proximal metatarsals. The apex of the arch is at the middle cuneiform and the second metatarsal base. All the metatarsals are connected to the cuneiforms and the cuboid forming Lisfranc's joint. The dorsal and plantar ligaments are more defined in the medial portion of the transverse arch, with the most important being the Lisfranc's ligament running from the lateral portion of the medial cuneiform to the medial portion of the base of the second metatarsal.

Several cutaneous nerves supply the foot (see Fig. 13–5). The main nerve to the plantar surface of the foot is the posterior tibial nerve. Its interdigital branches may pass below the transverse metatarsal ligament and become fibrotic under the repetitive weight of the body, leading to painful neuroma (Morton's neuroma), mainly third and

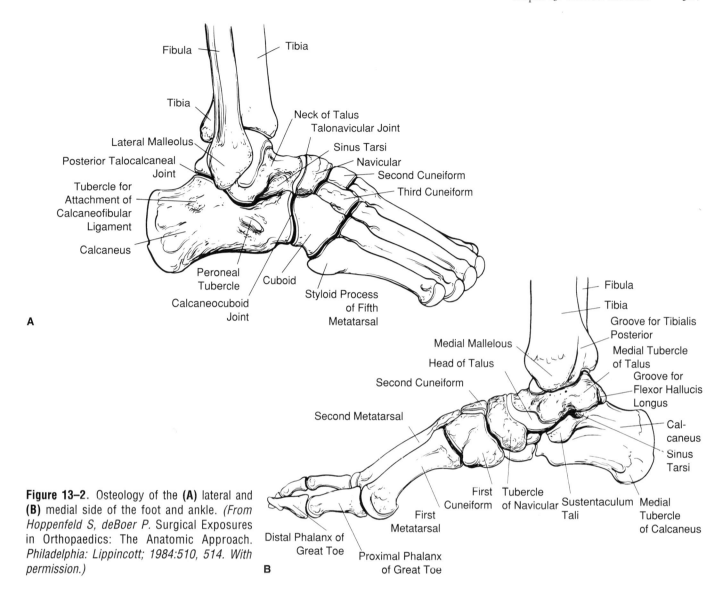

Figure 13-2. Osteology of the **(A)** lateral and **(B)** medial side of the foot and ankle. *(From Hoppenfeld S, deBoer P. Surgical Exposures in Orthopaedics: The Anatomic Approach. Philadelphia: Lippincott; 1984:510, 514. With permission.)*

fourth. The posterior tibial nerve also innervates the intrinsic muscles of the foot. The dorsal surface of the foot is innervated by the superficial peroneal nerve. The medial and the lateral borders of the foot are innervated by the saphenous nerve and the sural nerve, respectively. All three of these cutaneous nerves may be involved in painful conditions. Finally, the first web space is innervated by the deep peroneal nerve. Since the deep peroneal nerve innervates the muscles of the anterior tibial compartment, sensory changes in the first web space may be an indication of abnormality in the anterior tibial compartment.

BIOMECHANICS OF WALKING

Gait Cycle

The gait cycle is the period from initial contact of one foot to the following contact of the same foot. It consists of the stance phase and swing phase. The stance phase comprises 62 percent of the gait cycle and is subdivided into double limb support, single limb support, and a second double limb support. Stance is followed by the swing phase, which comprises 38 percent of the gait cycle. The stance phase starts with a heel strike, progresses to foot flat by 7 percent, ends double stance phase with opposite toe off at 12 percent, which begins single limb support from 12 to 50 percent. A second double limb stance begins with opposite heel strike at 50 percent, then ends with toe off at 62 percent. Finally, this foot enters the swing phase from 62 to 100 percent, completing the gait cycle (see Fig. 13-6 to 13-8).

Ground reaction forces (GRF) are the forces exerted by the ground on the foot during foot contact. Since the body is moving through a three-dimensional space, the ground reactive forces occur in three different planes: saggital, frontal, and transverse. The most significant of

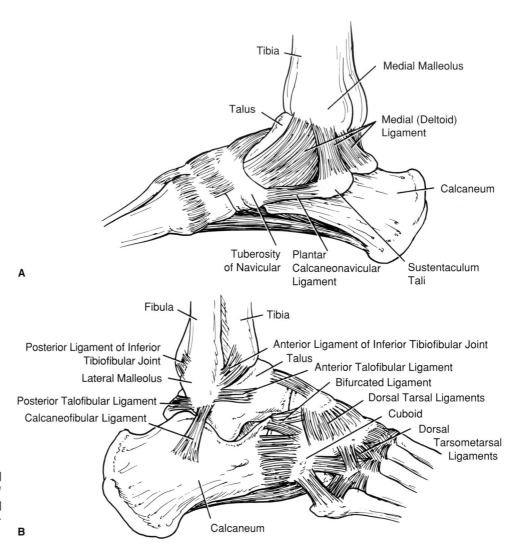

Figure 13–3. Ligaments of the medial **(A)** and lateral **(B)** ankle. *(From Snell RS.* Clinical Anatomy for Medical Students. *Boston: Little, Brown; 1992:676. With permission.)*

these forces is the vertical GRF. This force reaches its peak of 1.3 to 1.5 times body weight twice during the stance phase at 15 and 42 percent of the gait cycle.[5,6] The fore aft and medial lateral shear GFR exhibits much less force—10 to 15 percent and 5 percent of the body weight, respectively, during the stance phase.

The ankle joint is a single axis joint, oriented in an oblique axis with an average of 93 degrees from vertical (see Fig. 13–9).[5,6] This oblique ankle axis allows the foot to pronate in dorsiflexion and supinate in plantar flexion.[5] However, when the foot is fixed to the ground as in the stance phase, dorsiflexion of the ankle transmits its torque to the tibia causing the tibia to internally rotate.[5] Conversely, plantar flexion of the ankle causes external rotation of the tibia.[5] The subtalar joint is similar to the hinge-type single axis ankle joint and is offset, on the average, 41 degrees from the horizontal plane and 23 degrees from the long axis of the foot.[5] The metatarsal

break is an axis represented by a line drawn obliquely across the metatarsal heads.[6] The average angle of the metatarsal break is 53.5 degrees from the long axis of the foot.[7] This oblique break allows the distribution of the body weight among the metatarsal heads during the heel off portion of the stance phase. The midtarsal joint is also important in the ability to transmit motion to the forefoot. The calcaneal cuboid and the talonavicular joints articulate together with the movement of the subtalar joint (see Fig. 13–9). Eversion of the calcaneus causes a parallel calcaneal cuboid and talonavicular joints, resulting in flexibility of the midtarsal joints. Inversion of the calcaneus causes nonparallel joints, resulting in rigidity of the midtarsal joints, which helps form a stable platform for heel-rise and lift-off.

The gait function of muscles are stabilization, acceleration, and deceleration. All three must occur in normal gait. Joint motion and muscle activity during the walking cycle start with heel strike and result in flat foot in the first 15 percent of the walking cycle. The tibia internally rotates and the ankle undergoes plantar flexion to 7 percent of the cycle and dorsiflexion begins (see Fig. 13-9). The heel is everted, resulting in a flexible pronated forefoot adapting to the ground.[7] The pretibial muscles are actively undergoing eccentric contraction to control ankle plantar flexion. During midstance, from 15 to 40 percent of the walking cycle, the center of gravity passes over the weight-bearing portion of the leg at 35 percent of the cycle. The ankle undergoes progressive dorsiflexion and the subtalar joint demonstrates progressive inversion due to the external rotation of the tibia.[5] This stabilizes the forefoot for toe-off.[5] The posterior calf muscles become increasingly active, undergoing eccentric contraction to control the dorsiflexion and forward shift of the center of gravity. From late flat-foot to toe-off, 40 to 60 percent of the cycle, the ankle undergoes progressive plantar flexion with propulsion provided by concentric contraction of the calf muscles. The tibia and the subtalar joints reach their maximal external rotation and inversion just before toe-off. At this time, the forefoot is locked in rigid supination and the longitudinal arch is maximally stabilized by the "windlass mechanism."[5] The metatarsal break plays a role at the time of heel rise to toe-off by allowing the forefoot to be in a supinated position and by tightening the plantar fascia with dorsiflexion of the metatarsal phalangeal joints.[5] Finally, after liftoff all events reverse as the tibia internally rotates, subtalar joint everts, forefoot pronates, and the ankle dorsiflexes until the next heel strike, thereby completing a walking cycle.[5]

BIOMECHANICS OF RUNNING

Overuse injuries to runners occur as a result of one of three causes: training errors, anatomic variations, or shoes and surfaces. Clearly, biomechanical factors are implicated in all of these causes. Even large anatomic variations will not result in injury in the sedentary individual, but higher forces and the repetitious manner in which these forces are applied, often result in injury to an athlete when only minor anatomic variation exists. Consider that a 150-pound man who runs only 1 mile absorbs about 2.5 times his body weight with each step. This means that over 110 tons per leg must be absorbed.[8] Thus, a marathon runner with anything less than a biomechanically sound lower extremity, or whose musculoskeletal system is unaccustomed to these repetitive forces, is at a great risk for an overuse injury. Understanding the forces placed on the foot and ankle during athletic activities will enable the clinician

to more effectively prevent and possibly treat these injuries.

The mechanics in walking and running both have similar gait cycle events. The similarities end there, however. Authors often differentiate running from walking by velocity. The major difference is the presence of a float phase in running where neither foot is in contact with the ground.[9] The double support phase seen in walking is also absent (see Fig. 13-10). Runners will have a narrower base of support and even a crossover stride, where one foot may extend beyond the midline with heel strike placing a marked varus stress on the heel. Initial contact with the support foot will occur underneath the runner's center of gravity, rather than in front as in the walker.[10] This lessens impact forces and allows a more efficient forward progression of the body. In walking, the foot placement in front of the center of gravity actually serves as a braking mechanism, slowing forward progression. Normal walking gait will always consist of a heel-toe pattern. In the normal running gait, however, initial contact may occur with the forefoot, especially at the faster speeds.[10] Finally, as shown in Figure 13-10, the stance phase, which consumes approximately two thirds of the cycle in walking, makes up only one third of the gait cycle in running and even less in sprinters.[11] Mann and Hagy[11] feel that this decrease in stance phase is the major cause of injury to runners as all of the events of the stance phase, shock absorption, deceleration, foot stabilization, and acceleration, must occur in a very short time. Additionally, the ground reaction force that enters the lower extremities increases greatly with increasing speed.[12] The increased ground reaction force, with decreased time for the lower extremities to dissipate them, is illustrated in Figure 13-11.

Kinetics

Kinetics is the study of forces that produce motion in joints. These forces can include both external forces, primarily the ground reaction force (GRF), and internal forces, as a result of the muscle action in response to an external load.[9] Vertical GRF in the runner has been reported to be between 1.6 and 2.3 times body weight.[12] However, between individual runners, there is much variability in the vertical GRF and the loading rate due to differences in velocities and running styles. About 20 percent of runners will make initial contact near the forefoot.[13] This eliminates the initial spike in the vertical GRF and results in a slower loading rate of forces (see Fig. 13-11). This occurs at the expense of the gastrocnemius and soleus complex that must absorb most of the impact force, resulting in a slow descent of the heel. The tensile load on the Achilles tendon can increase to about

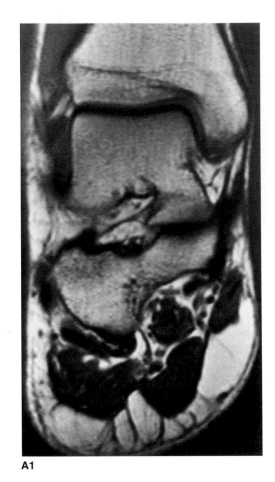

A1

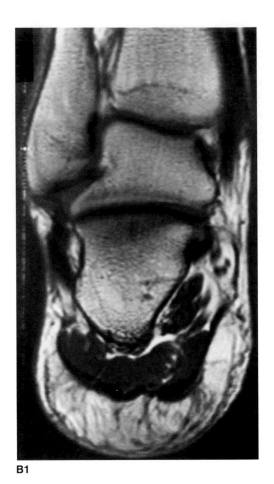

B1

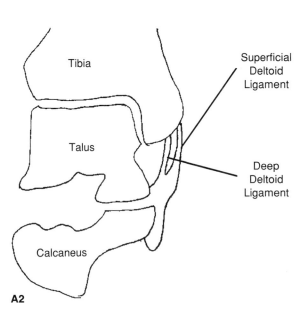

A2

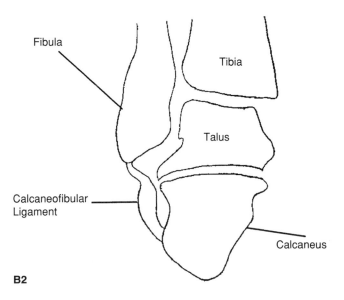

B2

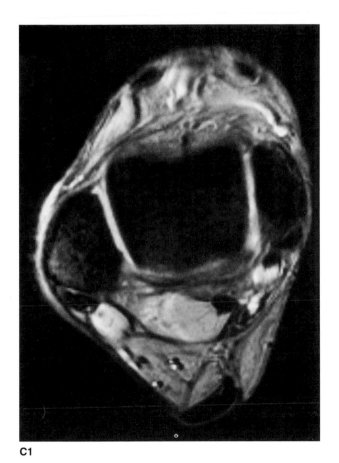

C1

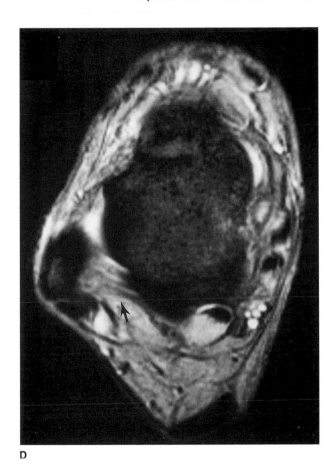

D

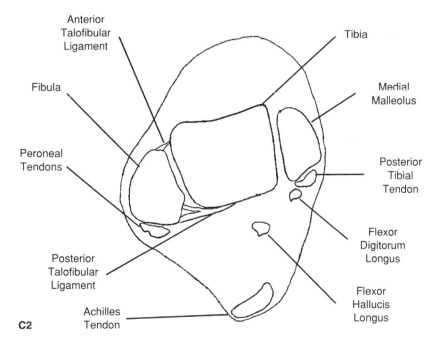

Anterior
Talofibular
Ligament

Tibia

Fibula

Medial
Malleolus

Peroneal
Tendons

Posterior
Tibial
Tendon

Posterior
Talofibular
Ligament

Flexor
Digitorum
Longus

Achilles
Tendon

Flexor
Hallucis
Longus

C2

Figure 13–4. MRI of ankle ligaments. **A1.** T1 coronal image of a normal deltoid ligament. **A2.** Corresponding line drawing of the deltoid ligament. **B1.** T1 coronal image of a normal calcaneofibular ligament. **B2.** Corresponding line drawing of the calcaneofibular ligament. **C1.** T2 gradient cross-sectional image of the ankle ligaments. **C2.** Corresponding line drawing of the of the ankle ligaments. **D.** Note the (*arrow*) thickness of the posterior talofibular ligament as compared to the anterior talofibular ligament.

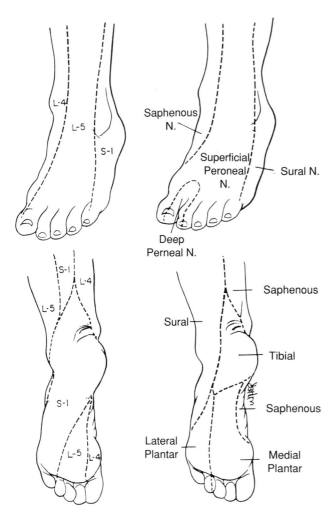

Figure 13–5. Illustration showing the peripheral nerve pattern of innervation of the surface of the foot and ankle (on the right) and dermatome innervation (on the left).

2 to 10 times the individual's body weight in the forefoot striker, greatly increasing the chance for injury.[14] It is generally not recommended, however, to attempt to change athletes' running styles, as they will naturally choose the optimal style for themselves. Modifications in running shoes, training, and running surfaces are more appropriate.

The most obvious kinematic changes, as one progresses from walking to running, is the increase in hip and knee motion. This is due to both the absorption of higher impact force during early stance and increased flexion in the swing leg caused by the rapid acceleration of the proximal limb after toe-off.[11] As individuals increase in speed, initial contact is made with the forefoot instead of the heel. Less obvious but significant changes also occur in the talocrural and subtalar joints. Starting with initial contact in walking, the moment the heel contacts the ground,

the talocrural joint undergoes a rapid plantar flexion that is controlled by the eccentric contraction of the anterior tibial muscles.[8] During running, kinematic studies have shown that talocrural dorsiflexion occurs predominately after initial contact.[10,15] This dorsiflexion continues through midstance. The amount of ankle dorsiflexion and total ankle motion depends on the speed of gait[11] and reaches a maximum of 20 degrees with running. This additional dorsiflexion is needed to more effectively absorb energy from the higher impact force that occurs in running.[11] There is evidence to show that the anterior tibialis actually accelerates the tibia forward to cause a more rapid dorsiflexion and forward progression of the body.[8,16] The posterior calf muscles control the dorsiflexion of the ankle through eccentric contractions. This muscle group begins activity during the last 25 percent of swing phase and continues to be active throughout the first 80 percent of stance phase, reaching its peak activity during the midstance phase.[8,17] The activity of the posterior calf muscles is markedly increased with increasing gait velocity. At increasing speeds, where there is a much shortened stance time, the posterior muscle groups must act with a rapid and forceful eccentric contraction, placing this muscle group at risk for injury.

Pronation of the ankle complex contributes greatly to the ability of the lower extremity to absorb shock and adapt to surfaces. Excessive or prolonged pronation is thought to be a common cause of overuse injuries in the lower extremity. Pronation normally occurs from initial contact to midstance but may extend further into the gait cycle dependent on individual anatomic and biomechanic factors.[18] External factors, such as shoes and orthotics, influence pronation. During running, pronation must occur at a much greater rate due to the shortened stance time with running. This value can be greater than 800 degrees per second.[18] This places tremendous demands on the muscles, primarily the posterior tibialis, to control this very rapid motion in a short period of time. This is consistent with the findings of Reber and colleagues,[17] who demonstrated the higher activity of the posterior tibialis in the early stance phase.

From midstance to toe-off, the lower extremity begins to externally rotate, which results in the supination of the ankle joint complex, thus stabilizing the midtarsal joints in preparation for push-off.[8] Heel rise produces passive dorsiflexion of the metacarpal and phalangeal joints. This tightens the plantar fascia and raises the longitudinal arch, which also increases the stability of the foot.[19] Muscle activity during the latter stance is markedly less compared to early stance phase. Reber and associates[17] showed that the tibialis anterior is active during late stance to clear the toes from the ground. The posterior tibialis also demonstrates some activity to assist in stabilization of the foot. Contrary to what many

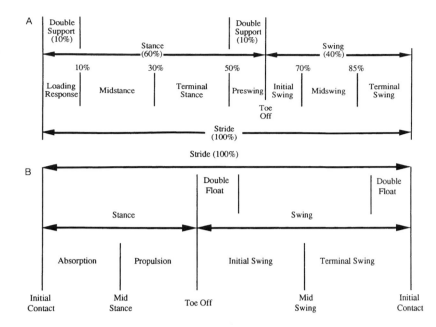

Figure 13–6. Gait cycle of **(A)** walking and **(B)** running. *(From Ounpuu S. The biomechanics of walking and running. Clin Sports Med. 1994;13:845. With permission.)*

clinicians believe, the gastrocnemius and soleus group is minimally active in the late stance phase.[17] Mann[8] feels the propulsion of the body forward comes from the swinging contralateral leg and arm motion. Others believe that this is only the case with steady state running, and that during acceleration, the calf muscles do contribute to the forward propulsion of the body. Mann and Hagy's[11] study of competitive sprinters demonstrated the calf muscles electrically active at toe-off. Thus, it appears the calf muscles function primarily as decelerators for the tibia in

steady state running and may also act as accelerators. These factors should be considered when designing a rehabilitation program for the calf musculotendinous complex.

Prolonged pronation from midstance to toe-off is implicated in a variety of overuse injuries in the lower extremity[20] and deserves special attention. When pronation continues beyond midstance, the midtarsal joints remain unlocked and hypermobile.[21] The posterior tibialis then must attempt to stabilize the hypermobile foot

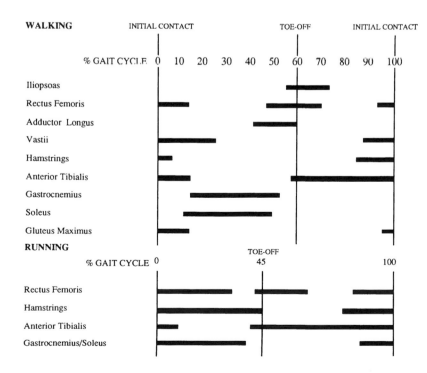

Figure 13–7. Muscle activity during gait cycle. *(From Ounpuu S. The biomechanics of walking and running. Clin Sports Med. 1994;13:847. With permission.)*

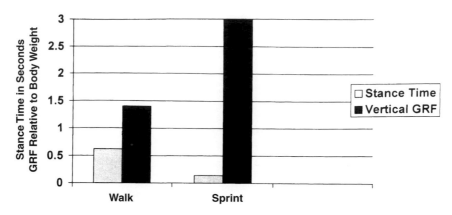

Figure 13–8. Graph showing the difference in ground reaction and stance time in walking versus running.

in an elongated position to prepare for toe-off. This additional stress, along with the eccentric contraction to decelerate pronation during the earlier phase of gait, places the posterior tibialis tendon and muscle at risk for injury. Clement and co-workers[22] proposed two mechanisms where excessive pronation may contribute to Achilles tendon injuries. First, the excessive pronation produces a whipping action or bowstring effect on the Achilles tendon causing microtears in the medial aspect of the Achilles tendon. Second, knee extension in the terminal phase of gait will begin to generate external tibial rotation, which will conflict with the exaggerated internal tibial rotation produced by the excessive pronation. These opposite rotary forces may "ring out" the blood vessels in the Achilles tendon and peritendon causing vascular impairment and subsequent degenerative changes. Finally, excessive pronation may contribute to plantar fasciitis by creating excessive traction on the medial plantar fascia.[23] Therefore, successful management of these types of overuse injuries must address biomechanical faults.

Progressing from terminal stance to early swing, the hip, knee, ankle, and toe flexors are activated to clear the foot as the lower extremity is pulled forward. Of interest in the foot, is the very high activity of the tibialis anterior. In a study of muscular control of the ankle during running, the tibialis anterior muscle showed the highest rate of sustained activity of all major muscles crossing the ankle.[17] Peak activity levels occurred during the mid and late swing phases. From these results, the authors concluded that the tibialis anterior may be more likely to experience fatigue and problems, such as cellular damage in muscle, subsequent edema, and increased compartmental pressure. All other ankle muscle groups are relatively inactive during the swing phase of running.

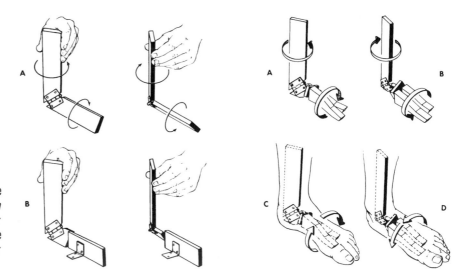

Figure 13–9. Schematic representation of the movement of the ankle and foot. *(From Mann R. Biomechanics of the foot and ankle. In: Mann RA, Coughlin MJ, eds. Surgery of the Foot and Ankle. 6th ed. St. Louis: Mosby; 1993:21. With permission.)*

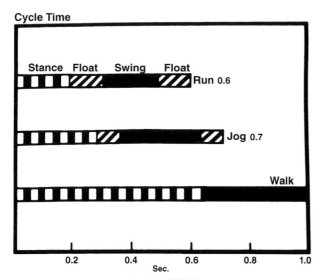

Figure 13–10. The cycle times for walking, jogging, and running. Note the marked decrease in stance time relative to other gait events as speed increases. *(From Mann RA, Hagy J. In: Bateman J, Trott A, eds. The Foot and Ankle. New York: Thieme; 1989. With permission.)*

Jumping

The athlete involved in a sport such as basketball or volleyball, that requires repetitive and forceful jumping, requires a stable foot on which to push off.[24] Thus, the athlete with a hyperflexible and pronated foot will probably be at a greater risk for injury. However, most of the stress in jumping occurs during the landing phase. Valian and Cavanagh[25] reported most individuals will land on their forefoot resulting in a ground reaction force of 4.1 times body weight. Individuals landing foot flat experienced ground reaction force 6.0 times their body weight. Hamill and associates[18] list some strategies for decreasing the impact force on the lower extremities during landing. Landing on both feet will distribute the stress over a greater area, and increasing the amount of flexion in the hip, knee, and ankle will allow the stress to be dissipated over a greater time period. An individual with a limitation of these motions will be less effective in dissipating impact forces.[18]

Multidirectional Activities

The demands on the foot and ankle are very different in multidirectional sports, as compared to forward running. With frequent and substantial lateral forces on the foot and ankle in multidirectional sports, there is a higher risk for lateral ankle sprains. The neuromuscular system must function optimally to maintain ankle stability during these activities. Athletes with residual weakness or proprioceptive deficits are at risk for reinjury. Athletes involved in multidirectional sports will often play on their forefoot, leaving the ankle in a plantar flexed position. The ankle is more unstable in the plantar flexed position, exposing the athlete to greater risk of a plantar flexion and inversion sprain.

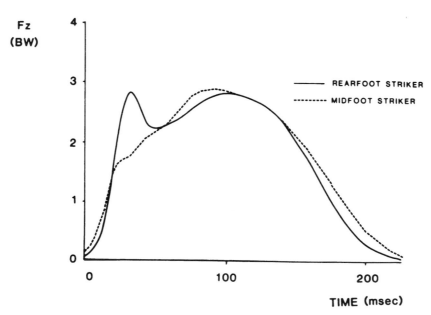

Figure 13–11. Vertical component of the ground reaction force (Fz) vs time for a rearfoot and a midfoot striker *(From Cavanagh PR, Valient GA, Misevich KW. In: Frederick EC, ed. Sports Shoes and Playing Surfaces. Champaign, IL: Human Kinetics; 1984. With permission.)*

Individuals with excessive rearfoot varus are also at risk for lateral ankle sprains. Taping or various types of orthoses are often used to lessen the chance of injury in multidirectional sports, especially for those with previous history of ankle sprains.

Most racquet sports and court activities, such as basketball and tennis, also require sudden accelerations forward. Just as in jumping, the athlete needs a stable platform on which to push off, and therefore must achieve a supinated position for optimal performance and least risk for injury. A supinated foot is also desirable for the same reasons while back peddling. The rapid forward accelerations also place great demands on the gastrocnemius and soleus muscles. Full ankle dorsiflexion is desirable during these rapid accelerations. If there is inadequate dorsiflexion at the talocrural joint, combined with incomplete supination, the midtarsal joints will compensate by dorsiflexing, placing additional strain on the plantar fascia.

Conclusion

The mechanism of injury to athletes may be obvious in traumatic injuries. In overuse injuries, the mechanism is often unclear but is usually related to physiologic, biomechanical, or training factors. Repetitive microtrauma will often lead to disruption of the normal structure of the involved muscle, tendon, or bone.[26] Without time for the musculoskeletal system to appropriately adapt, continual demands will eventually exceed the structural limits of the tissue, leading to failure and injury. The practitioner with an understanding of the motion and forces applied to the foot and ankle will be equipped to identify etiologic factors and modify them to allow tissue recovery and return to normal structure and function. Treating the symptoms of the injury will provide temporary relief and may allow the athlete to improve via a rehabilitation program. Treating the athlete with an understanding of the biomechanics will, ideally, eliminate the cause of the injury and lead to the best long-term result.

LATERAL ANKLE SPRAINS

Epidemiology

It is estimated that ankle inversion injuries occur at the rate of one per 10,000 persons each day. This correlates to about 27,000 ankle sprains every day in the United States alone.[27] In a study of West Point cadets by Jackson, inversion injury of the ankle was the most common injury at an incidence of 33 percent over 4 years.[28] Garrick has reported that ankle injuries account for 45 percent of injuries in basketball, 25 percent in volleyball, and 31 percent in soccer.[29] Other sports identified include football and racquetball.[30] Ankle sprains also account for 10 to 15 percent of all time lost to injuries in football at the professional, college, and high school levels.[31] Ankle sprains are more common in men overall, but there appears to be no gender difference in the incidence of ankle sprains when comparing injuries sustained from similar activities.[31] Previous ankle sprain predisposes the athlete to residual sprains and symptoms up to 40 percent of the time.[32]

Functional Anatomy and Mechanism

The ankle joint includes three major ligament groups: the tibiofibular ligaments, the deltoid ligament complex, and the lateral ligament complex. The lateral ligament complex is composed of three separate ligaments: the anterior talofibular ligament (ATFL), calcaneofibular ligament (CFL), and the posterior talofibular ligament (PTFL). Of these ligaments, the ATFL is the most frequently injured ligament, with isolated injury occurring about two thirds of the time.[33,34] The ATFL runs from the anterior inferior border of the fibula to the neck of the talus parallel to the long axis of the talus when the ankle is in neutral. With the ankle in plantar flexion, the ATFL is in line with the fibula and is under tension.[35] Strain gauge testing reveals the ATFL to have increased strain in internal rotation and inversion, and highest in plantar flexion.[36] Biomechanical testing of ankle ligaments have shown the ATFL to have the lowest maximum load to failure, 138.9 Newtons, plus or minus 23.5 Newtons.[37,38]

The CFL runs in a posterior inferior direction from the tip of the fibula to the tubercle of calcaneus under the peroneal tendons. The CFL appears to be extra-articular and crosses two joints, the tibial talar and the subtalar. The CFL is under maximum tension when the ankle joint is in neutral to dorsiflexion when it is in line with the fibula.[35] Strain gauge testing shows that CFL strain increases with inversion and the highest strain with full dorsiflexion.[36] Biomechanical studies have shown that the CFL has a higher ultimate strength than the ATFL, 345.7 Newtons plus or minus 55.2 Newtons.[37] Since the CFL crosses two joints, inversion and eversion of the subtalar joint results in movement of the CFL. As the subtalar joint inverts, the CFL rotates anteriorly. During eversion of the subtalar joint, the CFL rotates posteriorly.[35] This motion is important in reconstruction of the lateral ankle ligaments.

The PTFL runs from the posterior border of the distal fibula to the lateral tubercle of the talus. The PTFL has the greatest strain with the ankle in full dorsiflexion.[36] Biomechanical studies reveal that the PTFL has the highest ultimate strength of the lateral ligaments.[37]

The ankle in dorsiflexion is stable because of its bony anatomy, but in plantar flexion, stability is reduced as the narrow posterior portion of the talus is brought into the mortise.[39] In other words, the ankle depends more on ligamentous stability when the ankle is in plantar flexion. Isolated sectioning of the ATFL showed increased laxity in inversion and drawer in all positions of plantar flexion.[40] Sectioning of the CFL results in increased inversion with the talus in both dorsi and plantar flexion.[41] CFL tears also increase foot adduction through increase in subtalar joint motion.[41] Sectioning of the ATFL and the CFL results in increase anterior drawer, inversion, and internal rotation.[40,42,43] Sectioning of all the ankle lateral collateral ligaments also increases external rotation and dorsiflexion.[40,43]

The ATFL is the ligament most susceptible to injury and the first injured in an ankle sprain. At the time of operation (not injury), the ATFL is always torn,[44,45] the CFL is often torn in association with the ATFL (40 to 99 percent of the operative sprains),[44,46-48] and the stronger PTFL is rarely torn (0 to 9 percent of operative sprains).[47,49]

The common mechanism of acute lateral ankle injury is when the player lands on a plantar flexed and internally rotated ankle. There is decreased tibial talar contact and the ligament absorbs the stress. This happens when poorly executing a cutting maneuver or landing on a competitor's foot or an irregular surface.

History and Physical Exam

The history is helpful in determining the mechanism of injury. Many patients will remember the position of the foot at the time of injury, inversion, plantar flexion, or internal rotation. They may describe a popping or tearing sensation of the ankle. It is very important to ask about previous ankle sprains and history of ankle instability such as feeling the ankle "giving out."

The initial exam is often limited by pain produced by bleeding into the ankle joint or soft tissue.[50] Examination usually reveals a diffusely swollen ankle, plantar flexed foot, and possibly, ecchymotic and tender around the anterolateral ankle. Pain will limit the range of motion of the foot in all directions. Instability may be detected acutely.

Performing an exam on a chronic ankle injury or a delayed exam is more reliable and tolerated better by the patient because there is less reactive muscle guarding. First, general ligamentous laxity should be noted. The examiner should look for pes cavus or genu varum, which may predispose an athlete to recurrent ankle sprains. Palpation of the ankle will reveal maximal tenderness on the anterolateral aspect of the ankle. However, it will be difficult to tell the difference between an isolated ATFL tear or a combined ATFL and CFL tear by palpation. Comparison with the uninjured side may be helpful.

Stress tests are valuable to determine the degree of mechanical instability. The anterior drawer test mainly assesses the stability of the ATFL. The test is performed with the ankle plantar flexed making the ATFL tight, then applying anterior force on the calcaneus while stabilizing the tibia (see Fig. 13-12). The amount of

translation is compared to the contralateral normal ankle. Increased translation suggests ATFL injury. The talar tilt inversion stress test assesses the stability of the CFL. The ankle is placed in a neutral position relaxing the ATFL and placing more tension on the CFL. Then, the tibia is stabilized and a varus stress is applied to the ankle. Again, this is compared to the contralateral side. Increase in laxity suggests both ATFL and CFL ligament injuries, since isolated CFL injuries are very uncommon.

Also, it is important to rule out other causes of lateral ankle pain at this time (see Table 13-1). Fractures of the fibula, tibia, calcaneus, fifth metatarsal, talus, or cuboid can be checked by palpating these bones. Syndesmosis injury to the ankle can be diagnosed with the "squeeze test." The fibula and the tibia are squeezed at the midcalf, which causes pain distally in the syndesmosis or the ankle (see Fig. 13-13).[51] Sural nerve or superficial peroneal nerve injury can be diagnosed with a thorough neurologic sensory evaluation of the foot. The peroneal tendons can be subluxated or dislocated due to dorsiflexion injury and will have pain, subluxation, or dislocation with resisted inversion of a dorsiflexed and everted foot.[50]

Diagnostic Studies

Plain anterior, posterior, mortise, and lateral radiographs allow the physician to detect bone lesions. In some cases

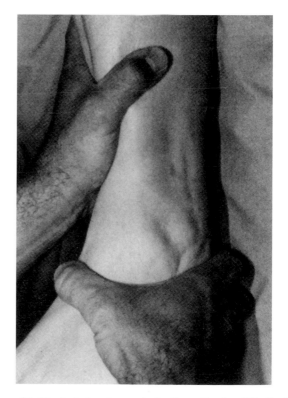

Figure 13–12. Anterior drawer test. *(From Trevino SG, Davis P, Hecht PJ. Management of acute and chronic lateral ligament injuries of the ankle.* Orthop Clin North Am. *1994;25:5. With permission.)*

TABLE 13–1. LATERAL ANKLE PAIN

Disorder	History	Physical Exam	Provacative Test	Plain Radiographs	Other Diagnostic Tests
Lateral ankle sprain	History of recurrent inversion injuries and ankle sprains	Tenderness and swelling anterior to the lateral malleolus	Anterior drawer and talar tilt test	Noncontributory	Stress views of the ankle. MRI may reveal ATFL or CFL ligament edema or tear
Subtalar sprain sinus tarsi syndrome	History of ankle sprain or inversion injury, difficulty walking on uneven ground	Pain over lateral side of sinus tarsi	Subtalar instability to varus stress	Noncontributory	Subtalar arthrogram and MRI shows rupture of talocalcaneal interosseous membrane stress subtalar views may show instability
Syndesmosis injury	History of external rotation and plantar flexion injury of the ankle	Tenderness of anterior syndesmosis and interosseous membrane	Squeeze test, external rotation,[a] cotton test[b]	May show widening of the ankle mortise	Stress x-ray in external rotation with foot in dorsiflexion and plantarflexion. Bone scan and MRI will show increased signal in the areas of tear
Osteochondral lesions of the talus	History of ankle sprain (popping, catching, or locking of ankle)	Tenderness medially or laterally with ROM of ankle	Diagnostic ankle injection	May show osteochondral fracture of the posterior medial dome or more often anterior lateral dome	Bone scan, MRI, or tomograms will help identify the lesions
Peroneal tendon injury	Patient unsure of mechanism of injury history of popping and snapping	Swelling and tenderness posterior to the lateral malleolus	Pain with resisted dorsiflexion and eversion of the ankle from an inverted plantar flexed position	May show boney avulsion from the posterior lateral malleolus near the origin of the SR	MRI may reveal tendinitis or subluxation of the peroneal tendons
Stress fx of fibula or calcaneus	Insidious onset of vague pain with activity	Tenderness of fx site, distal fibula or calcaneus		May show reactive bone sclerosis	Bone scan or MRI will reveal fracture site
Nerve injury sural nerve or superficial peroneal nerve	History of recurrent ankle sprains with burning or tingling sensation	Pain and hypersensitivity along distribution of sural and sup. peroneal nerve	Positive tinels over the nerves	Diagnostic injections of the sites of compression	EMG or nerve conduction study

[a] External rotation test. With knee flexed 90 degrees external rotation of the foot will give pain in anterior syndesmosis.
[b] Cotton test. Hold calcaneus and talus and try to move it from side to side within the mortise to check for widening.

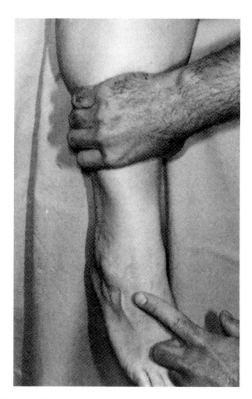

Figure 13–13. Squeeze test. *(From Trevino SG, Davis P, Hecht PJ. Management of acute and chronic lateral ligament injuries of the ankle.* Orthop Clin North Am. *1994;25:6. With permission.)*

with chronic lateral ankle pain and instability, stress radiographs may be valuable. The talar tilt stress radiograph is performed similar to the talar tilt stress test using manual stress or a commercially available jig. Local anesthesia or general anesthesia, may be helpful for this test according to the amount of pain. Interpretation of the result appears to be confusing as there is a great deal of variability in the range of normal values,[52-54] but most physicians agree that the CFL is torn when there is more than 10 degrees on one side or the side-to-side comparison difference is more than 5 degrees.[55]

The anterior drawer stress radiograph is performed much like the anterior drawer exam. It can also be performed with manual stress or using a jig. A lateral radiograph is obtained with the talus stressed undergoing anterior displacement. Again, the calculated normal values vary with different studies, but abnormality exists when there is more than 10 mm of translation or a side-to-side difference of 3 mm.[55,56]

An arthrogram is a radiograph taken with contrast inserted into the ankle joint. A recent prospective study comparing arthrography, stress radiographs, and clinical examinations in the diagnosis of acute injury to the lateral ankle ligaments showed that arthrography detected both ligament tears in about 85 percent of the cases, while clinical exams and stress radiographs

detected only about 50 percent of the injuries.[57] But, for various reasons, arthrograms are rarely performed to confirm lateral ligament disruption.

MRI accurately demonstrates the acute lateral ankle ligament injury when edema, irregular contour, and discontinuity of ligaments are present.[58,59] Also, associated soft-tissue pathology such as peroneal tendon injury or osteochondral defects can be identified.[58] In chronic ankle injuries, it is able to identify elongated or redundant ligaments.[50] However, due to its high cost, MRI is usually reserved for chronic pain associated with inversion sprains (see Figs. 13–14 and 13–15).

Surgical Treatment

Ankle sprains are graded from 1 to 3. Grade 1 sprain signifies an ATFL stretch with no ligamentous disruption. Grade 2 sprain signifies a moderate injury to the lateral ligaments, frequently with complete tear of the ATFL and partial tear of the CFL. Finally, grade 3 injury signifies both ATFL and CFL tears.[60]

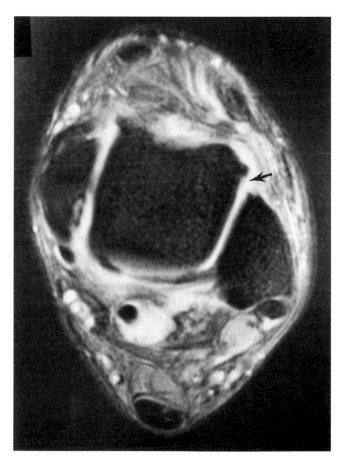

Figure 13–14. MRI of anterior talofibular ligament tear of the ankle. The T2 gradient cross-sectional image *(arrow)* demonstrates the absence of the anterior talofibular ligament indicating a complete tear.

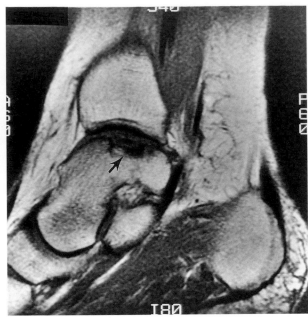

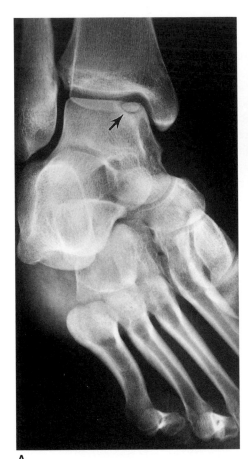

Figure 13–15. Osteochondral lesion of the talus. **A.** Radiograph of posterior medial osteochondral lesion of the dome of the talus. **B.** T1 MRI of the more common anterior lateral osteochondral lesion of the talus.

All sprains are initially treated nonsurgically with functional rehabilitation. Estimates are that 40 percent of third-degree sprains will result in chronic instability requiring further treatment.[32,60] Surgical stabilization is indicated for those patients who exhibit mechanical and functional instability.[55]

Reconstruction of the lateral ankle ligaments can be divided into two basic types, anatomic and nonanatomic. Anatomic reconstruction was first described by Brostrom. He found that it was possible to repair chronic ankle ligament injuries by direct repair of the ligaments years after injury (see Fig. 13–16A).[33] Most contemporary reports suggest the anatomic reconstruction should be the primary choice when surgery is indicated.[27] The advantages are that it is simple, biologically more stable than the nonanatomic reconstruction, and highly successful (87 percent).[61,62]

Nonanatomic or tenodesis procedures include Watson-Jones, Evans, and the most popular, Chrisman-Snook modification of the Elmslie procedure (see Fig. 13–16B). These involve harvesting the peroneus brevis tendon and routing it through the fibula. Watson-Jones requires a full-thickness peroneus brevis graft, routing it through the fibula to recreate the ATFL, but does not recreate the calcaneofibular ligament anatomically (see Fig. 13–16B).[60] The Evans procedure routes the full-thickness peroneus brevis tendon through the fibula in a vector that is the average of the ATFL and calcaneofibular ligaments.[62] The Chrisman-Snook modification uses a partial-thickness peroneus brevis tendon through the fibula to recreate the ATFL and calcaneofibular ligaments.[63] These nonanatomic reconstructions obtain stability with significant loss of subtalar motion.[62,64] Of the nonanatomic procedures, the Chrisman-Snook reconstruction appears to have the best stability, but according to biomechanical studies, is inferior to the anatomic reconstruction.[62,64] The current recommendation is to perform nonanatomic (Chrisman-Snook) reconstruction for failed primary repair.

CONSERVATIVE TREATMENT OF ANKLE SPRAINS

"It's just an ankle sprain" is, unfortunately, a common saying. For the number of athletes who sustain an ankle sprain and return to play in a few days, there are an equal number who complain of residual pain, stiffness, and instability. In a study of 84 high school basketball players, 80 percent of the players who sustained one ankle sprain went on to have a repeat injury[65]; 50 percent of

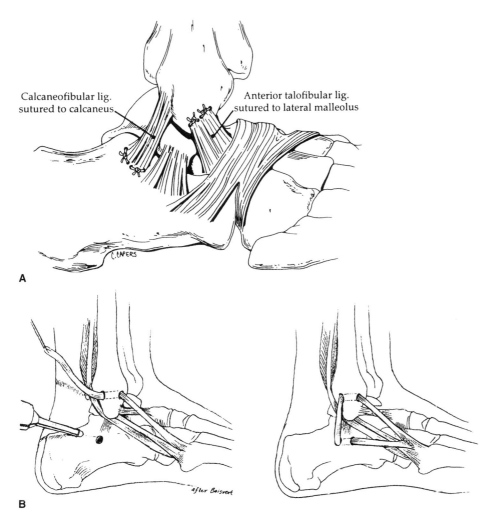

Calcaneofibular lig.
sutured to calcaneus

Anterior talofibular lig.
sutured to lateral malleolus

A

B

Figure 13–16. A. Brostrom procedure of anatomic lateral ankle ligament reconstruction. **B.** Chrisman-Snook procedure of nonanatomic lateral ankle ligament reconstruction. (**A** *from Liu SH, Baker CL. Comparison of lateral ankle ligamentous reconstruction procedures.* Am J Sports Med. *1994;22:314. With permission.* **B** *from Renstrom PAFH. Persis-tently painful sprained ankle.* J Am Acad Orthop Surg. *1994;2:273. With permission.)*

the players in this survey had residual symptoms. Numerous examples of residual problems following the ankle sprain can be found in the literature. Reasons for the continued disability are several; weakness of the surrounding muscles, particularly the peroneals, and kinesthetic deficits[66] are often cited. Thus, the goals of a rehabilitation program should include the restoration of strength and kinesthesia, in addition to full motion, to return of the athlete to competition, while minimizing risk for further injury.

The conservative treatment of inversion ankle sprains can be divided into acute treatment, rehabilitation phase, and functional activity phase. The acute stage of treatment should not just focus on the use of physical modalities to control pain and swelling, but also should include motion and functional training as soon as possible. The addition of early motion and functional activities ensures the most rapid return to sports. Just how rapidly the athlete can be progressed during rehabilitation is still argued despite the voluminous research. Some areas of consideration when designing a rehabilitation program include whether to mobilize or immobilize the ankle, weight-bearing status, and what, if any, external support will be used. The following discussion on rehabilitation of ankle sprains will address these issues and others.

Acute Phase

The principle of protection, rest, ice, compression, and elevation (PRICE) is inarguably the choice for immediate treatment for ankle sprains. In addition to PRICE, Sloan and co-workers[67] recommend high doses of nonsteroidal anti-inflammatory drugs within 6 hours of injury. In a double blind study, they reported that the administration of 1200 mg of ibuprofen within 6 hours of injury and 2400 mg daily thereafter, resulted in a better recovery than when administration of ibuprofen began at 48 hours. These procedures, and others, are necessary to control the deleterious effects of swelling, bleeding, and inflammation. Swelling not only limits the motion in the ankle joint, but can also hinder the healing of the injured ligament. The lateral ligaments of the ankle joint are part of the joint capsule; therefore any swelling within the joint may hinder the approximation of any stretched or torn ligament fibers.[68]

Cryotherapy and Edema Control

Cryotherapy refers to methods used to decrease tissue temperature in the area of injury. The effects of cryotherapy include vasoconstriction, decreased cellular waste, reduction in inflammation, decreased pain, and decreased muscle spasm.[69] The cooling of the tissues is also thought to decrease the metabolic requirements of the tissues, thus preventing any further hypoxic injury.[70] Not all studies demonstrate a reduction in swelling; moreover, some show an increase in edema.[71] Cote and colleagues[72] compared the effects of ice immersion, contrast baths, and heat treatments on ankle swelling following inversion sprains and found that all treatments produced an increase in swelling. The ice immersion treatment, however, produced the least increase in swelling. The increase in swelling may be explained in part by the ankles being dangled in a dependent position during treatment.

Other studies have shown dramatic positive effects of early cold therapy on ankle sprains. Hocutt and associates[73] treated 37 patients with ankle sprains with heat and cold. They found that patients treated with cold therapy within 36 hours of injury returned to full activity in 13 days. The group treated with cold 36 hours after injury did not reach full activity until 30 days. Numerous other studies and review articles have been published advocating the positive effects of cryotherapy.

Cryotherapy can be performed in a variety of ways, each having its advantages. Due to the bony architecture of the ankle, an inflexible ice pack or ice bag may or may not have total contact with the ankle, producing less effective cooling. A partially filled bag of crushed ice is more flexible, and when compressed around the joint with an elastic bandage, results in a more even application while providing the beneficial effects of compression. Further compression can be added by making a "horseshoe" out of felt to be placed on the soft tissues around the lateral malleolus (see Fig. 13–17). Following treatment in the training room, the athlete can continue to wear the horseshoe wrapped in an elastic bandage. There are commercially available U-shaped pads with a gel compartment that can be frozen to provide cold therapy and focal compression. One should use caution with any type of chemical ice pack, as these can sometimes reach temperatures below 0°C if not used properly. Finally, ice water immersion with the temperature between 13 and 18°C is also frequently used. This technique ensures coverage of the entire ankle and lower leg, but the

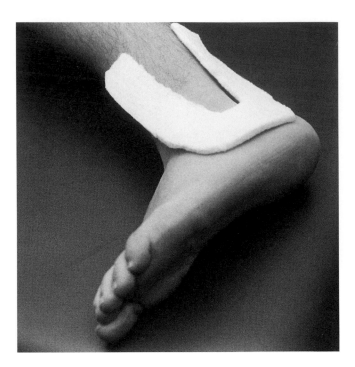

Figure 13–17. A felt pad can be held in place around the lateral malleolus with an elastic bandage to provide focal compression to minimize or decrease edema after an acute ankle sprain.

necessary dependent position of the foot may encourage edema.

Compression can easily be used in conjunction with cryotherapy. The primary benefit of compression is the increase in the interstitial fluid pressure, which decreases capillary outflow and facilitates lymphatic drainage.[70] Wilkerson[70] also reports that the compaction of the soft tissues with compression will increase perfusion of the hypoxic tissues by decreasing the diffusion distance from the capillaries. Sloan and associates,[67] in their study of induced superficial soft-tissue inflammation, found that cold and compression had synergistic effects. Cold or compression alone reduced the inflammatory reaction for 10 minutes after application, but the combination of cold and as little as 10 mm Hg of sustained pressure resulted in a reduced inflammatory reaction for as long as 60 minutes after application. Intermittent pneumatic compression (IPC) has also been found to be effective in reducing edema. Airaksinen and co-workers[74] studied 44 acute ankle sprains for 4 weeks. Half were treated with just an elastic bandage and the other half were treated with IPC daily for the first week. At 4 weeks after injury, the group treated with IPC had statistically significant less pain, improved perceived function, and less swelling compared to the elastic bandage group. Cold and IPC are often used simultaneously as shown in Figure 13–18. Cycling times (on and off times) should be 15 to 30

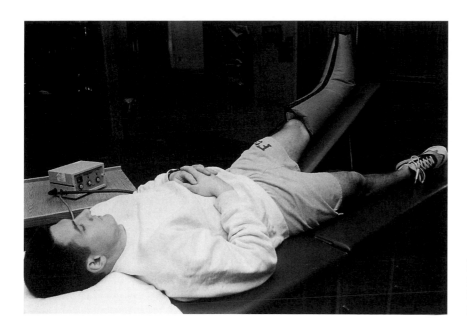

Figure 13–18. Intermittent pneumatic compression combined with elevation and an ice bag wrapped around the ankle is an effective method to control edema.

seconds with the pressure being approximately 60 mm Hg, but never greater than the athlete's diastolic blood pressure. During the deflation period, active motion exercises of the ankle and foot can be performed. Some commercial devices provide added convenience by circulating cold water through the boot to provide the simultaneous compression and cold therapy. Treatment time for this regime, in addition to other cryotherapy techniques, is 20 to 30 minutes. Cryotherapy can and should be repeated several times daily during the inflammatory stage of the injury.

Electromagnetic energy and therapeutic electricity have also been used extensively to decrease swelling in the acutely sprained ankle. In their double-blind study of 50 acute ankle sprains, Pennington and associates[75] reported that pulsed, nonthermal, high-frequency electromagnetic energy (diapulse) produced a swelling reduction four times that of a control after one treatment. Subjects treated with diapulse also had a greater reduction in pain than the controls. Various types of electrical stimulation are also recommended for edema reduction. Electrical stimulation can assist in the reduction of edema in two ways. One is by eliciting muscle contractions, which milk the tissue and promote drainage from the area.[69] With lack of sufficient musculature in the ankle, sensory level stimulation is used to assist edema reduction. Table 13–2 presents a recommended protocol for application of sensory level electrical stimulation to reduce edema.[76]

Thus, there are several methods for the reduction of swelling after an acute ankle sprain. Which method used depends on available resources, athlete preference, and the clinician's comfort and experience with the various procedures (see Table 13–2).

Gait and Exercise

The type of gait (nonweight-bearing versus weight-bearing), immobilization versus mobilization, and the type of exercise for treating the acutely sprained ankle are debated. Most clinicians will agree that weight bearing as tolerated can be performed immediately after grade I and II ankle sprains. The use of crutches is usually necessary to minimize pain and additional stress to the injured ankle, but their use should be discontinued as soon as possible. Bracing or elastic bandaging can provide additional protection and comfort for those with more severe sprains. Even in a severe ankle sprain, the athlete can attempt to simulate the normal heel-toe gait while bearing minimal weight on the affected ankle. Letting the ankle dangle in a plantarflexed position while ambulating encourages edema, loss of motion, and hinders ligament healing.

TABLE 13–2. DECREASING EDEMA FOLLOWING AN ANKLE SPRAIN

Waveform	High-voltage pulsed monophasic
Pulse rate	120 pulses per second
Pulse duration	50–100 microseconds
On/off time	Continuous
Interphase interval	65 to 75 microseconds
Amplitude	10 percent below motor threshold
Application	Monopolar technique with the ankle in a water bath with the negative electrode and the positive electrode proximal
Treatment duration	30 minutes
Frequency	Immediately after injury and 2 to 4 times daily

Adapted with permission from *Course Manual. Electrotherapy and Ultrasound Update.* International Academy of Physio Therapeutics; 1995.

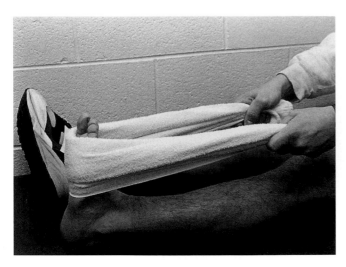

Figure 13–19. In the acute phase, stretching the gastrocnemius and achilles tendon in the open chain position is more comfortable than in the closed chain. Stretching should also be performed with the knee flexed to isolate the soleus.

It is common practice to treat the athlete with a grade I or II ankle sprain with early mobilization rather than casting. Early mobilization results in less pain and an earlier return to work than those treated with immobilization.[77,78] There is much controversy, however, over the treatment for a severe or grade III inversion sprain. In a retrospective study, Kay[79] reported that 60 percent of the grade III sprains were treated with immobilization with a plaster cast and 14 percent were treated with primary repair. In the study of 160 ankle injuries by Klein and co-workers,[80] the majority of the grade III sprains were treated surgically and most of the others were treated with functional rehabilitation. Overall, the surgical group had the best results in regard to pain, swelling, and subjective stability, but they were equal to the functional rehabilitation group in performance. The group treated with plaster immobilization had the poorest results. Konradsen and co-workers[81] compared mobilization versus immobilization treatment in patients with grade III sprains and followed them for 1 year. The mobilization group wore an aircast for 6 weeks. The immobilization group wore a plaster splint for 1 week, then a short-leg walking cast for an additional 5 weeks. The mobilization group returned to work and sports quicker than the immobilization group, while both had a similar number of residual symptoms at 1 year (9 percent for immobilization and 13 percent for mobilization treatment). In both groups, 95 percent of the ankles were mechanically stable after 1 year of treatment. Konradsen and co-worker[81] reported that the percentage of patients with residual symptoms in this study were equivalent to other studies evaluating surgical treatment. Additionally, they found that both groups of patients in this study had

greater stability than previous reports of surgically treated grade III sprains. It is difficult to compare all these studies as different criteria for entrance, definitions of stability, and outcome measures were used. However, it does appear that the long-term results in the three different forms of treatment (mobilization, immobilization, and surgery) are similar, while those treated with early, controlled mobilization returned to activity more quickly.

If not immobilized, exercise should be initiated as soon as possible after the ankle sprain. Goals of the exercise program in the acute phase are to increase range of motion (ROM), minimize muscle atrophy, and facilitate edema resolution. As early as the first day after the injury, the athlete can be instructed in gentle Achilles stretching (see Fig. 13-19) and active range-of-motion (AROM) exercises as tolerated. The Achilles stretch and AROM exercises are most easily performed in the open-chain position during the acute phase. However, if tolerable, the AROM can be performed in the closed-chain position, while seated, with the biomechanical ankle platform system (BAPS) (see Fig. 13-20). It is important that the athlete not be too aggressive and only perform the ROM exercises within the pain-free range. Progression to isometric exercises in all planes can be performed when the athlete can resist against moderate force without pain. Foot intrinsic muscle strengthening, such as towel

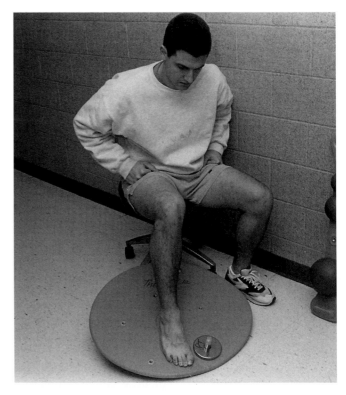

Figure 13–20. Use of the BAPS in a seated position allows early proprioceptive training. The size of the ball under the platform can be increased to challenge the patient as more motion is gained.

curling, can usually be tolerated. This gentle muscular exercise will not only help prevent muscle atrophy, but may also assist in edema resolution. Weight-bearing, as tolerated, can provide proprioceptive input. The addition of pool walking is an excellent method to provide proprioceptive input, while minimizing weight-bearing on the injured extremity.

Part of the initial exercise session should include patient education. The athlete should be instructed to keep the ankle in a neutral position and avoid prolonged positions of plantar flexion, which is usually the position of comfort. In addition, all exercise sessions should be followed with ice. The length of time the athlete is in the acute stage of treatment is dependent on the severity of the injury. For most grade I and II sprains, the period will be 1 to 3 days. For more severe sprains treated with mobilization, the athlete may not be ready to progress to the next level for up to 1 week. The patient treated with immobilization will progress through the same three phases but will need more emphasis on regaining ROM and less on edema control.

Early Rehabilitation Phase

The athlete can progress to the early rehabilitation phase when edema is under control, ROM is nearly full with minimal pain, and the use of crutches has been discontinued. New activities should be introduced gradually during this and the final phase. An increase in pain (other than nonspecific muscle soreness) or swelling with a new activity, may indicate that the activity was introduced too early or at too high an intensity. If this is the case, the athlete should rest from the offending activity for at least a day and attempt the activity at a reduced intensity when recovered. The goals of the early rehabilitation phase include the achievement of normal walking gait, full ROM, normal strength, and the maintenance of fitness. The additional stresses applied during this phase will also facilitate ligament healing by providing a stimulus for the reorientation of collagen structures in the ligament.[82] Transverse friction massage over the injured ligament may also promote healing and prevent adherence to adjacent tissue as collagen fibers are being laid down.[83] Cryotherapy, compression, and electrical modalities should continue for the resolution of swelling and pain.

As pain and swelling decrease, ROM exercise can be more aggressive. Greater ranges of motion can be achieved by increasing the size of the ball while using the BAPS. Stretching of the Achilles tendon and the gastrocnemius and soleus is essential as this musculotendinous group often becomes shortened with disuse. If the patient has difficulty achieving ROM, the manual assistance of the clinician may be indicated. The clinician should determine whether limitations of motion are primarily due to joint stiffness, muscle and tendon shortening, or pain and

guarding. If the limitation of motion is due to joint stiffness, various mobilization techniques can be employed (see Fig. 13-21). A detailed description of joint assessment and mobilization techniques can be found in various rehabilitation textbooks.

The athlete is able to discontinue crutches in the early rehabilitation stage. If an antalgic gait still persists, time should be spent in weight transfer and specific gait training. If available, a pool or parallel bars are valuable tools for this practice.

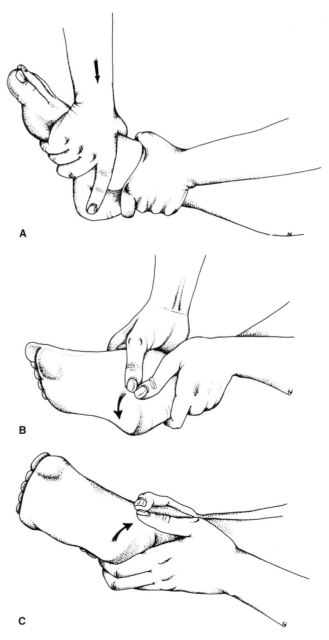

Figure 13–21. A. A posterior glide of the talus on the tibia is used to increase ankle joint dorsiflexion. **B.** A valgus tilt of the calcaneus is used to improve subtalar eversion. **C.** A varus tilt of the calcaneus is used to increase subtalar inversion.

The strengthening program can be progressed by discontinuing isometrics and starting resistive exercises through the available ROM with the use of rubber tubing or other forms of elastic resistance. The motions can be performed in straight plantar motions (dorsi and plantar flexion, inversion and eversion) or preferably, along the lines of muscle actions. These motions would be the combination of dorsiflexion and inversion to plantarflexion and eversion, and dorsiflexion and eversion to plantarflexion and inversion. Strengthening exercises on isokinetic equipment can also be performed. If the patient is in the subacute stage of the pathology, it is recommended that exercising begin at high speeds to minimize joint compressive forces.[84] The athlete can then progress to intermediate and then slow speeds to acquire strength at varying speeds of joint movement. This training throughout the range of speeds is termed the velocity spectrum rehabilitation program, and is commonly used in knee rehabilitation programs.[84] Modern isokinetic equipment also allows eccentric training. As mentioned in the biomechanics section, the muscles around the ankle experience strong and rapid eccentric contractions during running and other activities. Training eccentrically at high velocities may help prepare the musculotendinous units for this type of stress, but places great demands on the muscles and tendons and must therefore, be integrated into the program gradually.

Closed-chain strengthening exercises have the distinct advantage of allowing concomitant training of the proprioceptive system. One can begin closed-chain strengthening by adding weight to the BAPS. The athlete can progress as tolerated from a seated position, to partial weight-bearing, and finally, to a single leg stance on the injured extremity. Early strengthening exercises should emphasize a high number of repetitions with mild resistance to minimize stress on the ankle joint. As pain and swelling decrease, resistance can be increased as tolerated. Once an athlete can perform a single leg stance on the injured extremity without pain, he or she can begin a progression of balancing activities specifically designed to improve proprioception (see Table 13-3 and Fig. 13-22). The athlete only progresses to the next level when the current level is performed with control and is pain free (see Table 13-3). There are continual progressions of proprioceptive training in the functional

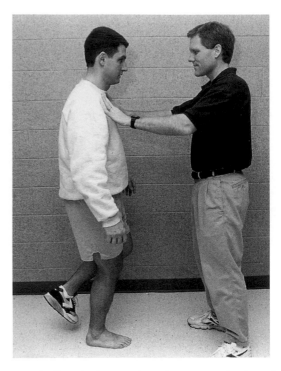

Figure 13–22. To train the proprioception system, the therapist can destabilize the athlete while standing on the affected extremity. The athlete attempts to recover to a stable position as quickly as possible. This is repeated in several different directions.

activity phase. This cannot be overemphasized, as poor proprio-ception is a major cause of repeat sprains and functional instability.[85]

Finally, the athlete must maintain total leg strength and cardiovascular fitness to ease the transition to full participation. A stationary bike, stair step machine, cross-country ski machine, and deep water pool running with a flotation vest can all be used to accomplish this goal. These activities also provide an excellent warm-up prior to each day's rehabilitation session.

Once the athlete has achieved full ROM, normal strength, minimal to no swelling, and has good control of balance, he or she is ready to progress to functional activities.

Functional Activities

The goal in this phase of rehabilitation is the final preparation for the return to play. With normal strength and ROM attained, emphasis is now placed on balance, agility, and gaining the functional skills necessary for the athlete's activity. The clinician must determine the stresses the athlete's ankle will experience when returned to play and design activities that will simulate these stresses to prepare the athlete to return to a high level of participation with minimal risk of reinjury. Naturally, this phase of rehabilitation

TABLE 13–3. PROGRESSION OF PROPRIOCEPTION EXERCISES

Balance with single leg stance (SLS)

Balance with eyes closed during SLS

SLS with weight shift and recovery in four directions

SLS with destabilization by therapist

Repeat of above with SLS on BAPS

will be different for a triple jumper than a basketball player. One common thread, however, is the continual progression of activities designed specifically to improve strength and proprioception. Now the athlete can practice balancing on the affected leg while performing various activities with the other leg or upper extremities (see Fig. 13-23).

Almost all sporting events require running. Before the athlete can progress to any agility or other sports-specific drills, he or she must be able to run forward comfortably. Once this goal is reached, numerous drills involving cutting, pivoting, lateral movement, and changes in direction can be designed for sports such as basketball. The athlete should begin by jogging slowly through these drills, gradually increasing speed and taking sharper angles as tolerated. As discussed in the biomechanics section, the stresses on the muscles and tendons are exaggerated with increasing speed. The very strong eccentric contractions to decelerate and absorb shock are responsible for additional stress. At this stage, progressive training that simulates these stresses should be performed. For the foot and ankle, jumping rope is an excellent activity to prepare the ankle for repetitive concentric and eccentric contractions. It is recommended the athlete begin with double stance jumping with equal weight on each leg with a slow rhythm, and low jumps. Intensity can be increased by increasing the jumping rate, height, and shifting weight over to the affected extremity and even alternating legs to allow some single leg jumps. At this stage, the clinician may use creativity to design functional drills that best simulate the athlete's sports activity.

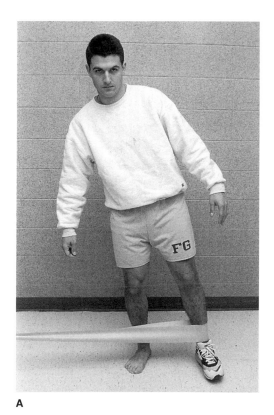

A

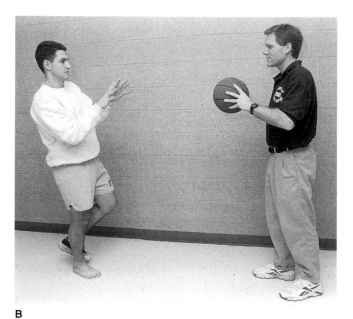

B

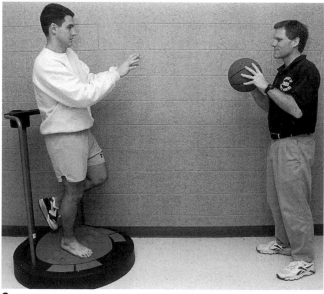

C

Figure 13–23. Various activities with the opposite leg and upper extremities can be performed to improve proprioception in the affected extremity. **A.** While balancing on the injured leg, hip abduction is performed against elastic resistance with the uninvolved leg. Hip flexion, extension, and adduction can also be performed against the elastic resistance. **B.** Playing catch while balancing on the affected extremity. **C.** Playing catch while balancing on the KAT balance system with the affected extremity.

The athlete is ready to return to play when pain and swelling are resolved, joint motion and strength are normal, and most importantly, the athlete has the ability to perform the sports-specific activities. Prior to returning to the sport, the athlete should simulate the activities that will be encountered at full speed. This not only gives the clinician an indication of the athlete's readiness for play, but if successful, gives the athlete confidence in his or her abilities. Another criteria for return to play is the athlete's perception of his or her abilities. The athlete can be asked at what percent he or she is currently functioning. This often proves to be very useful and accurate, with the exception of the motivated athlete who will exaggerate to get on the playing field.

Taping and Bracing

The use of taping or bracing is very common when treating foot, and particularly, ankle injuries. Tape or braces can be used at any stage in rehabilitation and are even used for the prevention of ankle sprains in healthy athletes. Surve and associates[86] studied the effect of a semirigid orthosis on the incidence of ankle injury of 258 soccer players during a single season. The players were divided into those with previous ankle sprains and those without previous ankle injury. The result showed that athletes with previous ankle sprains using the orthosis had significantly fewer sprains than the nonbraced, previously injured group. The athletes without previous injury did not benefit from wearing the brace. Tropp and co-workers found that an ankle foot orthosis was as effective as coordination training in preventing sprains in previously injured athletes. However, there were no differences between controls, the orthosis group, or the training group, in subjects without previous ankle injury. From these two studies, it appears that bracing may prevent recurrent injury in those with previous injury, but does not make a difference in those without previous injury. There are, however, some studies and clinicians that advocate the routine use of prophylactic taping or bracing even in athletes without previous ankle injuries. Because of the inconvenience, expense, and possible adverse effect on athletic performance, routine prophylactic taping of healthy athletes is not recommended. However, the clinician is encouraged to consider the consequences of an injury to an athlete and make the decision based on the individual athlete's sport or position, susceptibility to injury, and results of preseason evaluations.

Several studies were performed to compare the effectiveness of tape and different types of orthoses.[87-89] In general, this research shows that tape and orthoses provided similar stabilization prior to athletic participation. However, after exercise, the tape loosened and its ability to stabilize the ankle was markedly reduced compared to the orthoses. Other advantages of an orthosis over taping are that taping can be more expensive, requires a skilled trainer, and can sometimes cause skin irritation and blisters. If the clinician decides an orthosis is useful for an athlete, there are several to choose from. In a study of three different types of orthoses,[90] it was found that the ankle ligament protector (ALP) and Air-Stirrup provided more stability before and after exercise than the Swedo brace. However, the Air-Stirrup adversely affected base running times in softball players whereas the Swedo brace and ALP did not. Equally important is the comfort, fit, and the athlete's confidence and performance with the orthosis.

During the management of an athlete with an acute ankle sprain, the addition of an orthosis or taping can provide additional comfort and protection. The use of the external support is especially recommended for athletes with severe ankle sprains treated with early mobilization. The Air-Stirrup is the support most commonly used in the treatment of an acute ankle sprain. In addition, the Air-Stirrup provides a considerable amount of compression to assist in edema control. The Air-Stirrup's air bag lining allows compression of 25 mm Hg with weight bearing and up to 75 mm Hg with extreme dorsiflexion.[91]

To summarize, due to the expense, inconvenience, and research findings, the routine use of tape and bracing in healthy athletes is not justified. However, external support is recommended for competing athletes with previous ankle injuries. The semirigid orthoses, such as the Air-Stirrup and ALP, are preferred over tape for their longer lasting stability. Finally, the use of an external support provides comfort and edema control during the acute phase of an ankle sprain.

Rehabilitation After Lateral Ankle Ligament Surgery

Rehabilitation following lateral ankle ligament reconstruction does not differ significantly from the nonoperative rehabilitation program. Therapy is begun with emphasis on regaining ROM early on, then progressing to strengthening, proprioceptive exercises, and finally, functional activities. Modalities to assist in pain and swelling reduction are also used. The primary differences in the patient after surgery are soft-tissue and joint restrictions due to the period of immobilization after the surgery. This time period may vary from 3 to 6 weeks, depending on the type of surgery performed. Thus, the patient who requires more time to regain full ROM and inversion should be progressed cautiously to protect the ligament repair. Soft-tissue mobilization over the healed incision and adjacent areas will assist in the restoration of ROM. Patients having nonanatomic repairs (Watson-Jones, Chrisman-Snook, and others) are less likely than those patients who have had anatomic repairs to regain full rearfoot inversion.[92] Communication with the surgeon is helpful to gain insight on the potentials and precautions of the specific surgical procedure. Once the patient becomes more active, some form of protective tape or bracing is recommended.

TENDINITIS

The athlete with tendinitis may not have the most disabling injury, but has a persistent and challenging injury to effectively rehabilitate. A plethora of treatment regimes for tendinitis reflects the absence of a treatment program rigorously proven to be superior. Current treatment programs include rest, numerous physical therapy modalities, injections, stretching, strengthening, immobilization, surgery, orthotics, and other forms of support. There is little scientific research that demonstrates the efficacy of several of these treatment approaches. Most treatment programs include a combination of these treatments; however, determining when and how vigorously to apply them is challenging. At one end of the spectrum, if the athlete's musculotendinous unit and joints are immobilized, muscle and tendon atrophy, loss of soft-tissue extensibility, and joint contracture may result. On the other hand, if the athlete's rehabilitation program is too vigorous, healing is adversely affected and return to competition is delayed. Most will agree that some loading of the involved tendon is helpful. Animal studies demonstrated that imposing some mechanical tension to healing tendons results in a stronger tendon than in control animals and those immobilized.[93,94] In the following sections, some of the more common forms of tendinitis found in the foot and ankle and treatment will be discussed.

Achilles Tendinitis

Achilles tendinitis is a persistent overuse injury that challenges and often frustrates clinicians during the course of rehabilitation. Like most overuse injuries, its cause is multifactorial, and a thorough evaluation is essential to identify and address the etiologic factors. Training errors were cited as the main implicating factor in 75 percent of more than 100 runners studied by Clement and associates.[95] Varus alignment with functional pronation and insufficient gastrocnemius and soleus strength and flexibility were also implicated in this study. After addressing training errors and biomechanical factors, the most challenging aspect of rehabilitation is preparing the musculotendinous complex to withstand repetitive forces of up to 10 times body weight,[96] without traumatizing the tendon.

Acute Phase

In the first or acute phase of treatment, the clinician must modify activities, control pain and inflammation, and attempt to correct or lessen the effects of any biomechanical faults. The athlete must discontinue the training or competitive activities that contributed to the tendinitis. Pain and inflammation is controlled with various modalities. The application of these modalities should be performed several times daily. The frequent application of ice is practical and can be performed up to 20 minutes every waking hour. To decrease the tension on the Achilles tendon, a small heel lift (less than 10 mm thick) can be placed in both of the athlete's shoes. For insertional Achilles tendinitis, pain is often located on the medial aspect of the dorsal calcaneus. This may be the result of excessive tensile forces on the Achilles medial insertion due to a rearfoot valgus that accompanies excessive pronation. In this instance, a combination heel lift and medial wedge can be effective in minimizing tensile strain at the insertion site,[95] as shown in Figure 13–24. If tolerable, the athlete should begin alternative exercise for cardiovascular fitness. By the end of this phase, the patient should be able to move the ankle joint through most of the ROM with minimal discomfort.

Subacute Phase

In the subacute stage, tension must be applied to the Achilles tendon to stimulate collagen production and

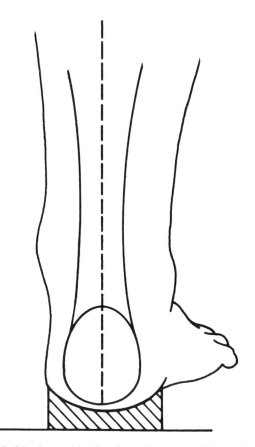

Figure 13–24. A combination heel lift and medial wedge can decrease strain on the medial insertion of the Achilles tendon.

proper orientation of the fibers along the lines of stress. Early on, this form of tension is applied through stretching the Achilles gastrocnemius soleus complex. The athlete should perform the stretching with both a straight and bent knee position to isolate the gastrocnemius and soleus, respectively (see Fig. 13-25). This stretching should be done after the athlete has done some form of general aerobic exercise (swimming, upper body ergometer), as tissues are much more extensible with an elevated temperature. Use of the BAPS is effective for improving multiplanar motion in the ankle. Since ankle ROM is usually not severely restricted in the athlete with Achilles tendinitis, a large ball under the BAPS is utilized for maximal motion. The BAPS ROM exercises are initially performed in a seated position to minimize stress to the tendon. The athlete can progress to a standing position, increasing weight bearing as tolerated. Physical modalities are continued during this phase with the aim of decreasing pain and inflammation.

Finally, strengthening of the proximal musculature is necessary in the subacute stage. This is because of potential atrophy due to disuse and the significant contribution these muscles make during loading after initial contact while running or landing from a jump. The lower extremity must be viewed as a linked system in the closed kinetic chain to completely understand the following concept. During initial contact from running, the hip and knee extensors contract eccentrically to absorb the impact of landing. The soleus is also very active during this phase to decelerate ankle dorsiflexion and knee flexion. If the more proximal muscles have weakened due to disuse, more of the work may be placed on the soleus and thus on the recovering Achilles tendon. The same concept holds true when landing from a jump, except in this case, the gastrocnemius is also very active to decelerate ankle dorsiflexion. Ideally, these muscles should be trained in the closed chain to simulate normal function. This is difficult, as the Achilles tendon may not yet be able to tolerate all encompassing closed kinetic chain exercise. The stress on the Achilles can be eliminated by having the athlete perform the leg press exercise with the force applied through the heel rather than the forefoot. Riding a stationary bike is usually tolerated at this stage and will help maintain the endurance of proximal muscles. The athlete is ready to progress into the next phase when full ROM is achieved with minimal or no pain at the end range of ankle dorsiflexion.

Rehabilitation Phase

In the rehabilitation phase, emphasis is placed on strengthening the Achilles gastrocnemius and soleus complex. The athlete should be able to tolerate moderate isometric resistance to plantar flexion before starting the strengthening exercises. Concentric and eccentric strengthening in the open-chain is least stressful and is begun with the use of an elastic band in both the bent and straight knee position (see Fig 13-26). Once the athlete has maximized the resistance provided by the elastic band, he or she can perform heel raises with the forefoot on a step, allowing the rearfoot to drop below the step into ankle dorsiflexion. This will allow strengthening throughout the range of motion. The athlete will begin this exercise in a double leg stance and as strength improves, weight should be shifted toward the affected extremity until the athlete is able to perform the exercise in a single leg stance. This exercise is performed with the knee straight, which strengthens the gastrocnemius muscle and its musculotendinous junction. The soleus is just as important as the gastrocnemius. As discussed in the biomechanics section, there are great demands on the soleus as it decelerates the forward progressing tibia between initial contact and midstance during running. The soleus can be strengthened in the bent knee position as shown in Figure 13-27.

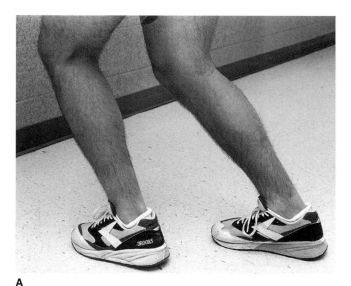

A

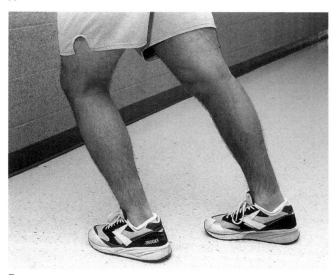

B

Figure 13–25. A. Stretching of the gastrocnemius/Achilles tendon. **B.** Stretching of the soleus/Achilles tendon.

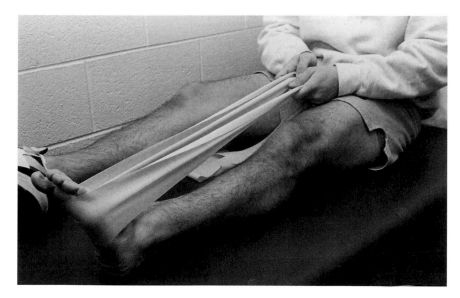

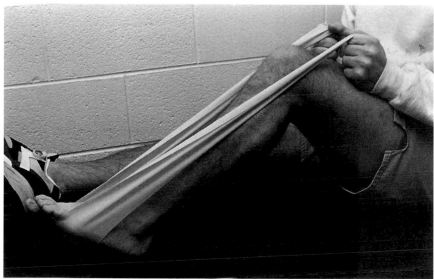

Figure 13–26. Strengthening of the gastrocnemius and soleus with elastic resistance.

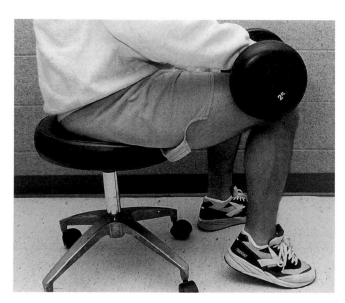

Figure 13–27. Isolation of the soleus for strengthening.

As strength improves, additional emphasis can be placed on the eccentric component. Both the heel raises and the soleus strengthening exercise can be progressed by increasing resistance. For the heel raises, this is done by holding dumbbells and for the soleus exercise, by simply increasing the weight on the machine. The athlete performs the concentric portion of the exercises (raising the heels) with double leg support, then the eccentric phase with single, involved leg support (see Fig. 13-28 and Table 13-4). Niesen-Vertommen and associates[97] demonstrated that an eccentric training program can be effective in the treatment of Achilles tendinitis. They found that a group of patients treated with an eccentric program had greater decreases in pain ratings and produced three times as many pain-free subjects than a group treated with a concentric program at the end of the 12 weeks. As emphasized earlier, because of the high demands on the musculotendinous unit with eccentric exercise, the athlete should be

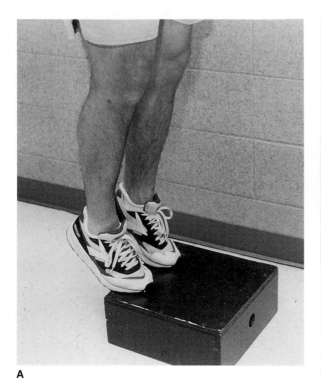
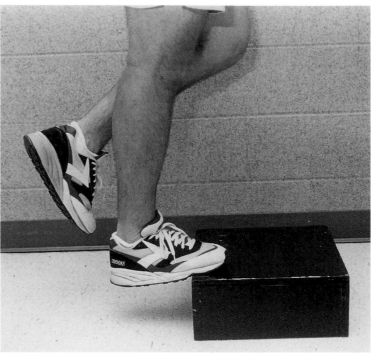

A   **B**

Figure 13–28. Strengthening the gastocnemius/soleus/Achilles complex through concentric **(A)** and eccentric **(B)** contraction. Performing the eccentric contraction with a single leg stance provides additional resistance.

slowly progressed and closely monitored. A thorough warm-up and stretching regime should precede this exercise. Stretching and cryotherapy at the completion of the exercise is recommended.

Once the above activities are well tolerated, more functional strengthening is performed. Here the clinician is invited to use his or her imagination to simulate activities the athlete will experience during sport activity. The Achilles tendon is often injured as a result of the repetitive demands placed on the tendon by rapid and forceful eccentric contractions. Thus, training should simulate these activities. Hopping is an excellent start. In hopping, the gastrocnemius and soleus complex first experiences a rapid eccentric contraction followed by a concentric contraction. The athlete can begin hopping with a double leg stance and gradually shift weight to the affected side until single leg stance hopping is tolerated. Prior to doing this on a firm surface, the hopping can be performed on a trampoline. Here, the gastrocnemius and soleus still undergoes the eccentric and concentric contractions, but it is much less demanding on the musculotendinous unit. Hopping on a firm surface can be further advanced by drop jumping. The athlete drops from a small platform, lands, and rebounds as quickly as possible onto another small platform. This is designed for the athlete involved in an explosive-type activity such as the basketball player or triple jumper. It is up to the clinician to design activities

that simulate the sport activity. It will inevitably involve the combination of eccentric and concentric contraction in a closed-chain position.

Functional Activities

The final phase of rehabilitation is return to activity. This phase is similar to that discussed for other overuse injuries. Before returning to a full training regime or competition, the athlete should have normal flexibility, strength, and endurance throughout the affected extremity. The athlete should pass all activities designed to simulate the sporting activities without pain. For runners, the return to a running program as outlined previously provides a gradual method to return to running. Finally, the athlete should also feel confident that he or she is ready to return to competition.

ACHILLES TENDON RUPTURES

Achilles tendon ruptures usually occur as a result of rapid, forceful eccentric loading as the foot and ankle are in dorsiflexion with the knee extended.[98] The treatment goal is to return to the activity that caused the original injury. Whether closed treatment or surgical repair is done, the rehabilitation process needed to achieve this goal is lengthy. Both the athlete and clinician must have patience.

TABLE 13–4. EXAMPLE OF AN ACHILLES TENDINITIS
REHABILITATION PROGRAM

Week	Days	Exercise	Activity Level
1	1 to 3	Slow drop, bilateral weight support	Cannot participate
	3 to 5	Moderate speed, bilateral support	
	6, 7	Fast drop, bilateral support	
2	1 to 3	Slow, increased weight on symptomatic leg	Cannot participate in sports
	3 to 5	Moderate, increased weight	
	6, 7	Fast, increased weight	
3	1 to 3	Slow, weight supported on symptomatic leg	Pain during rapid drop; active in sports, but limited
	3 to 5	Moderate, weight on one leg	
	6, 7	Fast speed	
4	1 to 3	Slow, add 10% of body weight	Pain during vigorous activity
	3 to 5	Moderate, same weight	
	6, 7	Fast speed	
5	1 to 3	Slow, increase by 5 to 10 lb	Pain only during exertion
	3 to 5	Moderate speed	
	6, 7	Fast speed	
6	1 to 3	Slow, increase 5 to 10 lb	Rarely experience pain
	3 to 5	Moderate speed	
	6, 7	Fast speed	

From Curwin S, Stanish WD. *Tendinitis: Its Etiology and Treatment.* New York: Macmillan; 1984. With permission.

Nonoperative Treatment

The nonoperative treatment of Achilles tendon ruptures is a battle between being overly conservative with prolonged immobilization and mobilizing the athlete too early. Prolonged mobilization results in numerous adverse effects including joint stiffness, muscle and tendon atrophy, cartilage degeneration, and others. Aggressive mobilization can result in rerupture. It is better to err on the conservative side and to be sure that adequate healing has occurred before advancing activity prematurely.

The early treatment of an Achilles tendon rupture involves some form of immobilization. The times and positioning of the lower extremity vary only slightly among clinicians. A long-leg cast is often used for the first 2 to 4 weeks followed by a short-leg cast for an additional 8 weeks.[99] During the period of the long-leg cast, the knee is flexed and the ankle is plantar flexed. The degree of plantar flexion is maximal initially and gradually brought closer to neutral during the immobilization period.[100] After the removal of the plaster, the addition of a heel lift or the wearing of cowboy boots for another month helps minimize the strain on the tendon. Clain[101] advises the use of a removable cast boot with a heel lift and a rocker sole during the month after cast removal. Heel lifts not only reduce the passive tension in the Achilles tendon, but also further reduce the tension by decreasing the activity of the gastrocnemius.[102]

Rehabilitation can begin as soon as the athlete is placed in the cast. During the period of cast immobilization, the athlete can train the uninvolved leg for cardiovascular endurance and also for the crossover effects of training. Since the athlete is nonweight-bearing for the first several weeks, the entire lower extremity will lose strength. Thus, proximal leg strengthening is needed. Hamstring stretching must also be performed during this time, especially if the athlete was placed in a bent long-leg cast during the first period of immobilization. Stretching and strengthening of the toe flexors and extensors are also done during this period.

Following removal of the cast, the primary goal is the restoration of ROM. Early on, the motion should be primarily active. The athlete can perform active inversion, eversion, plantar and dorsiflexion, ankle circles, and diagonal patterns. Passive stretching into ankle dorsiflexion is performed with a towel or elastic band the first 4 weeks out of the cast. Stretching should be done with both a straight and bent knee to isolate the gastrocnemius and soleus, respectively. As stated previously, a general body warm-up or heating modalities applied to the area prior to stretching, increases the extensibility of the tissues. Manual mobilization techniques performed on the joints of the foot and ankle can increase accessory motion. Since the athlete will be unable to dorsiflex the ankle, accessory motion needed to accomplish ankle dorsiflexion can be restored through manual techniques. The technique required is a dorsal glide of the talus in the ankle mortise. The subtalar motion and midtarsal joints should also be mobilized.

Gentle strengthening exercises can begin the first week after cast removal with elastic resistance in all planes of motion. The resistance should be light initially and increased as tolerated. The elastic band is safe to exercise with as it is difficult to apply a great amount of resistance with it. Toe flexors and extensors can be strengthened by performing toe curls and pushes using a towel and weight. The athlete should continue to perform total leg strengthening exercises, rather than just concentrating on the injured foot and ankle. Bicycling with a light resistance or swimming are performed to maintain fitness. Regaining a normal gait is facilitated with pool walking in waist deep water.

The safe and early ROM and gentle strengthening exercises are thought to assist healing by the reduction of adhesions, stimulation of the intrinsic tendon healing response, and promotion of nutrient transport.[98] Physical modalities can also assist in the healing of tendons. Ultrasound and electrical stimulation can be employed for this purpose. Transverse friction massage and soft-tissue mobilization around the ankle is also recommended after cast removal.

By 4 weeks after cast removal, the athlete should be able to ambulate in regular shoes, but may still require a heel lift. At this stage, begin heel raises starting in a neutral position with equal weight on both lower extremities. As strength increases, weight can be shifted toward the injured leg to add resistance. The athlete can progress to performing these heel raises starting from a dorsiflexed position while using an incline board. A proprioception training regime is begun as soon as the athlete is able to tolerate single leg stance. The proprioception regime described in the ankle sprain rehabilitation section can be followed. Running in waist-deep water may be tolerated during this stage. Exercise equipment such as a stair climber are effective conditioning and strengthening tools. The stair climber is particularly desirable, as it allows the gastrocnemius and soleus complex to be trained in a primarily concentric mode, protecting the tendon from the much higher stresses eccentric contractions bring.

Approximately 16 weeks after injury, much of the rehabilitation program can be followed as discussed under the Achilles tendinitis heading. Of course, the athlete with the Achilles tendon rupture will progress much more slowly. It is expected that the athlete with nonoperative treatment of an Achilles tendon rupture will be ready to run in 5 to 6 months. Vigorous activities involving rapid eccentric contractions, such as jumping and sprinting, may require 8 to 9 months of rehabilitation. The athlete must prepare and train with the ultimate goal of returning to the sport. Therefore, rehabilitation activities simulating that sport must be introduced into the program, but gradually.

Postoperative Rehabilitation

Acute Phase

The rehabilitation following repair of the Achilles tendon rupture can follow markedly different paths. Treatment after surgery can consist of cast immobilization, immediate free ankle motion, or a limited immobilization.[98,103–107] Return to full activity is generally faster than nonoperative treatment, but reports in the literature range from 5 to 12 months.[101,104] Traditional postoperative treatment of Achilles tendon repair consists of 6 to 8 weeks of immobilization with a plaster cast.[104,106] The advent of using early motion to rehabilitate patients after tendon and ligament

surgeries in other joints, prompted clinicians to question the necessity of subjecting the patient with an Achilles tendon repair to the same immobilization period. Solveborn[103] treated 17 patients with a patella tendon bearing plaster cast with a protecting frame under the foot. This orthosis made it possible for immediate weight bearing of the extremity proximal to the knee and unrestricted ankle motion. After 1 year, 88 percent of the patients had excellent results. The main drawbacks of this protocol are the cumbersome orthosis and the fact that a near-perfect fit is required for comfort and the prevention of skin breakdown around the patella tendon.

Carter[106] and Mandelbaum[107] used ankle foot orthoses to allow early, protected motion in their studies on rehabilitation after Achilles tendon repair. The orthosis used by Carter consisted of a plastizote dorsal orthosis that allowed unlimited plantar flexion and blocked dorsiflexion to neutral. The patient was placed in a bulky, compressive dressing for the first 3 to 5 days after surgery. The orthosis was then worn for the next 6 to 8 weeks. The patient was started on toe-touch weight bearing. Weight bearing was gradually increased according to the patient's tolerance. All patients were full weight bearing prior to the termination of the brace and no patients were required to wear heel lifts after removal of the brace. The rehabilitation program was not further described, but at the 2 year follow-up, patients had full ROM and plantar and dorsi flexor strength and endurance were normal. Unlimited activity was allowed when normal strength was reached, which was around the 3-month mark. No mention was made of the preinjury activity level of the patients in this study. There were no reports of rerupture.

Mandelbaum[107] studied 29 athletes with a mean age of 35. The hinged orthosis used in this study allowed full plantar flexion and dorsiflexion 10 degrees from neutral. The patient spent the first 2 weeks after surgery in a posterior splint. The hinged orthosis was then worn for the next 4 weeks. Patients progressed from partial to full weight bearing during the bracing period. Gentle ROM and strengthening exercises were initiated 1 week following surgery. Cycling and pool activities were started 2 to 3 weeks after surgery. Heel raises and jogging were initiated at 6 weeks after surgery. Patients returned to their normal activity level 4 months after surgery. At 6 months, strength deficits were only 2 to 3 percent compared to the uninvolved leg. There were no reruptures and all patients returned to their previous activity level.

Returning the athlete to competition as quickly as possible without risking reinjury is the goal for sports medicine practitioners. A rehabilitation protocol consistent with the prior discussion is preferred over prolonged immobilization. The rehabilitation team should have open communication with the surgeon.

POSTERIOR TIBIALIS TENOSYNOVITIS

Posterior tibialis tenosynovitis is a classic example of the need to treat the etiologic factors of the injury, rather than just the symptoms. Unlike other overuse injuries of the lower extremities where a multitude of etiologic factors are responsible, posterior tibialis tenosynovitis is largely due to excessive demands placed on the posterior tibial tendon during the muscle's eccentric contraction when controlling subtalar pronation. Environmental factors can increase this demand on the tendon. Running on a crowned road can increase the amount and time of pronation on the higher leg, thus making the posterior tibialis work harder and for a longer period of time. Wearing old or unsupportive shoes also places greater demands on the posterior tibialis to stabilize the foot and ankle.

Acute Phase

Treatment of posterior tibial tenosynovitis during the acute phase is as discussed in the general treatment of tendinitis, including the use of cryotherapy and physical modalities such as pulsed ultrasound and iontophoresis. Delcerda reported successful treatment of 18 cases of "shin splints" (ten were classified as posterior tibialis tendinitis) with iontophoresis. Xylocaine (2.5 percent) was used for three treatments followed by 0.5 percent hydrocortisone until pain was relieved (up to a maximum of ten treatments). Smith and co-workers[108] compared ice massage, continuous ultrasound, phonophoresis (mixture of decadron and lidocaine), and iontophoresis (mixture of dexamethasone and lidocaine) in the treatment of shin splints, which was defined in this study as medial tibial pain and tenderness. They found that all treatments were effective over the control group, but that none of the treatments were superior over the others.

Correcting any abnormal foot mechanics with temporary posting is also done during the acute phase of treatment. This may not only alleviate discomfort and minimize stress on the affected tendon, but will also give the clinician an idea if the athlete is a candidate for more permanent orthotic fabrication. As mentioned earlier, excessive or prolonged pronation is a common finding in those with posterior tendon problems. A medial heel wedge made of 0.5 to 1.0 cm felt can limit subtalar pronation. Compensatory subtalar pronation due to a forefoot varus can be controlled with 0.5 to 1.0 cm felt pad placed under the medial forefoot (just distal to the calcaneus to the first metatarsal head). These temporary posts can be secured under the inner pad of the athletic shoe that is removable. If these temporary measures appear to correct the biomechanical faults and lessen discomfort with ambulation, the athlete should be further evaluated and fitted with a permanent foot orthotic.

Subacute Phase

During the subacute phase of rehabilitation, any strength or flexibility deficits found in the exam should be addressed. Muscles that eccentrically control the internal rotation of the lower extremity occurring between the initial contact and midstance phase of gait should be strengthened. In closed-chain function, excessive and prolonged pronation is associated with excessive or prolonged internal rotation throughout the lower extremity. The posterior tibialis is active in decelerating internal rotation of the tibia. Thus, it is thought that strengthening other muscles that decelerate internal rotation of the lower limb may lessen the load on the posterior tibialis. Other muscles that decelerate lower extremity internal rotation include the flexor hallucis and digitorum longus, biceps, femoris, and hip external rotators. The anterior tibialis does not decelerate internal rotation of the tibia directly, but does assist the decelerating subtalar pronation and should also be strengthened specifically. During the subacute phase, strengthening these muscles is most tolerated in open-chain positions. Finally, during this phase, ankle ROM and stretching of the posterior tibialis tendon is beneficial as it facilitates movement of the tendon within the sheath and may assist in the prevention of adhesions between the tendon and sheath. Alternative exercise to maintain lower extremity strength and cardiovascular fitness may include bicycling, stair step machine, deep water running with a float vest, or swimming.

Rehabilitation Phase

The rehabilitative phase involves greater tensile loading of the posterior tibialis tendon. This can be accomplished through isolation of the posterior tibialis tendon through open-chain strengthening using elastic resistance. The pattern to isolate the posterior tibialis would be the plantar flexion and inversion diagonal pattern. The BAPS in a seated position can also be used safely during early strengthening. The weight placed on the medial side of the BAPS allows both concentric and eccentric strengthening of the decelerators of pronation. Resistance is increased through the addition of weights and increasing weight bearing. Progressing to standing will enhance the coordination of more proximal muscle groups involved in decelerating lower extremity internal rotation. Further resistance can be added by wrapping an elastic band around the leg and connecting it to a stationary object. The band wrapped in this manner while performing partial squats places additional demands on the internal rotation decelerators.

Athletes involved in court sports or those involving lateral movements spend much of the time on the forefoot. These athletes with a forefoot varus will compensate with excessive subtalar pronation, placing great tensile strain on the posterior tibialis tendon and causing early fatigue of the muscle. These patients must have an orthotic that extends the length of the forefoot to prevent the subtalar compensation. In addition, these athletes must train in activities that will simulate the foot and ankle positioning used in their sport. Before the athlete performs functional training of the ball of the foot, however, the tibialis posterior must be assessed to ensure adequate strength. Conti[109] reports that when the athlete raises up on the toes, the rear foot should invert. If it does not, the reason is due to pain, weakness, or a tendon tear. Athletes may also learn substitution patterns to prevent stress on the tendon. Thus, if the athlete's rear foot does not invert, further testing of the tibialis posterior is warranted prior to functional training.

Functional Activities

In the fourth phase, the athlete performs sport simulation activities and is gradually returned to competitive training. Many athletes with this problem are either runners or running is a large part of their activity. For long-distance runners, the return to running program previously presented in this chapter provides a guideline to ease the runner back to training. Hills and uneven surfaces should be avoided initially. Athletes in court sports or who spend much time on their forefoot should focus their training on activities like jump roping and lateral movements on the forefoot. Thorough warm-ups prior to training and ice afterwards to control inflammation are encouraged. In addition, muscles identified as inflexible or weak should continue to be specifically trained as part of the athlete's normal routine, even after symptoms are gone.

Rehabilitation After Surgery for Posterior Tibialis Tendon Problem

The type of surgeries performed for posterior tibialis problems include tenosynovectomy for a recalcitrant tendinitis and repair of a partial or complete rupture of the tendon. The general times of immobilization and expected return to activity are described by Conti[109] and are as follows. With tenosynovectomy, the first 3 postoperative weeks are spent in a nonweight-bearing, short-leg cast in slight inversion and plantarflexion. During the second 3 weeks after surgery, a weight-bearing, removable ankle walker boot in neutral is worn. ROM is begun after the first cast is removed at 3 weeks. The athlete can return to sports when full ROM is restored and strength is 80 percent. With the repair of a partially or completely ruptured tendon, the time period of initial immobilization and nonweight-bearing is 4 weeks. Then, instead of the walker boot, a short-leg, weight-bearing cast in neu-

tral is worn for 2 to 3 additional weeks. Return to competitive sports is predicted at 6 months after surgery for these patients.

The rehabilitation of these patients is not significantly different from rehabilitation after other surgical procedures in the foot and ankle. The athlete can participate in upper body, contralateral lower extremity, or ipsilateral proximal lower extremity exercise to maintain fitness during the period of immobilization. Both active and passive ROM should begin immediately after cast removal. The tendon's sliding action through its sheath and surrounding soft tissue will help prevent the formation of adhesions between the tendon and surrounding soft tissue, thus facilitating restoration of ROM. Soft tissue and joint mobilization will also assist in the return of full ROM. Strengthening with the use of isometrics can begin after cast removal and gradually progress. With posterior tibial tendon ruptures, strengthening of the posterior tibial tendon should progress slowly, with only light resistance until at least postoperative week[12]. Thereafter, strengthening can progress using the general guidelines for the rehabilitation of tendinitis, while carefully monitoring for pain and signs of increased inflammation. Orthotics to control pronation are worn to lower the demand on the posterior tibialis tendon.

PERONEAL TENDON INJURIES

Injury to the peroneal tendons often occur as a result of an acute dorsiflexion and eversion injury, a lax retinaculum due to chronic ankle instability, or from overuse.[110] In the first two cases, the peroneal tendons can sublux over the lateral malleolus. In these cases, the primary problem, either the eversion sprain or chronic instability, must be addressed initially. After appropriate rehabilitation, treatment can be focused on the peroneal tendons, should they still be a source of complaint.

Tendinitis and Tenosynovitis

The treatment for peroneal tendinitis and tenosynovitis does not differ from that outlined in the general treatment of tendinitis. This includes the use of physical modalities to control pain and inflammation, stretching, strengthening, foot orthotics if indicated, alternative activity, and a gradual return to competitive training when ready. Peroneal tendinitis may occur at two different sites, at the distal fibular groove or where the peroneus longus courses under the cuboid. Subotnick[110] terms the inflammation of the peroneal tendon or its sheath at the latter location the peroneal and cuboid syndrome. According to Subotnick, the cuboid may become everted or mildly subluxed during supination or inversion injuries. The pulling of the peroneal tendons may further accentuate this position and the altered position of the cuboid may further irritate the tendon. To restore its normal position, the cuboid can be manipulated as described by Newell and Woodan.[111] Following manipulation, the area can be stabilized with tape and padding. The pad should be placed on the plantar surface of the medial portion of the cuboid in an attempt to invert the cuboid. Tape is then applied starting from the dorsal lateral side of the foot going to the plantar, depressing the lateral portion of cuboid. A thorough biomechanical evaluation may also identify the need for custom foot orthotics to stabilize the foot in these patients.

Peroneal tendinitis is related to factors other than pure overuse, in particular, chronic lateral ankle instability, and these must be addressed. A rehabilitation program as described under the ankle sprain rehabilitation section of this chapter is initiated in such conditions. Another factor causing peroneal tendinitis is recurrent subluxation and dislocation of the peroneal tendons over the lateral malleolus. This is often associated with a shallow fibular groove, a lax or stretched retinaculum, and chronic ankle instability.[105] The chronic instability of the tendon is usually initiated with a traumatic dorsiflexion and eversion injury to the ankle, which will often avulse the peroneal retinaculum off the distal fibula.[110] In the case of the traumatic dislocation, rehabilitation is begun after a period of immobilization in a nonweight-bearing cast. Following cast removal, rehabilitation is similar to that described in the ankle sprain rehabilitation section. However, since ankle dorsiflexion and eversion encourages the forward subluxation of the peroneal tendon, this combined motion should be avoided the first few weeks after immobilization is discontinued. If chronic peroneal subluxation develops, taping the ankle to restrict ankle dorsiflexion and eversion may be beneficial.[112] A medial wedge may also provide the same effect.

Rehabilitation After Surgery for the Dislocating Peroneal Tendon

Due to the numerous operative procedures for this problem, it is imperative that the rehabilitation professional communicate with the surgeon to determine the type of procedure performed and the specific rehabilitation precautions. Following surgery, the patient is often immobilized for a period of up to 6 weeks, part of this time may be in a weight-bearing cast. During immobilization, cardiovascular conditioning is performed along with proximal muscle strengthening. Following immobilization, ROM exercises are initiated. Any motions that may markedly stress the peroneal tendons are avoided for 3 weeks. These motions would be dorsiflexion and inversion. Soft tissue mobilization around the scar site can be employed to increase the soft tissue mobility. With the exception of the motion precautions, rehabilitation can

proceed much like that of the chronic ankle sprain. However, the rehabilitation after surgery is likely to take more time to fully restore motion, strength, and function.

POSTERIOR TIBIAL TENDINITIS

Epidemiology

Inflammation of the posterior tibial tendon is a frequently encountered overuse syndrome, mostly in runners. Spontaneous rupture of the posterior tibial tendon in athletes is extremely rare. Woods and Leach have reported partial or complete posterior tibial tendon ruptures in only six athletic patients.[112a] Though posterior tibial tendon ruptures are very rare in athletes, tendinitis or tenosynovitis accounts for 0.6 to 3.6 percent of injuries among runners.

Functional Anatomy and Mechanism

The tibialis posterior muscle arises in the deep posterior compartment of the leg originating from the proximal third of the tibial, proximal two thirds of the fibula, and the interosseous membrane. It is innervated by the tibial nerve and runs distally behind the medial malleolus in a tendinous form through the tarsal tunnel. It inserts on the navicular tuberosity, the base of the second, third, and fourth metatarsal bases, all the cuneiforms, and the cuboid. The main action of this muscle is plantar flexion and inversion of the foot and opposes eversion. The normal excursion of the posterior tibial tendon is 2 cm. It works in conjunction with the flexor digitorium longus and the flexor hallucis longus as the dynamic stabilizer of the longitudinal arch together with the static restraints, spring ligament, and the deep plantar ligaments.

Funk has shown that, during gait, the foot will progressively invert after the initial heel strike, locking the midfoot to allow the gastrocnemius soleus complex to produce a more stable heel rise and efficient toe-off.[112b] With loss of the posterior tibial function, the force of the gastrocnemius soleus complex will act on the talonavicular joint, rather than the metatarsophalangeal joint, losing the moment arm of the metatarsals. This results in a less efficient toe-off.

History and Physical Exam

The patient will complain of pain just distal to the medial malleolus and weakness. The pain is made worse with activity and is relieved with rest or NSAIDs. It is important to ask about any change in training intensity, as this may precipitate tenosynovitis. Training errors, such as type of shoes or running on a banked oval track only in one direction, should be specifically questioned. A history of direct trauma may suggest edema within the tendon sheath. Finally, athletes may also have a systemic disease such as rheumatoid arthritis and seronegative arthropathies, which may incite inflammatory tenosynovitis, commonly along the posterior tibial tendon.

On physical exam, first observe for general abnormalities of the foot such as a prominent navicular tuberosity of a hyperpronated foot. Look for swelling behind or distal to the medial malleolus. Palpate the course of the tendon. The area of the maximum tenderness is usually in the area just posterior and distal to the medial malleolus or at the insertion site, usually associated with an accessory navicular bone. Pain and weakness can be elicited with the single heel rise test and the resisted inversion of the everted and plantar flexed foot.

A neurologic exam should be performed to rule out nerve entrapment in the tarsal tunnel. Ankle stability and subtalar motion should be checked to rule out painful joint abnormalities.

Diagnostic Studies

Plain radiographs of the foot anteroposterior, lateral and oblique, along with anteroposterior, lateral, and mortise views of the ankle are taken. These views are rarely helpful in diagnosing posterior tibial tenosynovitis; however, they are important in differentiating fractures or stress fractures and in identifying accessory navicular problems.

For cases failing functional rehabilitation, magnetic resonance imaging (MRI) is indicated. MRI may reveal abnormal signal and thickening of the surrounding sheath due to edema or abnormal signal or thickening within the tendon (see Figs. 13-29 and 13-30). The MRI is also useful to look for intra-articular pathology and stress fractures of the midfoot and hindfoot.

Functional Rehabilitation

The rehabilitation of tendinitis can be broken down into four stages: acute, subacute, rehabilitation, and return to activity. The goals of each of these stages are listed in Table 13-5. What stage of treatment is applicable to the athlete depends on several factors. Time, of course, is one factor. If the onset of symptoms is less than 48 to 72 hours, the injury is considered acute. With chronic tendinitis, however, the athlete experiences recurrent exacerbations and time alone is not a good indicator. In the acute phase, the athlete will complain of pain in the affected structure before the end of the ROM is reached. In the chronic stage, the end of the ROM will be reached before the athlete complains of pain. The additional application of passive overpressure will often be needed to reproduce the pain. The use of isometric resistance can similarly be used to determine the acuteness of an injury to the musculoskeletal unit. If the athlete complains of pain with minimal isometric resistance to the examiner's force, the patient is in the acute stage of injury. The ability to tolerate moderate to maximal iso-

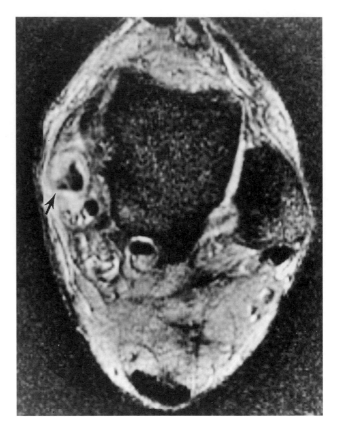

Figure 13–29. T2 gradient MRI of a partial tear of the posterior tibial tendon with surrounding tenosynovitis. Notice the increased signal within the tendon and surrounding tendon sheath (*arrow*).

metric resistance places the athlete in the subacute to chronic stage of tendinitis. Finally, if pain in the affected musculotendinous unit can only be elicited with a strong isometric contraction while in a lengthened position or with strong and rapid eccentric contractions, the athlete is in the chronic stage of the injury and closer to recovery.

Acute Phase

In the acute stage, which lasts approximately 72 hours after onset of symptoms, the athlete should stop all painful activities. Ice and other modalities are applied to decrease pain and inflammation. The administration of dexamethasone through iontophoresis is effective in decreasing pain in patients with musculoskeletal inflammatory conditions[113] and is recommended in the acute treatment of tendinitis. Low-voltage galvanic stimulation increased the tensile strength in tenotomized animal tendons,[114] as did the application of pulsed ultrasound.[115] The application of continuous ultrasound during the acute phase is not recommended as the thermal effects may exacerbate the inflammation. Support to the foot and ankle in the form of tap-

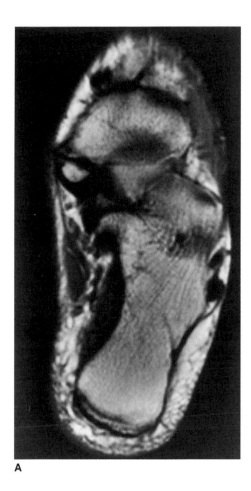

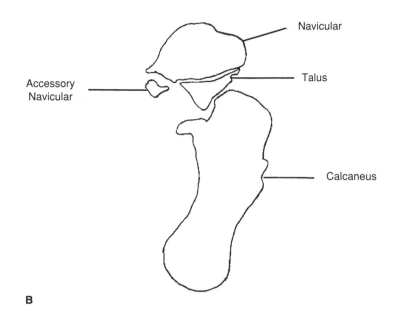

Figure 13–30. A. T1 MRI of accessory navicular with evidence of degeneration between accessory navicular and tarsal navicular. **B.** Corresponding line drawing.

ing, padding, or temporary posting to address any biomechanical faults should be performed during this phase. Alternative exercise can begin to maintain the athlete's fitness level and strength in the more proximal joints. In cases of severe pain, immobilization may be necessary for several days.

Subacute Phase

During this phase, the application of gentle tension to assist collagen production and remodeling[116] is begun. This is done primarily through gentle stretching and active ROM to tolerance. The ROM can be performed initially in the open-chain position and progressed to the closed-chain position using the BAPS with minimal weight-bearing in the seated position. Prior to stretching, a general total body warm-up is recommended to increase the elasticity of the musculotendinous units. The application of ice and other modalities to decrease pain and inflammation is continued during this phase. If not yet begun in the acute stage, alternative activities to maintain cardiovascular fitness and proximal lower extremity strength are initiated.

Rehabilitation Phase

During the third stage, rehabilitation, increased tensile loading of the affected musculotendinous unit is initi-

ated. The stretching program initiated during the subacute phase should be continued to maintain or increase extensibility of the involved musculotendinous group. Additional stress is provided through resistive exercises. The athlete should progress from isometric, isotonic, and then isokinetic exercise. Initially, low loads and more repetitions are performed, and then resistance is

TABLE 13–5. GENERAL GOALS IN THE REHABILITATION OF TENDINITIS

Acute phase	Control pain and inflammation. Maintain ROM. Maintain cardiovascular and proximal lower extremity strength.
Subacute phase	The above. Increase ROM. Promote appropriate collagen remodeling.
Rehabilitation phase	Promote appropriate collagen remodeling. Full and pain-free ROM. Normal strength and proprioception. Appropriate recruitment and coordination of synergist muscles during functional exercise.
Return to activity	Return to competition without recurrence.

increased gradually, as tolerated. With isokinetics, moderate speeds are performed, first with faster velocities to simulate functional speeds later.

Both open and closed-chain exercises should be performed. Though open-chain strengthening exercises do not simulate normal activity well, they do allow isolation of the involved musculotendinous unit. Neglecting this may allow other synergistic muscles to substitute for the involved muscle to produce the motion. This was shown in postoperative anterior cruciate ligament (ACL) reconstruction patients during stair climbing. In this study, knee extensor power was significantly decreased in the involved limb while stair climbing. To make up for this deficit, there was a significant increase in the hip extensor power in the same limb. Though this example does not involve the foot and ankle, similar substitution strategies are likely. Substituting a synergist for the involved musculotendinous unit is especially likely if the athlete experiences discomfort in the affected tendon while performing strengthening exercises in the full weight-bearing closed-chain position. Thus, open-chain strengthening exercises are performed initially to gain adequate strength. Once moderate to maximal resistance is tolerated without pain, the athlete is ready to move on to closed-chain strengthening exercises in a full weight-bearing, double stance position. As strength and tolerance improves, the athlete gradually shifts weight to the affected extremity to increase weight bearing on the leg until the exercise is performed in a single limb stance position. This progression may take days or weeks depending on the specific affliction. The concept of adequate strength in the open-chain position prior to beginning closed-chain exercises is in reference to full weight-bearing, strengthening exercises. Closed-chain exercises to improve strength, ROM, and propriocep-

TABLE 13–6. ECCENTRIC TRAINING PROGRAM

Begin with an alternate activity for a thorough warm-up and proceed to the following.

1. Stretch
   Static stretch
   Hold 15 to 30 seconds
   Repeat 3 or 4 times
2. Eccentric exercise
   Three sets of 10 repetitions
   Progression:
   Days 1 and 2: slow
   Days 3 to 5: moderate
   Days 6 and 7: fast
   Increase external resistance; after day 7, repeat cycle
3. Stretch, as prior to exercise
4. Ice over the tender or painful area

Eccentric training program as outlined by Curwin and Stanish.[120a]

tion in a partial weight-bearing position can begin very early in the rehabilitation program.

During the third phase, exercise is the area of emphasis, though modalities are continued. Other modalities, including heat, are often begun during this stage. Though various modalities are used in the treatment of tendinitis, little clinical research on patient populations is available that compares the effectiveness of different types of modalities. Ultrasound is commonly used in the treatment of tendinitis. In a study on rat Achilles tendons, application of continuous wave ultrasound increased collagen synthesis and breaking strengths of the tendons.[117] Continuous ultrasound can also produce a vigorous heating effect. This effect on contracted soft tissue prior to and during prolonged stretching is effective in increasing extensibility of muscles, ligaments, and tendons.[118] Another common technique used in the treatment of tendinitis is transverse friction massage. This technique can increase local blood flow, improve the mobility and extensibility of the ligament or tendon structures, and promote normal orientation of collagen fibers. Transverse friction massage can be taught to the patient for more frequent applications during the day and is also an effective way to warm up the tendon prior to activity or stretching. For each session of transverse friction massage, Gross[119] recommends starting the massage over an adjacent, nonpainful area of the tendon, progressing to the affected area, and then finishing in a nonpainful area. Finally, thorough assessment for permanent foot orthoses should be performed at this time.

Both the open and closed-chain strengthening exercises early in the third phase are performed with equal emphasis on concentric and eccentric contractions. The submaximal eccentric loading during this phase of rehabilitation probably provides no additional tensile stress on the musculotendinous unit than concentric exercise.[119] However, maximal, high-velocity eccentric contractions do provide a higher tensile load to the musculotendinous unit.[120] These high-velocity eccentric contractions occur in every athletic activity to decelerate rapid angular motions. Thus, before an athlete returns to competitive training, he or she must be able to withstand these stresses. Performing rapid, eccentric contractions for training results in increased tensile strength of the musculotendinous unit[116] and makes the musculotendinous unit less vulnerable to injury. Specifically, eccentric strengthening exercises in the functional, closed kinetic chain are most effective and have the additional benefit of neural adaptations to coordinate optimal performance (see Table 13–6). Pain, speed, and resistance are guides to therapy progression (see Fig. 13–31). The load on the musculotendinous unit is increased not only by increasing the resistance, but also by increasing the speed of con-

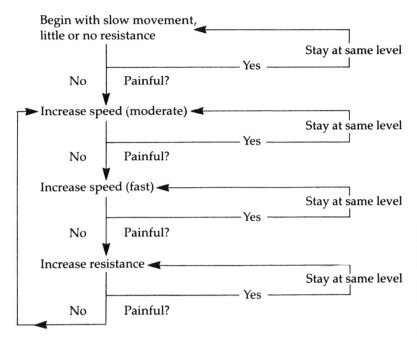

Figure 13–31. Progression of the eccentric training program. The load on the musculo-tendinous unit is not only increased by increased resistance, but also by increasing the speed of the exercise. *(From Curwin S, Stanish WD. In: Tendinitis: Its Etiology and Treatment. New York: Macmillan; 1984. With permission.)*

traction. While fast concentric contractions are associated with a relatively light demand, the faster the eccentric contraction, the greater the demand on the musculotendinous unit.[120] The athlete's progression is gauged by pain in this program. If there is no pain during 3 sets of 10 repetitions, the subject is not working hard enough. If pain is felt throughout the exercise period, there is either too much resistance or the speed of contraction is too rapid. The ideal load on the musculotendinous unit is one that produces some discomfort in the last set of 10 repetitions. Because of the high loads on tendons and muscle soreness associated with eccentric contractions, the athlete should progress cautiously and be monitored closely during this program.

Surgical Treatment

Patients unresponsive to functional rehabilitation after 3 to 4 months may undergo a surgical tenosynovectomy. The goal of the operation is to remove inflamed tissue and reduce the bulk of the tendon. This allows for improved function and prevents further degeneration. However, for patients with insertional tendinitis and associated accessory navicular, the accessory navicular is excised and the tendon is reattached to the medial side of the navicular.

ANTERIOR TIBIAL TENDINITIS

Anterior tibial tendinitis is an uncommon condition associated with overuse in running, hiking, or local irritation from ski boots.[121] The patient will have localized swelling, tenderness, and crepitus over the tendon.[121] The tibialis anterior muscle arises from the proximal two thirds of the tibia. The lateral tibial condyle and the interosseous membrane travels in a straight course under the superior extensor retinaculum and inserts on the dorsal medial navicular, medial cuneiform, and the base of the first metatarsal.[122,123] The muscle is innervated by the deep peroneal nerve and it provides 80 percent of the dorsiflexion power of the foot.[122] The tibialis anterior is a powerful tendon that is able to undergo repeated eccentric loading during heel strike to foot flat.[124] It is postulated that due to its straight line of pull without a bony fulcrum and its excellent blood supply, injury appears to be rare and usually transient.[121,125]

PERONEAL TENDON TENDINITIS, SUBLUXATION, AND DISLOCATIONS

Epidemiology

Peroneal tendinitis or tenosynovitis is a relatively rare source of significant disability for the athlete. Acute tendinitis or tenosynovitis occurs when an athlete returns to activity after a period of inactivity.[126] The original case of dislocated peroneal tendon was initially described by Monteggia in a ballet dancer in 1803.[127] The incidence of peroneal tendon dislocation is about 0.9 percent of lower extremity injuries in skiers.[128] Among reported cases, 97 percent are related to athletic activity; 71 percent in snow skiing, 7 percent in football, and the remainder in basketball, soccer, and ice skating.[129] However, asymptomatic congenital dislocation of the peroneal tendon appears to be more common. A 3.3 percent incidence of peroneal tendon dislocation was noted in neonates and infants with all of these cases resolving spontaneously without treatment.[130]

Functional Anatomy and Mechanism

The peroneus brevis and the longus muscle comprise the lateral compartment of the leg. The peroneus brevis muscle originates on the lower two thirds of the lateral aspect of the fibular and the intermuscular septa. The tendinous portion travels posterior to the lateral malleolus and anterior to the peroneus longus tendon. As it passes behind the lateral malleolus, it travels lateral to the calcaneofibular ligament and inserts on the fifth metatarsal styloid.[131] The peroneus longus muscle originates on the lateral tibial condyle, the upper two thirds of the lateral surface of the fibula. The long tendinous portion travels behind the lateral malleolus and the tendon of peroneus brevis. Then the tendon travels inferior to the peroneal tubercle on the calcaneus, entering its own tunnel and traveling beneath the cuboid. It travels under the long plantar ligament and inserts on the lateral side of the medial cuneiform and the base of the first metatarsal.[131] Both of these muscles are innervated by the superficial peroneal nerve and work to evert and plantar flex the foot (see Fig. 13–32).[131]

As the tendons of the peroneus brevis and longus pass behind the lateral malleolus, they are kept in position by the sulcus of the distal fibular and the superior peroneal retinaculum. The superior peroneal retinaculum is formed as a condensation of the superficial fascia of the leg and the sheath of the peroneal tendons, beginning about 2 cm proximal to the tip of the fibula on the posterior aspect. It then inserts on the fascia surrounding the Achilles tendon and is about 1 to 2 cm wide.[131,132]

The superior peroneal retinaculum is the principle structure injured in the acute peroneal tendon dislocation. The retinaculum separates from its origin on the fibula.[126,133,134] Also about 18 percent of fibulae exhibit convex of flat posterior sulcus, predisposing to dislocation.[135]

The mechanism of injury in tendinitis and tenosynovitis is primarily related to repetitive movement (overuse) and direct trauma.[129] Cavovarus deformity of the foot may increase peroneal stress, leading to tendinitis.[136] Chronic subluxation of the peroneal tendons during the toe-off phase of gait may predispose a person to tendinitis and tenosynovitis.[136] In dislocation of the peroneal tendon causing a superior peroneal retinaculum tear, the mechanism is a sudden dorsiflexion of the inverted foot with reflex contracture of the peroneal muscles.[127]

History and Physical Exam

Often the patient will give a history of returning to athletic activity after a period of inactivity or a history of trauma.[126,127] They will complain of pain and swelling behind and just distal to the fibula.[126] If the symptoms develop over a period of several weeks, it may represent chronic tendinitis due to overuse. However, if swelling and pain occur without activity, it may be associated with systemic inflammation such as rheumatoid arthritis. First, inspect and look for swelling posterior to the lateral malleolus and any cavovarus deformity of the foot. Palpation will reveal tenderness along the tendon sheath from the lateral malleolus distally.[127] Symptoms will be exacerbated by eversion of an inverted foot to resistance and passive inversion and plantar flexion.[127] The patient may also exhibit an antalgic gait and limited subtalar motion.

In athletes with acute subluxation or dislocation of the peroneal tendons, it may be difficult to differentiate from a lateral ankle sprain. They will complain of lateral

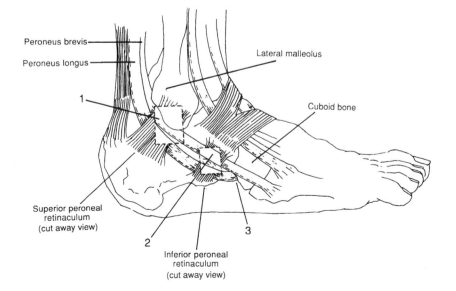

Figure 13–32. Regions of stenosis of the peroneal tendon. Stenosis occurs at regions of increased stress around fixed pulleys **(1)** posterior to the lateral malleolus; **(2)** peroneal trochlea; **(3)** peroneus longus tendon passing under the cuboid. *(From Trevino S, Baumhauer JF. Tendon injuries of the foot and ankle. Clin Sports Med. 1994;4:728. With permission.)*

ankle pain suffered during an athletic event. However, patients cannot explain the position of the foot during the injury. On exam, the point of maximal tenderness is posterior to the fibula, while in ankle sprains it is usually anterior to the fibula.[129] As in tendinitis, stressing the retinaculum by resisted dorsiflexion with eversion causes pain and may dislocate the tendons.[127]

In chronic subluxation or dislocation, a patient will complain of popping or a snapping sensation of the lateral ankle. This may or may not be associated with pain and swelling.[129] On examination, there may be mild swelling or tenderness of the posterior fibula. The ankle should be tested to rule out ligamentous injury. Stressing the retinaculum by resisted dorsiflexion with eversion may reproduce the dislocation or cause apprehension.[129]

Diagnostic Studies

Plain radiographs of the ankle in the anteroposterior, mortise, and lateral views will be helpful to look for a possible bony fragment off the posterior lateral border of the lateral malleolus. This fragment may be present in 15 to 50 percent of superior peroneal retinaculum avulsions.[137-139] In chronic cases, a MRI may be indicated. In tendinitis, a MRI will show edema around the tendon and possible edema within the tendon. In subluxation and dislocations, MRI will show a deficiency of the superior peroneal retinaculum near the posterior lateral fibular border, dislocated peroneal tendons, or tears within the peroneus brevis tendon at or above the lateral malleolus (see Fig. 13-33).[126]

Surgical Treatment

In recalcitrant chronic tendinitis, surgical debridement of the tendon and tenosynovectomy can be performed.[126,129]

In acute subluxation or dislocation of the peroneal tendon, controversy exists about its treatment. Nonoperative treatment can lead up to an 80 percent redislocation rate.[134,140] Acute surgical treatment may afford better results, with some reports of a 76 percent excellent results rate.[134] Many types of repairs are described, but the main goal is to anatomically reconstruct the superior peroneal retinaculum.[129,133]

In chronic subluxation or dislocation, surgery is indicated if the patient remains symptomatic. However, there are many surgical options with variable reported success rates. These can be divided into the following categories: (1) reattachment of the superior peroneal retinaculum with local tissue augmentation, (2) a bone block procedure, (3) reinforcement of the superior peroneal retinaculum with tissue transfer, (4) rerouting of the peroneal tendons, and (5) groove-deepening procedures.

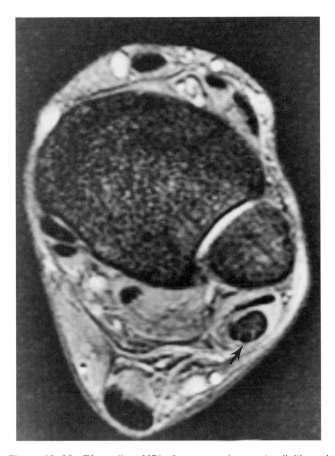

Figure 13–33. T2 gradient MRI of peroneus longus tendinitis and tenosynovitis. Arrow points to the thickening of the peroneus longus tendon with increased signal within the tendon and the surrounding tendon sheath.

ACHILLES TENDINITIS

Epidemiology

Injury to the Achilles tendon is common among athletes.[141] Achilles tendon injuries afflict runners with an incidence of injury from 6 to 18 percent.[142-144] Achilles injury is prevalent in any sport requiring vigorous repetitive plantar flexion of the foot such as football, track and field, basketball, gymnastics, running, bicycling, and skiing.[145] Repetitive motion leads to tendinitis, while forceful concentric or eccentric contraction of the gastrocsoleus complex leads to rupture.[146] However, acute rupture in an athlete less than age 30 is uncommon. They are associated with the over age 30, weekend athlete.[145-147] One study shows that 62 percent of the ruptures occurred in professionals and white collar workers with sedentary day jobs who participated in sports activities occasionally.[148]

Other factors that may lead to Achilles tendinitis are training errors, hyperpronation of the foot, poor gastrocsoleus flexibility, and improper shoe wear.[149] Tendinitis may be associated with anatomic impingement such as Haglund's deformity.[150] Systemic disorders such as seronegative arthropathy or gout can lead to tendinitis or rupture. Aging also predisposes a person to tendinitis and acute ruptures, as the Achilles tendon undergoes degeneration and loses its flexibility.[147] Males have a higher reported incidence of rupture.[151]

Functional Anatomy and Mechanism

The Achilles tendon is comprised of tissue from the gastrocnemius and the soleus muscles. The gastrocnemius originates from the medial condyle of the femur and the lateral femoral condyle and crosses the knee joint. The soleus originates on the posterior aspect of the proximal third of the fibula, soleal line on the tibia, and the interosseous membrane. The soleus lies deep to the gastrocnemius in the superficial posterior compartment of the lower leg and is innervated by the tibial nerve. The two tendons coalesce and insert on the distal aspect of the calcaneal tuberosity.[152,153] The fibers of the tendon twist one quarter turn as it inserts on the calcaneus. This leaves the soleus insertion more medial to the gastrocnemius insertion.[154]

The Achilles tendon lacks a true synovial sheath, but is encased by the paratenon, which enhances tendon gliding by minimizing friction between the tendon and the surrounding epitenon.[153]

The Achilles tendon receives its blood supply from the bony and muscular attachment.[155] A watershed area exists about 2 to 6 cm proximal to the bony insertion site[156] and is the clinically reported site of tendon degeneration and rupture.

Distally, the tendon is also surrounded by a retrocalcaneal bursa and a precalcaneal bursa.[157] These protective bursas may become inflamed and cause irritation.

It has been estimated an Achilles tendon force of 6 to 8 times the body weight is exerted during running, which approaches the ultimate strength of the cadaveric tendon.[157] Therefore, any jumping activity exceeding the ultimate strength of the Achilles tendon may lead to a rupture in the hypovascular area of the tendon.

During walking and running, the calcaneus pronates from heel strike to toe-off and slightly externally rotates with regard to the tibia. This motion subjects the medial portion of the Achilles tendon to a higher tensile load.[158] Therefore, hyperpronation of the foot will lead to increased tensile load on the medial Achilles tendon insertion.

The site of Achilles tendon pain is either at the calcaneal insertion (insertional tendinitis) or in the midportion of the tendon (noninsertional tendinitis).

History and Examination

Patients will complain of pain in the posterior calcaneus with insertional type tendinitis, or pain about 2 to 6 cm proximal to the insertion of the Achilles tendon in non-insertional Achilles tendinitis.[159] The patient will also complain of pain with activity, especially running uphill or during acceleration.[153,159] It is important to ask about changes in the patient's level of activity; change in mileage, degree of hill running, interval training, type of shoe wear, and running surface are important in the etiology of this condition.[150,153,157]

On physical exam, patients with insertional tendinitis may have an associated excessive superior prominence (Haglund's deformity) of the calcaneal tuberosity.[160] They will also exhibit tenderness of this area. In patients with noninsertional tendinitis, the area of maximal tenderness and swelling will be about 2 to 6 cm proximal to the insertion.[153] Nodular swelling within the tendon may signify chronic tendinitis.[153] They will also exhibit pain with passive dorsiflexion of the foot. Tenderness anterior to the Achilles tendon may signify retrocalcaneal bursitis, and tenderness posterior to the calcaneal tuberosity may signify precalcaneal bursitis due to irritating shoe wear.[153,159] It is important to look for general alignment of the lower extremity. Femoral anteversion, genu varum, tibia vara, and subtalar pronation can result in excessive Achilles tendon excursion and subsequent degeneration in noninsertional tendinitis.[153] Cavus foot may increase the symptoms of insertional tendinitis by bringing the bony prominence closer to the Achilles tendon and the heel counter of the shoe.[159]

Achilles tendon ruptures may or may not follow a prodrome of Achilles pain.[147,155] Patients often describe a sudden pop or snap in the lower extremity with immediate pain.[155] On examination, there will be a palpable gap between the ends of the Achilles tendon. However, diagnosis may be difficult due to edema and hematoma at the rupture site. The patient will not be able to perform a single limb heel rise. Thompson's test is performed by squeezing the calf. Failure of passive foot plantar flexion is a sign of tendon rupture. This test is 100 percent reliable in acute ruptures and 80 percent in chronic ruptures.[161]

Diagnostic Studies

Plain radiographs of the foot and ankle should be obtained. The bony contour of the calcaneus (radiograph of Haglund's deformity), calcification in the Achilles tendon, and soft-tissue swelling may be noted.[150]

MRI may be indicated in chronic Achilles tendinitis, partial tears of the Achilles tendon, and chronic tears of the Achilles tendon. MRI can differentiate between paratendinous adhesion and swelling versus true tendinous degeneration (see Fig. 13-34).[150,153]

Surgical Treatment

Patients who fail rehabilitation are candidates for surgical release of posterior fascia, excision of inflamed or scarred paratenon, and debridement of degenerative

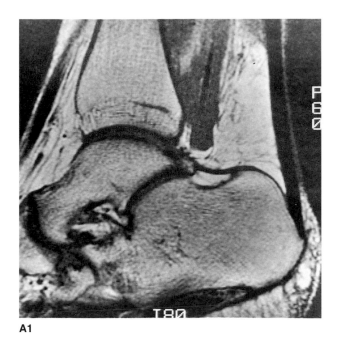

A1

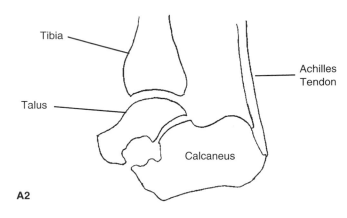

A2

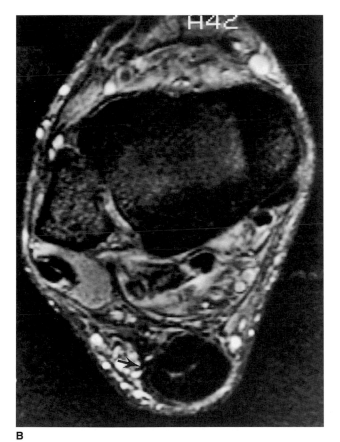

B

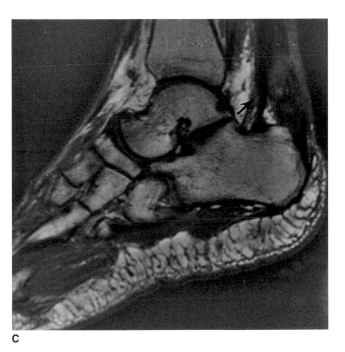

C

Figure 13–34. MRI of Achilles tendon and tendinitis. **A1.** T1 image of normal Achilles tendon. **A2.** Corresponding line drawing. **B.** T2 gradient image of Achilles tendinitis with partial tear. **C.** T1 image of a complete Achilles tendon rupture. Arrow points to the area of complete tear in the hypovascular zone of the Achilles tendon.

tendon with side-to-side repair of the tendon. With extensive debridement, reinforcing the remaining Achilles tendon by turn down flap, plantaris tendon weave, or flexor digitorum longus augmentation may be necessary.[153,159]

Patients who have failed nonoperative treatment for insertional tendinitis are candidates for surgical debridement.[159] If Haglund's deformity is present, it should be removed. Any detached portion of the Achilles tendon should be reattached to the calcaneus.

If a large defect is present, it may be augmented as in noninsertional tendinitis.

Partial Achilles tendon tears occur proximally in the avascular zone or distally near the insertion point on the calcaneus. In proximal tears, the tendon is incised and degenerated tissue excised. Then the tendon and paratenon are sutured. In distal tears, the tendon is incised, degeneration tissue is excised, bone is removed from the superior calcaneal tuberosity, and resection of the retrocalcaneal bursa is performed.

Complete rupture of the Achilles tendon in an athlete requires repair according to most authors. In early repair without wide gap (within 1 week of injury), direct end-to-end suturing is undertaken with or without augmentation. With chronic tears or acute tears with a large gap, end-to-end repair may not be possible and grafting techniques are applied.

STRESS FRACTURES

Epidemiology

As people have become more active with recreational sports, there has been an increase in the reported frequency of fatigue fractures. A fatigue fracture is defined as bone damage in normal bone subjected to repetitive loading. In contrast, insufficiency fractures develop in abnormal bone subjected to normal stress.[162]

The incidence of fatigue fractures has not been studied in the general population. Fatigue fractures may comprise up to 10 percent of all sports injuries and 25 percent of runners with chronic leg pain.[163,164] The incidence of fatigue fractures is higher in females and whites.[165,166]

The bones most commonly involved are the tibia, fibula, and the second, third, and fifth metatarsals. Calcaneus, tarsal navicular, and the sesamoids are less commonly involved. The athletes at risk are ones who participate in sprinting, jumping, and running activities (see Table 13-7).[162]

Pathogenesis and Mechanism

Bone is a living tissue constantly reacting and remodeling to the surrounding stresses to accommodate its biomechanical environment. The constant remodeling occurs through cells that lay down new bone and other cells, which resorb bone. Initial stress will cause microdamage, leading to the disruption of local cortical blood circulation to the metatarsals.[162] Then, bone remodeling begins with resorption of the necrotic bone by osteoclasts. Initially, osteoclast activity predominates, leading to weakened bone. Then osteoblast activity increases, leading to increased bone mass and strength. If during the weakened state the excessive stress level continues, the microfractures may lead to complete fracture.[162,163]

TABLE 13–7. STRESS FRACTURE OF THE FOOT/ANKLE

Tibia	Most common Site: Junction of the distal and middle third of the tibia; pronated foot has been implicated Comp: Delayed union/nonunion in anterior middle third tibia fx
Fibula	Third most common Site: 5 cm proximal to the tip of the lateral malleolus
Navicular	Uncommon Long delay in diagnosis
Calcaneus	Uncommon Associated with hindfoot varus
Metatarsal	Second most common Site: Second or third metatarsals Cavus and planus feet have been implicated
Jones Fx	Fracture of the proximal metaphyseal diaphyseal junction High rate of delayed union

Muscle activity plays an important role in stress fractures.[167] Muscles act to first absorb, then gradually release, energy to the bone. However, when muscles fatigue, the dampening capacity is diminished and more energy is transmitted directly to the bone. This change in the loading pattern may lead to fatigue fracture metatarsals.[162,163,167,168]

Bony imbalance may also lead to fatigue fractures by placing more stress on a particular bone. A hyperpronated foot may transfer increased stress on the medial portion of the foot, leading to tibia fatigue fractures.[162,169] A hypermobile first ray or a long second metatarsal may lead to increase stress on the second metatarsal.[169]

History and Physical Examination

The pain is usually insidious in onset and is typically associated with activity and resolves with rest. History often reveals change in the training program, increase in physical activity, change in the type of surface on which the activity occurs, or change in shoe wear.[162,167,169] In females, it is important to obtain a menstrual history, as amenorrheic athletes have a higher possibility of osteoporosis causing insufficiency fractures.[167]

Nearly 65 to 90 percent of athletes with fatigue fractures will have point tenderness of the area involved. About 25 to 45 percent of the time, there will be local swelling, possibly starting with ecchymosis.[170,171] Also, check the foot for deformities such as hypermobile first ray, hyperpronated foot, or long second toe.

Diagnostic Studies

Plain radiographs may be variable. Stress fracture may not be visible until 3 to 6 weeks after the onset of symptoms. At about 2 weeks, a stress fracture demonstrates periosteal new bone formation or a cortical break and by 6 weeks callus may finally be visible (see Fig. 13–35).[172]

If clinical findings are suggestive and plain radiographs are negative, a bone scan can be helpful. A bone scan may be positive as early as 3 days after the onset of fatigue fracture.[173] A positive bone scan will show an area of focal uptake, but it cannot distinguish between infection and possible tumor. Recently, MRI has been used to diagnose fatigue fractures. MRI will show increased edema at the fracture site. It can also identify possible tumors (see Fig. 13–36).

Functional Rehabilitation

Prevention is the best treatment for stress fractures. Prior to and throughout the season, the team trainer or therapist must educate the coaches and participants involved in high-risk sports. Proper foot wear, training methods, running surfaces, recognition of symptoms, and the maintenance of proper diet are important topics for discussion.

The treatment of a stress fracture depends on whether or not it is considered as a risk-fracture or a non-

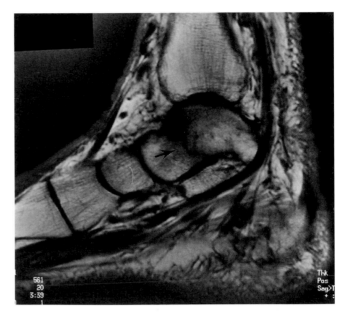

Figure 13–36. T1 MRI of a talar neck stress fracture (*arrow*).

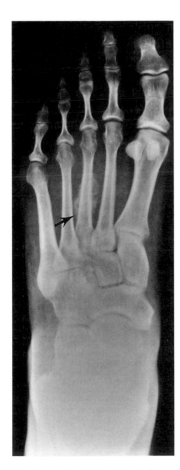

Figure 13–35. Radiograph of the foot demonstrating callus formation of the third metatarsal secondary to stress fracture (*arrow*).

critical stress fracture.[174] This categorization is based on the location of the stress fracture and the potential to develop complications. Stress fractures of the tarsal navicular, proximal second metatarsal, and base of the fifth metatarsal are considered critical stress fractures, while the distal fibula, distal metatarsal, and os calcis stress fractures are considered noncritical.[174] Athletes who have noncritical stress fractures are allowed to continue modified activity below the threshold of pain while waiting for the bone to heal.[174] Bicycling, underwater running, a stair stepper, or cross-country machine provide excellent means to maintain fitness. However, if basic activities of daily living, including walking, are painful, partial or nonweight-bearing ambulation with crutches may be necessary. Critical stress fractures are treated more aggressively, often requiring internal fixation or cast immobilization. Various bone stimulation devices are also available for the treatment of slow healing stress fractures. Treatment is highly individualized for each injury using the radiograph as a guideline.[174]

For effective long-term results, the causes of the stress fracture must be addressed. Contributory factors include lower extremity mechanics, shoes and playing surfaces, training errors, muscle weakness or fatigue, and insufficient diet with amenorrhea in the female athlete. Regarding lower extremity mechanics, both a rigid, cavus foot and flexible, pronated foot may contribute to a stress fracture. Athletes with cavus feet may benefit from a shock-absorbing insole, while those with the pronated foot will benefit from a custom foot orthotic to control the abnormal motion. The individual with a cavus foot may also benefit by training on a more forgiving surface. All athletes with these injuries should

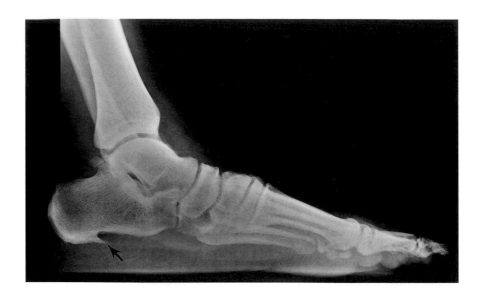

Figure 13–39. Radiograph of calcaneal spur.

the acute phase of rehabilitation, the use of physical modalities, medications, and relative rest are used to control the pain and inflammation. The second part of the rehabilitation is directed at correcting any biomechanical factors that contribute to the problem. The contributing factors proposed by various authors[187-192] are listed in Table 13-9. The evaluation and correction of biomechanical factors can certainly be initiated during the first visit. Only after the pain is well under control and potential etiologic factors are addressed in the rehabilitation program, should the athlete begin the gradual return to sports.

The Acute Phase: Controlling Pain and Inflammation

The primary goals during this phase are to protect the plantar fascia from excessive strain, decrease pain and

inflammation, and maintain the athlete's fitness level. There are numerous physical therapy modalities commonly used to treat pain and inflammation in athletes with plantar fasciitis and other overuse injuries. In the acute phase of plantar fasciitis, where there is significant pain to palpation and with weight bearing, aggressive heating modalities are not generally recommended. The vigorous heating may actually promote the inflammatory process. Instead, during this phase, the application of cold and nonthermal modalities such as pulsed ultrasound, sensory level electrical stimulation, and iotophoresis are recommended. Common medications used with iontophoresis include dexamethasone, salicylate, hydrocortisone, and lidocaine. These physical agents and medications are not to be solely relied on for treatment of overuse injuries. They are only an adjunct to decrease pain to help the athlete progress to the latter stages of rehabilitation.

Temporary support also alleviates much of the discomfort in the acute phase and can decrease the strain on the plantar fascia. Types of support recommended in the early phases of plantar fasciitis include the low-dye taping, arch supports, and felt pads strategically placed in the shoe to control abnormal foot motion. A thin (one-eighth inch) medial felt pad can be placed under a varus

TABLE 13–8. SUMMARY OF REHABILITATION PROGRAM FOR PLANTAR FASCIITIS

Acute Phase	Rehabilitation Phase
Physical Agents	
Pulsed ultrasound	Continuous ultrasound
Electrical stimulation	Ionto/phonophoresis
Iontophoresis	Cryotherapy
Cryotherapy	Friction massage
Exercise	
Achilles tendon stretching	Achilles tendon stretching
Foot mobilization	Foot mobilization
	Plantar fascia stretch
	Intrinsic foot strengthening
	Strengthen pronation decelerators
Support	
Arch taping	Custom foot orthotics
Temporary posting	

TABLE 13–9. MECHANICAL FACTORS ASSOCIATED WITH PLANTAR FASCIITIS

Forefoot varus strength	Decreased plantar flexion
Prolonged pronation	Worn-out shoes
Rigid, cavus foot	Low foot arch
Tight Achilles tendon	Loose heel counter
Leg length discrepancy	Excessive body weight
Decreased first ray mobility	

forefoot or under a varus rearfoot to control compensatory pronation.[193] If some of these supports decrease the patient's pain, it is often a good indication that long-term, custom-made orthoses will be beneficial. While taping for support, the first ray should be taped in plantar flexion to improve stability during propulsion, thus easing the strain on the plantar fascia.[194] During this early phase, the athlete is encouraged to have the support of a good shoe with a firm heel counter. Walking barefoot encourages flattening of the arch which places more tension on the inflamed plantar fascia. Finally, Wapner and Sharkey[195] have found the use of polypropylene ankle foot orthosis in 5 degrees of dorsiflexion useful in the treatment of plantar fasciitis. Nighttime use, to resist contraction of the plantar fascia and Achilles tendon shortening, help with maintaining a healthier length and tension relationship.

During both the early and later phases of treatment, the athlete needs to minimize weight-bearing demands of the foot. Non or minimal weight-bearing activities should be performed in place of the normal training regimen. Deep water running wearing a flotation device is an excellent conditioning regimen. Riding a stationary bike, using a stair step machine, or cross-country ski machine will also usually be tolerated and provides a satisfactory cardiovascular training session. If specific flexibility deficits have been identified in the evaluation, gentle stretching is usually tolerated well during the early stage of rehabilitation. Any joints in the foot or ankle where accessory joint motion is limited should also be mobilized for optimal function.[194]

Rehabilitation Phase: Focus on Etiologic Factors

Once the athlete has minimal tenderness and is able to bear weight and walk without pain, more aggressive rehabilitation is initiated. Physical agents continue to be used during this phase, including cryotherapy, which is particularly useful after a rehabilitation session to decrease any inflammation that may occur from new challenges introduced in the program. Deep heating modalities, such as continuous-wave ultrasound, are recommended to increase tissue extensibility prior to stretching the affected tissues. Soft-tissue mobilization and transverse friction massage across the plantar fascia can help decrease the patient's complaints.

Stretching and strengthening exercises are well under way at this stage of rehabilitation. Specific deficits, if not addressed in the earlier phase, are addressed now. In a study of athletes with plantar fasciitis, Kibler and associates[189] found significant deficits in ankle plantar flexor strength and ankle dorsiflexion ROM. From their study, one cannot assess whether these deficits were a contributing factor in the injury or an effect of the injury. However, Kibler and associates report that the lack of ankle dorsiflexion and weak plantar flexors manifests as a functional pronation. During running, this results in an excessive tensile strain on the plantar fascia. Thus, stretching the Achilles tendon by individually isolating the gastrocnemius and soleus is a key part of the rehabilitation program. To avoid further strain on the plantar fascia while stretching, the foot and ankle should be supinated by toeing-in or placing a support under the arch. The plantar flexors can be strengthened by simply performing heel raises, starting with weight bearing on both extremities and gradually shifting weight until they can be performed comfortably with a single leg stance heel raise. The foot should also remain in the supinated position while performing this exercise. Passive flexion and extension of the great toe is often limited in patients with plantar fasciitis.[196] Lack of dorsiflexion of the great toe could indicate a contracted plantar fascia. The athlete can easily stretch the plantar fascia by passively dorsiflexing the toes himself or herself. This should be preceded with a deep heating modality to increase the extensibility of the tissues. In those athletes where excessive or prolonged pronation is a contributing factor, specifically strengthening the muscles that control pronation or internal rotation of the leg through eccentric contraction may assist in the management of plantar fasciitis. These muscles include the anterior and posterior tibialis, flexor hallucis longus, and biceps femoris. Eccentric, closed-chain strengthening of these muscles is more specific to their function. These can be performed using the BAPS, as described in the ankle sprain rehabilitation section. Though the intrinsic ligaments and plantar fascia in the foot provide the primary support for the foot, intrinsic muscle strengthening may be beneficial. These muscles can be strengthened by performing the towel curl exercise, picking up marbles with the foot, and other similar methods. Finally, if absent from their sport for an extended period, the athlete involved in multidirectional activities should be evaluated for proprioceptive deficits, and if indicated, a proprioceptive exercise program should be initiated.

The use of orthotics is often necessary to control for abnormal foot and ankle mechanics that contribute to plantar fasciitis. The orthotic device accomplishes this by keeping the foot in as close to a neutral position as possible to encourage normal function of the leg and foot. There are a wide range of orthotic devices available. They differ in size, shape, costs, rigidity, and materials used in fabrication. Oddly, both a hypermobile, pronated foot and the rigid, cavus foot are cited in the literature as contributing factors to plantar fasciitis.[197] Generally speaking, the individual with a hypermobile pronated foot will need a rigid orthotic with a deep heel cup for maximum control of motion.[198] The athlete with a cavus foot will need a more yielding orthotic (soft or semirigid).[209] McPoil and McGarvey[197] recommend that the orthotic for the cavus foot be a total contact orthosis to support the medial longitudinal arch. For the less competitive athlete who needs only mild additional control, an off-the-shelf orthotic designed to control rearfoot motion may be effective. For the mildly symptomatic individual with a cavus foot, various off-the-shelf cushioning inserts may be beneficial. The more competitive athletes, or those with more extreme biomechanical problems, will need custom-made orthoses designed to correct specific biomechanical faults. Athletes should be referred to a clinician experienced in orthotic prescription for optimal treatment of an athlete's specific problem.

Once received by the athlete, a program of gradually introducing the orthotic should be started. Wearing the orthotic 1 hour in the morning and 1 hour in the afternoon is an appropriate beginning. The time is increased over a 2-week period. Once the orthotic feels comfortable, training in the orthotic can be initiated. It is advisable that the athlete begin training with the orthotic in a new shoe. The athletic shoe for the athlete recovering from plantar fasciitis should have a firm heel counter. The athlete with the cavus foot should look for a shoe with more cushioning than motion control, while the athlete who overpronates should look for a more stable shoe.

Return to Play

Before returning to sport activity, the athlete should have full ankle and foot ROM and strength, a nontender plantar fascia, and no pain with simple daily activities. The athlete should also have simulated the activities involved in his or her sport in a less demanding environment, for example, in the pool. Since most sporting activities involve running, this is the first activity that should be mastered (see Table 13–10). The long-distance runner will need to progress this program further. A general rule is that distance should be increased before speed, and that distance should not be increased more than 10 percent per week. Until the normal training regimen is reached, the athlete should only perform full weight-bearing training every other day. Hills and

hard surfaces should be avoided. Once forward running is performed comfortably, athletes involved in multidirectional sports can begin functional activities appropriate for their sport. These activities should begin at half speed, progress to full speed as tolerated, and then return to competition.

Rehabilitation After Fascial Release

It is recommended that patients be placed in a weight-bearing short-leg cast for 2 weeks after surgery to allow for tissue healing.[199] During this time and after cast removal, the athlete can perform an alternative activity to maintain cardiovascular fitness. Once the cast is removed, regaining ROM is the first priority. Most important is ankle dorsiflexion; therefore, Achilles tendon stretching is begun immediately. Gentle plantar fascia stretching and stretching of the long toe flexors and extensors is also performed. Soft-tissue mobilization around the healed incision will minimize soft-tissue contraction. Modalities to control pain and inflammation are also recommended. Many athletes will have difficulty restoring normal gait initially. The terminal stance phase, when the toes are passively dorsiflexed, is particularly uncomfortable. Walking in waist-deep water allows a more normal, pain-free gait and is an excellent way to train. Strengthening exercises are also performed immediately after the immobilization period. Athletes can perform ankle joint strengthening exercises as described in earlier sections of this chapter and towel curl exercises to strengthen the intrinsic muscles. Finally, the athlete should wear some type of firm arch support or custom foot orthotic to maintain the arch.

Prior to returning to normal training, the athlete will progress from strengthening and stretching exercises to more functional activities. These can be performed early in the pool or on a minitrampoline and advanced to the field, court, or track following similar guidelines discussed earlier in this chapter. Most athletes are able to start running in about 9 weeks and continue to improve up to 6 months.[199]

Surgical Treatment

Fortunately, nonoperative, empiric treatments for subcalcaneal pain syndrome are 95 percent successful.[183] However, in refractory cases that have failed conservative therapy for 6 to 12 months, surgery may help.[180] Prior to surgery, a definitive diagnosis should be made from the list of differential diagnoses. An accurate diagnosis limits the amount of surgical dissection.[180,187] The surgical list includes exploration of the tarsal tunnel, the medial calcaneal nerve, the nerve to the abductor digiti quinti, the medial and lateral plantar nerve, release of the central plantar fascia, and calcaneal spur excision.[180,183,200]

TABLE 13–10. SAMPLE RETURN TO RUNNING PROGRAM

Phase 1	Brisk walk for 30 minutes
Phase 2	Walk 5 minutes; jog 1 minute, walk 4 minutes (repeat 4 times); walk 5 minutes
Phase 3	Walk 5 minutes; jog 2 minutes, walk 3 minutes (repeat 4 times); walk 5 minutes
Phase 4	Walk 5 minutes; jog 3 minutes, walk 2 minutes (repeat 4 times); walk 5 minutes
Phase 5	Walk 5 minutes; jog 4 minutes, walk 1 minute (repeat 4 times); walk 5 minutes
Phase 6	Walk 5 minutes; jog 20 minutes; walk 5 minutes

CHRONIC EXERTION COMPARTMENT SYNDROME

Epidemiology

Chronic exertional compartment syndrome is due to abnormally high intramuscular pressure during exercise in a closed fibro-osseous space, which causes ischemia of muscles and nerves. Relative incidence in athletes is unclear, but it appears to be common in runners.[201] One study diagnosed 3 cases per year out of 40,000 students.[202] Clanton has reviewed 150 patients with exercise induced leg pain and found 33 percent with chronic compartment syndromes, 25 percent with stress fractures, 14 percent with muscle strains, 13 percent with medial tibial stress syndrome, 10 percent with nerve entrapment, 4 percent with venous pathology, and one patient with spinal stenosis.[203]

Compartment syndrome affects the anterior and deep posterior compartment most commonly and may occur in multiple compartments about one fourth of the time.[204]

Functional Anatomy and Mechanism

Traditionally, the lower leg is divided into four compartments: anterior, lateral, superficial posterior, and deep posterior (see Fig. 13-40). The anterior compartment contains the extensor digitorum longus, extensor hallucis longus, and the tibialis anterior. The lateral compartment contains the peroneus longus and brevis. The superficial posterior compartment contains the gastrocnemius and the soleus. Finally, the deep posterior compartment contains the flexor hallucis longus, tibialis posterior, and the flexor hallucis longus.

The four compartments are bounded by bone and thick, noncompliant fascial covering. When this is coupled with increased muscle bulk or muscle swelling, pressure increases within the compartment, resulting in decreased tissue perfusion and ischemia. Ischemia results in increased metabolic byproducts causing increased capillary permeability. The increased capillary permeability results in increased intra- and extracellular fluid. This fluid further increases compartment pressure.[205]

History and Physical Examination

The athlete with chronic leg pain could have a number of problems (see Table 13-11). The diagnosis of chronic compartment syndrome can be made with history, physical examination, and intracompartmental pressure measurements. The athlete with chronic compartment syndrome complains of pain during exercise and immediately after activity over the compartments involved.[203] The onset of pain is predictable, occurring at about the same time during exercise.[206] The pain will completely or partially resolve with rest, depending on the severity. Simultaneous bilateral involvement of the lower extremity may occur but presentation of one leg is more frequent.[205] The athlete may also complain of numbness,

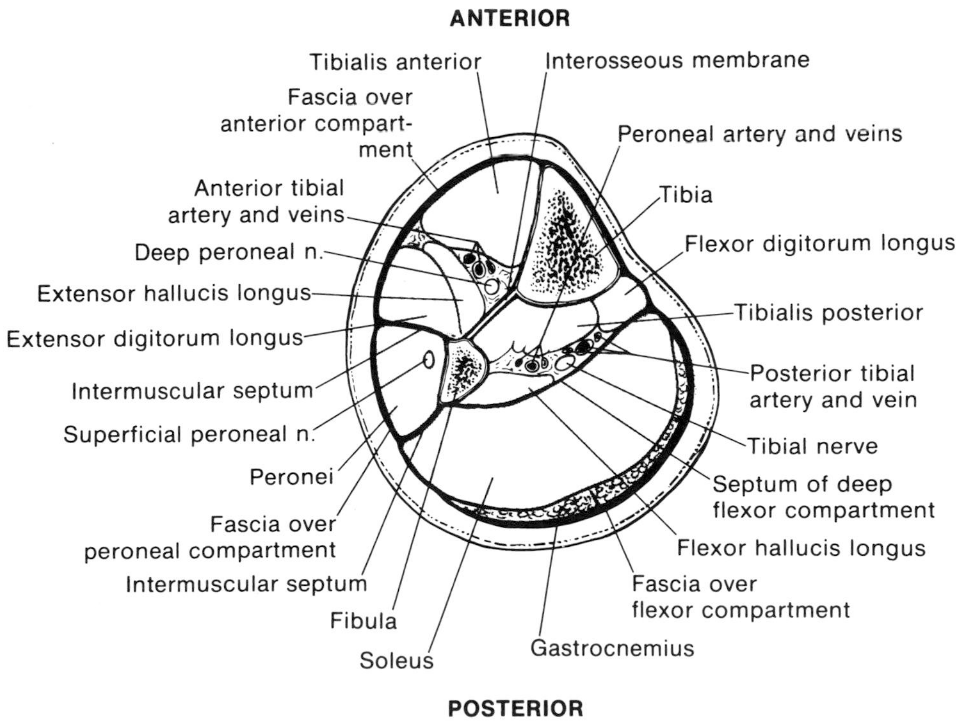

Figure 13–40. Contents of the compartments of the leg. *(From Hoppenfeld S, deBoer P. Surgical Exposures in Orthopaedics: The Anatomic Approach. Philadelphia: Lippincott; 1984:458. With permission.)*

TABLE 13–11. CHRONIC LEG PAIN

Chronic compartment syndrome (33%)	Activity-related pain, relieved with rest.
	Increased compartmental pressures.
	Treat with fasciotomy.
Stress fractures (25%)	Increase or change in workout routine with change in equipment and localized pain and tenderness.
	Bone scan reveals focal uptake.
	Rest with gradual return to activity.
Muscle strain (14%)	Sudden popping sensation and pain in the posterior leg with accompanying ecchymosis with eccentric loading of the gastrocnemius and soleus complex.
	Rest with stretching and strengthening.
Medial tibial stress syndrome (13%)	Pain with exercise along the medial border of the middle and distal tibia.
	Bone scan may show diffuse uptake along the posteromedial border of the tibia.
	Rest with stretching and strengthening.
Nerve entrapments (10%)	Pain, burning, tingling, usually along the superficial peroneal nerve distribution with a positive Tinel's sign at the site of compression.
	EMG may be diagnostic.
	NSAID, rest, injection.
Venous insufficiency (4%)	Vague pain over thrombosed vessels in repetitive throwing athletes.
	Distended superficial vessels with tenderness.
	Venogram is best to evaluate extent of disease.
	Anticoagulation.

shooting pain, tingling, or burning along the course of the nerve.[203,205,206] The athlete may also have a history of a previous stress fracture.[202]

The examination of the athlete at rest will provide little clues to the diagnosis. However, after exercise, the athlete may have tenderness and increased pressure in the involved compartment. Passive stretching of the muscles involved may cause pain.[206] Anterior and deep posterior compartments are most commonly involved. Examination of the anterior compartment after exercise may show reduced sensation in the first dorsal web space of the foot due to ischemia of the deep peroneal nerve.[206] Nerve compression of the posterior compartment is rare and the pain will be poorly localized.[207] The involvement of the lateral compartment fascial defect is relatively common.[206] After activity, a muscle bulge may be palpated in the distal third of the leg on the anterior lateral aspect. This herniation is through the opening in the fascia for the superficial peroneal nerve. Therefore, with the muscle herniation, compression of the superficial peroneal nerve may occur causing decreased sensation of the dorsum of the foot.[206]

Diagnostic Studies

Plain radiographs are taken of the tibia to check for stress fractures. If the plain radiographs are negative, a bone scan is obtained to rule out stress fractures.

The measurement of intracompartmental pressure can confirm the diagnosis. Various criteria are available to make the diagnosis at rest, during exercise, and after exercise. Pedowitz has modified Mubarak's criteria for

the diagnosis: a preexercise pressure greater than 15 mm Hg, a 1-minute postexercise pressure greater than 30 mm Hg, or a 5 minute postexercise pressure greater than 20 mm Hg.[208] However, compartment measurements also have limitations, as only one compartment can be measured at a time. The measurement of the deep posterior compartment pressure may be unreliable due to the uncertainty of the location of the needle tip.[206]

MRI has also been used as a safe, reproducible test for chronic exertional compartment syndrome.[209]

Functional Rehabilitation

If the athlete desires to continue with high-level performance, true chronic compartment syndrome may only be completely alleviated by surgery. However, a trial of conservative care is warranted, especially if the athlete plans on reducing or modifying activities. As in all overuse injuries, the conservative care begins with a thorough evaluation to identify the precipitating factors. These factors are often related to training errors, training surfaces and terrain, or biomechanical factors.

The conservative rehabilitation of the athlete with chronic compartment syndrome differs little from rehabilitation of other overuse injuries. Emphasis is placed on stretching inflexible muscles, eliminating training errors, and correcting biomechanical faults to reduce the load on the muscles in the affected compartment. For example, an inflexible gastrocnemius and soleus can increase the work performed by the ankle dorsiflexor muscles during the swing phase of gait. Excessive downhill running similarly increases the load on the ankle dorsiflexors while decelerating the foot after heel strike. Finally, in an athlete with excessive pronation, the muscles decelerating pronation are overworked. The long-term demands on these muscles result in hypertrophy and, while in use, the muscle compartment develops high pressures and thus, compartment syndrome. In both training and rehabilitation, excessive demands on the affected muscles and their compartment must be minimized. Unless specific weaknesses are found in the exam, strengthening of the muscles in the affected compartment is not a key component in conservative management as hypertrophy in a restricted compartment can be a contributing factor. Alternative activity, such as bicycling, swimming, or deep water running, allows the athlete to maintain cardiovascular fitness when the athlete is unable to train symptom-free.

Once the precipitating factors are addressed, the athlete is ready to gradually resume training. For most athletes with compartment syndrome, the symptoms present at a fairly consistent time into the training session, enabling the athlete to easily gauge the intensity and duration of the training. The athlete must know when this occurs and train below the threshold. Slowing the running pace and avoiding hills may allow an increased training time. The sample return to running program previously mentioned allows a progressive, gradual return. If the athlete is involved in a multidirectional sport, functional activities are also initiated at this time beginning with very low-intensity activity and gradually progressing to activities simulating their sport. Beginning with jumping or lateral activities on a trampoline or in waist deep water provide a low-stress means to begin functional training. Early in the return to training, frequent, but short-duration training sessions often allow good quality training without bringing on symptoms.

Rehabilitation After Compartment Release

The goals of rehabilitation in the first several days after surgery are to reduce pain and swelling and to maintain ROM. Compressive dressings surrounding the leg and foot, and elevation, are usually sufficient to achieve these goals. Partial weight bearing to tolerance with crutches is allowed during the first 2 days, but the athlete should avoid long periods with the leg in the dependent position. Finally, gentle stretching and active and passive ROM are performed as early as tolerated.

If swelling is minimal, the athlete is able to progress in the rehabilitation program approximately 1 week following surgery. At this time, the athlete should already be walking with a normal gait without any assistive device. Strengthening with gentle resistance is initiated to tolerance. An elastic band provides a smooth and effective form of resistance. When the athlete is able to withstand a moderate amount of resistance,

strengthening and proprioceptive exercises are performed in a closed-chain position. With residual strength losses up to 20 percent after surgery,[210,211] emphasis is placed on strengthening the muscles in the involved compartment. Once the incisions are healed, swimming, deep water running, or functional activities in waist deep water are initiated. Some athletes can start running at 2 weeks if full ROM is present. However, before the athlete begins running, he or she must be pain free with basic daily activities including walking, stair climbing, and squatting. If available, the athlete should be comfortable running in place on a minitrampoline or in waist-deep water. When running is initiated, the program should involve a walk and jog program and progress gradually as described.

Once the athlete has full ROM and flexibility, is able to withstand moderate to maximal resistance of the affected muscles, and can run comfortably, more functional activities are begun. If the athlete is a runner, distance and intensity of the training runs are increased. Work on hills is initiated gradually if the runner competes in cross-country. Running downhill is avoided initially, however, as the strong, eccentric contractions in this activity are significantly more stressful than uphill running. Athletes involved in multidirectional sports begin lateral and sports-specific activities in this stage. The progression is similar to the rehabilitation procedures described for other overuse injuries.

Surgical Treatment

If an athlete can reduce activity to a tolerable symptom level, then surgery is not recommended. However, if the decreased level of activity continues to cause pain, then fasciotomy of the involved compartments is recommended. The main concern of the fasciotomy is the release of the involved compartments without causing injury to neurovascular structures or muscle. Release of muscle compartments may reduce work efficiency of that group of muscles.

With the release, about 90 percent of athletes have significant clinical improvement or resolution of symptoms.[203] There are reports of up to 20 percent strength loss in the released compartment, but the weakness is offset by the improvement in pain.[210,211] Poor surgical results are usually attributable to incorrect diagnosis, inadequate release, or neurovascular damage.[203]

TURF TOE

Epidemiology

Acute flexion and extension injury to the first metatarsophalangeal joint (MTP) has become increasingly more common in sports since 1976.[212] Bowers and Martin coined the term "turf toe" for the injury of the first metatarsophalangeal joint attributed to hard artificial turf playing surfaces and flexible shoe wear.[213]

The incidence of turf toe has been established on the collegiate football level. At West Virginia University and the University of Arkansas, an average of 5.4 and 6 injuries per season respectively were noted.[213,214] One survey of professional football players revealed that 45 percent of 80 active players had sustained a turf toe injury.[215] With turf toe injury, the athlete missed an average of 6 days.[216] Though the number of ankle sprains in football players reported by Coker at the University of Arkansas are four times more common, the number of practice days missed were less than the days missed due to turf toe.[214] In the same study, there were more games missed due to turf toe than due to ankle sprains.

Functional Anatomy and Mechanism

The first metatarsophalangeal joint is composed of a capsuloligamentous complex, tendons of the abductor and adductor hallucis, long and short flexor and extensor tendons, the proximal phalanx, and the metatarsal head. The stability of the joint is obtained by the capsuloligamentous complex and the short tendon, with the first metatarsophalangeal bony articulation and the long tendons playing a minor role.[212] The stability of the first MTP joint capsule is augmented in the medial and lateral sides by the strong collateral ligaments.[212] The plantar plate is a thickened fibrous portion of the capsule that blends in with the sesamoid bones and the tendons of the flexor hallucis brevis, adding to the strength and stability to the joint. The plantar plate is firmly anchored to the base of the proximal phalanx and loosely attached to the neck of the metatarsal.[212]

The range of motion of the first MTP joint is somewhat variable ranging from 3 to 43 degrees of passive plantar flexion and 40 to 100 degrees of passive dorsiflexion.[217] In walking barefoot, at least 60 degrees of dorsiflexion is considered normal.[218]

Biomechanically, the great toe typically supports about 40 to 60 percent of the body weight in normal walking increasing up to 8 times body weight in running or jumping.[212,219] The center of motion for the first MTP joint falls within the metatarsal head, resulting in some sliding motion between the metatarsal head and the proximal phalanx.[220] The gliding motion gives way to compression of the dorsal articular surface of the metatarsal head and proximal phalanx.[216]

The main mechanism of injury is a hyperextension to the first MTP joint. The toes are typically in a dorsiflexed position with the forefoot fixed on the ground and the heel raised. Then an external force drives the first MTP joint further into dorsiflexion. This tears the weaker joint capsule attachment at the metatarsal neck.

Also, compression injury to the dorsal articular surface may occur.[212]

History and Physical Examination

The athlete will initially complain of mild pain with or without swelling, worsening over the course of the next 24 hours. Another presentation is to complain of persistent toe pain, swelling, MTP joint stiffness, and worsening pain with running months after the event.[221]

The severity of the sprain can be assessed on physical examination. A grade 1 sprain is a minor tearing of the capsuloligamentous complex of the first MTP joint. There is minimal swelling, localized plantar or medial tenderness, and minimal restriction in the range of motion. The athlete can bear weight with minimal symptoms and can participate in competition. A grade 2 sprain is a partial tear of the capsuloligamentous complex. There is moderate swelling and ecchymosis with moderate restriction in range of motion. The athlete walks with an antalgic gait on a supinated forefoot and is unable to compete. Grade 3 is a complete tear of the capsuloligamentous complex and an impaction of the proximal phalanx. This may be associated with a sesamoid fracture. There is severe ecchymosis, swelling, and tenderness on both the plantar and dorsal aspect of the joint, with severe decrease in range of motion.[212]

Diagnostic Studies

Plain radiographs are recommended following the acute sprain. Anterior and posterior, lateral, and oblique views are taken to rule out bony pathology such as capsular avulsion, sesamoid fracture, impaction injury of the dorsal articular surface, or proximal migration of the sesamoid.[212]

Functional Rehabilitation and Preventive Measures

Neglected treatment and rehabilitation of turf toe, in the long-term, can result in a disabling injury. Some of the sequela of turf toe include calcification of the periarticular soft tissue, hallux valgus, and hallux rigidus.[222-224] The loss of motion in the first metatarsophalangeal joint, either due to pain or joint contracture, often results in gait compensation that compounds the problem and results in a loss of performance.[225] Thus, early and complete rehabilitation is necessary to restore to the athlete optimal function with the least chance of long-term morbidity.

The basic principles in the rehabilitation of turf toe are similar to that of other lower extremity injuries. This includes controlling pain and swelling, increasing ROM and strength, maintaining cardiovascular fitness, and preparing the athlete to return to play. The initial phase of rehabilitation includes modification of activities, ice, compression, and elevation. Since the injury is usually the result of hyperextension, controlling hyperextension is desirable to allow the injured soft tissues to heal. Controlling this motion is accomplished by having the athlete wear a shoe with a stiff sole in the forefoot,[223] wearing an orthosis,[224,226] or taping.[222] In severe cases, the use of crutches is necessary for several days.[226]

After the acute pain has subsided, modalities such as pulsed ultrasound or iontophoresis can be used to control inflammation and assist the healing of the soft tissues. Gentle joint mobilization in the form of distraction and dorsal and proximal glides of the proximal phalanx on the first metatarsal can assist in restoring normal joint ROM and mechanics. Active exercises such as curling up a towel with the toes or moving the toes in a bucket of sand are helpful in restoring motion and strength. Running in waist deep water can provide a cardiovascular workout, in addition to functional training of the lower extremity.

When the athlete returns to competition is dependent on the severity of the injury. Table 13-12 displays an injury classification developed by Clanton and coworkers[224] that predicts the time loss from sports. In general, the athlete is ready to return to competitive training when swelling is minimal, ROM is full and painless (up to 90 degrees), and there is no tenderness.[222] Upon the return to competition, some protection to prevent hyperextension of the MTP joint should continue to be used by the athlete for an extended period. This protection can be in the form of taping,[222] wearing a shoe with a stiff forefoot,[224,226] or a custom-made orthosis with a Morton extension.[226]

Surgical Treatment

The mainstay of treatment for turf toe is rehabilitation and preventive protection. However, in persistent cases with loose body within the joint, sesamoid fracture, or separation of bipartite sesamoid, surgical resection and repair of the damaged capsule may allow return to activity.[212]

TABLE 13–12. GRADES OF TURF TOE INJURY WITH PREDICTED TIME LOSS FROM THE SPORT

Classification	Findings	Time Loss from Sport
Grade I	Localized tenderness Minimal, if any swelling No ecchymosis	Continues to participate
Grade II	Diffuse tenderness Mild to moderate swelling Ecchymosis Decreased ROM	1 to 2 weeks
Grade III	Severe tenderness Marked effusion Ecchymosis Severe decrease in ROM Severe	3+ weeks

REFERENCES

Anatomy of the Foot

1. Sarrafian SK. *Anatomy of the Foot and Ankle.* Philadelphia: Lippincott; 1993:37-112.
2. Inman VT. *The Joints of the Ankle.* Baltimore: Williams & Wilkins; 1976.
3. American Academy of Orthopaedic Surgeons. *Joint Motion Method of Measuring and Recording.* Chicago: AAOS; 1965:69-85.
4. Chan CW, Rudins A. Foot biomechanics during walking and running. *Mayo Clin Proc.* 1994;69:448-461.

Biomechanics of Walking

5. Chan CW, Rudins A. Foot biomechanics during walking and running. *Mayo Clin Proc.* 1994;69:448-461.
6. Inman VT. *The Joints of the Ankle.* Baltimore; Williams & Wilkins; 1976.
7. Isman RE, Inman VT. Anthropometric studies of the human foot and ankle. *Bull Prosthet Res.* 1969;97:10-11.

Biomechanics of Running

8. Mann RA. Biomechanics of running. In: Mack RP, ed. *Symposium on the Foot and Leg in Running Sports.* St. Louis; Mosby; 1982:1-63.
9. Ounpuu S. The biomechanics of walking and running. *Clin Sports Med.* 1994;13:843-863.
10. Aston JW, Carollo JJ. Normal patterns of walking and running. In: Subotnick SI, ed. *Sports Medicine of the Lower Extremity.* New York: Churchill Livingstone; 1989:171-178.
11. Mann RA, Hagy J. Biomechanics of walking, running, and sprinting. *Am J Sports Med.* 1980;8:345-350.
12. Munro CF, Miller DI, Fuglevand AJ. Ground reaction forces in running: A reexamination. *J Biomech.* 1987; 20:147-155.
13. Bates BT. Course notes. San Diego: Medithon; 1985.
14. Nigg BM, Denoth J, Kerr B, et al. Load, sport shoes, and playing surfaces. In: Frederick EC, ed. *Sport Shoes and Playing Surfaces.* Champaign, IL: Human Kinetics; 1984:1-23.
15. Vaughan CL. Biomechanics of running gait. *Crit Rev Biomech Eng.* 1984;12:1-48.
16. Nuber GW. Biomechanics of the foot and ankle during gait. *Clin Sports Med.* 1988;7:1-13.
17. Reber L, Perry J, Pink M. Muscular control of the ankle in running. *Am J Sports Med.* 1993;21:805-810.
18. Hamill J, Holt KG, Derrick TR. Biomechanics of the foot. In: Sammarco GJ, ed. *Rehabilitation of the Foot and Ankle.* St. Louis: Mosby; 1995:25-44.
19. Sammaarco GJ. Biomechanics of the foot. In: Nordin M, Frankel VH, eds. *Basic Biomechanics of the Skeletal System.* Philadelphia: Lea & Febiger; 1980:193-220.
20. James SL, Bates BT, Osternig LR. Injuries to runners. *Am J Sports Med.* 1978;6:40-45.
21. Subotnick SI. Clinical biomechanics. In: Subotnick SE, ed. *Sports Medicine of the Lower Extremity.* New York: Churchill Livingstone; 1989:171-178.

22. Clement DB, Taunton JE, Smart GW. Achilles tendinitis and peritendinitis: Etiology and treatment. *Am J Sports Med.* 1984;12:179–184.

23. Winter DA, Bishop PJ. Biomechanical factors associated with chronic injury to the lower extremity. *Sports Med.* 1992;14:149–156.

24. Subotnick SI. Sports-specific biomechanics. In: Subotnick SE, ed. *Sports Medicine of the Lower Extremity.* New York: Churchill Livingstone; 1989:203–216.

25. Valian GA, Cavanagh PR. A study of landing from jump: Implications for the design of a basketball shoe. In: Winter DA, ed. *Biomechanics IX.* Champaign, IL: Human Kinetics; 1983.

26. Hart LE. Exercise and soft tissue injury. *Balliere's Clin Rheumatol.* 1994;8:137–148.

Lateral Ankle Sprains

27. Renstrom PAFH. Persistently painful sprained ankle. *J Am Acad Orthop Surg.* 1994;2:270–280.

28. Jackson DW, Ashley RD, Powell JW. Ankle sprains in young athletes: Relation of severity and disability. *Clin Orthop.* 1974;101:201–215.

29. Garrick JM. The frequency of injury, mechanism of injury epidemiology of ankle sprains. *Am J Sports Med.* 1977; 5:241–242.

30. Demaio M, Paine R, Drez D. Chronic lateral ankle instability-inversion sprains, 1. *Orthopaedics.* 1992;15:87–96.

31. Garrick JG, Requa RK. Role of external support in prevention of ankle sprains. *Med Sci Sports.* 1973;5:200–203.

32. Reeman M. Instability of the foot after injury to lateral ligaments of the ankle. *J Bone Joint Surg.* 1965;47B:669–677.

33. Brostrom L. Sprained ankles VI: Surgical treatment of "chronic" ligament ruptures. *Acta Chir Scand.* 1966;132: 551–565.

34. Garrick JG. The frequency of injury, mechanism of injury and epidemiology of ankle sprains. *Am J Sports Med.* 1977;5:242–242.

35. Mann RA. Chronic lateral instability of the ankle. In: Chapman M, ed. *Operative Orthopaedics.* 2nd ed. Philadelphia: Lippincott; 1993:2279–2285.

36. Colville MR, Marder RA, Boyles JJ, et al. Strain measurements in lateral ankle ligament. *Am J Sports Med.* 1990;18:196–200.

37. Siegler S, Block J, Schnede CD. Mechanical characteristics of collateral ligaments of human ankle joint. *Foot Ankle.* 1988;8:234–242.

38. Attarian DE, McCrackin HJ, Devito DP, et al. Biomechanical characteristics of human ankle ligament. *Foot Ankle.* 1985;6:54–58.

39. Wilkerson L. Ankle injury in athletes. *Prim Care.* 1992;19:377–392.

40. Johnson EE, Markolf KL. The contribution of the anterior talofibular ligament to ankle laxity. *J Bone Joint Surg.* 1983;65:81–88.

41. Kjaersgaard-Anderson D, Wethelund JO, Nielson S. Lateral talocalcaneal instability following sectioning of CFL: A kinesiologic study. *Foot Ankle.* 1986;7:355–361.

42. Leonard MH. Injuries of lateral ligament of ankle. *J Bone Joint Surg.* 1949;31:373–377.

43. Siegler S, Block J, Schneck CD. The mechanical characteristics of collateral ligament of human ankle. *Foot Ankle.* 1988;8:234–242.

44. Brostrom L, Liljedahl S, Lindvall N. Sprained ankle II. Arthrographic diagnosis of recent ligament ruptures. *Acta Chir Scand.* 1965;129:485–499.

45. Brank RL, Collins MD, Templeton T. Surgical repair of ruptured lateral ankle ligament. *Am J Sports Med.* 1981;9:40–44.

46. Cass JR, Morrey BF, Kutoh Y, Chao EY. Ankle instability: Comparison of primary repair and delayed reconstruction after long term follow-up study. *Clin Orthop.* 1985; 198:110–117.

47. Juskulka R, Fisher G, Schedl R. Injury of the lateral ligament of the ankle joint: Operative treatment and long term results. *Ach Orthop Trauma Surg.* 1988;107:217–221.

48. Korkala O, Rusanen M, Jokipii P, et al. A prospective study of the treatment of severe tears of the lateral ligament of the ankle. *Int Orthop.* 1987;11:13–17.

49. Gronmark T, Johnsen O, Kogstad O. Rupture of the lateral ligament of the ankle: A controlled clinical trial. *Injury.* 1980;11:215–218.

50. Trevino SG. Management of acute and chronic lateral ligament injuries of the ankle. *Orthop Clin North Am.* 1994;25:1–16.

51. Hopkinson WJ, St. Pierre P, Ryan JB, et al. Syndesmosis sprains of the ankle. *Foot Ankle.* 1990;10:325–330.

52. Cox JS. "Normal" talar tilt angle. *Clin Orthop Rel Res.* 1979;140:37–41.

53. Rubin G, Witten M. The talar tilt angle and the fibular collateral ligaments. *J Bone Joint Surg.* 1960;42:311.

54. Grace DL. Lateral ankle ligament injuries: Inversion and anterior stress radiographs. *Clin Orthop.* 1984;183: 153–159.

55. Peters JW, Trevino SG, Remstrom PA. Chronic lateral ankle instability. *Foot Ankle.* 1991;12:182–191.

56. Johannsen A. Radiological diagnosis of lateral ligament lesion of the ankle. A comparison between talar tilt and anterior drawer sign. *Acta Orthop Scand.* 1978;49: 295–301.

57. Raatikainen T, Putkonan M, Puramen J. Arthrography, clinical examination and stress radiographs in the diagnosis of the acute injury to thc lateral ligaments of the ankle. *Am J Sports Med.* 1992;20:2–6.

58. Schneck CD, Mesgarzadeh M, Bonakdarpour A. MR imaging of the most commonly injured ankle ligament. *Radiology.* 1992;184:507–512.

59. Verhaven EFC, Shahabpour M, Handelberg FWJ, et al. The accuracy of 3-D MRI in diagnosis of ruptures of the lateral ligaments of the ankle. *Am J Sports Med.* 1991;19:583–587.

60. Liu SH, Jason WJ. Lateral ankle sprain and instability problems. *Clin Sports Med.* 1994;13:793–809.

61. Karlsson J, Bergsten T, Lansinger O, et al. Surgical treatment of chronic lateral instability of the ankle joint: A new procedure. *Am J Sports Med.* 1989;17:268–274.

62. Colville MR, Marder RA, Zarins B. Reconstruction of lateral ankle ligament: A biomechanical analysis. *Am J Sports Med.* 1992;20:594–600.

63. Chrisman OD, Snook GA. Reconstruction of lateral ligament tears of the ankle. *J Bone Joint Surg.* 1969;51: 904–912.

64. Liu SH, Baker CL. Comparison of lateral ankle ligamentous reconstruction procedures. *Am J Sports Med.* 1994;22:313-317.

Conservative Treatment of Ankle Sprains

65. Smith RW, Reischl S. Treatment of ankle sprains in young athletes. *Am J Sports Med.* 1986;14:465-471.
66. Garn SN, Newton RA. Kinesthetic awareness in subjects with multiple ankle sprains. *Phys Ther.* 1988;68:1667-1671.
67. Sloan JP, Giddings P, Hain R. Effects of cold and compression on edema. *Phys Sports Med.* 1988;16:116-120.
68. Mascaro TB, Swanson LE. Rehabilitation of the foot and ankle. *Orthop Clin North Am.* 1994;25:147-160.
69. Starkey C. *Therapeutic Modalities for Athletic Trainers.* Philadelphia: Davis; 1993:53-96.
70. Wilkerson GB. Treatment of the inversion ankle sprain through synchronous application of focal compression and cold. *Athletic Training.* 1991;26:220-237.
71. Matsen FA, Quested K, Matsen AL. The effects of local cooling on post fracture swelling. *Clin Orthop.* 1975;109:201-206.
72. Cote DJ, Prentice WE, Hooker DN, Shields EW. Comparison of three treatment procedures for minimizing ankle sprain swelling. *Phys Ther.* 1988;68:1072-1076.
73. Hocutt JE, Jaffe R, Rylander CR, Beebe JK. Cryotherapy in ankle sprains. *Am J Sports Med.* 1982;10:316-319.
74. Airaksinen O, Kolari PJ, Miettinen H. Elastic bandages and intermittent pneumatic compression for treatment of acute ankle sprains. *Arch Phys Med Rehabil.* 1990;71:380-383.
75. Pennington GM, Danley DL, Sumko MH, et al. Pulsed, nonthermal, high frequency electromagnetic energy (diapulse) in the treatment of grade I and grade II ankle sprains. *Mil Med.* 1993;158:101-104.
76. Castel C. Course manual. *Electrotherapy and Ultrasound Update.* Topeka: International Academy of Physiotherapeutics; 1995.
77. Dettori JR, Pearson BD, Basmania CJ, Lednar WM. Early mobilization, I. The immediate effect on acute, lateral ankle sprains (a randomized clinical trial). *Mil Med.* 1994;159:15-24.
78. Eiff MP, Smith AT, Smith GE. Early mobilization versus immobilization in the treatment of lateral ankle sprains. *Am J Sports Med.* 1994;22:83-88.
79. Kay DB. The sprained ankle. Current therapy. *Foot Ankle.* 1985;6:22-28.
80. Klein J, Hoher J, Tiling T. Comparative study of therapies for fibular ligament rupture of the lateral ankle joint in competitive basketball players. *Foot Ankle.* 1993;14:320-324.
81. Konradsen L, Holmer P, Sondergaard L. Early mobilizing treatment for grade III ankle ligament injuries. *Foot Ankle.* 1991;12:69-73.
82. Howell D. Therapeutic exercise and mobilization. In: Hunt GC, ed. *Physical Therapy of the Foot and Ankle.* New York: Churchill Livingstone; 1986:257-285.
83. Kessler RM, Hertling D. *Management of Common Musculoskeletal Disorders.* Philadelphia: Harper & Row; 1983:192-201.
84. Davies GJ. *A Compendium of Isokinetics in Clinical Usage.* La Crosse, WI: S & S Publishers, 1984:82-86.
85. Tropp H, Asklin C, Gillquist J. Prevention of ankle sprains. *Am J Sports Med.* 1985;13:259-262.
86. Surve I, Schwellnus MP, Noakes T. A fivefold reduction in the incidence of recurrent ankle sprains in soccer players using the sport-stirrup orthosis. *Am J Sports Med.* 1994;22:601-606.
87. Gross MT, Bradshaw MK, Ventry LC, Weller KH. Comparison of support provided by ankle taping and semirigid orthosis. *J Orthop Sports Phys Ther.* 1987;9:33-39.
88. Shapiro MS, Kabo JM, Mitchell PW, et al. Ankle sprain prophylaxis: An analysis of the stabilizing effects of braces and tape. *Am J Sports Med.* 1994;22:78-82.
89. Myburgh KH, Vaughan CL, Isaacs SK. The effects of ankle guards and taping on joint motion before, during and after a squash match. *Am J Sports Med.* 1984;12:441-446.
90. Greene TA, Wright CR. A comparative support evaluation of three ankle orthoses before, during and after exercise. *J Orthop Sports Phys Ther.* 1990;11:453-466.
91. Stover CN. Air Stirrup management of ankle injuries in the athlete. *Am J Sports Med.* 1980;8:360-365.
92. Davis PF, Trevino SG. Ankle injuries. In: Baxter DE, ed. *The Tendinitis Foot and Ankle in Sport.* St. Louis: Mosby; 1995:147-170.
93. Enwemeka CS, Spieholz NI, Nelson AJ. The effect of early functional activities on experimentally tenotomized Achilles tendons in rats. *Am J Phys Med Rehabil.* 1988;69:264-269.
94. Loitz B, Zernicke R, Salem G, et al. Influence of continuous passive motion on the mechanical properties of tendon in rabbit. *Phys Ther.* 1988;68:843. Abstract.
95. Clement DB, Taunton JE, Smart GW. Achilles tendinitis and peritendinitis: Etiology and treatment. *Am J Sports Med.* 1984;12:179-184.
96. Burdett RG. Forces predicted at the ankle during running. *Med Sci Sports.* 1982;14:308-316.
97. Niesen-Vertommen SL, Tautnon JE, Clement DB, Mosher RE. The effect of eccentric versus concentric exercise in the management of Achilles tendinitis. *Clin J Sports Med.* 1992;2:109-113.
98. Soma CA, Mandelbaum BR. Achilles tendon disorders. *Clin Sports Med.* 1994;13:811-823.
99. Landvater SJ, Renstrom P. Complete Achilles tendon ruptures. *Clin Sports Med.* 1992;11:741-758.
100. Lea RB, Smith L. Non-surgical treatment of tendo-Achilles rupture. *J Bone Joint Surg.* 1972;54A:1398-1407.
101. Clain MR. The Achilles tendon. In: Baxter DE, ed. *The Foot and Ankle in Sports.* St. Louis; Mosby; 1995:71-80.
102. Lee KH, Matteliano A, Medige J, Smiehorowski T. Electromyographic changes of left muscles with heel lift: Therapeutic implications. *Arch Phys Med Rehabil.* 1987;68:298-301.
103. Solveborn S, Moberg A. Immediate free ankle motion after surgical repair of acute Achilles tendon ruptures. *Am J Sports Med.* 1994;22:607-610.
104. Feder KS. Rehabilitation of volleyball injuries. In: Sammarco GJ, ed. *Rehabilitation of the Foot and Ankle.* St. Louis: Mosby; 1995:305-310.
105. Sammarco GJ. Peroneal tendon injuries. *Orthop Clin North Am.* 1994;25:135-145.

106. Carter TR, Fowler PJ, Clokker C. Functional postoperative treatment of Achilles tendon repair. *Am J Sports Med.* 1992;20:459-462.

107. Mandelbaum BR, Myserson MS, Forster R. Achilles tendon ruptures: A new method of repair, early range of motion, and functional rehabilitation. *Am J Sports Med.* 1995;23:392-395.

108. Smith W, Winn F, Parette R. Comparative study using four modalities in shin-splint treatments. *J Orthop Sports Phys Ther.* 1986;8:77-80.

109. Conti SF. Posterior tibial tendon problems in athletes. *Orthop Clin North Am.* 1994;25:109-121.

110. Subotnick SI. Foot injuries. In: Subotnick SI, ed. *Sports Medicine of the Lower Extremity.* New York: Churchill Livingstone; 1989:223-270.

111. Newell SG, Woodle A. Cuboid syndrome. *Phys Sports Med.* 1981;9:71-75.

112. Schroeder JK. Support for strained and subluxed peroneal tendons. *Athletic Training.* 1988;23:45.

112a. Woods L, Leach RE. Posterior tibial tendon rupture in athletic people. *Am J Sports Med.* 1991;5:495-498.

112b. Funk DA, Cass JR, Johnson RA. Acquired adult flat foot secondary to posterior tibial-tendon pathology. *J Bone Joint Surg.* 1986;1:95-102.

113. Harris PR. Iontophoresis: Clinical research in musculoskeletal inflammatory conditions. *J Orthop Sports Phys Ther.* 1982;4:109-112.

114. Owoeye I, Spielholz NI, Fetto J, et al. Low intensity pulsed galvanic current and the healing of tenotomized rat Achilles tendons. Preliminary report using load to breaking measurements. *Arch Phys Med Rehabil.* 1987;68:415-418.

115. Nwachukwu LN. Effect of two different periods of early pulsed ultrasound application on the tensile strength of ruptured Achilles tendons in rats. Doctoral dissertation, New York University, 1985.

116. Fyfe I, Stanish WD. The use of eccentric training and stretching in the treatment and prevention of tendon injuries. *Clin Sports Med.* 1992;11:601-625.

117. Jackson BA, Schwane JA, Starcher BC. Effect of ultrasound therapy on the repair of Achilles tendon injuries in rats. *Med Sci Sports Exerc.* 1991;23:171-176.

118. Warren CG, Lehman JF, Koblanski JN. Elongation of rat tail tendon. Effect of load and temperature. *Arch Phys Med Rehabil.* 1971;52:465-474.

119. Gross MT. Chronic tendinitis: Pathomechanics of injury, factors affecting the healing response, and treatment. *J Orthop Sports Phys Ther.* 1992;16:248-261.

120. Petersen FB. Muscle training by static, concentric and eccentric contractions. *Acta Physiol Scand.* 1960;48.

120a. Curwin S, Standish WD. *Tendinitis: Its Etiology and Treatment.* Lexington: DC Health; 1984:45-67.

Anterior Tibial Tendinitis

121. Trevino S, Baumhauer JF. Tendon injury of the foot and ankle. *Clin Sports Med.* 1992;11:727-739.

122. Jones DC. Tendon disorders of the foot and ankle. *J Am Acad Orthop Surg.* 1995;1:87-94.

123. Hoppenfeld S, deBoer P. *Surgical Exposures in Orthopaedics. The Anatomical Approach.* 2nd ed. Philadelphia: Lippincott; 1994:502-504.

124. Morrissy RT. *Pediatric Orthopaedics.* 3rd ed. Philadelphia: Lippincott; 1990:73-74.

125. Scheller AD, Kasser JR, Quigley TB. Tendon injuries about the ankle. *Clin Sports Med.* 1983;2:631-641.

Peroneal Tendon

126. Sammarco GJ. Peroneal tendon injury. *Orthop Clin North Am.* 1994;25:135-145.

127. Trevino S, Baumhauser JF. Tendon injuries of the foot and ankle. *Clin Sports Med.* 1992;11:727-739.

128. Leach RE, Lower G. Ankle injuries in skiing. *Clin Orthop.* 1985;198:127.

129. Clanton TO, Schon LC. Athletic injuries to the soft tissues of the foot and ankle. In: Mann RA, Coughlin MJ, eds. *Surgery of the Foot and Ankle.* 6th ed. St. Louis: Mosby; 1993:1167-1177.

130. Kojima Y, Kataoka Y, Suzuki S, Akagi M. Dislocation of the peroneal tendons in neonates and infants. *Clin Orthop.* 1991;266:180-184.

131. Hoppenfeld S, deBoer P. *Surgical Exposures in Orthopaedics. The Anatomic Approach.* 2nd ed. Philadelphia: Lippincott; 1994.

132. Sarrafian SK. *Anatomy of the Foot and Ankle. Descriptive, Topographic, Functional.* Philadelphia: Lippincott; 1983.

133. Jones DC. Tendon disorders of the foot and ankle. *J Am Acad Orthop Surg.* 1993;1:87-94.

134. Eckert WR, Davis EA. Acute rupture of the peroneal retinaculum. *J Bone Joint Surg.* 1976;58:670-673.

135. Zoellner G, Clancy W. Recurrent dislocation of peroneal tendon. *J Bone Joint Surg.* 1979;61:292-294.

136. Baxter DE, Zingas C. The foot in running. *J Am Acad Orthop Surg.* 1995;3:136-145.

137. Rask MR, Steinberg LH. The pathognostic sign of tendoperoneal subluxation: Report of a case treated conservatively. *Orthop Rev.* 1979;8:65-68.

138. Church CC. Radiographic diagnosis of acute peroneal tendon dislocation. *Am J Radiol.* 1977;129:1065-1068.

139. Moritz JR. Ski injuries. *Am J Surg.* 1959;98:493-505.

140. Escalas F. Dislocation of peroneal tendons. Long-term results of surgical treatment. *J Bone Joint Surg.* 1980;62A:451-453.

Achilles Tendinitis

141. Scheller AD, Kasser JR, Quigley TB. Tendon injuries about the ankle. *Orthop Clin North Am.* 1980;11:801.

142. Krissoff WB, Ferris WD. Runners' injuries. *Phys Sports Med.* 1979;7:55-64.

143. James SL, Bates BT, Osternig LR. Injuries to runners. *Am J Sports Med.* 1978;6:40-50.

144. Clement DB, Taunton JE, Smart GW, et al. A survey of overuse running injuries. *Phys Sports Med.* 1981;9:47-58.

145. Clanton TO, Schon LC. Athletic injuries to the soft tissues of the foot and ankle. In: Mann RA, Coughlin MJ, eds. *Surgery of the Foot and Ankle.* 6th ed. St. Louis: Mosby; 1993:1181-1182.

146. Krist M. Achilles tendon injuries in athletes. *Ann Chir Gynaecol.* 1991;80:188.

147. Landvater SJ, Renstrom PAFH. Complete Achilles tendon ruptures. *Clin Sports Med.* 1992;11:741-758.
148. Jozsa L, Kvist M, Balint BJ, et al. The role of recreational sport activity in Achilles tendon rupture. *Am J Sports Med.* 1989;17:338-343.
149. Clement DB, Founton JE, Smart GW. Achilles tendinitis and eritendinitis: Etiology and treatment. *Am J Sports Med.* 1984;12:179-184.
150. Scioli MW. Achilles tendinitis. *Orthop Clin North Am.* 1994;25:177-182.
151. Carden DG, Noble J, Chalmers J, et al. Rupture of the calcaneal tendon. *J Bone Joint Surg.* 1987;69B:416-420.
152. Hoppenfeld S, deBoer P. *Surgical Exposures in Orthopaedics. The Anatomic Approach.* 2nd ed. Philadelphia: Lippincott; 1994:506.
153. Galloway MT, Jokl P, Dayton OW. Achilles tendon overuse injury. *Clin Sports Med.* 1992;11:771-782.
154. Turco VJ, Spinella AJ. Achilles tendon ruptures peroneus brevis transfer. *Foot Ankle.* 1987;7:253-259.
155. Jones DC. Tendon disorders of the foot and ankle. *J Am Acad Orthop Surg.* 1993;1:87-94.
156. Lagergen C, Lindholm A. Vascular distribution in Achilles tendon: An angiographic and microangiographic study. *Acta Chir Scand.* 1958;116:491-495.
157. Allenmark C. Partial Achilles tendon tears. *Clin Sports Med.* 1992;11:759-769.
158. Lundberg A, Croldie I, Kalin B, et al. Kinematics of the ankle foot complex. *Foot Ankle.* 1989;9:194-200.
159. Baxter DE, Zingas C. The foot in running. *J Am Acad Orthop Surg.* 1995;3:136-145.
160. Schepsis AA, Leach RE. Surgical management of Achilles tendinitis. *Am J Sports Med.* 1987;15:308-315.
161. Beskin JL, Saunders RA, Hunter SC, et al. Surgical repair of Achilles tendon ruptures. *Am J Sports Med.* 1987; 15:1-8.

Stress Fractures

162. Mcyer SA, Saltzman CL, Albright JP. Stress fractures of the foot and leg. *Clin Sports Med.* 1993;12:395-413.
163. McBryde AM. Stress fractures in athletes. *J Sports Med.* 1976;3:212.
164. Clanton TO, Solcher BW. Chronic leg pain in the athlete. *Clin Sports Med.* 1994;13:743-759.
165. Prozman RR, Griffis CG. Stress fractures in men and women undergoing military training. *J Bone Joint Surg.* 1977;59A:835.
166. Brudvig TJ, Gudger TD, Obermeyer L. Stress fractures in 295 trainees: A one year study as related to age, sex, and race. *Mil Med.* 1983;148:666.
167. Eisele SA, Sammarco GJ. Fatigue fractures of the foot and ankle in the athlete. *Instr Course Lect.* 1993; 42:175-183.
168. Baker J, Frankel VH, Burnstein A. Fatigue fractures: Biochemical considerations. *J Bone Joint Surg.* 1972; 54A:1345-1346.
169. Clanton TO, Schon LC. Athletic injuries to the soft tissue of the foot and ankle. In: Mann RA, Coughlin MJ, eds. *Surgery of the Foot and Ankle.* 6th ed. St. Louis: Mosby; 1993:1229-1231.
170. Matheson GO, Clement DB, McKenzie DC, et al. Stress fractures in athletes: A study of 320 cases. *Am J Sports Med.* 1987;15:46.
171. Sullivan D, Warren RF, Pavlov H. Stress fractures in 51 runners. *Clin Orthop.* 1984;187:188.
172. Santi M, Sartpros DG. Diagnostic imaging approach to stress fracture of the foot. *J Foot Surg.* 1991;30:85.
173. Markey KL. Stress fractures. *Clin Sports Med.* 1987;6:405.

Fracture Rehabilitation

174. McBryde AM Jr. Stress fractures in runners. *Clin Sports Med.* 1985;4:737-752.

Subcalcaneal Pain Syndrome

175. Lapidus PW, Gudotti FP. Painful heel: Report of 323 patients with 3643 painful heels. *Clin Orthop.* 1965;39:179-186.
176. McBryde AM. Plantar fasciitis. *Instr Course Lect.* 1984;33:278-282.
177. Jahss MH, Kummer F, Michelson JD. Investigations into the fat pads of the sole of the foot: Heel pressure studies. *Foot Ankle.* 1992;13:227-232.
178. Jahss MH, Michelson JD. Investigations into the fat pads of the sole of the foot: Anatomy and histology. *Foot Ankle.* 1992;13:233-242.
179. Paul IL, Munro MB, Abernathy PJ, et al. Musculoskeletal shock absorption: Relative contribution of bone and soft tissues at various frequencies. *J Biomech.* 1978; 11:237-239.
180. Karr SD. Subcalcaneal heel pain. *Orthop Clin North Am.* 1994;25:161-175.
181. Sarrafian SK. Functional characteristics of the foot and plantar aponeuroses under tibiotalar loading. *Foot Ankle.* 1987;8:4-18.
182. Hicks JH. The mechanism of the foot: The plantar aponeuroses and the arch. *J Anat.* 1954;88:25-31.
183. Bordelon RL. Heel pain. In: Mann RA, Coughlin MJ, eds. *Surgery of the Foot and Ankle.* 6th ed. Louis: Mosby; 1993:837-847.
184. Kwong PK, Kay D, Voner RT, et al. Imaging study of the painful heel syndrome. *Foot Ankle.* 1988;7:119-126.
185. Williams PL, Smibert JG, Cox R, et al. Imaging study of the painful heel syndrome. *Foot Ankle.* 1987;7:345-349.
186. Eastmond CJ, Rajah SM, Tovey D, et al. Seronegative pauciarticular arthritis and HLA-B27. *Ann Rheum Dis.* 1980;39:231-234.

Plantar Fasciitis

187. Tanner SM, Harvey JS. How we manage plantar fasciitis. *Phys Sports Med.* 1988;16:39-47.
188. Kwong PK, Kay D, Voner RT, White MW. Plantar fasciitis. *Clin Sports Med.* 1988;7:119-126.
189. Kibler WB, Goldberg C, Chandler TJ. Functional biomechanical deficits in running athletes with plantar fasciitis. *Am J Sports Med.* 1991;19:66-71.
190. Warren BL. Plantar fasciitis in runners. *Sports Med.* 1990;10:338-345.
191. Karr SD. Subcalcaneal heel pain. *Orthop Clin North Am.* 1994;25:161-174.

192. Middleton JA, Kolodin EL. Plantar fascitis-heel pain in athletes. *J Ath Training.* 1992;27:70-75.

193. Marshall P. The rehabilitation of overuse foot injuries in athletes and dancers. *Clin Sports Med.* 1988;7:175-191.

194. Seto JL, Brewster CD. Treatment approaches following foot and ankle injury. *Clin Sports Med.* 1994;13: 695-718.

195. Wapner KL, Sharkey PF. The use of night splints for treatment of recalcitrant plantar fascitis. *Foot Ankle.* 1991; 12:135-137.

196. Creighton DS, Olson VL. Evaluation of range of motion of the first metatarsophalangeal joint in runners with plantar fasciitis. *Orthop Sports Phys Ther.* 1987;8:357-361.

197. McPoil TG, McGarvey TC. The foot in athletics. In: Hunt GC, ed. *Physical Therapy of the Foot and Ankle.* New York: Churchill Livingstone; 1986:199-230.

198. Brody DM. Rehabilitation of the injured runner. In: Murray JA, ed. *Instructional Course Lectures.* St. Louis: Mosby; 1984:268-277.

199. Leach RE, Seavey MS, Salter DK. Results of surgery in athletes with plantar fasciitis. *Foot Ankle.* 1986;7:156-161.

200. Baxter DE. The heel in sports. *Clin Sports Med.* 1994;13:683-693.

Chronic Extertional Compartment Syndrome

201. Detmer DE. Chronic shin splints: Classification and management of medial tibial stress syndrome. *Sports Med.* 1986;3:436-446.

202. Detmer DE, Sharpe K, Sufit RL, et al. Chronic compartment syndrome: Diagnosis, management and outcomes. *Am J Sports Med.* 1985;13:162-170.

203. Clanton TO, Solcher BW. Chronic leg pain in the athlete. *Clin Sports Med.* 1994;13:743-759.

204. Martens MA, Backaert M, Vermaut G, et al. Chronic leg pain in the athlete due to a recurrent compartment syndrome. *Sports Med.* 1990;9:62-68.

205. Clanton TO, Schon LC. Athletic injuries to the soft tissue of the foot and ankle. In: Mann RA, Coughlin MJ, eds. *Surgery of the Foot and Ankle.* 6th ed. St. Louis: Mosby; 1993:1105-1121.

206. Eisele DA, Sammarco GJ. Chronic exertional compartment syndrome. *Instr Course Lect.* 1993;42:213-217.

207. Matsen FA, Clawson DK. The deep posterior compartmental syndrome of the leg. *J Bone Joint Surg.* 1975; 57A:34-39.

208. Pedowitz RA, Hargens AR, Mubarak SJ, et al. Modified criteria for the objective diagnosis of chronic compart-

ment syndrome to the leg. *Am J Sports Med.* 1990: 18:35-40.

209. Amendola A, Rorabeck CH, Vellett D, et al. The use of magnetic resonance imaging in exertional compartment syndromes. *Am J Sports Med.* 1990;18:29-34.

210. Garfin SR, Tipton CM, Mubarak SJ, et al. The role of fascia in maintenance of muscle tendon and pressure. *J Appl Physiol.* 1981;51:317-210.

211. Mozan LC, Keagy RD. Muscle relationship in functional fascia. *Clin Orthop.* 1969;76:225-230.

Turf Toe

212. Clanton TO, Ford JJ. Turf toe injury. *Clin Sports Med.* 1994;13:731-741.

213. Bowers KD, Martin RB. A shoe related football injury. *Med Sci Sports Exerc.* 1976;8:81-83.

214. Coker TP, Arnold JA, Weber DL. Traumatic lesions of the metatarsophalangeal joint of the great toe in athletes. *Am J Sports Med.* 1978;6:326-334.

215. Rodeo SA, O'Brien S, Warren RF, et al. Turf-toe: An analysis of metatarsal joint sprains in professional football players. *Am J Sports Med.* 1990;18:280-285.

216. Clanton TO, Butler JE, Eggert A. Injury to the metatarsophalangeal joint in athletes. *Foot Ankle.* 1986;7:162-176.

217. Joseph J. Range of movement of the great toe in men. *J Bone Joint Surg.* 1954;36B:450-457.

218. Bojsen-Moller F, Lamorequx L. Significance of free dorsiflexion of the toes in walking. *Acta Orthop Scand.* 1979;50:471-479.

219. Stroke IAF, Hutton WC, Scott JRR. Forces under the hallux valgus foot before and after surgery. *Clin Orthrop.* 1979;142:64-72.

220. Sanmarco GJ. *Biomechanics of the Foot. Biomechanics of the Skeletal System.* Philadelphia: Lea & Febiger; 1980:193-219.

221. Sammarco GJ. Turf toe. *Instr Course Lect.* 1993;42: 207-212.

222. Sammarco GJ. How I manage turf toe. *Phys Sports Med.* 1988;16:113-118.

223. Cooker TP, Arnold JA, Weber DL. Traumatic lesions of the metatarsophalangeal joint of the great toe in athletes. *Am J Sports Med.* 1978;6:326-334.

224. Clanton TO, Butler JE, Eggert A. Injuries to the metatarsophalangeal joints in athletes. *Foot Ankle.* 1986; 7:162-176.

225. Herrmann TJ. The foot and ankle in football. In: Sammarco GJ, ed. *Rehabilitation of the Foot and Ankle.* St. Louis: Mosby; 1995:259-268.

226. Clanton TO, Ford JJ. Turf toe injury. *Clin Sports Med.* 1994;13:731-741.

Index